Headache

in Clinical Practice

Second edition

Stephen D Silberstein MD FACP

Jefferson Headache Center, Thomas Jefferson University Hospital,
Philadelphia, USA

Richard B Lipton MD

Department of Neurology, Epidemiology and Social Medicine,
Albert Einstein College of Medicine,
New York, USA

and

Peter J Goadsby MD PhD

Institute of Neurology, The National Hospital for
Neurology and Neurosurgery, London, UK

**Supported as an unrestricted
educational grant
from AstraZeneca**

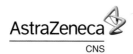

CNS

MARTIN DUNITZ

© 1998, 2002 Martin Dunitz Ltd, a member of the Taylor & Francis group

First edition published in the United Kingdom in 1998 by Isis Medical Media Ltd, 58 St Aldgates, Oxford OX1 1ST

Second edition published in the United Kingdom in 2002 by Martin Dunitz Ltd, The Livery House, 7–9 Pratt Street, London NW1 0AE
Tel.: +44 (0) 20 74822202
Fax.: +44 (0) 20 72670159
E-mail: info.@dunitz.co.uk
Website: http://www.dunitz.co.uk

A CIP record for this book is available from the British Library.

ISBN 1-901865-88-6

Cover illustration: 'Headache' by Rebekah Raye of Deer Isle, Maine, USA (© 1991, Sandoz Pharmaceuticals Corporation.)

Although every effort has been made to ensure that all owners of copyright material have been acknowledged in this publication, we would be glad to acknowledge in subsequent reprints or editions any omissions brought to our attention.

Distributed in the USA by
Fulfilment Center
Taylor & Francis
7625 Empire Drive
Florence, KY 41042, USA
Toll Free Tel.: +1 800 634 7064
E-mail: cserve@routledge_ny.com

Distributed in Canada by
Taylor & Francis
74 Rolark Drive
Scarborough, Ontario M1R 4G2, Canada
Toll Free Tel.: +1 877 226 2237
E-mail: tal_fran@istar.ca

Distributed in the rest of the world by
Thomson Publishing Services
Cheriton House
North Way
Andover, Hampshire SP10 5BE, UK
Tel.: +44 (0)1264 332424
E-mail: salesorder.tandf@thomsonpublishingservices.co.uk

Composition by Wearset Ltd, Boldon, Tyne and Wear
Printed and bound in the United States of America

Contents

Preface

Headache is an almost universal human experience. For some, it is an occasional, episodic nuisance symptom, while for others it may be a manifestation of a disabling chronic disease or the first manifestation of a life-threatening condition. The etiology, frequency, severity, and life consequences of headache vary widely. To put our current concepts in perspective, the book begins by reviewing the history and epidemiology of headache.

Although headache is a highly variable experience, the first step to successful management is a confident, credible, specific diagnosis. Patients often fear that their headaches are symptomatic of a serious underlying disorder. Fortunately, we can usually reassure patients that they have a primary headache disorder, such as migraine or tension-type headache, rather than a secondary headache due to a brain mass lesion, an infection, a metabolic derangement, or some other potentially life threatening cause.

Following a chapter on diagnosis, this book focuses on the major primary and secondary headache disorders. The pain mechanisms of the secondary headache disorders are well understood. Inflammation, traction, or nerve root irritation of intracranial or extracranial processes may cause headache. We are beginning to gain insight into the pain mechanisms of the primary headache disorders. In fact, the molecular basis of one variety of migraine (familial hemiplegic migraine) has been shown to be an abnormality of a calcium channel, suggesting that migraine may be a channelopathy. The book reviews the mechanisms of primary and secondary headache disorders.

Stephen P Silberstein
Richard B Lipton
Peter J Goadsby

Acknowledgements

Stephen Silberstein would like to thank his "brain trust," Lynne Kaiser and Linda Kelly, for their dedication, hard work, and unique talents, and Marsha Silberstein for her encouragement, love, and support.

chapter 1

Historical introduction

Headache has troubled mankind from the dawn of civilization. Signs of trepanation, a procedure wherein the skull was perforated with an instrument, are evident on neolithic human skulls dating from 7000 BC.[1] The procedure may have been done to release the demons and evil spirits[1] that were believed to cause headaches, madness, and epilepsy, but recent evidence suggests that it was done for medical reasons (Figures 1.1 and 1.2).[2] In the 19th century, Paul Broca showed that only 30–45 minutes were required to remove a slice of bone from the cranium and proved that a human being could survive trepanation.[3] Some 17th century physicians recommended trepanning to treat migraine. In 1660, William Harvey recommended trepanation to a patient with intractable migraine.[4] Trepanation continues to be practised today, without anesthesia, by some African tribes. It is primarily done for relief of headache or removal of a fracture line after head injury.[5]

For millennia, the medical and popular literature has described headache triggers, relieving factors, and the signs and symptoms of the migraine complex, including headache, aura, prodrome, nausea or vomiting, and familial tendency.[6,7] References to headache are found as far back as 3000 BC. The earliest published reference is a Sumerian epic poem,[8] an early description of the 'sick headache':

> The sick-eyed says not
> 'I am sick-eyed'
> The sick-headed not
> 'I am sick-headed'.[9]

The Ebers Papyrus, an ancient Egyptian prescription for headache dated circa 1200 BC and said to be based on medical documents from 2500 BC, describes migraine, neuralgia, and shooting head pains. (Figure 1.3).[10] The Egyptians, like other ancients, believed the gods could cure their ailments and followed the instructions on the Papyrus. For example, a clay crocodile holding grain in its mouth was firmly bound to the patient's head by a strip of linen that bore the names of the gods.[4,9] This technique

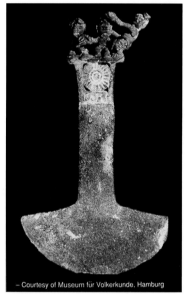

Figure 1.2
Neolithic instrument used for trepanation. (Courtesy of Museum für Völkerkunde, Hamburg.)

– Courtesy of Museum für Volkerkunde, Hamburg

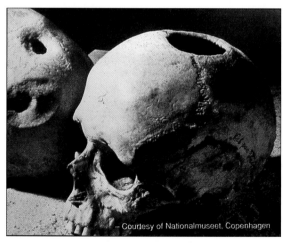

– Courtesy of Nationalmuseet, Copenhagen

Figure 1.1 Neolithic skull showing trepanation hole (c. 7000 BC). (Courtesy of Nationalmuseet, Copenhagen.)

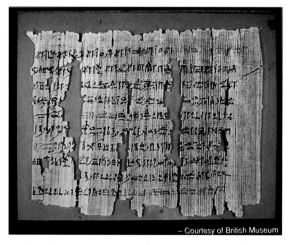

– Courtesy of British Museum

Figure 1.3 An ancient Egyptian headache prescription on papyrus (c.1200 BC). (Courtesy of The British Museum.)

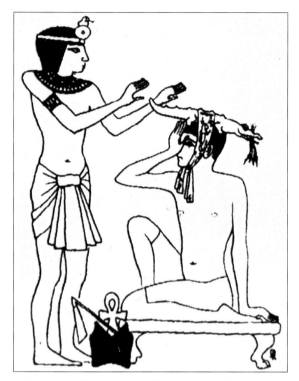

Figure 1.4 The treatment of headache in 1200 BC.

may have produced headache relief by compressing and cooling the scalp (Figure 1.4).[4] A later report from Mesopotamia describes a headache with associated visual disturbance, in which '. . . the head is bent with pain gripping his temples . . . and his eyes are afflicted with dimness and cloudiness'. Hippocrates (Figure 1.5), in

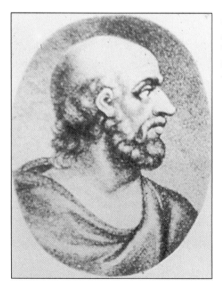

Figure 1.5 Hippocrates, who described migraine in 400 BC.

400 BC, described both the visual aura that can precede the migraine headache and its relief by vomiting.[11] Hippocrates described a shining light, usually in the right eye, followed by violent pain that begins in the temples and eventually reaches the entire head and neck area.[4,9]

The medical and intellectual climate strongly influenced belief in the causes and triggers of headache. Hippocrates believed that headache could be triggered by exercise or intercourse,[9] that migraine resulted from vapours rising from the stomach to the head, and that vomiting could partially relieve the pain of headache.[4,9] Plato believed that preoccupation with the body triggered headaches:[11]

> 'Yes, indeed', he said, 'this excessive care for the body that goes beyond simple gymnastics is about the greatest of all obstacles . . . It is troublesome in household affairs and military service and . . . it puts difficulties in the way of any kind of instruction, thinking, or private meditation – forever imagining headaches and dizziness and attributing their origins to philosophy . . . It makes the man always fancy himself sick and never cease from anguishing about his body'.

In the Platonic dialogue, 'Charmides', the elements of holistic care are delineated in terms that manage to sound both modern and timeless:[12]

> You must begin by curing the soul . . . The cure . . . has to be effected by use of certain charms, and these charms are fair words, and by them temperance is implanted in the soul, and when temperance comes and stays, there health is speedily imparted . . . This is the great error of our day in the treatment of human beings . . . Men try to be physicians of health and temperance separately.

Gobel et al[13] assert that St. Paul's thorn in the flesh was migraine that met International Headache Society criteria. They believe that the spell that St. Paul suffered on the way to Damascus, which resulted in his conversion to Christianity, can be attributed to an episode of migraine with aura. The Talmud, a collection of rabbinic discussions and commentaries on Biblical law compiled from 200 to 600 AD, considers the blowing away of the froth or foam of beverages such as beer to be one cause of headache. Headache was also believed to be inflicted by divine decree as a punishment for sins and cured by repentance and good deeds.[14] Celsus (215–300 AD) believed 'drinking wine, or crudity [dyspepsia], or cold, or heat of a fire or the sun' could trigger migraine. Because of his classic descriptions, Aretaeus of Cappodocia (2nd century AD) is credited with discovering migraine headache. Clearly, migraine was well known in the ancient world.[10]

The term 'migraine' itself is derived from the Greek word hemicrania, introduced by Galen in approximately 200 AD. He mistakenly believed it was caused by the ascent of vapours, either excessive, too hot, or too cold. Popular names that evolved over the years for this uncomfortable, sometimes disabling, disorder include sick headache, blind headache, and bilious headache.[7,10,15]

In the 12th century, Abbess Hildegarde of Bingen described her visions, later attributed to her migraine aura, in terms that are both mystical and apocalyptic (Figure 1.6):[16]

> I saw a great star, most splendid and beautiful, and with it an exceeding multitude of falling sparks with which the star followed southward . . . and suddenly they were all annihilated, being turned into black coals . . . and cast into the abyss so that I could see them no more.

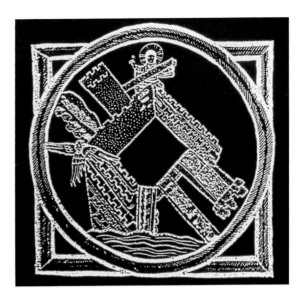

Figure 1.6 *'Vision of the Heavenly City' from a manuscript of Hildegard's* Scivias *written at Bingen (c.1180 AD).*

Timothy Bright tells us in his 1586 essay, 'A Treatise of Melancholy', 'Melancholic humor is . . . settled in the spleane and with his vapour annoyeth the harte and passing up to the brayne, countersetteth terrible objects to the fantasie'.[17]

Thomas Willis in 1683 brilliantly described a woman with severe, periodic, migrainous headache preceded by a prodrome and associated with vomiting:[10]

> . . . beautiful and young woman, imbued with a slender habit of body, and an hot blood, was wont to be afflicted with frequent and wandering fits of headache . . . On the day before the coming of the spontaneous fit of this disease, growing very hungry in the evening, she eat a most plentiful supper, with an hungry, I may say a greedy appetite; presaging by this sign, that the pain of the head would most certainly follow the next morning; and the event never failed this augury . . . she was troubled also with vomiting.

The medical text, 'Incipit epistula vulturus', written around 500 AD was still in use 500 years later: 'The bones from the head of the vulture, wrapped in deerskin, will cure any headache; its brain, mixed with the best of oil and put up the nose will expel all ailments of the head'.[18]

Opium and vinegar solutions applied to the skin were widely used as headache remedies in Europe during the 13th century. The vinegar probably allowed the opium to be absorbed more quickly through the skin.[4] Vinegar compresses alone have been used as a headache treatment. Leo Tolstoy, in *War and Peace*, describes a countess who lay down in the new sitting room with a vinegar compress on her head to treat a headache that was brought on by noise and turmoil.

Shakespeare discusses headache treatment: Desdemona binds her husband's head with the handkerchief (a remedy still used by many migraineurs) that will later be her undoing.[19]

> OTHELLO: I have a pain upon my forehead here. DESDEMONA: Faith, that's with watching; twill away again. Let me but bind it hard, within this hour. It will be well.

In King John, a similar remedy is described:[20] 'When your head did but ache, I knit my handkerchief about your brows'. This suggests it was a popular treatment in Elizabethan times.

Migraine was distinguished from common headache by Tisso in 1783, who ascribed it to a supraorbital neuralgia,[15] '. . . provoked by reflexes from the stomach, gallbladder, or uterus'. Over the next century, DuBois Reymond, Mollendorf, and, later, Eulenburg proposed different vascular theories for migraine. In the late 1700s, Erasmus Darwin, grandfather of Charles Darwin, suggested treating headache by centrifugation. He believed headaches were caused by vasodilation, and suggested placing the patient in a centrifuge to force the blood from the head to the feet.[4,9] Fothergill in 1778 introduced the term 'fortification spectra' to describe the typical visual aura or disturbance of migraine. Fothergill used the term 'fortification'[9] because the visual aura resembled a fortified town surrounded with bastions.[7,21]

Airy, in 1870, quoted the 19th century poet, Alfred, Lord Tennyson whom he felt depicted a fortification spectra in suitably stately fashion. '. . . (A)s yonder walls rose slowly to a music slowly breathed, a cloud that gathered shape'.[22] (Figure 1.7).

In the 18th century, Alexander Pope offers this account of migraine in 'The Rape of the Lock':[23]

> When screen'd in shades from day's detested glare,
> Spleen sighs forever on her pensive bed,
> Pain at her side, and megrim at her head.

James Ware (1814) described bouts of visual aura without accompanying headache, which he termed 'muscae voli-

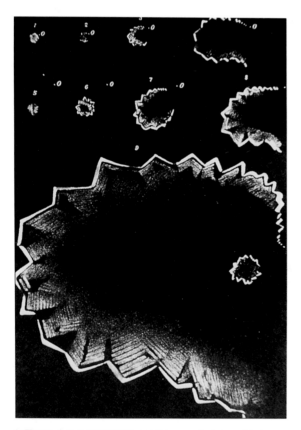

● **Figure 1.7** A fortification spectra seen during a migraine aura (as quoted by Airy in 1870 from Tennyson '. . . as yonder walls rose slowly to a music slowly breathed, a cloud that gathered shape'. (Courtesy of the Royal Society of London.)

tantes' and which are now called migraine equivalents.[10] Liveing, in 1873, wrote the first monograph[24] on migraine, entitled 'On Megrim, Sick-headache, and some Allied Disorders: a Contribution to the Pathology of Nerve-storms', and originated the neural theory of migraine. He ascribed the problem to '. . . disturbances of the autonomic nervous system', which he called 'nerve storms'.[7]

William Gowers, in 1888, published an influential neurology textbook, *A Manual of Disease of the Nervous System*.[21] Gowers emphasized the importance of a healthy lifestyle and advocated using a solution of nitroglycerin 1% in alcohol, combined with other agents, to treat headaches. The remedy later became known as the 'Gowers mixture'. Gowers was also famous for recommending Indian hemp (marijuana) for headache relief.[4,9]

In 1900, Deyl[25] suggested that migraine, including menstrual migraine, resulted from intermittent swelling of the hypophysis, with compression of the trigeminal nerve. Spitzer, in 1901,[25] suggested that headache was produced by recurrent interventricular foramen blockage causing lateral ventricle dilation.

These theories may sound odd, but even Proust tells us of a physician who believes that everything, '. . . whether headache or colic, heart disease or diabetes, was a disease of the nose that had been wrongly diagnosed'.[26] Sinclair Lewis introduces us to Almus Pickerbaugh, a doctor with dubious clinical skills, who says that his wife has 'sick headaches . . . [due to] . . . early neglect of her diet'.[27,28]

> 'Yes', said Mary, beginning to feel faint . . . The pain in her head was setting the room afire. Chairs and tables were developing lurid nimbuses. But she would not give way; not this time. She stared at Willie; he seemed to be standing pale and serene, at the center of a mandala of flame . . . all morning she had felt as if she might, at any moment, be struck by The Headache, which she feared more than death. When the clamp of fire went round her head, she could not see for the pain and often, she would end up flat on the floor, vomiting from the pain. The Headache, as she always thought of it, to differentiate it from ordinary headaches, had begun many years earlier . . . Her behavior [during an attack] . . . could be . . . like that of a mad woman.

Modern writers often link headache and depression, a connection that has been observed in modern epidemiological studies. In her civil war diaries, Mary Chesnutt mentioned headaches and being 'nervous and depressed' in the same breath.[29] In *The Razor's Edge*, by Somerset

Maugham, Gray Maturin's headaches follow in the wake of severe financial difficulties: 'His frenzied efforts to stave off the disaster that finally overwhelmed him, the burden of anxiety, the humiliation, resulted in a nervous breakdown, and he began to have headaches so severe that he was incapacitated for twenty-four hours and as limp as a wet rag when they ceased'.[30] Gore Vidal, in detailing the agony of Mary Lincoln, describes not only the visual phenomena that can be associated with migraine, but also the attendant pain and behavior.[31]

Stephen King, the 'horror' novelist, vividly describes the pain, sensory hyperresponsiveness, and feeling of prostration associated with migraine:[32]

> *The headache would get worse until it was a smashing weight, sending red pain through his head and neck with every pulsebeat. Bright lights would make his eyes water helplessly and send darts of agony into the flesh just behind his eyes. Small noises magnified, ordinary noises as loud as jackhammers, loud noises insupportable. The headache would worsen until it felt as if his head were being crushed inside an inquisitor's lovecap. Then it would even off at that level for six hours. He would be next to helpless.*

Stephen King also gives us a contemporary account of exertional headache:[33]

> *Lobsterlike, Richards humped backwards on his knees. His breath came in sharp, doglike gasps. The air was hot, full of the slick taste of oil, uncomfortable to breathe. A headache surfaced within his skull and began to push daggers into the backs of his eyes.*

Lewis Carroll described migrainous phenomena in *Alice in Wonderland* and *Through the Looking Glass*, depicting instances of central scotoma, tunnel vision, phonophobia, vertigo, distortions in body image, dementia and visual hallucinations.

Joan Didion, in her 1968 essay, 'In Bed', describes a mundane reality with which most headache sufferers can probably identify:[34]

> *We have reached a certain understanding my migraine and I. It never comes when I am in real trouble. Tell me that my house is burned down, my husband has left me, that there is gunfighting in the streets and panic in the banks, and I will not respond by getting a headache. It comes when I am fighting not an open but a guerilla war with my own life, during weeks of small household confusions, lost laundry, unhappy help, cancelled appointments, on days when the telephone rings too much and I get no work done and the wind is coming up. On days like that my friend comes uninvited.*

Analgesic overuse is not new. Faulkner's Jason Compson prefers inhaling camphor fumes to more traditional remedies: '. . . there's not a damn thing in that aspirin except flour and water for imaginary invalids'.[35] Caffeine is a popular remedy contained in many over-the-counter analgesics. In *The Woman in White*, Laura Fairlie is dosed with 'restorative tea' for 'that essentially feminine malady, a slight headache'.[36] Many headache sufferers, in literature as in life, have experimented and discovered their own, often bizarre, remedies. Emmett Smith, the Vietnam veteran in Bobbie Ann Mason's *In Country*, is plagued by headaches that his family and friends believe are linked to his exposure to Agent Orange. He is found 'sitting up in bed, his hair crammed into his Pepsi cap, drinking from the Coke can, chasing away that pain in his head'.[37] However, the protagonist of Raymond Carver's 'Viewfinder' looks for dietary help: 'I had a headache. I know coffee's no good for it, but sometimes Jello helps'.[7,38]

Ruth Rendell has one of her characters recommend feverfew, only to have the migraine sufferer respond, 'What the hell is feverfew?'.[39] A physician in David Williams' *Prescription for Murder* defines it as 'a white flowering hedgerow plant which has substances that may well inhibit the release of natural serotonin in the body'.[7,40]

Emotional well-being can effect great change in headache intensity. One dramatic example is found in the *Personal Memoirs of U.S. Grant*.[41] The general describes a 'sick headache' he suffered on 9 August, 1865. He attempts to cure it by 'bathing [his] feet in hot water and mustard and putting mustard plasters on [his] wrists and the back of [his] neck'. He gets complete relief, however, only when he receives word that Robert E. Lee agrees to discuss terms of surrender; '. . . the instant I saw the contents of the note I was cured'.[7,41]

Unfortunately, the most pervasive element running through the appearance of headaches in literature is not a general consensus on causes or treatment, but rather an underlying tone of skepticism. Headache is the Rodney Dangerfield of medical maladies – it gets no respect. Joan Didion puts it most bluntly when discussing the attitudes of those around her:[34] 'For I had no brain tumor, no eyestrain, no high blood pressure, nothing wrong with me at all. I simply had migraine headaches, and migraine headaches were, as everyone who did not have them knew, imaginary'.

In defining the elements of the 'migraine personality', Joan Didion's physician focuses on two areas that are considered, for the most part, to be areas of feminine concern: personal appearance and housework:[7]

> 'You don't look like a migraine personality . . . Your hair's messy. But I suppose you're a compulsive housekeeper'.

> Actually my house is kept even more negligently than my hair, but the doctor was right nonetheless; perfectionism can also take the form of spending most of a week writing and rewriting a paragraph.

> But not all perfectionists have migraine, and not all migrainous people have migraine personalities.[34]

In 1938, John Graham and Harold Wolff[42] demonstrated that the drug ergotamine worked by constricting blood vessels and used this as proof of the vascular theory of migraine.[4] Greek and Roman ancient writings include references to 'blighted grains' and 'blackened bread', and to the use of concoctions of powdered barley flower to hasten childbirth. During the Middle Ages, written accounts of ergot poisoning first appeared. Epidemics were described in which the characteristic symptom was gangrene of the feet, legs, hands, and arms, often associated with burning sensations in the extremities. The disease was known as 'Ignis Sacer' or 'Holy Fire' and, later, as 'St. Anthony's Fire', in honor of the saint at whose shrine relief was obtained. This relief probably resulted from the use of a diet free of contaminated grain during the pilgrimage to the shrine (Figure 1.8).[43]

The term 'ergot' is derived from the French word argot meaning 'rooster's spur' (Figure 1.9). It describes the small, banana-shaped sclerotium of the fungus. Louis René Tulasne of Paris in 1853 established that ergot was not a hypertrophied rye seed, but a fungus having three stages in one life cycle, and he named it *Claviceps purpurea*. Once infected by the fungus, the rye seed was transformed into a spur-shaped mass of fungal pseudotissue, purple-brown in colour – the resting stage of the fungus, known as the 'sclerotium' (derived from the Greek skleros, meaning hard).[43]

In 1831, Heinrich Wiggers, a pharmacist of Göttingen, Germany, tested ergot extracts in animals. Among his models was the 'rooster comb test' – a rooster, when fed ergotin, became ataxic and nauseous, acquired a blanched comb, and suffered from severe convulsions, dying days later. The 'rooster comb test' continued to be used into the following century by investigators studying the physiological properties of ergot.[43] Later, Woakes, in 1868, reported the use of ergot of rye in the treatment of neuralgia.[44]

The earliest reports in the medical literature on the use of ergot in the treatment of migraine were those of Eulenberg in Germany in 1883, Thomson in the United States in 1894, and Campbell in England in 1894. Stevens' *Modern Materia Medica* mentioned the use of ergot for the treatment of migraine in 1907.[45] The use of ergot was romanticized by Alfred, Lord Tennyson (1809–97):

> He gently prevails on his patients to try
> The magic effects of the ergot rye.

The first pure ergot alkaloid, ergotamine, was isolated by Stoll in 1918 and used primarily in obstetrics and gynaecology until 1925, when Rothlin successfully treated a case of severe and intractable migraine with a subcuta-

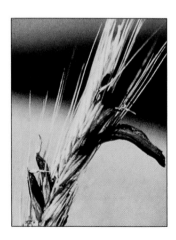

Figure 1.8 *Ergot fungus on rye.*

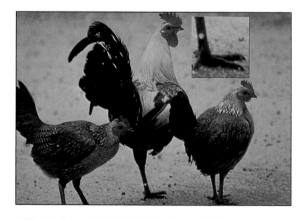

Figure 1.9 *Rooster spur which gave ergot its name.*

Table 1.1 *A brief history of ergot therapy (ET)*

Year	Study	Therapy
1883	Eulenberg (Germany)	Injections of ergot extract
1894	Thompson (USA)	Oral ergot extract
1894	Campbell (England)	Mentioned antimigraine effect of ergot in headache book
1918	Stoll (Basel)	Isolated ergotamine and named it Gynergan. Original use OB/GYN
1925	Rothlin (Basel)	First used subcutaneous ET for migraine
1926	Maier (Zurich)	Reported use of ET at Paris Neurological Society
1927	Tzanck (France)	First systemic study of oral ET
1928	Trautman (Germany)	Good results with oral ET
1934	Lenox (Boston) Brock, O'Sullivan and Towne (NY) Logan and Allen (Mayo Clinic)	First controlled ET studies in USA
1937	Graham and Wolff (NY)	Effect of ET on blood vessels. Scientific clinical investigation
1943	Stoll and Hofmann (Basel)	Synthesized DHE
1945	Horton, Peters and Blumenthal (Mayo Clinic)	Used DHE to treat migraine

DHE: dihydroergotamine.

neous injection of ergotamine tartrate. This indication was pursued vigorously by various researchers over the following decades (Table 1.1) and was reinforced by the belief in a vascular origin for migraine and the concept that ergotamine tartrate acted as a vasoconstrictor. Lennox in Boston, and others working independently, conducted the first controlled studies of ergotamine tartrate in 1934. Graham and Wolff, in 1937, demonstrated the effects of ergotamine tartrate on blood vessels.[42]

Dihydroergotamine (DHE) was synthesized by Stoll and Hofmann in 1943 and was used to treat migraine by Horton, Peters, and Blumenthal at the Mayo Clinic.[45] The earliest ergot formulations were simple fluid extracts – some were very potent while others were practically inert, owing to differential extraction of active substances and the instability of the compounds in alkaline solution. The extract was injected or given orally, although the superiority of parenteral administration was noted even then.[45]

The modern approach to treating migraine began with the development of sumatriptan by Pat Humphrey and his colleagues. Based on the concept that serotonin can relieve headache, they designed a chemical entity that was similar to serotonin, although more stable and with fewer side effects. This development led to the modern clinical trials for acute migraine treatment and to the elucidation of the mechanism of action of what are now called the triptans.

We are at the threshold of an explosion in the under-

standing, diagnosis, and treatment of migraine and other headaches. Many new triptans have been developed and many more will soon be, or are already, available, including zolmitriptan, naratriptan, eletriptan, frovatriptan, rizatriptan, and almotriptan. Modern preventive treatment began with the belief that migraine was due to excess serotonin. Sicuteri helped develop methysergide, a serotonin antagonist for the prophylactic treatment of migraine and cluster headache.[46] After a long hiatus, new drugs are being tested and developed for the preventive treatment of migraine. The antiepileptic drugs have been tested and some have already been proven to be effective for migraine. Concomitant with the development of new treatments is the development of the basic sciences of headache and the renewed dedication of clinicians to headache treatment and teaching.

The gene for familial hemiplegic migraine has been cloned, and putative brainstem centres for migraine and cluster have been identified. Let us hope that future headache sufferers will not relate to this refrain from Iolanthe:[47]

> *When you're lying awake with a dismal headache*
> *And repose is taboo'd by anxiety,*
> *I conceive you may use any language you choose*
> *To indulge in without impropriety.*

References

1. Lyons A, Petrucelli RJ. Medicine: an illustrated history. New York: Harry N. Abrams, Incorporated, 1978.
2. Venzmer G. Five thousand years of medicine. New York: Taplinger Publishing Co, 1972, 19.
3. Thorwald J. Science and secrets of early medicine. London: Thames and Hudson Ltd, 1962, 300–7.
4. Edmeads J. The treatment of headache: a historical perspective. In: Gallagher RM, ed. Therapy for headache. New York: Marcel Dekker Inc., 1990, 1–8.
5. Rawlings CE, Rossitch E. The history of trepanation in Africa with a discussion of its current status and continuing practice. Surg Neurol 1994; 41: 507–13.
6. McHenry LC. Garrison's history of neurology. Springfield: Charles C. Thomas, 1969.
7. Patterson SM, Silberstein SD. Sometimes Jello helps: perceptions of headache etiology, triggers and treatment in literature. Headache 1993; 33: 76–81.
8. Alvarez WC. Was there sick headache in 3000 BC? Gastroenterology 1945; 5: 524.
9. Lance JW. Mechanisms and management of headache. 4th edn. London: Butterworth Scientific, 1982.
10. Critchley M. Migraine: from Cappadocia to Queen Square. In: Smith R, ed. Background to migraine. London: Heinemann, 1967.
11. Plato. The Republic. In: Hamilton E, Cairns H, eds. The collected dialogues of Plato. New York: Pantheon Books, 1961, 651–2.
12. Plato. Charmides. In: Hamilton E, Cairns H, eds. The Collected dialogues of Plato. New York: Pantheon Books, 1961, 103.
13. Gobel H, Isler H, Hasenfratz HP. Headache classification and the Bible: Was St. Paul's thorn in the flesh migraine? Cephalalgia 1995; 15: 182–90.
14. Rosner F. Headache in the writings of Moses Maimonides and other Hebrew sages. Headache 1993; 33: 315–19.
15. Sachs O. Migraine: understanding a common disorder. Berkeley: University of California Press, 1985.
16. Singer C. The visions of Hildegarde of Bingen. In: From magic to science. New York: Dover, 1958.
17. Bright T. A treatise of melancholie. In: Ober WB, ed. Bottoms up!: a pathologist's essay on medicine and humanities. New York: Harper and Row, 1987, 179.
18. Giammarco R, Edmeads J, Dodick D. Critical decisions in headache management. London: B.C. Decker, 1998.
19. Shakespeare W. Othello, the Moor of Venice, Act III, Scene iii. In: The complete works of William Shakespeare. Stamford: Longmeadow Press, 1990, 1132.
20. Shakespeare W. King John Act IV, scene i: 41–2.
21. Gowers WR. A Manual of Diseases of the Nervous System, 1888. Philadelphia: P Plakiston, Son and Co.
22. Airy H. On a distinct form of transient hemianopsia. Philos Trans R Soc Lond 1870; 160: 247–70.
23. Pope A. The rape of the lock. In: Swallow A, ed. The Rinehart book of verse. New York: Holt, Rinehart, and Winston, 1962, 148–9.
24. Liveing E. On Megrim, Sick-headache, and some Allied Disorders: a Contribution to the Pathology of Nerve-storms. Churchill, 1873.
25. Bille B. Migraine in school children. Acta Pediatr Scand 1962; 51: 1–151.
26. Proust M. The Guermantes Way. New York: Vintage Books, 1982.
27. Lewis S. Arrowsmith. New York: American Library, 1952.
28. Vidal G. Lincoln. New York: Ballantyne Books, 1990.
29. Chesnutt M. Mary Chesnutt's Civil War. New Haven: Yale University Press, 1981.
30. Maugham WS. The Razor's Edge. New York: Penguin Books, 1984.
31. Plant GT. The fortification spectra of migraine. Br Med J 1986; 293: 1613–17.
32. King S. Firestarter. New York: Viking Press, 1980.
33. King S. The Running Man. New York: New American Library, 1982.
34. Didion J. In bed. In: Didion J, ed. The white album. New York: Farrar, Straus, and Giroux, 1979.
35. Faulkner W. The Sound and the Fury. New York: The Modern Library, 1929.
36. Collins W. The Woman in White. New York: Penguin Books, 1985.
37. Mason BA. In Country. New York: Harper and Row, 1989.
38. Carver R. Viewfinder. In: Carver R, ed. What we talk about when we talk about love. New York: Vintage Books, 1981, 13
39. Rendell R. Going Wrong. New York: The Mysterious Press, 1990.
40. Williams D. Prescription for Murder. New York: St. Martin's Press, 1991.
41. Grant US. Personal Memoirs of U.S. Grant. New York: The DaCapo Press, 1952.
42. Graham JR, Wolff HG. Mechanisms of migraine headache and action of ergotamine tartrate. Arch Neurol Psychiatry 1938; 39: 737–63.
43. Bové FJ. The Story of Ergot. New York: Karger, 1970.
44. Woakes E. On ergot of rye in the treatment of neuralgia. Br Med J 1868; 2: 360–1.
45. Silberstein SD. The pharmacology of ergotamine and dihydroergotamine. Headache 1997; 37: S15–S25
46. Silberstein SD. Methysergide. Cephalgia 1988; 18: 421–35.
47. Gilbert WS. Love, Unrequited, Robs Me of My Rest (The Nightmare Song). From Iolanthe, 1882.

section 1

Pathophysiology and epidemiology of headache

chapter 2

Classification and diagnosis of headache

Introduction

Headache, like back pain or abdominal pain, is a symptom that can have many causes. It can be a disorder unto itself, such as tension-type headache, part of a symptom complex, such as migraine, or a symptom of an evolving intracranial disorder, such as a brain tumour. Since a range of disorders can produce headache, a systematic approach to headache classification and diagnosis is an essential prelude to its management and treatment.

Before 1988, the headache classification systems that were available had no operational rules and nomenclature was not uniform. In 1988, the International Headache Society (IHS) instituted a classification system that has become the standard for headache diagnosis, particularly for clinical research.[1] The system identifies 12 major categories of headache, which can be divided into two broad groups: the primary headache disorders (Categories 1–4), and the secondary headache disorders (Categories 5–12) (Table 2.1). In secondary headache disorders, the headache is attributable to another condition, such as a brain tumour, stroke or metabolic state. In primary headache disorders there is no attribution; the headache itself is the problem. Thus, for the secondary disorders, the IHS criteria provide an aetiological system that classifies headaches based on their causes. For the primary headache disorders, the IHS criteria provide a descriptive system that classifies headaches based on their symptom profiles. A true aetiological classification is not yet possible for primary headaches because their fundamental causes and mechanisms remain uncertain.

The IHS criteria have received broad international support. They have been endorsed by the World Health Organization (WHO), and the principles of the system have been incorporated into the International Classification of Diseases (ICD-10). The criteria have been translated into German, French, Italian, Spanish, Chinese, Greek, Arabic, Turkish, Slovenian, Danish, Swedish, Thai, Japanese and Portuguese. Thus, the IHS criteria have done much to establish uniform terminology and consistent diagnostic criteria for a range of headache disorders around the world. This has facilitated epidemiological studies and the multinational clinical trials that provide the basis for the current research and treatment guidelines.[2] The IHS criteria are currently undergoing revisions based on what we have learned in the last 10 years.

Table 2.1(A) outlines the four major categories of primary headache: migraine, tension-type headache, cluster headache and a miscellaneous group. The eight secondary categories (summarized in Table 2.1(B)) include headache associated with head trauma, vascular disorders, non-vascular disorders, substances, non-cephalic infection, metabolic disorders, disorders of the face and neck, and cranial neuralgias. Finally, there is a 13th category: headache that is not classifiable elsewhere.

Using the IHS system

Because an individual patient may have more than one headache disorder, the IHS criteria were established to diagnose headache types. If a patient has more than one headache type, each receives its own diagnosis. A careful history is needed to determine how many headache types are present and to characterize each one.[3]

It is not possible or necessary to diagnose each individual headache attack. Single episodes may be difficult to diagnose if the patient does not recall the symptoms, if treatment has attenuated the full expression of symptoms, or if the attack has characteristics that do not fall neatly into a given category. Patients should be asked to describe typical, preferably untreated, attacks and, if necessary, keep diary records of attacks. The diagnosis should be based on the pattern of pain, the associated symptoms, and the physical findings and sometimes laboratory tests.[4]

The IHS criteria use both clinical features and laboratory tests to provide criteria of inclusion (features needed to establish a particular diagnosis) and exclusion (features that prevent assigning a particular diagnosis). The physical examination and laboratory investigations serve to exclude secondary disorders; they also may provide evidence to support the diagnosis of a secondary headache disorder. Thus, the diagnosis of primary headache disorders is based on the patient's report of symptoms of previous attacks, and accurate diagnosis requires explicit rules about the required symptom features. Each major category of primary headache has subtypes that are differentiated based on the symptom profile (i.e. migraine with aura versus migraine without aura), the temporal profile, or the attack frequency (i.e. episodic versus chronic tension-type headache, episodic versus chronic cluster headache). Details about subtyping are presented in subsequent chapters about each major headache category.

The IHS classification system was modelled, in part, on the DSM III system developed by the American Psychiatric

● **Table 2.1** *The IHS classification system*[1]

A Primary headache disorders

1 Migraine
  1.1 Migraine without aura
  1.2 Migraine with aura
  1.3 Ophthalmoplegic
  1.4 Retinal migraine
  1.5 Childhood periodic syndromes that may be precursors to or associated with migraine
  1.6 Complications of migraine
  1.7 Migrainous disorder not fulfilling above criteria

2 Tension-type headache
  2.1 Episodic tension-type headache
  2.2 Chronic tension-type headache
  2.3 Headache of the tension-type not fulfilling above criteria

3 Cluster headache and chronic paroxysmal hemicrania
  3.1 Cluster headache
    3.1.1 Cluster headache periodicity undetermined
    3.1.2 Episodic cluster headache
    3.1.3 Chronic cluster headache
  3.2 Chronic paroxysmal hemicrania
  3.3 Cluster headache-like disorder not fulfilling above criteria

4 Miscellaneous headaches unassociated with structural lesion
  4.1 Idiopathic stabbing headache
  4.2 External compression headache
  4.3 Cold stimulus headache
  4.4 Benign cough headache
  4.5 Benign exertional headache
  4.6 Headache associated with sexual activity

B Secondary headache disorders

5 Headache associated with head trauma
  5.1 Acute post-traumatic headache
  5.2 Chronic post-traumatic headache

6 Headache associated with vascular disorders
  6.1 Acute ischaemic cerebrovascular disease
  6.2 Intracranial haematoma
  6.3 Subarachnoid haemorrhage
  6.4 Unruptured vascular malformation
  6.5 Arteritis
  6.6 Carotid or vertebral artery pain
  6.7 Venous thrombosis
  6.8 Arterial hypertension
  6.9 Headache associated with other vascular disorder

7 Headache associated with non-vascular intracranial disorder
  7.1 High cerebrospinal fluid pressure
  7.2 Low cerebrospinal fluid pressure
  7.3 Intracranial infection
  7.4 Intracranial sarcoidosis and other non-infectious inflammatory diseases
  7.5 Headache related to intrathecal injections
  7.6 Intracranial neoplasm
  7.7 Headache associated with other intracranial disorder

8 Headache associated with substances or their withdrawal
  8.1 Headache induced by acute substance use or exposure
  8.2 Headache induced by chronic substance use or exposure
  8.3 Headache from substance withdrawal (acute use)
  8.4 Headache from substance withdrawal (chronic use)
  8.5 Headache associated with substances but with uncertain mechanism

9 Headache associated with non-cephalic infection
  9.1 Viral infection
  9.2 Bacterial infection
  9.3 Headache related to other infection

10 Headache associated with metabolic disorder
  10.1 Hypoxia
  10.2 Hypercapnia
  10.3 Mixed hypoxia and hypercapnia
  10.4 Hypoglycaemia
  10.5 Dialysis
  10.6 Headache related to other metabolic abnormality

11 Headache or facial pain associated with disorder of cranium, neck, eyes, ears, nose, sinuses, teeth, mouth or other facial or cranial structures
  11.1 Cranial bone
  11.2 Neck
  11.3 Eyes
  11.4 Ears
  11.5 Nose and sinuses
  11.6 Teeth, jaws and related structures
  11.7 Temporomandibular joint disease

12 Cranial neuralgias, nerve trunk pain and deafferentation pain
  12.1 Persistent (in contrast to tic-like) pain of cranial nerve origin
  12.2 Trigeminal neuralgia
    12.2.1 Idiopathic trigeminal neuralgia
    12.2.2 Symptomatic trigeminal neuralgia
  12.3 Glossopharyngeal neuralgia
  12.4 Nervus intermedius neuralgia
  12.5 Superior laryngeal neuralgia
  12.6 Occipital neuralgia
  12.7 Central causes of head and facial pain other than tic douloureux
  12.8 Facial pain not fulfilling criteria in groups 11 or 12

13 Headache not classifiable

● **Table 2.2** *Diagnostic criteria for migraine without aura*[1]

A At least five attacks fulfilling B–D	**D** During headache at least one of the following: 1 Nausea and/or vomiting 2 Photophobia and phonophobia
B Headache attacks lasting 4 to 72 hours (untreated or unsuccessfully treated)	
C Headache has at least two of the following characteristics: 1 Unilateral location 2 Pulsating quality 3 Moderate or severe intensity (inhibits or prohibits daily activities) 4 Aggravation by walking stairs or similar routine physical activity	**E** At least one of the following: 1 History, physical and neurological examinations do not suggest one of the disorders listed in groups 5–11 2 History and/or physical and/or neurological examinations do suggest such disorder, but it is ruled out by appropriate investigations 3 Such disorder is present, but migraine attacks do not occur for the first time in close temporal relation to the disorder

Association.[5] For example, Table 2.2 sets out the criteria to diagnose migraine without aura. The requirements under each lettered heading must be met. Some headings (i.e. A and B) have a single mandatory feature. Other headings include several alternative characteristics. For example, in C, only two of four pain features are required. No single 'pain' feature under heading C is absolutely required for diagnosis. The exclusion criteria are provided under category E. They eliminate other headache disorders based on the history, physical and neurological examinations (E1) or laboratory tests (E2). Alternatively, a secondary headache disorder may be present if the onset of the primary and secondary disorders are separated in time (E3).

Clinical approach: an overview

When evaluating a headache patient, the first task is to identify or exclude a secondary headache disorder. This decision is based on the history and the general medical and neurological examinations (Figure 2.1). Important features in the headache history are summarized in Table 2.3. If suspicious features are present, diagnostic testing may be necessary. Once secondary headaches are excluded, the task is to diagnose one or more specific primary headache disorders. In the initial evaluation, the experienced physician looks for 'headache alarms' that suggest the possibility of a secondary headache disorder. Table 2.4 summarizes these alarms, suggests a partial differential diagnosis, and outlines a possible work-up.

Recent studies have demonstrated that computed tomography (CT) and magnetic resonance imaging (MRI) of the head yield extremely few abnormal findings in headache patients if alarms are absent. If patients do not fit neatly into the IHS diagnostic categories or if response to treatment is atypical, the physician should re-evaluate the patient for secondary headache.[6,7]

Headache history

Overview

Most headache patients have normal medical and neurological examinations. Therefore, a comprehensive history is the most important tool for accurate diagnosis. The headache history should provide a comprehensive picture of the patient's headaches as well as any associated conditions or problems that could influence diagnosis or treatment (Table 2.3).

Taking the headache history provides an opportunity to establish a rapport with the patient that will serve as a basis for an ongoing relationship. Headache sufferers often fear that they are afflicted with some terrible malady. We generally let patients give an unstructured account of their problem ('Tell me about your headaches') and then

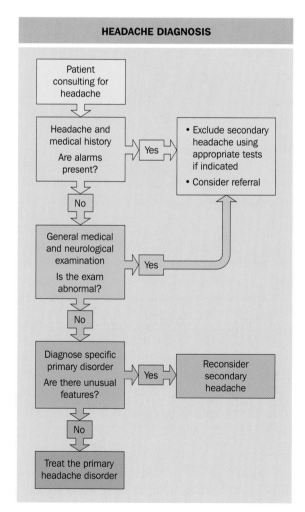

HEADACHE DIAGNOSIS

● *Figure 2.1* Core algorithm for headache diagnosis.

● **Table 2.3** Headache history

Attack onset
Pain location
Attack duration
Attack frequency and timing
Pain severity
Pain quality
Associated feature
Aggravating or precipitating factors
Ameliorating factors
Social history
Family history
Past headache history
Headache impact

● **Table 2.4** *Diagnostic alarms in the evaluation of headache disorders*

Headache alarm	Differential diagnosis	Possible work-up
Headache begins after the age of 50 years	Temporal arteritis, mass lesion	Erythrocyte sedimentation rate, neuroimaging
Sudden-onset headache	Subarachnoid haemorrhage, pituitary apoplexy, bleed into a mass or AVM, mass lesion (especially posterior fossa)	Neuroimaging, lumbar puncture
Accelerating pattern of headaches	Mass lesion, subdural haematoma, medication overuse	Neuroimaging, drug screen
New-onset headache in a patient with cancer or HIV	Meningitis (chronic or carcinomatous), brain abscess (including toxoplasmosis), metastasis	Neuroimaging, lumbar puncture
Headache with systemic illness (fever, stiff neck, rash)	Meningitis, encephalitis, Lyme disease, systemic infection, collagen vascular disease	Neuroimaging, lumbar puncture, blood tests
Focal neurological symptoms or signs of disease (other than typical aura)	Mass lesion, arteriovenous malfunction, stroke, collagen vascular disease (including antiphospholipid antibodies)	Neuroimaging, collagen vascular evaluation
Papilloedema	Mass lesion, pseudotumour, meningitis	Neuroimaging, lumbar puncture

systematically explore various features. Many patients have more than one type of headache or a change in headache pattern over time. We begin with the headache that is the greatest concern to the patient, the one that motivated the person to seek care. We then explore other current headaches and their evolution. When possible, patients complete a written questionnaire prior to consultation. This tool helps patients to focus on their symptoms and course, improving the reliability and efficiency of the history. One such questionnaire, the Headache Evaluation Questionnaire, is shown in Figure 2.2.

Headache onset

The age and context of headache onset provides important diagnostic clues. Primary headaches usually begin in childhood or early adult life, but when headaches begin after the age of 55 years, a serious disorder, such as a mass lesion or giant cell arteritis, is much more likely. The hypnic headache syndrome is a benign form of headache

that usually begins after the age of 60. Events associated with the headache onset may also give clues to diagnosis. A headache that begins after a head injury suggests a post-concussive headache disorder or intracranial pathology (however, head trauma may trigger both migraine and cluster). Headaches that occur in the peripartum period may be due to cortical vein or sagittal sinus thromboses. Fever in association with headache onset suggests an infectious aetiology. Exertion (i.e. weight lifting) may precipitate subarachnoid haemorrhage or benign exertional headache.

Location and duration of pain

Because many headaches follow typical pain patterns, pain localization at onset and the pattern of spread assist diagnosis. A unilateral, hemicranial headache usually suggests migraine or cluster headache. Many migraineurs report that the pain changes sides from attack to attack, although one side may be affected more often than the other. Cluster headaches are almost always unilateral, with the pain centred in or around the eye, temple, cheek or adjacent areas. In contrast to migraine, only 10–15% of cluster patients note a change in the side of pain from one bout of cluster to another. Tension-type headache pain is typically bilateral.

Localized pain may also occur with organic diseases. The trigeminal nerve is the major source of innervation to the pain-producing structures in the supratentorial space. Infratentorial pain-producing structures receive innervation from the upper cervical, glossopharyngeal and vagus nerves. Supratentorial lesions often cause frontal headaches, while infratentorial lesions often produce pain in the occipital region, although overlap in the distribution of neurons projecting to the trigeminocervical complex leads to referral outside this strict pattern (see Chapter 5). When headache is strictly limited to the periorbital region, ocular pathology or ophthalmic zoster before the rash should be considered. Trigeminal neuralgia may cause pain in any area of the face innervated by the trigeminal nerve. Over half of patients with brain tumours complain of headache, and the site of pain is on the same side as the tumour in 80%. Headaches associated with cerebrovascular disease may be global or lateralized. When lateralized, the headaches are ipsilateral to the lesion only half of the time.

Pain duration also provides clues for diagnosis. Migraines typically last from 4 to 72 hours. When they persist for more than 72 hours, the term 'status migrainosus' is applied. Cluster headaches usually last an average of 15–180 minutes; they may, however, be as short as 10 minutes or as long as several hours. The headaches of paroxysmal hemicrania typically last 5–20 minutes, with a

HEADACHE EVALUATION QUESTIONNAIRE

Instructions: This questionnaire helps evaluate the headaches you have had in the *past 3 months*.
Please answer every question as best you can in the space provided.

Name _____ Age _____ Sex: Female _____ Male _____ Today's date: _____

1 What would you like us to know about your headaches? (Tick all the answers that apply.)
a _____ I want you to know about my headaches, but I don't need help right now.
b _____ I would like help about my headaches this visit.
c _____ My headaches are the main reason for this visit.
d _____ I am very worried about my overall health because of my headaches.
e _____ Other _____ Please describe: _____

2 Has your doctor ever told you what kind of headache you have?
If Yes, what did you doctor call your headache? _____ Cluster _____ Migraine _____ Tension _____ Other: _____
If No, what kind of headache do you think you have? _____ Cluster _____ Migraine _____ Tension _____ Other: _____

3 During the *past 3 months*, how many days did you have headache? _____ Days

4 During the *past 3 months*, how many days did your headaches limit you from working, studying, or carrying on your usual activities? _____ Days

5 During the *past 3 months*, how many days have you taken the following drugs?
(Please write '0' for none.)

Over-the counter (OTC) drugs		Drugs prescribed by a doctor			
Advil®	_____ Days	Amerge®	_____ Days	Vicodin®	_____ Days
Aleve®	_____ Days	Cafergot®	_____ Days	Wigraine®	_____ Days
Aspirin®	_____ Days	Fioricet®	_____ Days	Zomig®	_____ Days
Excedrin®	_____ Days	Fiorinal®	_____ Days	Other prescription drugs	_____ Days
Motrin®	_____ Days	Imitrex®	_____ Days	Specify _____	
Nuprin®	_____ Days	Maxalt®	_____ Days		
Tylenol®	_____ Days	Midrin®	_____ Days		
Other OTC drugs	_____ Days	Tylenon® with codeine	_____ Days		
Specify _____					

6 During the *past 3 months*, has the pain, number of your headaches, or concern about your headaches changed? _____ Yes _____ No
If yes, tick the answers that apply to the *past 3 months*, as compared with other times before:
a The pain of my headaches has: _____ Decreased _____ Remained the same _____ Increased _____ Significantly increased
b The number of my headaches has: _____ Decreased _____ Remained the same _____ Increased _____ Significantly increased
c The worry, trouble, or anxiety
caused by my headaches has: _____ Decreased _____ Remained the same _____ Increased _____ Significantly increased

7 For *each* of the following statements, tick how often each type of pain was associated with your headaches during the *past 3 months*.

	Never	Rarely	Less than half the time	More than half the time
a The pain was worse on just one side	☐	☐	☐	☐
b The pain was pounding, pulsing, or throbbing	☐	☐	☐	☐
c The pain was moderate or severe	☐	☐	☐	☐
d The pain was made worse by routine activities such as walking or climbing stairs	☐	☐	☐	☐

8 For *each* of the following statements, tick how often you felt discomfort with your headaches during the *past 3 months*.

	Never	Rarely	Less than half the time	More than half the time
a You felt nauseated or sick to your stomach	☐	☐	☐	☐
b You saw spots, stars, zig-zags, lines, or grey areas continuously for several minutes or more during or before you headaches	☐	☐	☐	☐
c Light bothered you (a lot more than when you don't have headaches)	☐	☐	☐	☐
d Sound bothered you (a lot more than when you don't have headaches)	☐	☐	☐	☐

● **Figure 2.2** *Headache evaluation questionnaire.*

range from 1 to 120 minutes. Episodic tension-type headaches tend to last from 30 minutes to 7 days. Headaches of organic origin do not have a characteristic duration; a change in attack duration suggests the need for diagnostic evaluation.

Frequency and timing of attacks

The frequency and timing of headaches help to determine both diagnosis and treatment. We ask patients how often their attacks occur and what is the longest headache-free period they have had in the last 6 months. Migraine attacks may occur at random, in association with the menstrual cycle, or with specific temporal patterns (on weekends, on vacation, or upon relaxing after stress). Episodic cluster headaches typically occur in a regular pattern. During the cluster period, which usually lasts between 2 weeks and 6 months, headaches may occur as rarely as once every other day or as often as 8 times a day. The attacks tend to recur at similar times of the day or night, often waking the patient during rapid eye-movement (REM) sleep. Episodic tension-type headaches recur less than 15 times a month. If they recur more frequently, they are classified as chronic tension-type headaches. Headache patterns may lead to a useful preventive treatment strategy. For example, menstrual migraines may respond to perimenstrual nonsteroidal antiinflammatory medications (NSAIDs). Nocturnal cluster attacks may be prevented by administering ergotamine at bedtime. Organic headaches may be episodic or daily and continuous. Organic headaches do not occur with any set pattern and may mimic the known primary headaches, but if headache frequency increases or if the headaches change in character, diagnostic evaluation is needed.

Pain severity and quality

Pain severity and the rapidity of onset and resolution are important diagnostic clues. We advise using a 1–10 scale, wherein 1 represents minimal discomfort and 10 represents the most excruciating pain the patient can imagine. While these numbers may not be completely comparable across patients, they are very useful for charting improvement in an individual attack. Because most headaches vary in intensity during an attack and across different attacks, it is also useful to inquire about the range of pain experienced during a headache. Headaches of very sudden onset are worrisome. The headache of subarachnoid haemorrhage or pituitary apoplexy typically have a sudden, explosive onset.

Pain quality often provides diagnostic clues. Migraine pain is characteristically throbbing or pulsatile, but it often begins as a dull, steady ache that slowly evolves; it may

not acquire a throbbing quality until the pain becomes moderate or severe in intensity. The pain of cluster headaches is usually deep, boring or piercing. It is sometimes likened to having a red-hot poker thrust into an eye. Patients often describe their tension-type headaches as dull, band-like, or vice-like. The characteristic headache of a brain tumour resembles tension-type headache. The headache from a rupture of an aneurysm or arteriovenous malformation is most often a continuous, intense, aching or throbbing pain.

Associated features

Associated symptoms or features may occur prior to, during, or following the headache. The details of associated features of specific headache types are discussed in the appropriate subsequent chapters. We highlight a few points about history-taking here. We generally ask: 'When you get this headache, are there other features that come before, during, or after the pain? Is there anything else you note?' If the patient does not volunteer these features, the physician should inquire, taking care not to elicit false-positive responses. It is important to distinguish symptoms associated with the attack from symptoms that are always present. For example, if someone is always sensitive to light and the sensitivity does not change during the headache, photosensitivity is not an associated feature of the headache attack. Headache-associated photophobia refers to an unusual or heightened sensitivity to light during a headache attack.

Secondary headache disorders often have associated features. Neurological deficits may accompany the headache of organic disease, depending upon the localization of the lesion. Intracranial mass lesions are associated with nausea and vomiting or vomiting (projectile) without nausea in half the cases. Giant cell arteritis may be associated with localized scalp tenderness, malaise, arthralgias or myalgias (polymyalgia rheumatica), low-grade fevers, depression or other constitutional symptoms, and visual disturbances or stroke. Jaw claudication, if present, is virtually pathognomonic for giant cell arteritis. Fever and stiff neck typify the headache of meningitis.

Aggravating or precipitating factors

Identifying factors that precipitate or aggravate headache attacks may be useful in establishing a diagnosis or in implementing a treatment programme. Recognizing triggers helps patients avoid precipitants.

The pain of migraine can be influenced by internal or external factors. The most frequently reported triggers include menstruation, stress, relaxation after stress, fatigue, too much or too little sleep, skipping a meal, weather changes, high humidity, high altitude, exposure to glare or flickering lights, loud noises, perfumes or chemical fumes, postural changes, physical activity, or coughing. Food triggers occur in many adult migraineurs and most often include chocolate, cheeses, alcoholic beverages (especially red wine), citrus fruits, and foods containing monosodium glutamate, nitrates and aspartate. Some believe that the desire to eat chocolate is part of the pro-drome of migraine. Cocaine use and cocaine withdrawal may also trigger a migraine-like headache. Cluster headaches are usually triggered within 30 minutes by ingesting alcohol. During the remission phase of a cluster headache, alcohol consumption may not precipitate an attack. Cluster headache pain is often aggravated by lying down. Tension-type headaches are said to be aggravated by the stresses of everyday life and so may be worse toward the end of the day. Patients with trigeminal neural-gia have trigger points on the face and the mucous mem-branes of the mouth. Slight stimulation of these trigger points by eating, speaking, exposure to cold air, brushing the teeth, stroking, shaving, or washing the face may provoke an attack.

Headaches caused by brain tumours are intensified by exertion, postural changes, bending over or coughing. Aneurysmal rupture may be precipitated by exertion, including exercise or sex.

Ameliorating factors

Identifying the factors, both non-pharmacological and pharmacological, that ameliorate the discomfort of both the headache and the associated symptoms provides useful diagnostic and therapeutic information. Migraineurs commonly say that they must retire to a dark, quiet room and lie motionless to obtain relief; many patients find that sleep will clear their attacks. Relief often occurs when the patient applies hot or cold compresses or presses on the superficial temporal artery (but only during the period of compression). Migraine frequency and severity often decrease during the last two trimesters of pregnancy or with the onset of menopause, and this is probably also true of cluster headache. Cluster headache patients note that sitting upright, rocking in a chair, pacing to and fro, or engaging in vigorous movement seems to lessen the pain. Tension-type headache may be alleviated by relaxation, rest or sleep.

If medications have been used, determine their dosage, frequency, efficacy and side-effects. Inquire how long the prescription has been used. The patient may be using the drug erroneously, either taking a subtherapeutic dosage or taking the medication too infrequently. Conversely, he or she may be overusing or abusing the medications. Often patients will not recognize how much analgesic they are using until you ask 'How long does a bottle of 100 pills last?'

Social history

Social factors may play a significant role in headache. Explore the patient's marital and family status, education, occupation, outside interests and friendships. Are any of these areas a source of stress? Has the patient recently had a major life change such as marriage, divorce, separa-tion, a new job, retirement, or a death in the family? Is work satisfying or merely drudgery? Is there conflict in the workplace? What is the patient's employment? Exposure to drugs or toxins in the workplace may trigger headaches. For example, workers in munitions factories may develop nitroglycerin headaches or have migraine triggered. Carbon monoxide exposure can occur in the workplace or at home due to poor ventilation. Inquire about other habits, such as the use of alcohol, tobacco, caffeine or illicit drugs.

A history of unprotected sex should prompt a search for a potential infectious cause of the headache. Sleep habits may be significant. Sleep apnoea is not uncommon, espe-cially in the overweight, and may cause morning headache. Depression may be manifested as difficulty in falling asleep, difficulty staying asleep or early morning awakening. Likewise, trouble falling asleep may occur with anxiety. Careful questioning about the above possible stressors may uncover a source of conflict or a psychologi-cal component to the headache.

Family history

Because some headache disorders are familial, it is useful to obtain a family history. Attempt to get a description of the headache and associated features, rather than accept the patient's diagnosis of a relative's headache. It would be ideal to get a brief description of the headache from the affected relative because third-party reports of symp-toms are often unreliable. Approximately 50–60% of migraineurs have a parent with the disorder, and as many as 80% have at least one first-degree relative with migraine. Cluster headaches rarely occur within the same family. Forty percent of patients with tension-type headaches have family members with similar headaches.

Familial headaches do not necessarily imply a genetic basis, although genetic factors play a role in migraine, tension-type headache and cluster headache. Shared environmental exposures may contribute to familial headaches. For example, a leaky furnace may cause carbon monoxide-induced headaches in an entire family.

Past headache history

It is useful to be aware of medications that were previously prescribed and the dosages in which they were given because: (1) treatment response may support a diagnosis, and (2) a detailed history may help explain past treatment failures. Unsuccessful treatment is often the result of incorrect dosing strategies or not allowing enough time to obtain a potential benefit (e.g. discontinuing a beta-blocker after only a 1-week trial). (3) Knowing the history of benefits and side-effects will guide future treatment plan. Ascertain the benefits or side-effects of each past and current medication and the reason for its discontinuation. Inquire about the use and efficacy of prior non-drug therapies such as psychotherapy, biofeedback, acupuncture or chiropractic care.

Review the patient's current approach to headache treatment. Many headache sufferers overuse medications, knowingly or unwittingly. Many over-the-counter pain relievers contain caffeine with acetaminophen (paracetamol) or aspirin or NSAIDs. The excessive use of these agents, as well as narcotics, barbiturates, and ergots, can produce withdrawal or rebound headaches. Again, determine the dosages and the frequency of drug use. Correcting a subtherapeutic regimen may lead to better headache control. Abuse or overuse of medications must be addressed and may require hospitalization for detoxification.

Many patients with long-standing headaches have had a multitude of diagnostic procedures and have taken a variety of medications. Every reasonable effort should be made to verify prior test results. Obtain a copy of the test report or, better still, a copy of the test itself.

Impact and disability of headache

Diagnosis alone does not provide enough information about the primary headache disorders to optimize therapy. Headaches differ in severity within a diagnostic category. Some patients seek help primarily because they are concerned that the headache is symptomatic of a serious underlying disease. For these patients, reassurance may be the most important intervention. More often, patients have severe pain and disability and require a programme of care for improving their lives. It is therefore important to ask patients how their headaches affect their lives and establish what they were hoping for in seeking medical care.

We recommend a more formal approach to assessing headache severity. Figure 2.3 contains a version of a self-administered instrument called the Migraine Disability Assessment (MIDAS) questionnaire. The questionnaire assesses the impact of headache on work and school, chores and household work, as well as social, family, and leisure activity. It measures actual days of missed activity (i.e. work absenteeism as well as days with high levels of activity limitations). It can help doctors and patients focus on how headaches affect a patient's life. Formal validation studies have established the reliability, validity, and clinical utility of the MIDAS questionnaire. Migraine is the likely diagnosis when patients have high levels of disability due to episodic primary headache.

Physical and neurological examinations

A thorough physical examination should include vital signs, examination of the heart and lungs, and auscultation of the carotid and perhaps vertebral arteries for bruits. Palpate the head and neck, looking for trigger points, other tender areas, masses, bruises or thickened blood vessels. Examine the temporomandibular joint for tenderness, decreased mobility, asymmetry, or 'clicking'.

A few key signs on the neurological examination bear emphasis. Evidence of papilloedema suggests increased

This form can help you and your doctor improve the management of your headaches

Do You Suffer From

headaches?

MIDAS QUESTIONNAIRE

INSTRUCTIONS: Please answer the following questions about ALL your headaches you have had over the last 3 months. Write your answer in the box next to each question. Write zero if you did not do the activity in the last 3 months.

1	On how many days in the last 3 months did you miss work or school because of your headaches?	days
2	How many days in the last 3 months was your productivity at work or school reduced by half or more because of your headaches? (Do not include days you counted in question 1 where you missed work or school)	days
3	On how many days in the last 3 months did you not do household work because of your headaches?	days
4	How many days in the last 3 months was your productivity in household work reduced by half or more because of your headaches? (Do not include days you counted in question 3 where you did not do household work)	days
5	On how many days in the last 3 months did you miss family, social or leisure activities because of your headaches?	days
	TOTAL	days
A	On how many days in the last 3 months did you have a headache? (If a headache lasted more than 1 day, count each day)	days
B	On a scale of 0-10, on average how painful were these headaches? (Where 0 = no pain at all, and 10 = pain as bad as it can be)	

©Innovative Medical Research 1997

Once you have filled in the questionnaire, add up the total number of days from questions 1-5 (ignore A and B).

Grading system for the MIDAS Questionnaire:		
Grade	Definition	Score
I	Little or no disability	0-5
II	Mild disability	6-10
III	Moderate disability	11-20
IV	Severe disability	21+

⚡MIDAS

The MIDAS programme is sponsored by

AstraZeneca

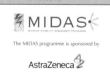

● *Figure 2.3* Migraine Disability Assessment (MIDAS) Questionnaire.

intracranial pressure and warrants an imaging procedure to rule out a mass lesion. Nuchal rigidity due to meningeal irritation is seen with meningitis, intracerebral mass lesions, and intraparenchymal or subarachnoid haemorrhages, and mandates a rapid work-up. Focal neurological deficits may indicate structural brain disease and therefore require neuroimaging. A thickened or nodular temporal artery, diminished or absent temporal artery pulsations, reddened, tender scalp nodules, or necrotic lesions of the scalp or tongue suggest giant cell arteritis and should prompt an erythrocyte sedimentation rate and perhaps a temporal artery biopsy. Horner's syndrome may be seen with cluster headaches, chronic paroxysmal hemicrania, or carotid or intracranial lesions.[7,8]

While most patients with a chief complaint of headache will have an entirely normal examination, this portion of the consultation must not be overlooked, for it will help guide subsequent diagnostic and treatment strategies.

History after the initial visit

On occasion, a diagnosis may not be established on the first visit, or the initial assessment may be incorrect. It is useful to have the patient keep a headache diary for both diagnostic and treatment purposes. The patient logs the headache frequency, severity and duration, the medications that were used and the possible headache triggers. On subsequent visits, reviewing the diary may uncover previously unrecognized patterns that can provide clues in diagnosis. The headache triggers that are identified may suggest behavioural interventions.

Conclusions

Obtaining a complete and accurate history is an art that takes practice. Though taking a headache history can be time-consuming and frustrating, time invested at the initial assessment facilitates diagnosis and provides a good opportunity to establish a relationship with the patient. The use of diaries and other patient-completed questionnaires can improve the accuracy of the history and save time. Table 2.5 summarizes features of the various headache disorders discussed in this chapter and throughout the text.

● **Table 2.5** *Differential diagnosis of selected headache disorders*

Headache type	Typical age of onset (years)	Usual location	Duration	Frequency/ timing	Severity	Quality	Associated Features
Migraine	5–40	Hemicranial	Several hours to 3 days	Variable	Moderate –severe	Throbbing > steady ache	Nausea, vomiting, photo/phono/ osmophobia, scotomata, neurological deficits
Tension type	10–50	Bilateral	30 min to 7 days +	Variable	Dull ache may wax/ wane	Vise-like, band-like pressure	Generally none
Cluster	15–40	Unilateral peri/retro-orbital	30–120 min	1–8 times per day, nocturnal attacks	Excruciating	Boring piercing	Ipsilateral conjunctival injection, lacrimation, nasal congestion, rhinorrhea, miosis, facial sweating
Mass lesion	Any	Any	Variable	Intermittent, nocturnal, upon arising	Moderate	Dull steady/ throbbing	Vomiting, nuchal rigidity, neurological deficits
Subarachnoid haemorrhage	Adult	Global, often occipitonuchal	Variable	Not applicable	Excruciating	Explosive	Nausea, vomiting, nuchal rigidity, loss of consciousness, neurological deficits
Trigeminal neuralgia	50–70	2nd–3rd > 1st division's trigeminal nerve	Seconds, occur in volleys	Paroxysmal	Excruciating	Electric shock-like	Facial trigger facial points, spasm of muscles ipsilaterally (Tic)
Giant cell arteritis	>55	Temporal, any region	Intermittent, then continuous	Constant, ? worse at night	Variable	Variable	Tender scalp arteries, polymyalgia rhematica, jaw claudication

References

1. Headache Classification Committee of the International Headache Society. Classification and diagnostic criteria for headache disorders, cranial neuralgia, and facial pain. Cephalalgia 1988; 8: 1–96.

2. Pryse-Phillips WEM, Dodick DW, Edmeads JG et al. Guidelines for the diagnosis and management of migraine in clinical practice. Can Med Assoc J 1997; 156: 1273–87.

3. Silberstein SD. Evaluation and emergency treatment of headache. Headache 1992; 32: 396–407.

4. Dalessio DJ, Silberstein SD. Diagnosis and classification of headache. In: Dalessio DJ, Silberstein SD, eds. Wolff's headache and other head pain. Sixth ed. New York: Oxford University Press, 1993, 3–18.

5. American Psychiatric Association. Diagnostic and statistical manual of mental disorders. Fourth ed. Washington: American Psychiatric Association, 1994.

6. Quality Standards Subcommittee of the American Academy of Neurology. Practice parameter: the utility of neuroimaging in the evaluation of headache in patients with normal neurologic examinations (summary statement). Neurology 1994; 44: 1353–4.

7. Frishberg B, Rosenberg JH, Matchar DB et al. Evidence-based guidelines in the primary care setting: Neuroimaging in patients with nonacute headache. http://www.aan.com.

8. Edmeads J. Emergency management of headache. Headache 1988; 28: 675–9.

chapter 3

Epidemiology and impact of headache disorders

Introduction

Epidemiologic studies describe the scope and distribution of headache disorders and their impact on individuals and on society.[1,2] These studies can facilitate clinical decision-making and help support the view that headache should be a treatment priority.[1–3] Understanding sociodemographic, familial, and environmental risk factors helps identify those groups at highest risk for headache and ultimately may provide clues to preventive strategies or disease mechanisms. Epidemiologic studies have identified a number of conditions that are comorbid (that is, occurring at a higher frequency than would be expected by chance) with migraine. Thus, comorbidity must be considered in formulating treatment plans and may provide insights into the mechanisms of disease.[3,4]

Epidemiologic studies evaluate individuals in the population, whether or not they seek care, to identify their headache disorders. This approach to research is important, since less than half of active migraine sufferers actually see a doctor each year for headache and consultation rates are even lower for tension-type headache.[5,6] As a consequence, substantial selection bias occurs in clinic-based studies, where factors that predispose individuals to consult may be mistaken for attributes of the disease.

Recent epidemiologic and health services research studies have employed the criteria of the International Headache Society (IHS), which are more complete, explicit, and rigorous than the criteria that were used in past studies.[1,2,7–13] In this chapter, we will review the epidemiology of headache, emphasizing the population-based studies of primary headache disorders that use the IHS criteria.

Epidemiology

Epidemiologic principles (Table 3.1)
For clinical practice and epidemiologic research, precise case definitions facilitate reliable and valid diagnosis.[1,2] There is no true diagnostic gold standard for the primary headache disorders, which makes it difficult to study validity. The gold standard used in most research is a diagnosis assigned after a careful clinical assessment applying the IHS criteria.[7] The validity of IHS-based diagnosis is sup-

ported by the creation of relatively homogeneous diagnostic groups with a consistent risk factor profile, natural history, pattern of treatment responses, and biological markers.

Epidemiologic studies often focus on prevalence or incidence. Prevalence is defined as the proportion of a given population that has a disease over a defined period. As the period selected for study increases, prevalence increases. Incidence refers to the rate of onset of new cases of a disease in a given population over a defined period. Prevalence is determined by the product of average incidence and average duration of disease. For example, migraine prevalence may increase because either incidence or duration of disease is increasing.

Epidemiologic studies require clearly-defined diagnostic boundaries. In headache, the most difficult boundary to identify is the one between migraine and tension-type headache. While some view these two disorders as distinct entities, others favor the 'spectrum' or 'continuum' concept, the idea that migraine and tension-type headache exist as polar ends on a continuum of severity, varying more in degree than in kind.[14–17] For example, Waters examined the associations among his key migraine features (warning, unilateral pain, nausea, or vomiting) in women between the ages of 20 and 64 years and found that as headache intensity increased, migrainous symptoms occurred together more frequently.[16,17] He concluded: 'The

● **Table 3.1** Definitions of epidemiological terms

Reliability:	Independent diagnostic evaluations yield consistent diagnostic results.
Validity:	The assigned diagnosis is related to the underlying biology of the disorder.
Prevalence:	The proportion of a given population that has a disorder over a defined period of time.
Lifetime prevalence:	The proportion of individuals who have ever had the condition.
Period prevalence:	The proportion of individuals who have had at least one attack within a defined interval, usually within one year of the time of ascertainment.
Incidence:	The onset of new cases of a disease in a defined population over a given period of time

distribution of the headache severity extends as a continuous spectrum from mild attacks, which usually have neither unilateral distribution nor warning nor nausea, to severe headaches which are frequently accompanied by the three migraine features'. Other authors have provided some empirical support for the continuum concept.[14,18]

There is ongoing debate regarding the relationship between migraine and tension-type headache.[7,15,18,19] Much of the available data supports the spectrum concept and the notion that the disorders are distinct. The Spectrum Study demonstrates that people with migraine have migraine, migrainous, and tension-type headaches and that all three headache types respond to sumatriptan.[19] The fact that 'pure tension-type' headache is unresponsive to sumatriptan supports the view that in pure form, tension-type headache and migraine are distinct.[19] Much of the epidemiologic work assumes that migraine is a distinct disorder. If the continuum concept is correct, the current literature describes the epidemiology of the upper tail of a distribution of severity rather than the epidemiology of a distinct disorder.

Epidemiology of primary and secondary headache

Using the IHS criteria, Rasmussen and coworkers examined the population distribution of all headache disorders using in-person clinical assessment in a large, representative community sample in the greater Copenhagen area.[2,8] The lifetime prevalence of various headache disorders is summarized in Table 3.2.

Tension-type headache was a far more common primary headache than migraine. Of the secondary headaches, fasting headache (a headache precipitated by hunger) was the most common, followed by the headache of nose/sinus disease and head trauma. Nonvascular

intracranial disease, which includes infections and brain tumours, is extremely rare. The rest of the chapter will focus on migraine, tension-type headache, and cluster headache.

Migraine incidence studies

Although migraine incidence is best evaluated in longitudinal studies of persons at risk for migraine, cross-sectional data can be used to derive incidence estimates. Stewart et al[20] estimated migraine incidence using prevalence data (Figure 3.1). In males, the incidence of migraine with aura peaked around 5 years of age at 6.6/1000 person-years; the peak for migraine without aura was between ages 10 and 11 years (10/1000 person-years). New cases of migraine were uncommon in men in their twenties. In females, the incidence of migraine with aura peaked between ages 12 and 13 (14.1/1000 person-years); migraine without aura peaked between ages 14 and 17 (18.9/1000 person-years). Thus, migraine begins earlier in males than in females and migraine with aura begins earlier than does migraine without aura.

Stang et al[21] used the linked medical records system in

● **Table 3.2** *Lifetime prevalence of headache*

Type	Prevalence (%)
Primary headache	
Tension-type headache	78
Migraine	16
Secondary headache	
Fasting	19
Nose/sinus disease	15
Head trauma	4
Non-vascular intracranial disease (including brain tumor)	0.5

After Rasmussen et al.[8]

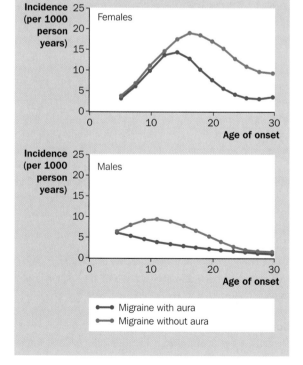

● **Figure 3.1** *Age- and sex-specific incidence of migraine.[20]*

Olmstead County, Minnesota, US, to identify migraine sufferers who sought medical care for headaches. Their incidence was lower (probably because many people with migraine do not consult doctors or receive a medical diagnosis)[5,6,22] and their peaks later than those identified by Stewart et al[20] (because medical diagnosis may occur long after the age of onset).

Migraine prevalence studies

The published estimates of migraine prevalence have varied widely (see reviews).[1,2,23] In 1995, a meta-analysis of 24 studies that met inclusion criteria included only five that used IHS criteria.[23] A meta-analysis revealed that the case definition, along with age and gender distribution of the study samples, explained 70% of the variation in migraine prevalence among studies. Rasmussen et al conducted the first epidemiologic study using the operational diagnostic criteria of the IHS[8] in Copenhagen. For men, the lifetime prevalences were 93% for any kind of headache, 8% for migraine and 69% for tension-type headache. For women, the lifetime prevalences were 99% for all headache, 25% for migraine and 88% for tension-type headache. The 1-year period prevalence of migraine was 6% in men and 15% in women; the 1-year period prevalence of tension-type headache was 63% and 86%, respectively.

The first American Migraine Study, conducted in 1989, used questionnaires mailed to 15 000 households selected to be representative of the US population.[9] Migraine diagnosis differed from the IHS criteria in that the headache duration and the lifetime number of previous migraine attacks were not considered. Migraine prevalence was 17.6% for women and 6% for men, closely paralleling the estimates of Rasmussen et al.[8] A follow-up study, the American Migraine Study II, used virtually identical methodology 10 years later and demonstrated very similar prevalence estimates.[13]

In France, Henry et al reported that the prevalence of IHS migraine was 11.9% in women and 4.0% in men.[10] In this study, diagnoses were assigned based on lay interviews using a validated algorithm. For the group that included 'borderline migraine', prevalence estimates were 17.6% for females and 6.1% for males, remarkably close to the findings of Stewart et al. A number of other recent studies in Western Europe and the United States have examined the prevalence of migraine.[11,12,24–26]

Sociodemographic variables

Migraine prevalence varies by age and gender. Before puberty, migraine prevalence is higher in boys than in girls; prevalence then increases more rapidly in girls than in boys as adolescence approaches.[27–33] Prevalence increases until approximately age 40, after which it declines (Figure 3.2).[1,2,9,13] These dramatic age effects account for some of the variation in previous studies.

The gender ratio (ratio of migraine prevalence in females over the prevalence in males) also varies with age (Figure 3.3).[9,13] Cyclical hormonal changes associated with menses may account for some aspects of the migraine prevalence ratio.[34] However, hormonal factors cannot account for all of the gender differences; prevalence remains substantially higher in women than men, even at

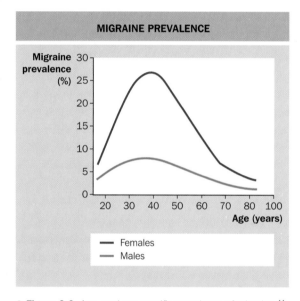

● *Figure 3.2* Age- and sex-specific prevalence of migraine.[44]

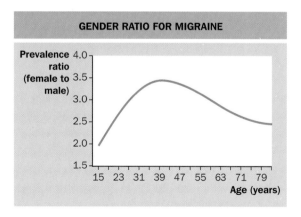

● *Figure 3.3* Female-to-male prevalence ratio of migraine by age.[27]

the age of 70 years, well beyond the time that cyclical hormonal changes can be considered a factor.[9,13]

Physician- and clinic-based studies have suggested that migraine is associated with high intelligence and social class. Bille did not demonstrate an association between migraine prevalence and intelligence in school children.[27,28] Epidemiologic studies in adults using intelligence testing and occupation as measures of socioeconomic status do not confirm a direct relationship between migraine and social class or intelligence.[35] In both the American Migraine Study I and II, migraine prevalence was inversely related to income[9,13] (i.e. migraine prevalence fell as household income increased) (Figure 3.4). The National Health Interview Study confirmed that migraine prevalence is highest in low-income groups;[36] prevalence was lowest for middle-income groups and began to rise in the high-income group. Since this study relied on self-reported migraine, and migraine awareness rises with income, differential ascertainment by income may account for this relationship in higher income groups. A population-based study in Kentucky[25] and a managed care-based study[36] have confirmed this inverse relationship in the US.

Individuals from high income groups were much more likely to report a medical diagnosis of migraine than were those with lower income.[5,22] Migraine appears to be a disease of persons with high income in the doctor's office, because of who seeks care, but migraine is not associated with high income in the community. As Waters suggested, people from higher income households are more likely to consult physicians and are therefore disproportionately included in clinic-based studies.[35]

The higher migraine prevalence in the lower socioeconomic groups may be a consequence of a circumstance associated with low income and migraine, such as poor diet, poor medical care, or stress.[1,9,13] It may also reflect social selection; i.e. migraineurs may have lower incomes because migraine interferes with educational and occupational function, causing a loss of income or the ability to rise from a low-income group. The relationship of migraine and socioeconomic status requires further study. Since migraine prevalence appears unrelated to social class in a number of studies from Europe and elsewhere, it may be influenced by patterns of medical consulting behavior and access to medical care in different countries.[2,8,11,12,37]

Is migraine prevalence increasing?

Some reports suggest that migraine prevalence may be increasing.[38] According to the Centers for Disease Control, self-diagnosed migraine prevalence in the United States increased 60%, from 25.8/1000 to 41/1000 persons, between 1981 and 1989. Medical records data from Olmstead County also suggest prevalence is increasing.[21] The stability of prevalence in studies in the US over the past decade does not support the view that prevalence is increasing.[9,13] We have suggested instead that the demonstrable increases in medical consultation and diagnosis may have caused an apparent rather than a real increase.[5,22,39]

Comorbidity of migraine

Why study comorbidity?

The term 'comorbidity', originally coined by Feinstein,[40] is now used to refer to the greater than coincidental association of two conditions in the same individual.[4] Migraine is comorbid with a number of neurologic and psychiatric disorders, including stroke, epilepsy, depression, and anxiety disorders. Understanding the comorbidity of migraine is potentially important from a number of different perspec-

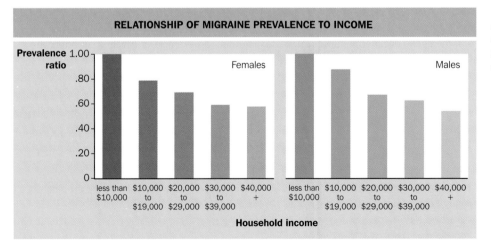

RELATIONSHIP OF MIGRAINE PREVALENCE TO INCOME

● *Figure 3.4*
Relationship of migraine prevalence to household income.

tives.[4] First, the occurrence of comorbidity has implications for headache diagnosis. Migraine has substantial symptomatic overlap with several of the conditions that are comorbid with it. For example, both migraine and epilepsy can cause transient alterations of consciousness as well as headache. This problem of differential diagnosis is well recognized. Less well recognized is the problem of concomitant diagnosis. When two conditions are comorbid, the presence of migraine should increase, not reduce, the index of suspicion for disorders such as epilepsy, depression and anxiety disorders. Second, comorbidity has important implications for treatment. Comorbid conditions may impose therapeutic limitations, but may also create therapeutic opportunities. For example, when migraine and depression occur together, an antidepressant may successfully treat both conditions. For example, the antimigraine antiepileptic agent, divalproex sodium (sodium valproate), may prevent attacks of both migraine and epilepsy. Finally, the study of comorbidity may provide epidemiologic clues to the fundamental mechanisms of migraine.

Migraine and stroke

Both migraine and stroke are chronic neurologic disorders associated with focal neurologic deficits, alterations in cerebral blood flow and headache. The relationships between migraine and stroke, are complex. Headaches have been associated with stroke as ictal, preictal or postictal phenomena.[41] The association between migraine and stroke is stronger for migraine with aura and for stroke within the posterior circulation.[42–44] Migraine aura, if prolonged, may give rise to stroke, a condition termed 'true migrainous infarction'.[7,41]

A number of hospital series have attempted to estimate the proportion of all strokes attributable to migraine using case-by-case clinical review. In patients under 50 years of age, 1–17% of strokes were attributed to migraine.[40–42] Bougousslavsky et al reported that among patients with stroke, if the stroke occurred during the migraine attack, only 9% had arterial lesions; if the stroke occurred remote from the migraine attack, 91% had an arterial lesion.[45] Mechanisms other than traditional arterial disease may underlie migrainous infarction.

A number of case–control studies have examined migraine as a risk factor for stroke. The Collaborative Group for the Study of Stroke in Young Women compared hospitalized stroke patients with both hospital-based and community controls.[46] There was a twofold increase in the risk of stroke for women with migraine when compared with community controls but not relative to hospital controls.[46] Henrich and Horowitz found an association between migraine and stroke in a hospital-based

case–control study, but differences disappeared after adjusting for stroke risk factors.[47]

Tzourio et al[48,49] reported that migraine was associated with a fourfold increased risk of stroke in women under 45 years of age, with an even greater risk in women who smoked. These studies did not examine the relationship between migraine and stroke at the time of the attack, making inferences about causal mechanisms difficult.

In a longitudinal study, Henrich et al estimated that the incidence of cerebral migrainous infarction was 3.36/100 000; if subjects with other stroke risk factors are excluded, estimates fall to 1.44/100 000.[50] Overall rates of ischaemic stroke in the population under age 50 range from 6.5/100 000 to 22.8/100 000.[51] To interpret these data, we need to estimate the relative risk in migrainous and nonmigrainous populations, stratified by migraine type (with and without aura) and adjusted for potential confounders.

To better understand the relationship between migraine and stroke, Welch has proposed a classification system that recognizes four types of relationships between migraine and stroke: coexistent stroke and migraine, stroke with clinical features of migraine, migraine-induced stroke and uncertain classification (Table 3.3).[41]

For stroke and migraine to be coexistent, '. . . a clearly defined stroke syndrome must occur remotely in time from a typical migraine attack'.[41] It may not be possible to establish the presence or absence of a causal relationship in an individual case. At least some cases may be coincidentally related. Some cases may be linked by underlying risk factors, such as mitral valve prolapse or an antiphospholipid antibody syndrome.

In stroke with clinical features of migraine, Welch[41] indicates that '. . . a structural lesion that is unrelated to migraine pathogenesis presents with clinical features of a migraine attack'. He identifies two subtypes: symptomatic and migraine mimics. In the symptomatic group, an established structural disease causes episodes typical of migraine with aura, an example of which is an arteriove-

● **Table 3.3** Classification of migraine-related stroke

Category	Feature
I	Coexisting stroke and migraine
II	Stroke with clinical features of migraine A Symptomatic migraine B Migraine mimic
III	Migraine-induced stroke A Without risk factors B With risk factors
IV	Uncertain

nous malformation that masquerades as migraine. For migraine mimic, stroke is accompanied by headache and other neurologic symptoms and signs that resemble migraine.

In migraine-induced stroke, the neurologic deficit of the stroke must be identical to the neurologic symptoms of prior migraine attacks. In addition, the stroke must occur in the course of a typical migraine attack and other causes of stroke must be excluded.

In the group with uncertain classification, migraine and stroke appear related, but causal attribution is difficult. For example, a patient may have a typical migraine with aura, take a vasoactive drug such as ergotamine, and then have a cerebral infarction. When this rare sequence occurs, it is not clear if the stroke is a consequence of the migraine itself, the treatment, or an interaction of the two. To clarify the causal mechanisms, we would need to compare the rates of stroke in close proximity to migraine with aura with and without vasoactive treatment. Migraine-like headaches and stroke may be associated with systemic vasculitides, antiphospholipid antibody syndrome, mitochondrial encephalopathies and oral contraceptive use. The classification of stroke and migraine in these settings may be difficult.

Migraine and epilepsy

Migraine and epilepsy are comorbid. Andermann and Andermann[52] reported a median epilepsy prevalence of 5.9% (range: 1–17%) in migraineurs, which greatly exceeds the population prevalence of 0.5%.[53] The reported migraine prevalence in epileptics ranges from 8% to 23%.[52] Problems of methodology make these studies difficult to interpret.[52]

Ottman, Lipton and coworkers[54–56] explored the comorbidity of migraine and epilepsy using Columbia University's Epilepsy Family Study. Among the subjects with epilepsy (probands), the prevalence of a migraine history was 24%. Among relatives with epilepsy, 26% had a history of migraine. In the control relatives without epilepsy, the prevalence of a migraine history was 15%. Epilepsy increases the relative risk of migraine by 2.4, both in probands and their epileptic relatives (Figure 3.5).

Migraine risk was not related to age of epilepsy onset, but was higher in patients with partial and generalized seizures and was highest in posttraumatic epileptics (relative risk = 4.1).

Migraine risk is elevated both before and after seizure onset; therefore it cannot be accounted for solely as a cause or solely as a consequence of epilepsy. Because migraine risk is elevated among posttraumatic epileptics, and head injury is also a risk factor for both disorders,

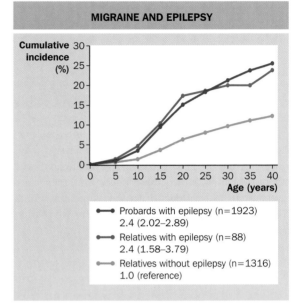

MIGRAINE AND EPILEPSY

Probands with epilepsy (n=1923)
2.4 (2.02–2.89)

Relatives with epilepsy (n=88)
2.4 (1.58–3.79)

Relatives without epilepsy (n=1316)
1.0 (reference)

● *Figure 3.5* Cumalitive incidence of migraine headache by age, in probands with epilepsy, relatives with epilepsy and relatives without epilepsy.

shared environmental risk factors may contribute to their comorbidity.[57,58] However, known environmental risk factors cannot fully account for this comorbidity, because migraine risk is also elevated in individuals with idiopathic epilepsy. Shared genetic risk factors cannot completely account for comorbidity, as migraine risk is elevated in probands with and without a positive family history of epilepsy.

Perhaps an altered brain state increases the risk of both migraine and epilepsy and thus accounts for the comorbidity of these disorders.[54] Genetic or environmental risk factors may increase neuronal excitability or decrease the threshold to both types of attack. A reduction in brain magnesium or alterations in neurotransmitters provide plausible potential substrates for this alteration in neuronal excitability.[59–61]

The association between migraine and epilepsy has implications for clinical practice. When treating patients for one disorder, it is important to maintain a heightened index of suspicion for the other disorder. Differentiating migraine and epilepsy can be difficult[52,62] as both conditions are characterized by episodes of neurologic dysfunction. Headache without other neurologic features is rare as a manifestation of epilepsy. The most difficult diagnostic issue is differentiating migraine with aura from partial complex seizure. If the aura is brief (<5 min) and associated with alteration of consciousness, automatisms and other positive motor features (tonic–clonic move-ments), epilepsy is more likely. If the aura is of long dura-tion (>5 min) and has a mix of positive (scintillations, tingling) and negative features (visual loss, numbness), migraine is more likely.

Treatment strategies for patients with comorbid migraine and epilepsy should be governed by the presence of comorbid disease. For example, in the treatment of migraine, drugs that lower seizure threshold should be used cautiously. Examples of such drugs include tricyclic antidepressants, selective serotonin re-uptake inhibitors and neuroleptics. On the other hand, it is sometimes advantageous to treat both migraine and epilepsy with a single drug. Sodium valproate has well-established efficacy in this setting.[63]

Migraine, major affective disorders and anxiety

Several population-based studies have examined the comorbidity of migraine, major depression, panic disorder and other psychiatric disorders.[24,64–67] Stewart et al reported on the relationships of migraine with panic dis-order and panic attacks.[65] Migraine headache in the 1-week period prior to a study telephone interview was higher in persons with a history of panic disorder. The rela-tive risk was 7.0 for men and 3.7 in women.

Stewart et al[66] found that 14.2% of women and 5.8% of men with a headache in the previous 12 months had consulted a doctor for headache. An unexpectedly high proportion of those who had consulted a physician for headache had a history of panic disorder. Of those who had recently seen a physician, 15% of women and 12.8% of men between the ages of 24 and 29 years had panic disorder. Comorbid psychiatric disease is apparently asso-ciated with seeking care for headache disorders.

In Zurich, Switzerland, Merikangas et al[64] found that anxiety and affective disorders were more common in migraineurs. The odds ratios were 2.2 for depression, 2.9 for bipolar spectrum disorders, 2.7 for generalized anxiety disorder, 3.3 for panic disorder, 2.4 for simple phobia and 3.4 for social phobia. Major depression and anxiety dis-orders were commonly found together. In persons with all three disorders, the onset of anxiety generally precedes the onset of migraine, whereas the onset of major depres-sion usually follows the onset of migraine.

Breslau and coworkers[24,68–70] studied the psychiatric comorbidity of IHS-defined migraine in young adults in southeast Michigan. Lifetime rates of affective and anxiety disorders were elevated in migraineurs. After adjusting for sex, the odds ratios were 4.5 for major depression, 6.0 for manic episode, 3.2 for any anxiety disorder and 6.6 for panic disorder. Migraine with aura was more strongly asso-ciated with the various psychiatric disorders than was migraine without aura.

Breslau et al[70] also prospectively studied migraine and major depression. Comparing subjects with and without migraine, the relative risk for the first onset of major depression during the follow-up period was 4.1. Compar-ing subjects with and without major depression, the rela-tive risk for the first onset of migraine during the follow-up period was 3.3. This bidirectional influence of each con-dition on the risk for the other is incompatible with simple unidirectional causal models.[70] Migraine is neither simply a cause nor simply a consequence of depression. Further-more, the association is not bidirectional between other severe headache and depression or other severe headache and panic disorder, suggesting some specificity for migraine and not a general association with headache.[71,72]

In summary, recent population-based studies demon-strate an association between migraine and major depres-sion. The longitudinal studies show a bidirectional influence, from migraine to subsequent onset of major depression, and from major depression to first migraine attack. Furthermore, these epidemiologic studies indicate that migraineurs have increased prevalence of bipolar dis-order, panic disorder and anxiety disorders.[71–73]

Migraine and personality characteristics

The relationships between migraine and personality characteristics have been discussed far more often than they have been systematically studied.[73] The idea of a migraine personality first grew out of clinical observations of the highly selected patients seen in subspecialty clinics. Many early authors have described migraineurs as perfec-tionistic, rigid, competitive, frustrated and overly sensitive (see review).[73]

Many investigators use personality scales, such as the Minnesota Multiphasic Personality Inventory (MMPI) or the Eysenck Personality Questionnaire (EPQ), to study migraine and personality characteristics.[74–76] These studies have been limited by several factors.[65,73] Most have used historical norms instead of concurrent controls. Many have not used explicit diagnostic criteria for migraine. Because the MMPI studies are usually clinic-based, their findings are of limited generalizability and are subject to selection bias. Despite these limitations, most studies show eleva-tion of the neurotic triad, although this is often not statisti-cally significant (Figure 3.6).[73]

In the first population-based, case–control study of personality in migraine, Brandt et al[77] used the EPQ in the Washington County Migraine Prevalence Study sample. The EPQ is a well-standardized measure that includes four

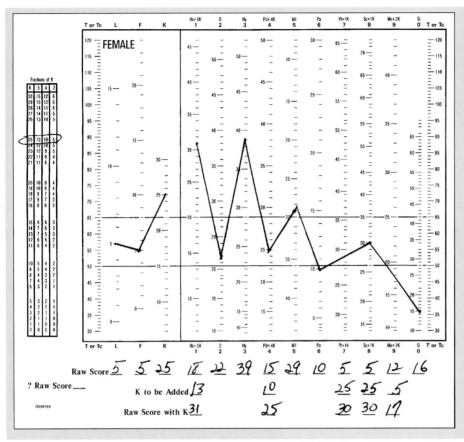

Figure 3.6 MMPI showing conversion-V. (© 1989 Regents of the University of Minnesota.)

scales: psychoticism (P), extroversion (E), neuroticism (N) and lie (L). Migraineurs had higher scores than controls on the EPQ N scale, indicating that they were more tense, anxious and depressed than the control group. Women with migraine scored significantly higher than controls on the P scale, indicating that they were more hostile, less interpersonally sensitive, and out of step with their peers.

Merikangas et al[67] investigated the cross-sectional association between personality, symptoms, and headache subtypes as part of a prospective longitudinal study of 19- and 20-year olds in Zurich, Switzerland. Migraineurs scored higher on neuroticism indicators than did non-migraine subjects.

Even the population-based studies of migraine and personality have generally not controlled for drug use, headache frequency and headache-related disability. Nor have they controlled for major psychiatric disorders (such as major depression or panic disorder), which, as discussed above, occur more commonly in migraineurs. Because major psychiatric disorders are associated with both migraine and personality disorders, confounding may alter the measured associations between these disorders and migraine.[73]

Migraine and public health

Migraine is a public health problem of enormous scope that has an impact on both the individual sufferer and on society.[2,5,9,13] The American Migraine Study II estimates that 28 million US residents have severe migraine headaches.[13] Nearly one in four US households has someone with migraine.[13] Twenty-five percent of women in the US who have migraine experience four or more severe attacks a month; 35% experience one to four severe attacks a month; 38% experience one, or less than one, severe attack a month.[13] Similar frequency patterns were observed for men.[13]

In the American Migraine Study II, 92% of women and 89% of men with severe migraine had some headache-related disability.[13] About half were severely disabled or needed bedrest.[19] In addition to the attack-related disability, many migraineurs live in fear, knowing that at any time an attack could disrupt their ability to work, care for their families or meet social obligations.

Migraine has an enormous impact on society. Recent US studies have evaluated both the indirect and direct costs of migraine.[78-80] Indirect costs include the aggregate effects of migraine on productivity at work (paid employment), for household work and in other roles. The largest component of indirect costs are the productivity losses that take the form of absenteeism and reduced productivity while at work. Hu et al estimated that productivity losses due to migraine cost American employers 13 billion dollars per year.[79] These issues have been recently reviewed in more detail elsewhere.[79-81]

Migraine's impact on healthcare utilization is marked as well. The National Ambulatory Medical Care Survey, conducted from 1976 to 1977, found that 4% of all visits to physicians' offices (over 10 million visits a year) were for headache.[82] Migraine also results in major utilization of emergency rooms and urgent care centers.[5,83] Vast amounts of prescription and over-the-counter medications are taken for headache disorders.

Migraine is a lifelong disorder. Bille followed a cohort of children with severe migraine for up to 37 years.[27,28] As young adults, 62% were migraine-free for more than 2 years, but only 40% continued to be migraine-free after 30 years, suggesting that migraine is often a lifelong disorder. For 15 years, Fry collected information on migraine patients in his general practice in Kent, UK.[84] His data showed a tendency for the severity and frequency of attacks to decrease as the patients got older. After 15 years, 32% of the men and 42% of the women no longer had migraine attacks. Waters noted a similar decrease in migraine prevalence.[16,35]

There is a subgroup of migraine sufferers afflicted with a syndrome variously called chronic daily headache evolving from migraine, transformed migraine or malignant migraine, in which attacks increase in frequency over a number of years until a pattern of daily or near-daily headache evolves.[34,85-87] In subspecialty clinics, about 80% of patients with this disorder are overusing acute headache medication. Medication overuse is believed to contribute to the accelerating pattern of pain through a mechanism that has been termed 'rebound headache'. When the cycle of medication overuse is broken, the headaches often improve.[88] However, in subspecialty clinics, this process of acceleration occurs without medication overuse in about 20% of patients, suggesting that there is a subgroup of migraine sufferers with a progressive condition. The epidemiology of frequent or chronic daily headache is discussed in the chapter on that subject.

Genetics of migraine

Introduction

The familial aggregation of migraine was first noted by Tissot in 1790.[89] Since then, numerous studies have examined the transmission of migraine within families, the concordance for migraine among twins, and the linkage of migraine to particular chromosomal loci (see reviews).[90-92] With the demonstration of a genetic locus for familial hemiplegic migraine (FHM) on chromosome 12,[93] and the discovery of a candidate gene product from that locus,[94] the study of migraine genetics has truly entered the molecular era. Since most people suffer rare vascular headaches over their entire life span, it is the tendency for recurrent attacks that defines migraine. This tendency is generally attributed to a lower threshold to migraine.[90]

Studies of familial aggregation

Many studies have examined the risk of migraine among relatives of migraine probands and nonmigrainous controls.[90-92] The controlled studies show an increased family risk of migraine among the relatives of migraine probands.[91,92] In the early studies, relative risks ranged from 1.5 to 19.3.[91] Variation in the family relative risk in the early studies is accounted for, at least in part, by methodological differences among studies.

The recent population-based migraine family studies avoid many of the limitations of earlier studies. Russell and Olesen used IHS criteria and directly interviewed first-degree relatives by telephone to determine migraine status.[95] First-degree relatives of probands who had migraine with aura had a fourfold increased risk of migraine with aura. The relatives of probands who had migraine without aura had a 1.9-fold increased risk of migraine without aura. Transmission of migraine type within families appears to be specific. In another population-based family study, the migraine probands with the greatest level of disability had the highest relative risk of family aggregation.[96] In this study, genetic factors accounted for about half of the risk of migraine.[96]

The familial studies strongly support the familial aggregation of migraine. Unfortunately, the evidence from segregation analysis does not provide consistent evidence for any single mode of inheritance.[90-92] The inconsistent results may reflect the genetic heterogeneity of migraine. Some families show apparent autosomal dominant transmission, while others show autosomal recessive transmission with incomplete penetrance.

Twin studies

Clinic-based twin studies have consistently shown that monozygotic (MZ) twins are more concordant for migraine than are dizygotic (DZ) twins, a finding that supports an etiological role for genetic factors. Recent twin studies using IHS case definitions and systematic ascertainment strategies support a genetic basis for migraine.[97–101]

For example, in the Australian study of 5844 twins,[97] proband-wise concordance for female same-sex twins was 0.44 for MZ twins and 0.24 for DZ twins. In males, the MZ concordance rate was 0.31 and the DZ concordance rate was 0.18. In most studies, about half of the variation in migraine prevalence was attributable to the additive effect of genetic factors, a finding similar to estimates from population-based familial aggregation studies.[96] Thus, the twin studies support the importance of genetic as well as risk factors for migraine. These data also demonstrate that nongenetic factors must play a role as the MZ concordance rate was well below 1.0. If genetic factors fully accounted for migraine, MZ twins would be fully concordant (i.e. both twins would always have migraine or always be free of the approximal chromosal locations of pathogenic genes).

Linkage studies and familial hemiplegic migraine (FHM)

Linkage studies have been conducted with great success to FHM, a rare autosomal dominant disorder with hemiplegia as one component of the aura. FHM is linked to chromosome 19 in about half of families[90,92,94,102–105] and to chromosome 1[104,105] in other families. In some families, FHM is linked to neither chromosome 19 nor chromosome 1, indicating at least three gene loci.[104,105] Thus, even this autosomal dominant, relatively stereotyped disorder is genetically heterogeneous.

The Dutch group has identified a neuronal calcium channel protein believed to be the product of the pathogenic gene on chromosome 19.[94] This gene codes for the alpha-1-A subunit of a voltage gated P/Q type calcium channel (CACNAIA). Several different missense mutations have been identified in association with FHM.[90,92,94]

The relationship between this chromosome 19 linkage marker/gene product and more common types of migraine is not clear.[104,105] Several studies report involvement of the CACNAIA gene in the usual forms of both migraine with and without aura[90–92] although results vary. Mutations of the CACNAIA gene have also been associated with episodic ataxia type 2 and spinocerebellar ataxia type 6.[90–92] The heterogeneity of FHM underscores the likely heterogeneity of the more common types of migraine. The implications of these genetic findings for the mechanisms of migraine have been discussed elsewhere[90–92] and are considered in Chapter 5.

Tension-type headache

Estimates of the prevalence of tension-type headache have varied widely. In Western countries, 1-year period prevalence ranges from 28% to 63% in men and from 34% to 86% in women.[8,11,26,106] This variation is explained, in part, by differences in case definition, sampling methods, and the procedures that were used to elicit histories. Few tension-type headache studies have been conducted outside the Western world. Wong et al[105] found very low prevalences in a study he conducted in mainland China. Several studies reported a prevalence of 2–3% for chronic tension-type headache.[8,106,107]

Tension-type headache is more common in women, with gender ratios ranging from 1.04 to 1.8.[8,106,108] Prevalence peaks between the ages of 20 and 50 years and then declines. Schwartz et al[106] reported a direct relationship between the prevalence of episodic tension-type headache and education. Pryse-Phillips et al[26] reported an increased prevalence in higher income groups, although the results were not consistent.

Tension-type headaches often interfere with activities of daily living. Eighteen percent of tension-type headache sufferers have to discontinue normal activity, while 44% experience some limitation of function. Attacks occur with a mean frequency of 2.9 days a month or 35 days a year: most sufferers have less than one attack a month and about one-third have two or more attacks a month.

Like migraine, tension-type headache is a disorder of middle life, striking individuals early in life and continuing to affect them through their peak productive years. Most migraineurs and 60% of tension-type headache sufferers have a diminished capacity for work or other activities. Despite prominent disability, nearly 40% of migraineurs and more than 80% of tension-type headache patients have never consulted their general practitioner because of headache.

In a Danish study, 43% of employed migraineurs and 12% of employed tension-type headache sufferers missed 1 or more days of work because of headache.[107] Migraine caused at least 1 day of missed work in 5% of sufferers while tension-type headache caused 1 day of missed work in 9%. Annually, per 1000 employed persons, 270 lost work-days were owing to migraine and 820 were because of tension-type headache.[107]

Individuals with frequent episodic tension-type headache may be at increased risk for chronic tension-type headache. When migraine and tension-type headache coexist, tension-type headache may be more frequent and more severe. The process whereby headache frequency increases and an episodic disorder becomes chronic is sometimes referred to as transformation. Overuse of ergotamine and/or analgesics is the most common factor leading to transformation. If analgesics are not withdrawn, these patients may be refractory to prophylactic therapy and have a very poor prognosis.

Genetics of tension-type headache

Although tension-type headache is often attributed to external factors, recent studies support a role for familial aggregation of chronic tension-type headache. Russell et al[108] examined the family relative risk of chronic tension-type headache in first-degree relatives and in spouses. Over 1 year, the relative risk was 3.2 in first-degree relatives and 1.23 in spouses.[109] These findings support a role for genetic factors as spouses share some environmental, but not genetic, risk factors. Complex segregation analysis suggests multifactorial inheritance for chronic tension-type headache.[109]

Conclusion

Using the IHS criteria, large population-based epidemiologic studies in Denmark, the United States, France, Canada and elsewhere have shed light on the descriptive epidemiology of migraine. While migraine is a remarkably common cause of temporary disability, many migraineurs, even those with disabling headache, have never consulted a physician for the problem. Prevalence is highest in women, in persons between the ages of 25 and 55 years, and, at least in the United States, in individuals from low-income households. Nonetheless, prevalence is high in groups other than these high-risk groups. Migraine prevalence may be increasing in the United States, but this has not been proven. Longitudinal studies are required to better determine the incidence and natural history of migraine as well as the life course of comorbid conditions.

References

1. Scher AI, Stewart WF, Lipton RB. Migraine and headache: a meta-analytic approach. In: Crombie IK, ed. Epidemiology of Pain. Seattle, Washington: IASP Press, 1999, 159–70.
2. Rasmussen BK. Epidemiology of headache. Cephalalgia 1995; 15: 45–68.
3. Lipton RB, Amatniek JC, Ferrari MD et al. Migraine: identifying and removing barriers to care. Neurology 1994; 44(suppl 6): 56–62.
4. Lipton RB, Silberstein SD. Why study the comorbidity of migraine? Neurology 1994; 44: 4–5.
5. Lipton RB, Diamond S, Reed M et al. Migraine diagnosis and treatment: results from the American Migraine Study II. Headache 2001; 41: 638–45.
6. Stang PE, Osterhaus JT, Celentano DD. Migraine: patterns of health care use. Neurology 1994; 44(suppl 4): 47–55.
7. Headache Classification Committee of the International Headache Society. Classification and diagnostic criteria for headache disorders, cranial neuralgias, and facial pain. Cephalalgia 1988; 8(suppl 7): 1–96.
8. Rasmussen BK, Jensen R, Schroll M, Olesen J. Epidemiology of headache in a general population – a prevalence study. J Clin Epidemiol 1991; 44: 1147–57.
9. Stewart WF, Lipton RB, Celentano DD, Reed ML. Prevalence of migraine headache in the United States. JAMA 1992; 267: 64–9.

10. Henry P, Michel P, Brochet B et al. A nationwide survey of migraine in France: prevalence and clinical features in adults. Cephalalgia 1992; 12: 229–37.
11. Gobels H, Petersen-Braun M, Soyka D. The epidemiology of headache in Germany: a nationwide survey of a representative sample on the basis of the headache classification of the International Headache Society. Cephalalgia 1994; 14: 97–106.
12. Launer LJ, Terwindt GM, Ferrari MD. The prevalence and characteristics of migraine in a population-based cohort: the GEM Study. Neurology 1999; 53: 537–42.
13. Lipton RB, Stewart WF, Diamond S et al. Prevalence and burden of migraine in the United States: data from the American Migraine Study II. Headache 2001; 41: 646–57.
14. Featherstone HJ. Migraine and muscle contraction headaches: a continuum. Headache 1985; 24: 194–8.
15. Raskin NH. Headache, 2nd edition. New York: Churchill-Livingstone, 1988.
16. Waters WE. Headache (Series in Clinical Epidemiology). Littleton, MA: PSG Co. Inc., 1986.
17. Waters WE. Headache and Migraine in General Practitioners, the Migraine Headache and Dixarit. Proceedings of a symposium held at Churchill College. Cambridge: Boehringer Ingelheim Brachnell, 1972.
18. Celentano DD, Stewart WF, Linet MS. The relationship of headache symptoms with severity and duration of attacks. J

Clin Epidemiol 1990; 43: 983–94.
19. Lipton RB, Stewart WF, Cady R et al. Sumatriptan for the range of headaches in migraine sufferers: results of the Spectrum Study. Headache 2000; 40: 783–91.
20. Stewart WF, Linet MS, Celentano DD et al. Age and sex-specific incidence rates of migraine with and without visual aura. Am J Epidemiol 1993; 34: 1111–20.
21. Stang PE, Yanagihara T, Swanson JW et al. Incidence of migraine headaches: a population-based study in Olmstead County, Minnesota. Neurology 1992; 42: 1657–62.
22. Lipton RB, Stewart WF, Celentano DD, Reed ML. Undiagnosed migraine: a comparison of symptom-based and self-reported physician diagnosis. Arch Int Med 1992; 152: 1273–8.
23. Stewart WF, Simon D, Schechter A, Lipton RB. Population variation in migraine prevalence: a meta-analysis. J Clin Epidemiol 1995; 48: 269–80.
24. Breslau N, Davis GC, Andreski P. Migraine, psychiatric disorders and suicide attempts: an epidemiological study of young adults. Psychiatry Res 1991; 37: 11–23.
25. Kryst S, Scherl E. A population-based survey of the social and personal impact of headache. Headache 1994; 34: 344–50.
26. Pryse-Phillips W, Findlay H, Tugwell P et al. A Canadian population survey on the clinical epidemiologic and societal impact of migraine and tension-type

headache. Can J Neurol Sci 1992; 19: 333–9.

27. Bille B. Migraine in school children. Acta Paediatr Scand 1962; 51(suppl 136): 1–151.

28. Bille B. Migraine in children: prevalence, clinical features, and a 30-year follow-up. In: Ferrari MD, Lataste X eds. Migraine and other headaches. New Jersey: Parthenon, 1989.

29. Sillanpaa M. Prevalence of migraine and other headache in Finnish children starting school. Headache 1976; 15: 288–90.

30. Sillanpaa M. Prevalence of headache in prepuberty. Headache 1983; 23: 10–14.

31. Sillanpaa M. Changes in the prevalence of migraine and other headaches during the first seven school years. Headache 1983; 23: 15–19.

32. Sillanpaa M, Piekkala P, Kero P. Prevalence of headache at preschool age in an unselected child population. Cephalalgia 1991; 11: 239–42.

33. Sillanpaa M. Headache in children. In: Olesen J, ed. Headache Classification and Epidemiology. New York, Raven Press 1994; 273–81.

34. Silberstein SD, Merriam GR. Sex hormones and headache. In: Goadsby P, Silberstein SD, eds. Blue Books of Practical Neurology: Headache. Boston: Butterworth Heinemann, 1997, 143–76.

35. Waters WE. Migraine: intelligence, social class, and familial prevalence. Br Med J 1971; 2: 77–81.

36. Stang PE, Sternfeld B, Sidney S. Migraine headache in a pre-paid health plan: ascertainment, demographics, physiological and behavioral factors. Headache 1996; 36: 69–76.

37. D'Alessandro R, Benassi G, Lenzi PL et al. Epidemiology of headache in the Republic of San Marino. J Neurol Neurosurg Psychiatry 1988; 51: 21–7.

38. No authors listed. Prevalence of chronic migraine headaches – United States, 1980–89. MMWR Morb Mortal Wkly Rep 1991; 40: 331–8.

39. Lipton RB, Stewart WF, Simon D. Medical consultation for migraine: results from the American Migraine Study. Headache 1998; 38: 87–96.

40. Feinstein AR. The pretherapeutic classification of comorbidity in chronic disease. J Chronic Dis 1970; 23: 455–68.

41. Welch KMA. Relationship of stroke and migraine. Neurology 1994; 44(suppl 7): 33–6.

42. Tatemichi TK, Mohr JP. Migraine and stroke. In: Barnett HJM, Stein BM, Mohr JP, Yarsu FM, eds. Stroke: Pathophysiology, Diagnosis and Management. New York: Churchill Livingstone, 1986, 845–63.

43. Bougousslavsky J, Regli F. Ischemic stroke in adults younger than 30 years of age: cause and prognosis. Arch Neurol 1987; 44: 479–82.

44. Rothrock J, North J, Madden K et al. Migraine and migrainous stroke: risk factors and prognosis. Neurology 1993; 43: 2473–6.

45. Bougousslavsky J, Regli F, Van Melle G et al. Migraine stroke. Neurology 1988; 38: 223–7.

46. Collaborative Group for the Study of Stroke in Young Women. Oral contraceptives and stroke in young women. JAMA 1975; 281: 718–22.

47. Henrich JB, Horowitz RI. A controlled study of ischemic stroke risk in migraine patients. J Clin Epidemiol 1989; 42: 773–80.

48. Tzourio C, Tehindrazanarivelo A, Iglesias S et al. Case–control study of migraine and risk of ischaemic stroke. Br Med J 1993; 307: 289–92.

49. Tzourio C, Tehindrazanarivelo A, Iglesias S et al. Case–control study of migraine and risk of ischaemic stroke in young women. Br Med J 1995; 310: 830–3.

50. Henrich JB, Sandercock PAG, Warlow CP, Jones LN. Stroke and migraine in the Oxfordshire Community Stroke Project. J Neurol 1986; 233: 257–62.

51. Kittner SJ, McCarer RJ, Sherwin RW et al. Black–white differences in stroke risk among young adults. Stroke 1993; 24(suppl 1): 113–15.

52. Andermann E, Andermann FA. Migraine–epilepsy relationships: epidemiological and genetic aspects. In: Andermann FA, Lugaresi E, eds. Migraine and Epilepsy. Boston: Butterworths, 1987, 281–91.

53. Hauser WA, Annegers JF, Kurland LT. Prevalence of epilepsy in Rochester, Minnesota: 1940–1980. Epilepsia 1991; 32: 429–45.

54. Ottman R, Lipton RB. Comorbidity of migraine and epilepsy. Neurology 1994; 44: 2105–10.

55. Lipton RB, Ottman R, Ehrenberg BL, Hauser WA. Comorbidity of migraine: the connection between migraine and epilepsy. Neurology 1994; 44(suppl 7): 28–32.

56. Ottman R, Lipton RB. Is the comorbidity of epilepsy and migraine due to a shared genetic susceptibility? Neurology 1996; 47: 918–24.

57. Schechter A, Stewart WF, Celentano DD et al. An epidemiologic study of migraine and head injury (abstract). Neurology 1990; 40(suppl 1): 345.

58. Annegers JF, Grabow JD, Groover RV et al. Seizures after head trauma: a population study. Neurology 1980; 30: 683–9.

59. Welch KMA. Migraine: a behavioral disorder. Arch Neurol 1987; 44: 323–7.

60. Welch KMA, Barkley GL, Tepley N, D'Andrea G. Magnetoencephalographic studies of migraine: evidence for central neuronal hyperexcitability. In: Rose FC, ed. New Advances in Headache Research, Volume 2. London: Smith Gordon, 1991, 127–30.

61. Olesen J. Synthesis of migraine mechanisms. In: Olesen J, Tfelt-Hansen P, Welch KMA, eds. The Headaches. New York: Raven Press, 1993, 247–53.

62. Marks DA, Ehrenberg BL. Migraine-related seizures in adults with epilepsy, with EEG correlation. Neurology 1993; 43: 2476–83.

63. Jensen R, Brinck T, Olesen J. Sodium valproate has a prophylactic effect in migraine without aura. Neurology 1994; 44: 647–51.

64. Merikangas KR, Angst J, Isler H. Migraine and psychopathology. Results of the Zurich cohort study of young adults. Arch Gen Psychiatry 1990; 47: 849–53.

65. Stewart WF, Linet MS, Celentano DD. Migraine headaches and panic attacks. Psychosom Med 1989; 51: 559–69.

66. Stewart WF, Schechter A, Liberman J. Physician consultation for headache pain and history of panic: results from a population-based study. Am J Med 1992; 92: 35–40.

67. Merikangas KR, Stevens DE, Angst J. Headache and personality: results of a community sample of young adults. J Psychiat Res 1993; 27: 187–96.

68. Breslau N, Davis GC. Migraine, major depression and panic disorder: a prospective epidemiologic study of young adults. Cephalalgia 1992; 12: 85–9.

69. Breslau N, Davis GC. Migraine, physical health and psychiatric disorders: a prospective epidemiologic study of young adults. J Psychiatric Res 1993; 27: 211–21.

70. Breslau N, Davis GC, Schultz LR et al. Migraine and major depression: a longitudinal study. Headache 1994; 7: 387–93.

71. Breslau N, Schultz LR, Stewart WF et al. Headache and major depression: is the association specific to migraine? Neurology 2000; 54: 308–13.

72. Breslau N, Schultz LR, Stewart WF et al. Headache types and panic disorder: directionality and specificity. Neurology 2001; 56: 350–54.

73. Silberstein SD, Lipton RB, Breslau N. Migraine: association with personality characteristics and psychopathology. Cephalalgia 1995; 15: 1–15.

74. Kudrow L, Sutkus GJ. MMPI pattern specificity in primary headache disorders. Headache 1979; 19: 18–24.

75. Weeks R, Baskin S, Sheftell F et al. A comparison of MMPI personality data and frontalis electromyographic

readings in migraine and combination headache patients. Headache 1983; 23: 75–82.

76. Invernizzi G, Gala C, Buono M et al. Neurotic traits and disease duration in headache patients. Cephalalgia 1989; 9: 173–8.

77. Brandt J, Celentano D, Stewart WF et al. Personality and emotional disorder in a community sample of migraine headache sufferers. Am J Psychiatry 1990; 147: 303–8.

78. Ziegler DK. Headache: public health importance. Neurol Clin 1990; 8: 781–91.

79. Hu XH, Markson LE, Lipton RB et al. Burden of migraine in the United States: disability and economic costs. Arch Intern Med 1999; 159: 813–18.

80. Osterhaus JT, Gutterman DL, Plachetka JR. Health care resources and lost labor costs of migraine headaches in the United States. Pharmacoeconomics 1992; 2: 67–76.

81. Lipton RB, Hamelsky S, Stewart WF. Epidemiology and impact of headache. In: Silberstein SD, Lipton RB, Dalessio DJ, eds. Wolff's Headache and Other Head Pain. Oxford University Press 2001, 85–107.

82. National Center for Health Statistics. Vital and Health Statistics of the United States. D.H.E.W., PHS Publication No. 53. Advance data. Hyattsville, MD: National Center for Health Statistics, 1979.

83. Celentano DD, Stewart WF, Lipton RB, Reed ML. Medication use and disability among migraineurs: a national probability sample. Headache 1992; 32: 223–8.

84. Fry J. Profiles of Disease. Edinburgh: Livingstone, 1966.

85. Mathew NT, Stubits E, Nigam MP. Transformation of episodic migraine into daily headache: analysis of factors. Headache 1982; 22: 66–8.

86. Mathew NT, Reuveni U, Perez F. Transformed or evolutive migraine. Headache 1987; 27: 102–6.

87. Silberstein SD, Lipton RB, Solomon S, Mathew NT. Classification of daily and near daily headaches. Proposed revisions to the IHS criteria. Headache 1994; 34: 1–7.

88. Silberstein SD, Silberstein JR. Chronic daily headache: long-term prognosis following inpatient treatment with repetitive IV DHE. Headache 1992; 32: 439–45.

89. Tissot S. Nervous traits and diseases [in French]. In: The Works of M.Tissot, vol. 13, Lausanne, 1790, pp. 92–3.

90. Ferrari MD, Han J. Genetics of headache. In: Silberstein SD, Lipton RB, Dalessio DJ, eds. Wolff's Headache and Other Head Pain. Oxford University Press 2001, 85–107.

91. Russell MB. Genetics of migraine without aura, migraine with aura, migrainous disorder, head trauma migraine without aura and tension type headache. Cephalalgia 2001; 21: 778–80.

92. Ferrari MD, Russell MB. Genetics of migraine. Is migraine a genetically determined channelopathy? In: Olesen J, Tfelt-Hansen P and Welch KMA, eds. The Headaches, 2nd edn. New York: Raven Press, 241–50.

93. Joutel A, Bousser MG, Biousee V et al. A gene for familial hemiplegic migraine maps to chromosome 19. Nat Genet 1993; 5: 40–5.

94. Ophoff RA, Terwindt GM, Vergowe MN et al. Familial hemiplegic migraine and episodic ataxia type-2 are caused by mutations in the calcium channel gene CACNLIA4. Cell 1996; 87: 543–52.

95. Russell MB, Olesen J. Increased familial risk and evidence of genetic factor in migraine. Br Med J 1995; 311: 541–4.

96. Stewart WF, Staffa J, Lipton RB et al. Familial risk of migraine: a population-based study. Ann Neurol 1997; 41: 166–72.

97. Merikangas KR, Tierney C, Martin NG et al. Genetics of migraine in the Australian Twin Registry. In: Rose CF, ed. New Advances in Headache Research, 4. London: Smith-Gordon, 1994, 27–8.

98. Honkasalo ML, Kaprio J, Winter T et al. Migraine and concomitant symptoms among 8167 adult twin pairs. Headache 1995; 35: 70–8.

99. Larsson B, Bille B, Pederson N. Genetic influence in headaches: a Swedish twin study. Headache 1995; 35: 513–19.

100. Ziegler DW, Hur YM, Bouchard TJ et al. Migraine in twins raised together and apart. Headache 1998; 38: 417–22.

101. Ulrich VM, Gervil KO, Kyvik C et al. Evidence of a genetic factor in migraine with aura: a population-based Danish twin study. Ann Neurol 1999; 45: 241–6.

102. May A, Ophoff RA, Terwindt GM et al. Familial hemiplegic migraine locus on 19p13 is involved in the common forms of migraine with and without aura. Hum Genet 1995; 96: 604–8.

103. Ophoff RA, Van Eijk R, Sandkuijl LA et al. Genetic heterogeneity of familial hemiplegic migraine. Genomics 1994; 22: 21–6.

104. Ducros A, Joutel A, Vahedi K et al. Mapping of a second locus for familial hemiplegic migraine to 1q21–q23 and evidence for further heterogeneity. Ann Neurol 1997; 42: 885–90.

105. Wong TW, Wong KS, Yu TS, Kay R. Prevalence of migraine and other headaches in Hong Kong. Neuroepidemiol 1995; 14: 82–91.

106. Schwartz BS, Stewart WF, Simon D, Lipton RB. Epidemiology of tension-type headache. JAMA 1998; 279: 381–3.

107. Rasmussen BK, Jensen R, Olessen J. Impact of headache on sickness absence and utilization of medical services: a Danish population study. J Epidemiol Comm Health 1992; 46: 443–6.

108. Russell MB, Iselius L, Ostergaard S et al. Inheritance of chronic tension-type headache investigated by complex segregation analysis. Hum Genet 1998; 102: 138–40.

109. Ostergaard S, Russell MB, Berndtsen E et al. Comparison of first-degree relatives and spouses of people with chronic tension headache. Br Med J 1998; 314: 1092–3.

chapter 4

Diagnostic testing and ominous causes of headache

Headache diagnosis is based on a complete and thorough history supplemented by general physical and neurological examinations (see Chapter 2). Testing (see Table 4.1) serves to:

- exclude organic causes of headache,
- rule out comorbid and coexistent diseases that could complicate headache diagnosis and treatment,
- establish a baseline for and exclude contraindications to drug treatment, and
- measure drug levels to determine compliance, absorption or medication overuse.

Diagnostic testing is often recommended for other reasons. These include:

- the quest for diagnostic certainty,
- a shortcut for a thorough evaluation,
- patient expectations,
- financial incentives,
- professional peer pressure where tests are expected, and
- medicolegal issues.

The attitudes and demands of patients and families and the practice of defensive medicine are especially important.[1]

A lack of controlled trials hinder decisions about which headache studies are appropriate for the patient. Furthermore, managed care systems often dictate which studies can be performed on their members, a decision often based on economic, not medical, considerations. However, omitting a test for economic reasons can have grave consequences for the patient and the physician. Lack of funds and underinsurance continue to be barriers for appropriate diagnostic testing for many patients.[1–3] Therefore, the cost–benefit ratio of performing a study must be considered, as must the medical/legal implications of omitting it.

Few guidelines have existed for headache (particularly migraine) investigation.[1,2] One expert[4] states that '. . . magnetic resonance imaging (MRI) should be reserved for those patients in whom the diagnosis of migraine cannot be made unequivocally on clinical grounds', and another[5] says that '. . . in practice the recurrent pattern of migraine is so characteristic that it is rarely necessary to undertake any investigation'. We do not know if the diagnosis of migraine is always valid if it satisfies the criteria established by the International Headache Society (IHS),[6] nor do we know how many 'migraine mimics' are falsely diagnosed.

Validity depends on the sensitivity and the specificity of the diagnostic test:

- sensitivity is defined as the ability of a test to identify correctly those who have the disease (high sensitivity will have few false-negatives).
- specificity is defined as the ability of a test to identify correctly those who do not have the disease (high specificity will have few false-positives).

Additional indicators of benign migraine might include:

- regular or near-regular perimenstrual or periovulatory timing of the headache,
- its appearance after sustained exertion,
- its abatement with sleep, and
- acquisition of food-, odour-, or weather-change-induced headache occurring concurrently with unprovoked headache.

● **Table 4.1** *Why do headache studies?*

Study*	Diagnosis	Baseline	Compliance/toxicity
Complete blood cell count, differentiation	✓	✓	✓
Sedimentation rate	✓		
Chemistry profile	✓	✓	✓
Electrocardiogram		✓	✓
Blood gases	✓		
Drug screen	✓		✓
Drug level			✓
Lyme disease, HIV, VDRL	✓		
ANA, lupus anticoagulant, anticardiolipin antibodies	✓		

*HIV = human immunodeficiency virus;
VDRL = venereal disease research laboratory;
ANA = antinuclear antibody.

However, these criteria have not been tested and have not been used to screen patients to improve the yield of diagnostic testing. For example, the IHS criteria for migraine require exclusion of secondary organic causes of headache. It is uncertain how specific the IHS criteria are and how many 'migraine mimics' meet the IHS criteria. This is the fundamental problem. Most studies performed to investigate organic disease (neuroimaging or electroencephalography (EEG)) use the more imprecise ad hoc criteria or even more vague headache definitions, making the studies very difficult to interpret. If the prevalence of the suspected organic disorder increases (by using additional indications of benign and malignant headache), the diagnostic test yield improves. Thus, the presence of any atypical feature increases the yield of organic diagnostic testing.

Studies to establish a cost–benefit analysis in the area of headache diagnosis are just beginning. In a typical healthy migraineur, laboratory tests may not be necessary for diagnosis, but are often recommended prior to treatment, for example, an electrocardiogram in the older migraineur prior to the use of sumatriptan, dihydroergotamine or ergotamine.

Refractory headache patients who attend tertiary referral centres usually undergo a greater number of studies than do those patients seen in specialists' or primary care physicians' offices. Since secondary causes of headache frequently are not apparent on physical examination, laboratory tests are sometimes performed on the initial visit to facilitate their diagnosis. A complete blood count and differential may rule out anaemia or infection. The antinuclear antibody test screens for autoimmune conditions. An erythrocyte sedimentation rate not only acts as a screen for serious diseases, such as a malignancy or collagen vascular disease, but can also establish the diagnosis of temporal arteritis, a cause of headache in the elderly. Thyroid function studies are performed to rule out thyroid disease such as thyrotoxicosis, a condition that may exacerbate headache and is a relative contraindication to ergot administration. Unexpected or overused medication that has a direct impact on headache and its treatment can be identified by a drug screen and toxicology studies. Specific studies (such as electrolytes and liver or kidney function studies) may be needed before starting drug treatment.

Methods of investigation

Electroencephalography

The EEG is a non-invasive and relatively low-cost study. It lacks specificity and sensitivity, however, and while it

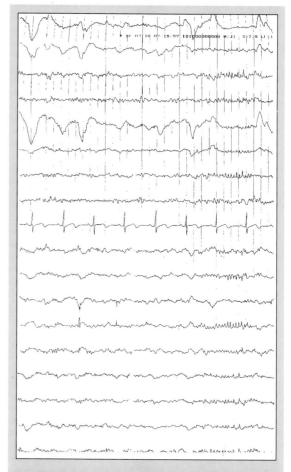

● **Figure 4.1** Normal EEG variant with 14 and 6 positive spikes.

reveals different rates of abnormality in headache subtypes, it is not helpful in distinguishing between subtypes (Figure 4.1). Between 12% and 15% of healthy adults who have no history of head injury, seizures, headaches, or other neurological diseases have nonspecific EEG abnormalities.[7] Earlier studies have reported EEG abnormalities in migraine. Slater[8] found posterior quadrant, bilateral but asymmetric, slow-wave abnormalities in 82 of 184 migraine patients. He also observed abnormal responses to photic stimulation and hyperventilation. He concluded that migraine causes a disorder of cerebral functioning that produces EEG changes. Smyth and Winter[9] found that 43% of 202 migraineurs had abnormal interictal records, with slowing in either the theta or delta range. The incidence of delta rhythm was related to headache severity, disease duration and a positive family history of migraine. Lauritzen et al[10] found no EEG abnormalities on hyperventilation or photic stimulation, during attacks or interictally, in 11 patients with migraine without aura or in eight of 10 patients with migraine with aura. Two patients who had migraine with aura had frontal slowing between and during attacks. While the interictal EEG may reveal diffuse or focal abnormalities to be more common in migraineurs, there is no migraine-specific pattern. The American Academy of

Neurology (AAN) has reviewed the use of EEG in headache diagnosis and found that many studies suffer from major flaws.[11] These include referral bias (studies not population-based) and poor controls (studies usually uncontrolled and, when controlled, not age- or sex-matched). The studies are frequently non-blinded and have high intraobserver variability. In addition, archaic criteria for normalcy

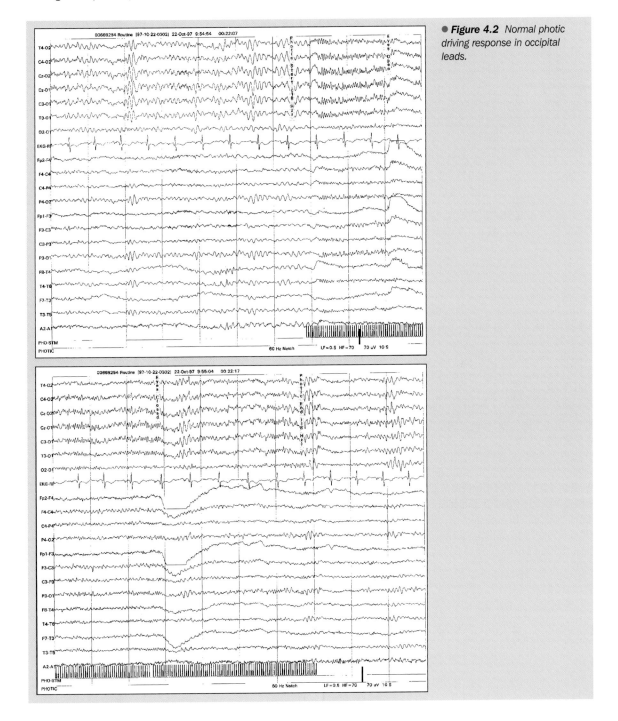

● **Figure 4.2** *Normal photic driving response in occipital leads.*

are employed (patterns originally considered abnormal are now considered normal, e.g. posterior slow waves of youth).

Studies designed to determine if headache patients have an increased prevalence of EEG abnormalities give conflicting results. In migraineurs, prominent photic driving at high flash frequencies (H-response) is the most consistently reported difference between headache patients and controls. The reported sensitivity of the H-response varied from 26–100%, the specificity from 80–91% (Figure 4.2).

Literature addressing the question of whether or not EEG can identify a structural cause for headache is scarce, suggesting that the EEG does not effectively identify or screen out underlying lesions in headache patients.

Since the EEG does not identify headache subtypes, nor does it screen for structural causes of headache, the AAN has concluded that EEG is not useful in the routine evaluation of patients presenting with headache. Indications for performing an EEG are outlined in Table 4.2.

Computed tomography and magnetic resonance imaging

Computed tomography (CT) will detect many, but not all, abnormalities that can cause headache. CT is generally preferable to magnetic resonance imaging (MRI) for the evaluation of acute subarachnoid haemorrhage, acute head trauma, and bony abnormalities. However, a number of disorders may be missed on routine CT of the head; these include vascular disease, neoplastic disease, cervicomedullary lesions, and infections (Table 4.3[12]). MRI is more sensitive than CT in detecting posterior fossa and cervicomedullary lesions, ischaemia, white matter abnormalities, cerebral venous thrombosis, subdural and epidural haematomas, neoplasms (especially in the posterior fossa), meningeal disease (such as carcinomatosis, diffuse meningeal enhancement in low cerebrospinal fluid (CSF) pressure syndrome, and sarcoid), and cerebritis and brain abscess. Pituitary pathology is more likely to be detected on a routine MRI of the brain than on a routine CT.[13]

Table 4.2 Indications for ordering EEG

- Alteration or loss of consciousness
- Transient neurological symptoms without ensuing headache
- Suspected encephalopathy
- Residual persisting neurological defects
- Baseline EEG prior to the institution of medicines or procedures which could induce seizures

Table 4.3 Causes of headache that can be missed on routine CT scan of the head

Vascular disease
    Saccular aneurysms
    Arteriovenous malformations (especially posterior fossa)
    Subarachnoid haemorrhage
    Carotid or vertebral artery dissections
    Cerebral infarctions
    Cerebral venous thrombosis
    Vasculitis
    Subdural and epidural haematomas
Neoplastic disease
    Neoplasms (especially in the posterior fossa)
    Meningeal carcinomatosis
    Pituitary tumour and haemorrhage
Cervicomedullary lesions
    Chiari malformations
    Foramen magnum tumours
Infections
    Paranasal sinusitis
    Meningoencephalitis
    Cerebritis and brain abscess

From Evans[12]

MRI is now preferred to CT for the evaluation of headaches. The yield depends on the field strength of the magnet, the use of paramagnetic contrast, the selection of acquisition sequences, and the use of magnetic resonance angiography and venography.[13]

Mitchell and Osborn[14] used CT scanning with contrast enhancement to evaluate 350 headache patients. Patients were included in the study regardless of the presence or absence of physical or neurological signs or findings. Seven patients (2%) had CT findings that were felt to be clinically significant, including multiple metastases, epidural abscesses, frontal meningiomas and subdural haematomas. Three of these patients (1%) had abnormalities on physical or neurological examination. Another four patients (1%) had unusual clinical symptoms in addition to headache. Twenty-five (7%) had scans that were interpreted as abnormal but incidental to the headache complaint (e.g. atrophy, sinus disease and arachnoid cysts). Mitchell and Osborn concluded that routine CT has a low likelihood of uncovering significant intracranial disease in headache patients who have normal physical and neurological examinations.[14]

Cala and Mastaglia[15] studied 46 patients who exhibited increasing headache frequency or severity or whose headaches were associated with neurological symptoms. Abnormal CT scans were found in 37 (80%). Abnormalities included:

- mild white matter oedema in one or both hemispheres, thought to be owing to increased fluid content on the basis of regional cerebral ischaemia due to vasospasm or alternatively due to reduced cerebral blood flow, 17 (45%),
- cerebral atrophy, eight (17%),
- occipital infarctions, six (9%), of whom four had homonymous haemianopsia, and
- unexpected tumours, two (4%), both of whom had abnormal neurological examinations.

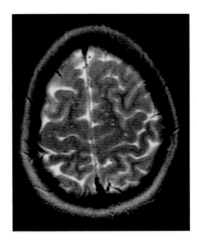

● **Figure 4.3** *MRI abnormalities that may be a consequence of migraine.*

Dorfman et al[16] described four migraineurs who had cerebral infarct: two had persistent neurological defects and one had transient weakness associated with the headache.

Kaplan and Solomon[17] suggested that MRI may be superior to CT scanning in headache evaluation. Nine patients with different headache types had both CT and MRI. In five patients with a normal CT, MRI demonstrated cerebral infarction in two cases, and in one case, a 24-year-old woman with a diagnosis of 'migraine equivalent', a high-intensity signal focus in the medulla that proved to be an astrocytoma.

Robbins and Friedman[18] compared the MRI of 46 migraineurs to sex-matched controls. Thirteen percent of the migraineurs had white matter lesions, compared to 4% of the controls. This finding may not be clinically significant.

Igarashi et al[19] found that 36 of 91 (31%) migraineurs had small foci of high intensity, predominantly in the centrum semiovale and frontal white matter, on T2-weighted MRI and proton density-weighted images. This was significantly more than the 11% seen in the age-matched controls. There was no correlation between MRI abnormalities and migraine type, ergotamine consumption, or frequency, duration or intensity of headaches. These abnormalities may be a consequence of migraine (Figure 4.3).

Forsyth and Posner[20] identified 111 patients with primary and metastatic brain tumours, and headache was found in 48%. The features of the headache were similar to tension-type headache in 77%, to migraine in 9%, and to other types of headache in 9%. The 'classic' presentation of early morning headache was seen in only 14%. Patients with a history of prior headache were more likely to have headache associated with brain tumours than were those with no previous history. Thirty-six percent of these patients with severe headache had pain identical to

previous headache, but it was associated with seizures, confusion, prolonged nausea, hemiparesis, or other abnormal neurological signs. The authors concluded that a change in headache symptoms is an indication for neuroimaging, but did not specify criteria for imaging.

The AAN has reviewed the role of neuroimaging in evaluating a headache patient whose neurological examination is normal. The AAN position paper is based on an analysis of 16 CT and MRI studies, most of which were retrospective case reports. It concluded that CT and MRI are not likely to produce substantial benefit and their routine use is not warranted in patients whose headaches fit a broad definition of recurrent migraine and who have had no recent change in headache pattern, no history of seizures, and no focal neurological findings.[21] Indications for CT or MRI in headache investigation are outlined in Table 4.4.

The US Headache Consortium has concluded that neuroimaging is not usually warranted in migraine patients who have a normal neurological examination; however, it should be considered when neuroimaging risk factors for intracranial pathology exist, as when a patient with a non-acute headache that lasts more than 4 weeks has an unexplained neurological examination, an atypical headache or headache features, or an additional risk factor, such as immune deficiency.[22] In the acute headache setting, which was outside of the original guidelines, risk factors for intracranial pathology include an acute onset, occipitonuchal location, age greater than 55 years, associated symptoms, and an abnormal neurological examination.[23]

In patients in whom an aneurysmal subarachnoid haemorrhage (SAH) is suspected, both CT and MRI have been utilized.[1] MRI is not as reliable as CT in detecting an acute SAH in the first 24 hours. Since CT scan without contrast provides a rather high initial sensitivity, it is the

- The first or worst headache of the patient's life, particularly if it is of rapid onset (thunderclap headache)
- A change in the frequency, severity, or clinical features of the headache attack
- A progressive or new daily persistent headache
- Neurologic symptoms that do not meet the criteria of migraine with typical aura or that themselves warrant investigation
- New-onset headache in patients who have cancer or who test positive for HIV infection
- New-onset headache after age 50
- Patients with headache and seizures
- An abnormal neurological examination

neuroimaging study of choice in the detection of acute SAH. In a cooperative series of 3521 patients, findings on the first CT scan after rupture of a saccular aneurysm were as follows: normal, 8.3%; decreased density, 1.1%; mass effect, 6.1%; aneurysm, 5%; hydrocephalus, 15.2%; intraventricular haematoma, 16.7%; intracerebral haematoma, 17.4%; subdural haematoma, 1.3%; and SAH, 85.2%. CT scan detected aneurysmal SAH in 92% of patients on day 0, decreasing to 58% on day 5. The percentage of scans that were normal on day 0 was 3.3%; on day 1, 7.2%; and on day 5, 27.3% (Table 4.5).[24,25] In detecting a SAH, MRI is not the equal of CT during the first 24 hours. From 24 to 72 hours, MRI was slightly superior to CT and from 3 to 14 days MRI was superior to CT.[26]

Cerebral angiography

Unless aneurysm, vasculitis, or arteriovenous malformation (AVM) is suspected, there is little reason to perform angiography when a patient has a normal neurological examination, a normal CT or MRI, and a history consistent with a benign primary headache disorder.[27] Earlier case reports suggest that complications may occur when

● **Table 4.5** *Approximate probability of recognizing an aneurysmal haemorrhage on computed tomographic scan after the initial event*[20,21]

Time post-initial event	Probability (%)
Day 0	95
Day 3	74
One week	50
Two weeks	30
Three weeks	Almost 0

angiography is performed in migraineurs, particularly during an attack.[28,29] However, Schuaib and Hachinsky have concluded that migraine does not increase the risk of complication, even if performed during the attack. Transient neurological symptoms, however, are not infrequent, especially in patients with migraine with aura.[30]

Magnetic resonance angiography

Although magnetic resonance angiography (MRA) allows for detection of aneurysms as small as 3–4 mm in the vicinity of the circle of Willis, this study has limitations:

- small aneurysms may be better visualized than larger, thrombosed aneurysms, and
- a high signal intensity thrombus within an aneurysm could be mistaken for slow blood flow.

As with conventional arteriography, vasospasm (with its diminished blood flow) may result in poor visualization of the aneurysm. If SAH is detected on CT, one should proceed to conventional angiography.

Aneurysms that occur in the supraclinoid internal carotid artery (ICA) or the parasellar area, or outside the circle of Willis, are more difficult to detect. If an acute SAH is suspected, CT scan would be the imaging method of choice.

MRA is a safe and non-invasive tool that is particularly useful for screening for a suspected aneurysm or AVM in patients who have not had an SAH.[31,32]

Lumbar puncture

The lumbar puncture (LP) is crucial in four distinct clinical situations. These include the patient who presents with:

- the first or worst headache of their life,
- a severe, rapid-onset, recurrent headache,
- a progressive headache, and
- an atypical chronic intractable headache.[33]

An LP should be performed if neuroimaging is normal, non-diagnostic or suggestive of a disorder that can only be diagnosed by measuring CSF pressure, cell count and chemistries. It should be performed first if imaging is not available and meningitis is suspected.

Patients who present with sudden-onset severe headache must always be considered to have an acute neurological event, even though migraine can present in this manner. Focal neurological signs or symptoms or a change in consciousness or mental status suggest an intracranial process. It is almost impossible to differentiate between severe, acute-onset migraine and SAH.[34] A brain image should be performed, if possible, prior to LP.

The best way to detect xanthochromia is by spectrophotometry, since it cannot be detected by the naked eye in about half of all cases.[35] The probability of detecting xanthochromia by spectrophotometry at various times after SAH is: 12 hours, 100%; 1 week, 100%; 2 weeks, 100%; 3 weeks, > 70%; and after 4 weeks, > 40% (Table 4.6). Other causes of xanthochromia include: jaundice, usually with a total plasma bilirubin of 10–15 mg/dl; CSF protein > 150 mg/dl; dietary hypercarotenaemia; malignant melanomatosis; and oral intake of rifampin.[36]

An LP is crucial to rule out an intracranial infection in the patient who presents with a confusional state, fever, or meningeal signs (with or without headache). If CT is readily available, it should be performed first. However, if an imaging procedure is not readily available, an LP should be performed when there is a strong suspicion of meningitis. Delaying the LP and thus the diagnosis may lead to increased morbidity and mortality. If the headache has the characteristics of a postural (orthostatic) headache and there is no obvious cause, an LP will establish the diagnosis of CSF hypotension.

Many disorders are associated with the syndrome of increased intracranial pressure. Patients who have papilloedema and are suspected of having increased intracranial pressure should have an initial neuroimaging procedure (MRI or CT) to rule out a mass lesion. If these studies are normal, a tentative diagnosis of idiopathic intracranial hypertension can be made. Identical symptoms can be caused by chronic meningitis, however, so it is crucial to perform an LP to document increased intracranial pressure, rule out chronic meningitis (particularly in patients who are immunosuppressed), and ascertain the therapeutic effect of drugs given to decrease intracranial pressure.

Patients with intractable chronic daily headache commonly fail to respond to the usual treatment modalities, and it is often assumed that their problems are not organic in origin. A frequently overlooked cause of head pain is increased intracranial pressure without papilloedema. An LP is necessary to make the diagnosis.

● **Table 4.6** *The probability of detecting xanthochromia with spectrophotometry in the cerebrospinal fluid at various times after a subarachnoid haemorrhage*[32]

Time post-haemorrhage	Probability (%)
12 hours	100
One week	100
Two weeks	100
Three weeks	>70
Four weeks	>40

Patients with daily headaches of subacute onset can also have a chronic fungal meningitis (particularly those who are immunosuppressed), the meningitis of Lyme disease or carcinomatous meningitis, all of which require an LP to diagnose.

Unless a diagnosis of meningitis, SAH, or high- or low-pressure syndrome is suspected, there is no reason to perform a spinal tap during a headache.[37] CSF pleocytosis may occur; it is rare, however, in migraine with or without aura and is more frequently seen in complicated migraine.[38]

Thermography

Abnormal thermograms have been described in headache patients. Temperature asymmetry is the most prominent finding in migraineurs. In patients with cluster headache and chronic paroxysmal hemicrania, a cold spot along the supraorbital area, or the inner orbit and canthus, is noted. The Therapeutics and Technology Assessment Subcommittee of the AAN reviewed the use of thermography in headache in 1990 and concluded that it had not been shown to provide sufficiently reliable information and data were insufficient to recommend it as a diagnostic test.[39]

Electromyography

Increased activity in the neck and scalp muscles occurs in some patients with migraine and tension-type headache, but there is no correlation between increased EMG activity and pain or tenderness. Relaxation of these muscles does not relieve headache. Sophisticated EMG studies measuring reflex muscular contraction in response to painful electrical stimulation of the face demonstrate changes in some patients with frequent headache, but EMG abnormalities do not have sufficient sensitivity or specificity for diagnostic testing.

Investigating specific headache types

Migrainous infarction and migraine with prolonged or atypical aura

Migrainous infarction always warrants investigation. When a migraineur presents with weakness, numbness, speech difficulty, or a persistent visual field defect, investigation for an organic aetiology such as stroke, tumour, subdural haematoma, or AVM should be undertaken. If there is a strong suspicion of carotid disease, vasculitis, or large artery dissection, MRA or arteriography should be performed promptly. Carotid duplex scanning, transcranial Doppler, EKG and Holter monitoring may be necessary. Antiphospholipid antibodies, protein S, protein C and occasionally antithrombin III levels may need to be determined in younger patients (under 55 years). Without an obvious cause of stroke, a more thorough diagnostic evaluation, including clotting factor analysis, should be undertaken.

Basilar migraine

Basilar migraine should be suspected in the presence of syncope, diplopia, vertigo, ataxia, change in mental state, and confusion. EEG should be performed to determine if epileptiform activity is present, and MRI or CT should be performed to exclude brainstem AVM or a space-occupying lesion. When vertebrobasilar disease is suspected, especially in older patients, MRA and transcranial Doppler may be necessary. If there is uncertainty about vascular disease, an angiogram may be necessary. Cardiac causes of cerebral vascular disease should also be excluded.

Migraine aura without headache

The disorder that was previously known as 'acephalic migraine' is now called 'migraine aura without headache'; in the elderly, it is known as 'late-life migraine equivalent.'[40] Diagnostic criteria for late-life migrainous equivalents are outlined in Table 4.7.

The headaches are either totally absent or mild, if present at all. Neuroimaging and arteriogram, if performed, are normal. Cerebral thrombosis, embolism, dissection, subclavian steal syndrome, epilepsy, thrombocytopenia, polycythemia, hyperviscosity syndrome, and antiphospholipid antibody must be excluded.[41]

Dennis and Warlow[41] defined transient ischaemic attacks (TIA) as the acute loss of focal cerebral or monocular function with symptoms lasting less than 24 hours, which, after adequate investigation, is presumed to be embolic or thrombotic vascular disease. Dennis and Warlow[41] compared a group of patients with migraine aura without headache with a group with TIA and found that 98% of the patients with migraine aura without headache had visual symptoms. These visual symptoms were binocular in 71%. Seventy-one percent described positive visual features, and 30% had other aura symptoms, including sensory disturbances, aphasia or dysarthria. Patients who had migraine aura without headache had longer attacks than did those with TIA. Symptoms lasted between 15 minutes and 1 hour in 74% of patients with migraine aura without headache.

The manifestations of migraine aura without headache are variable in extent, duration, severity, and quality. Diagnosis is more difficult when the condition occurs for the first time in a patient over the age of 40 years. The diagnosis should still be made by exclusion unless the symptoms are 'classic' (e.g. scintillating scotoma lasting 30 minutes).

Headache of sudden onset

Headache of sudden onset and extended duration may indicate an SAH or a sentinel headache without haemorrhage. More benign causes of this condition include migraine of sudden onset and coital cephalalgia (Table 4.8).

Thunderclap headache and subarachnoid haemorrhage

Thunderclap headache is the sudden onset of a severe headache that reaches maximum intensity within 1 minute. Benign thunderclap headache can be further defined by the absence of a SAH and other organic pathology.

The first or worst attack of migraine may be very difficult to differentiate from an SAH, particularly if the pain is acute in onset. The classical presentation of an aneurysmal SAH is an acute-onset, severe headache associated with a stiff neck, photophobia, nausea, vomiting and perhaps obtundation or coma; it is easily differentiated from migraine. This catastrophic presentation is often preceded by a minor haemorrhage that can signal the likelihood of a major rupture. An extensive neurological evaluation, including CT and LP, is indicated in patients presenting with their first or worst headache, particularly one associated with focal neurological signs, stiff neck, or changes in cognition. Computed tomography, which would be performed by most physicians under these clinical cir-

---

● **Table 4.7** *Late-life migrainous equivalents*

- The gradual appearance of focal neurological symptoms, spreading or intensifying over a period of minutes, not seconds
- Positive visual symptoms characteristic of 'classic' migraine, even if these come on abruptly, specifically fortification spectra (scintillating scotoma), flashing lights, dazzles, or a 'march' of paraesthesias
- Previous similar symptoms associated with 'classic' migraine or a more severe headache
- Serial progression from one accompaniment to another, such as a visual aura progressing to an aura with paraesthesias
- The occurrence of two or more identical spells
- A duration of 15–25 minutes (transient ischaemic attacks, TIAs, usually last less than 15 minutes)
- The occurrence of a 'flurry' of accompaniments (these generally occur in the 50–60-year-old age group)
- A generally benign course without permanent sequelae

● **Table 4.8** *Headache of sudden onset*

Primary headache disorders
• Crash migraine
• Cluster
• Benign exertional headache
• Benign orgasmic cephalgia
Secondary headache disorders
• Associated with vascular disorders
Unruptured saccular aneurysm
Subarachnoid haemorrhage
Internal carotid artery dissection
Cerebral venous thrombosis
Acute hypertension
pressor response
phaeochromocytoma
• Associated with non-vascular intracranial disorders
Intermittent hydrocephalus
Benign intracranial hypertension
Pituitary apoplexy
Cephalic infection
meningoencephalitis
acute sinusitis
Acute mountain sickness
Disorders of eyes
acute optic neuritis
acute glaucoma

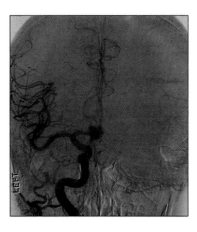

● **Figure 4.4** *Unruptured aneurysms.*

cumstances, can miss subarachnoid blood in as many as 25% of cases, particularly if it is not performed until days after the onset of headache.[24] An MRI may be more sensitive after 24 hours, but only with the LP can one unerringly diagnose SAH.

Day and Raskin[42] have stated that all patients who present with severe, sudden-onset headache should be evaluated for an aneurysm with angiography, even if CT, MRI, and LP do not show evidence of SAH.[43] Several prospective studies[44,45] have suggested that thunderclap headache is usually benign and angiography probably is not necessary if neurological examination, CSF examination, and CT or MRI are normal. However, Hughes[46] reported two cases of thunderclap headache due to unruptured aneurysms. Ng and Pulst[47] reported a 53-year-old woman who presented with the acute onset of the worst headache of her life. Examination, CT, and LP were normal. An angiogram showed a distal right ICA aneurysm. Raps et al[48] looked at the clinical spectrum of unruptured intracranial aneurysms. Acute, severe thunderclap headache, comparable to SAH but without nuchal rigidity,

was seen in seven of 111 patients (6.3%) with unruptured aneurysms, most of which were located in the anterior circle of Willis. Since the true frequency of unruptured aneurysm among patients with thunderclap headache is unknown, all patients in whom unruptured aneurysm is a possibility should undergo at least an MRA. The routine use of cerebral angiography is proscribed by the risk of permanent (0.1%) and transient (1.2%) deficits in this low-yield population (Figure 4.4).[49]

Coital headache (Table 4.9)

The coital headache, which usually begins at or shortly before or during orgasm, is of high intensity, is frontal or occipital in location, is explosive or throbbing in nature, and persists for a few minutes to 48 hours.[50] A second, less ominous, type of headache begins earlier in intercourse, is occipital or diffuse in location, is characterized as dull and aching, and is most severe at orgasm. For a coital headache of sudden onset, a CT scan should be performed and even if this is negative, an LP should be obtained. The question of whether to carry out angiography, even when the CSF is bloodless, is controversial; Day and Raskin,[42] however, advocate angiography. Aneurysm without rupture has presented as coital headache. Again, MRA may be a reasonable alternative.

● **Table 4.9** *International Headache Society diagnostic criteria for coital headache*

4.6 Headache associated with sexual activity	
A	Precipitated by sexual excitement
B	Bilateral in onset
C	Prevented or eased by ceasing sexual activity before orgasm
D	Not associated with an intracranial disorder such as aneurysm

Exertional and cough headaches

Originally described by Tinel[51] in 1932 ('la céphalée a l'effort') and later by Symonds,[52] exertional headache mainly affects middle-aged men; it runs its course over a few years and is not commonly encountered in the clinic. Transient, severe head pain upon coughing, sneezing, lifting, bending, straining at stool, or stooping defines exertional headache. MRI must be performed to rule out hindbrain abnormalities, which include Arnold–Chiari malformation, posterior fossa meningioma, midbrain cyst, basilar impression, and acoustic neurinoma (Figure 4.5). Other causes of brief severe headache are listed in Table 4.10.

Spontaneous internal carotid artery (ICA) dissection

Spontaneous ICA dissection is an uncommon but not altogether rare cause of headache and acute neurological deficit in younger patients. Headache, the most common symptom, is often unilateral and located in the orbital, periorbital and frontal regions. It may be accompanied by neck pain. The pain is usually moderate to severe and steady or throbbing in nature. A bruit or Horner's syndrome is often present. Focal cerebral symptoms, such as TIA or stroke, may either precede the headache or follow it by up to 2 weeks. The gold standard test for dissection was arteriography. High-resolution MRI and MRA, especially in the axial planes, can demonstrate the vessel lumina and changes in the arterial wall (Figure 4.6).

● **Table 4.10** Headache of sudden onset

Bilateral	Unilateral
Idiopathic, stabbing headache	Idiopathic stabbing headache
Benign cough and exertional headache	Trigeminal neuralgia
Coital headache	SUNCT
Headaches due to structural disease	Chronic and episodic paroxysmal hemicrania
Colloid cyst of IIIrd ventricle and other IIIrd ventricular tumours	Cluster headache
Pineal region tumours and masses	
Arnold–Chiari malformation	
Platybasia/basilar impression	
Phaeochromocytoma	

SUNCT = short-lasting unilateral neuralgiform headache with conjunctival injection and tearing.

Summary

The routine use of neuroimaging and other diagnostic testing is not warranted in adult patients with recurrent headaches that have been defined as migraine if there has been no recent change, no history of seizures, and no other focal neurological signs or symptoms. Some testing is appropriate prior to beginning treatment or if there are clinical features that suggest an organic aetiology for the disorder. In patients who have atypical headache patterns, such as chronic daily headache, or a history of seizures or focal neurological signs or symptoms, additional testing, including CT or MRI, is often indicated.

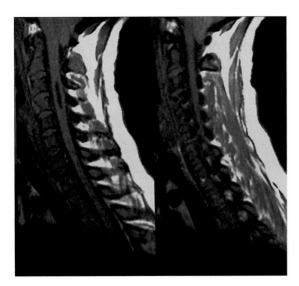

● **Figure 4.5** Arnold–Chiari malformation seen at MRI showing low-lying cerebellar tonsils and associated syrinx.

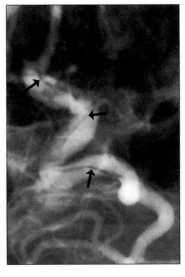

● **Figure 4.6**
Internal carotid artery dissection. Reproduced with permission.[53]

References

1. Evans RW. Diagnostic testing for the evaluation of headaches. Neurol Clin 1996; 14: 1–26.
2. Adams RD, Victor M. Principles of neurology. New York: McGraw-Hill, 1989.
3. Ziegler DK, Friedman AP. Intermittent or paroxysmal disorders, migraine. In: Rowland LP, ed. Merritt's Textbook of Neurology. New York: McGraw-Hill, 1993: 773–80.
4. Raskin NH. Migraine: clinical aspects. In: Raskin NH, Appenzeller O, eds. Headaches. New York: Churchill-Livingstone, 1988, 35–98.
5. Lance JW. Mechanism and management of headache. London: Butterworth Scientific, 1993.
6. Headache Classification Committee of the International Headache Society. Classification and diagnostic criteria for headache disorders, cranial neuralgia, and facial pain. Cephalalgia 1988; 8: 1–96.
7. Selby G. Assessment and investigation of the patient with migraine. In: Selby G, ed. Migraine and its variants. Australia: Adis Press, 1983, 74–93.
8. Slater KH. Some clinical and EEG findings in patients with migraine. Brain 1968; 91: 85–98.
9. Smyth VOG, Winter AL. The EEG in migraine. Electroenceph Clin Neurophysiol 1964, 194–202.
10. Lauritzen M, Trojaborg, Olesen J. The EEG in common and classic migraine attacks. In: Rose FC, ed. Advances in migraine research and therapy. New York: Raven Press, 1982: 79–84.
11. American Academy of Neurology Quality Standards Subcommittee. Practice parameter: the electroencephalogram in the evaluation of headache (summary statement). Report of the Quality Standards Subcommittee. Neurology 1995; 45: 1411–13.
12. Evans RW. Headaches. In: Evans RW, ed. Diagnostic testing in neurology. Philadelphia: W.B. Saunders, 1999, 2.
13. Evans RW, Rozen TD, Adelman JU. Neuroimaging and other diagnostic testing in headache. In: Silberstein SD, Lipton RB, Dalessio DJ, eds. Wolff's Headache and other Head Pain. Seventh edn. New York: Oxford University Press, 2001.
14. Mitchell CS, Osborn REG Sr. Computed tomography in the headache patient: is routine evaluation really necessary? Headache 1993; 33: 82–6.
15. Cala LA, Mastaglia FL. Computerized axial tomography findings in a group of patients with migrainous headaches. Proceedings of the Australian Association of Neurologists. 1976; 35: 41
16. Dorfman LJ, Marshall WH, Enzmann DR. Cerebral infarction and migraine: clinical and radiological correlations. Neurology 1979; 29: 317–22.
17. Kaplan Solomon
18. Robbins L, Friedman H. MRI in migraineurs. Headache 1992; 32: 507–8.
19. Igarashi H, Sakai F, Kan S et al. Magnetic resonance imaging of the brain in patients with migraine. Cephalalgia 1991; 11: 69–74.
20. Forsyth PA, Posner JB. Headaches in patients with brain tumors. A study of 111 patients. Neurology 1993; 43: 1678–83.
21. Frishberg BM. The utility of neuroimaging in the evaluation of headache in patients with normal neurologic examinations. Neurology 1994; 44: 1191–7.
22. Frishberg B, Rosenberg JH, Matchar DB et al. Evidence-based guidelines for neuroimaging in patients with nonacute headache. 1999 http://www.ann.com
23. Ramirez-Lassepas M, Espinosa CE, Cicero JJ et al. Predictors of intracranial pathologic findings in patients who seek emergency care because of headache. Arch Neurol 1997; 54: 1506–9.
24. Adams HP, Kassell NF, Torner JC, Sahs AL. CT and clinical correlations in recent aneurysmal subarachnoid hemorrhage: a preliminary report of the cooperative aneurysm study. Neurology 1983; 33: 981–8.
25. van Gijn J, van Dongen KG. The time course of aneurysmal hemorrhage on computed tomograms. Neuroradiology 1982; 23: 153–6.
26. Ogawa T, Inugami A, Shimosegawa E et al. Subarachnoid hemorrhage: evaluation with MR imaging. Radiology 1993; 186: 345–51.
27. Silberstein SD, Saper JR. Migraine: diagnosis and treatment. In: Dalessio DJ, Silberstein SD, eds. Wolff's Headache and other Head Pain. Sixth edn. New York: Oxford University Press, 1993: 96–170.
28. Kwentus J, Kattah J, Koppicar M, Potolicchio SJ. Complicated migraine and cerebral angiography: a report of an unusual adverse reaction. Headache 1985; 25: 240–5.
29. Dalessio DJ. Migraine. In: Dalessio DJ, ed. Wolff's Headache and other Head Pain. New York: Oxford University Press, 1980: 56–130.
30. Schuaib A, Hachinsky VC. Migraine and the risks from angiography. Arch Neurol 1988; 45: 911–12.
31. Glicklich M, Ross JS. MR angiography: clinical applications. Appl Radiol 1992; 10: 77–83.
32. Bosmans H, Marchal G, VanHecke P, Vanhoenacker P. MRA review. Clin Imaging 1992; 16: 152–67.
33. Silberstein SD, Corbett JJ. The forgotten lumbar puncture. Cephalalgia 1993; 13: 212–13.
34. Silberstein SD. Evaluation and emergency treatment of headache. Headache 1992; 32: 396–407.
35. Vermeulen M, VanGijn J. The diagnosis of subarachnoid hemorrhage. J Neurol Neurosurg Psychiatry 1990; 53: 365–72.
36. Vermeulen M, Hasan D, Blijenberg BG et al. Xanthochromia after subarachnoid hemorrhage needs no revisitation. J Neurol Neurosurg Psychiatry 1989; 52: 826–8.
37. Kovacs K, Bors L, Jelencsik I et al. Cerebrospinal fluid (CSF) investigations in migraine. Cephalalgia 1989; 9: 53–7.
38. Schraeder PL, Burns RA. Hemiplegic migraine associated with an aseptic meningeal reaction. Arch Neurol 1980; 37: 377–9.
39. American Academy of Neurology Quality Standards Subcommittee. Assessment: thermography in neurologic practice. Report of the Therapeutics and Technology Assessment Subcommittee. Neurology 1990; 40: 523–5.
40. Fisher CM. Late-life migraine accompaniments – further experience. Stroke 1986; 17: 1033–42.
41. Dennis M, Warlow C. Migraine aura without headache: transient ischaemic attack or not? J Neurol Neurosurg Psychiatry 1992; 55: 437–40.
42. Day JW, Raskin NH. Thunderclap headache: symptom of unruptured cerebral aneurysm. Lancet 1986; 1247–8.
43. Kassell NF, Torner JC, Haley EC et al. The international cooperative study on the timing of aneurysm surgery. Part I: overall management results. J Neurosurg 1990; 73: 18–36.
44. Wijdicks EFM, Kerkhoff H, VanGijn H. Long-term follow-up of 71 patients with thunderclap headache mimicking subarachnoid haemorrhage. Lancet 1988; 2: 68–70.
45. Harling DW, Peatfield RC, VanHille PT, Abbott RJ. Thunderclap headache: is it migraine? Cephalalgia 1989; 9: 87–90.
46. Hughes RL. Identification and treatment of cerebral aneurysms after sentinel headache. Neurology 1992; 42: 1118–19.
47. Ng PK, Pulst SM. Not so benign 'thunderclap headache'. Neurology 1992; 260: 42.
48. Raps EC, Rogers JD, Galetta SL et al. The clinical spectrum of unruptured intracranial aneurysms. Arch Neurol 1993; 50: 265–8.

49. Leow K, Murie JA. New information on several painful conditions: thunderclap headache mimicking subarachnoid hemorrhage. Neurology Alert 1988; 7: 5–6.

50. Johns DR. Benign sexual headache within a family. Arch Neurol 1986; 43: 1158–60.

51. Tinel J. Un syndrome d'algie veineuse intracranienne. La céphalée à l'effort. Prat Med Fr 1932; 13: 113–19.

52. Symonds C. Cough headache. Brain 1956; 79: 557–68.

53. Mokri B et al. Headache in spontaneous carotid and vertebral artery dissections. In: Goadsby PJ, Silberstein SD (eds), Headache. Boston: Butterworth-Heinemann 1997. pp 327–54.

chapter 5

The pathophysiology of primary headache

Headache is a common human experience, diverse in its expression, complex in its manifestation, and difficult to understand by any simple mechanism. While the biology may seem daunting, there are important common threads that can illuminate the difficult areas. The basic anatomy of the pathways responsible for head pain applies to most manifestations of the problem independent of cause. Pain control systems modulate headache of all causes and may be primarily involved in some headache syndromes. A genetic predisposition seems in some way pivotal to the headache phenotype. In this chapter we shall present the common themes as illustrated by migraine in detail. Because we take the view that migraine has both a clearly episodic form and a more persistent chronic form (chronic migraine), issues relevant to frequent headache, in the context of migraine, are included. Much of the fundamental anatomy and physiology has implications for all primary headaches. The pathophysiology of the other primary headaches is expanded in the relevant clinical chapters. It is our clinical experience that patients value an explanation of their problem, and value clinicians who provide the explanation.

Headache genetics: the predisposition

Migraine is predominantly an affliction of young people. The strong familial association and early onset of the disorder suggest that there is an important genetic component. It is extremely helpful in clinical practice to establish the familial aspects of headache when present as they provide a causal explanation for patients that can foreshorten anxiety over the need for investigation. We find this a particularly rewarding strategy in paediatric practice where one or other parent can often illustrate the principle during the consultation.

Migraine is a feature of some of the mitochondrial disorders, such as MELAS (mitochondrial encephalopathy lactic acidosis stroke-like episodes). This association, and the very many observations of clinicians over time, drew attention to the possible genetic basis for migraine. The first genetic locus for a migrainous disease was found on chromosome 19p13 for familial hemiplegic migraine (FHM).[1] This was the beginning of an extensive effort to

unravel the fundamental defect(s) that leads to migraine. The gene for FHM has been mapped to chromosome 19p13 in some, but not all, families (Figure 5.1). This region may also be involved in more common forms of migraine.[2,3] The defect in FHM has been found to be owing, in five families, to four different missense mutations in a P/Q Ca^{2+} channel alpha-1-subunit gene CACNAIA covering 300 kb with 47 exons.[4] This is the same gene associated with episodic ataxia with cerebellar vermal atrophy.[5] P/Q-type neuronal Ca^{2+} channels mediate 5-hydroxytryptamine (5-HT) release. Dysfunction of these channels may impair 5-HT release and predispose patients to migraine attacks or impair their self-aborting mechanism. Magnesium deficiency occurs in the cortex of migraineurs,[6] and magnesium interacts with Ca^{2+} channels. Ca^{2+} channels are important in spreading depression, which may initiate the migraine aura. Impaired function may predispose to more frequent and severe attacks. This suggests that migraine may be part of the spectrum of channelopathies.

FHM can be compared with other so-called channelopathies, such as hyperkalaemic periodic paralysis, paramyotonia congenita, hypokalaemic periodic paralysis, myotonia congenita, and episodic ataxia with myokymia.[7] In some of these episodic disorders patients are normal

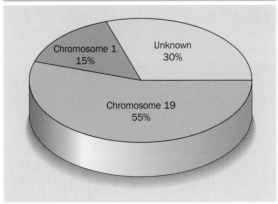

CHROMOSOMAL ALLOCATION OF GENES FOR FAMILIAL HEMIPLEGIC MIGRAINE (FHM)

● *Figure 5.1 Chromosomal allocation of genes for familial hemiplegic migraine (FHM). About 55% of families can be located on chromosome 19[3] and 15% on chromosome 1[8,9] with the remaining 30% unaccounted for at the present.*

between attacks yet may have profound disability during the attack. To account for a further 15% of families with FHM, a recent locus on chromosome 1 has been identified.[8,9] Of interest, the genotype–phenotype correlations among families with FHM seem rather weak.[10] A headache sufferer probably inherits a diathesis or constitution that makes them liable to headache. Triggers can bring on an attack owing to the individual's increased susceptibility. This is the basic neurobiology of migraine. The female predominance and the association with menstruation does not assist in differentiating the site of the problem, since the hormonal changes described[11] could affect either neural or vascular structures and probably act to further lower the threshold to migraine. However, linkage in some families to the X chromosome may explain in part the female preponderance.[12] Thus far, candidate linkage studies have not proved fruitful so that endothelial nitric oxide synthase[13] and 5-HT$_{2A}$ receptor[14] gene polymorphisms are not increased in migraine. Equally interesting is a possible genetic contribution[15-17] to cluster headache. Modern biology is only beginning to clarify this relationship.

Migraine: a sum of the parts

Migraine is a syndrome that is most easily recognized when all parts are present, but is no less debilitating nor valid if only one element predominates. The migraine attack consists of three essential elements: the beginning, the attack, and the resolution. From a biological point of view how the attack starts and how it stops are the most interesting and the least well understood, while the actual attack is the most important element to the sufferer and is becoming better understood. Does the brain institute a process to terminate the attack as soon as it starts? Are the premonitory features and the aura really mechanistically similar? We shall examine these questions below.

Stage 1. Premonitory features of migraine – the attack begins

About 25% of patients report symptoms of elation, irritability, depression, hunger, thirst, or drowsiness during the 24 hours preceding headache. These manifestations suggest a hypothalamic site for their origin.[18] The suprachiasmatic nucleus of the hypothalamus[19] is one of two primary oscillators that generates the circadian rhythms,[20] and could be responsible for the periodicity of migraine that is such an important clinical feature. Patients frequently may report that they are vaguely aware of the beginning of the attack, and while the neurobiology of the premonitory phase is as yet unexplored it is crucial to understanding migraine.

Stage 2A. The attack proper – migraine aura

Most patients never have aura,[21] so clinical and theoretical models that assign a unique sequential stage for migraine aura cannot be truly generalizable. The experience of visual disturbances, such as the scintillating scotoma (flashing lights that move across the visual field), paraesthesias, or other focal neurological signs, are so dramatic that they have been been a focus of attention.

The migraine aura is associated with a reduction in cerebral blood flow (CBF) that moves across the cortex at a rate of 2–3 mm/min (Figure 5.2).[22] The blood flow

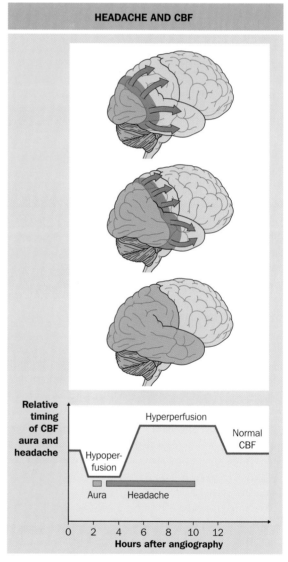

● **Figure 5.2** Line drawing (panel A) of the spreading oligemia observed with studies of cerebral blood flow during aura after Lauritzen[28]. Panel B illustrates the variable time course and relationship of the changes in cerebral blood flow and the symptomatology of migraine.[22]

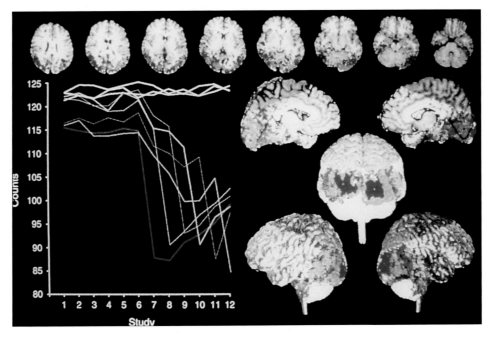

changes usually begin in the occipital region but generally are anterior to the occipital pole. The area of CBF reduction enlarges and may involve the whole hemisphere. The spreading oligaemia does not respect vascular territories and is unlikely to be due to vasoconstriction.[23] The oligaemia may be preceded by a phase of focal hyperaemia.[24] Such a change is what would be expected were a phenomenon similar to cortical spreading depression[25–27] involved.[28] Following the passage of the oligaemia, the cerebrovascular response to hypercapnia is blunted while autoregulation is intact: the cerebral blood vessels do not dilate normally in response to high CO_2 but do respond to changes in blood pressure.[29] This pattern is also seen in spreading depression.[28] Olesen's group observed migraine triggered by carotid angiography, but similar changes occur in spontaneous migraine attacks studied with single-photon emission computed tomography (SPECT).[30] Some have argued that spreading oligaemia is a SPECT scan artefact owing to Compton scatter; however, positron emission tomography (PET) has clearly demonstrated spreading oligaemia during a migraine attack. Woods et al[31] reported measurements of regional CBF from the start of a spontaneous migraine attack in a 21-year-old female migraineur without aura who was a volunteer for a PET CBF study (Figure 5.3). The patient never had a clear neurological deficit either before, during, or after the PET study. Bilateral decreases in CBF began in the occipital cortex and spread anteriorly. Since the patient had transient visual blurring but no aura, it is possible that blood flow changes occur in both migraine with and without aura. It is remarkable that spreading oligaemia can occur and clinically be relatively silent.

Lashley,[32] who suffered from migraine, calculated that the growth of his own migrainous fortification spectrum corresponded to an event moving across the cortex at a rate of 2–3 mm/min (Figure 5.4). Leao[25] found that noxious stimulation of the exposed cerebral cortex of a rabbit produced a spreading decrease in electrical activity

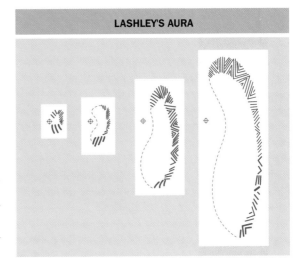

LASHLEY'S AURA

● *Figure 5.4* Line drawings of Lashley's aura moving across his visual field.[32]

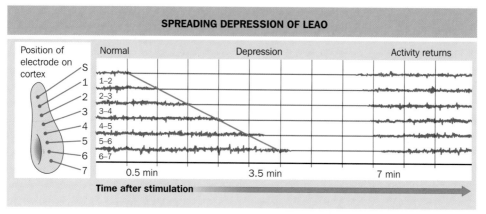

● **Figure 5.5**
Recordings from the rabbit cortex illustrating spreading depression of EEG activity.[25]

that moved at a rate of 2–3 mm/min (spreading depression of Leao) (Figure 5.5). The rates of progression of spreading oligaemia, migrainous scotoma and spreading depression are equal, suggesting that these phenomena may be related. Magnetoencephalography measures changes in the magnetic activity of the cerebral cortex. Some signals found in migraine patients are not found in control subjects. This is felt to be consistent with changes seen with spreading depression in rabbits and provides indirect evidence that this phenomenon exists in humans.[33] Migraine with aura may be associated with a state of neuronal hyperexcitability including the excitatory amino acids: glutamate and possibly aspartate.[34] A low brain magnesium concentration (measured by ^{31}P-NMR spectroscopy) may enhance the responsiveness of the N-methyl-D-aspartate (NMDA) receptor that may be involved in the genesis of both spreading depression and neuronal sensitization.[35] Headache may begin while cortical blood flow is still reduced[22,36,37] and bilateral flow changes can occur making the likelihood that the pain arises from a primary vascular abnormality untenable. We do not know just how common the described blood flow changes are. Do patients with a clouded sensorium or patients just feeling odd have similar focal blood flow changes in areas of cortex that are clinically less eloquent? Do other changes take place that do not cause tightly coupled changes in CBF, and if so, will those changes only be demonstrated in studies of brain metabolism? These are some of the testable hypotheses we will see examined in the next decade.

Most clinicians now believe that the migraine aura is due to neuronal dysfunction, not ischaemia, and that ischaemia rarely, if ever, occurs during the aura. The neurological changes that occur during aura parallel those that occur when the brain is directly stimulated and resemble what might be predicted if ocular dominance columns were sequentially activated. Spreading depression or its human homologue is likely to be the neurobiological basis for the migraine aura.[38]

Stage 2B. The attack – headache
Anatomy
The trigeminal innervation of pain-producing intracranial structures surrounding the large cerebral vessels, pial vessels, large venous sinuses, and dura mater is a plexus of largely unmyelinated fibres that arise from the trigeminal ganglion and in the posterior fossa from the upper cervical dorsal roots.[39,40] Tracing studies have shown that fibres innervating cerebral vessels arise from within the trigeminal ganglion from neurons that contain substance P and calcitonin gene-related peptide (CGRP).[41] Substance P and CGRP are released when the trigeminal ganglion is stimulated either in humans or cats.[42] The cell bodies in the trigeminal ganglion are pseudo-unipolar neurons that innervate the large cerebral arteries and dura mater and arise from the first or ophthalmic division of the trigeminal nerve. Stimulation of the cranial vessels, such as the superior sagittal sinus, is certainly painful in humans,[43,44] and in experimental animals causes cranial release of CGRP.[45] Human dural nerves that innervate the cranial vessels largely consist of small-diameter myelinated and unmyelinated fibres that subserve a nociceptive function[46,47] (Table 5.1).

Physiology: potential sources of pain in migraine
Wolff[44] believed that the aura of migraine was caused by intracerebral vasoconstriction and the headache pain was caused by reactive vasodilatation of the carotid artery. This explained the throbbing quality of the pain, its varied localizations, and its relief by ergot administration.[48]

● **Table 5.1** *Processing of craniovascular pain*

Order	Structures	Comments
1st	Trigeminal ganglion	Located in middle cranial fossa
2nd	Trigeminocervical complex (via quintothalamic tract)	Trigeminal nucleus caudalis and dorsal horns of C_1 and C_2 cervical spinal cord (laminae I/IIo)
3rd	Thalamus	Ventrobasal complex
		Medial nuclei
Final	Cortex	Site unknown

The 'vascular theory' runs into certain difficulties because:

- it failed to explain the premonitory features of a migraine attack;
- some of the drugs used to treat migraine have no effect on blood vessels;
- the theory has not been supported by evidence from recent blood-flow studies; and
- most patients do not have aura.

Some studies have suggested that the headache of migraine could result from dilatation of the large conductance intracerebral arteries. If the carotid artery is occluded on the headache side then two-thirds of migraineurs will experience relief; however, the other one-third do not respond at all.[49] Since the resistance vessels would not be affected, there would be no change in CBF, although balloon inflation of the middle cerebral artery (MCA) in humans produces focal headache, referred to the ophthalmic division of the trigeminal nerve.[50] The relevance of this unphysiological painful dilatation to headache is uncertain. MCA dilatation, as measured by transcranial Doppler during a migraine attack, is not a constant finding.[51] Moreover, while nitrates induce migraine,[52] the immediate clearly vasodilator headache is mild and not migrainous.[53] These powerful clinical observations render a purely 'vascular theory of migraine' implausible.

Neuropharmacology of migraine treatment: what can we learn?

Serotonin and migraine

Several lines of indirect evidence suggest a relationship between serotonin and migraine. It was observed more than three decades ago that urinary excretion of 5-hydroxyindoleacetic acid, the main metabolite of serotonin, is increased in association with migraine attacks,[54] and that platelet 5-HT drops rapidly during the onset of the migraine attack.[55] Furthermore, 5-HT depletion can induce a migraine attack,[56] while intravenous 5-HT can abort acute migraine attacks.[56,57] Headaches similar to migraine can be triggered by serotonergic drugs, such as reserpine (a 5-HT releaser and depleter), and m-chlorophenylpiperazine (m-CPP) (a serotonergic agonist).[58,59] In the years following the intravenous 5-HT observations, Humphrey and his colleagues clarified the 5-HT receptor responsible for selective cranial vasoconstriction,[60] and this led to the development of sumatriptan.[61] 5-HT receptors consist of at least three distinct types of molecular structures: guanine nucleotide G protein-coupled receptors, ligand-gated ion channels, and transporters. There are at least seven classes of 5-HT receptors: 5-HT$_1$, 5 HT$_2$, 5-HT$_3$, 5-HT$_4$, 5-HT$_5$, 5-HT$_6$, and 5-HT$_7$ (Table 5.2).[62] In humans there are at least five 5-HT$_1$ receptor subtypes: 5-HT$_{1A}$, 5-HT$_{1B}$, 5-HT$_{1D}$, 5-HT$_{1E}$, and 5-HT$_{1F}$,[63] and the various triptans are active at a number of these subtypes (Table 5.3). The 5-HT$_{1B/1D}$ receptor agonist actions seem most relevant to the action of the triptans, with some data that might clarify the role of the 5-HT$_{1D}$ and 5-HT$_{1F}$ receptors.

A specific, highly selective 5-HT$_{1D}$ receptor agonist[64] has been tested in acute migraine and was no better than placebo,[65] although some patients complained of chest symptoms,[66] in the absence of the compound having any vascular effects. While the compound may have not been

● **Table 5.2** *Classification of serotonin receptors*

5-HT receptor class	Second messenger	Antagonist	Function
1	↓Adenylate cyclase		See Table 5.3 for details
2	↑Phosphoinositide turnover	Methysergide Pizotifen	Contraction of smooth muscle Central nervous system excitation Subtypes: 2A, 2B, 2C
3	K+, CA^{2+}, Na$^+$	Ondansetron Granisetron	Membrane depolarisation
4	↑Adenylate cyclase	GR113808	Stimulates GI contraction
5	—		Subclasses a & b
6	↑Adenylate cyclase	—	Single receptor
7	↑Adenylate cyclase	—	Splice variants Role in circadian rhythms

*Modified from Hoyer and colleagues.[62]

● **Table 5.3** *Classification of serotonin (5-HT) subclass 1 receptors.**

Subtype of 5-HT$_1$ receptor	Agonist	Antagonist	Function
A	8-OH-DPAT† Dihydroergotamine	WAY100165†	Hypotension Behavioural (satiety)
Rat B Human B (previously known as 1$_{D\beta}$)	CP-93,129† Sumatriptan Dihydroergotamine Almotriptan Eletriptan Naratriptan Rizatriptan Zolmitriptan	GR127935†	Central autoreceptor (rat) Craniovascular receptor
D (previously known as 1$_{D\alpha}$)	Sumatriptan Dihydroergotamine Almotriptan Eletriptan Naratriptan Rizatriptan Zolmitriptan	GR127935†	Trigeminal neuronal receptor
E	—	?	
F	Sumatriptan Dihydroergotamine Almotriptan Eletriptan Naratriptan Zolmitriptan LY334370**	—	?

*Modified from Hartig and colleagues.[63]
**Currently in early development.
†8-OH-DPAT (8-hydroxy-2-(di-n-propylamino)tetralin), WAY100165, CP-93,129 and GR127935 are all compounds used in the laboratory for pharmacological purposes and have no current clinical indications.

interact with the blood vessel wall, producing dilatation, plasma extravasation, and sterile inflammation (Figure 5.6). Electron micrographs of the interior of these blood vessels show platelet activation.[72] Thus, platelet activation occurring during migraine may be an epiphenomenon produced by neurogenic inflammation. The sterile inflammatory process is also thought to sensitize nerve fibres to respond to previously innocuous stimuli, such as blood vessel pulsations (Figure 5.7).[73] Neurogenic inflammation results in the leakage of plasma proteins into the dura mater, which can be quantified by measuring the leakage of radiolabelled albumin.

Administration of either sumatriptan or dihydroergotamine, or newer 5-HT (5-HT$_{1B/1D}$) agonists, such as almotriptan, eletriptan, naratriptan, rizatriptan, and zolmitriptan, prevent the leakage of albumin (see below; Figure 5.6).[74] Furthermore, neurogenic plasma protein extravasation (PPE) can be blocked by ergot alkaloids,[71] indomethacin, acetylsalicylic acid,[75] GABA agonists, such as valproate and benzodiazepines,[76,77] neurosteroids,[78] substance P antagonists,[79] and the endothelin antagonist bosentan.[80] These models do not always predict antimigraine efficacy.[81] The lack of clinical effect in acute

ideal in pharmacological terms,[66] it is remarkable that without vasoconstriction chest symptoms still occur. Some data suggest that 5-HT$_{1F}$ receptor agonists[67] may be effective in acute migraine,[68] although relatively high doses were used in the dose-ranging study. These targets offer the possibility of nonvasoconstrictor treatments of acute migraine, an exciting and promising option for migraine sufferers and their physicians.

Neurogenic plasma protein extravasation

Moskowitz and Cutrer have provided an elegant series of experiments to suggest that the pain of migraine may be a form of sterile neurogenic inflammation.[69] The trigeminal sensory C-fibres contain substance P and other neuropeptides, including CGRP and neurokinin A. Antidromic stimulation of the trigeminal nerve releases substance P, CGRP, and neurokinin A from the sensory C-fibres,[70] resulting in neurogenic inflammation.[71] The released neuropeptides

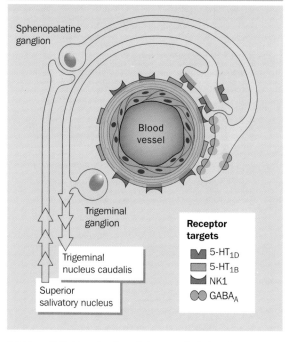

NEURALLY-INDUCED PLASMA PROTEIN EXTRAVASATION MODEL SYSTEM FOR MIGRAINE

● **Figure 5.6** *Line drawing of the neurally-induced plasma protein extravasation model system for migraine.[159]*

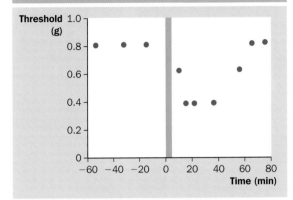

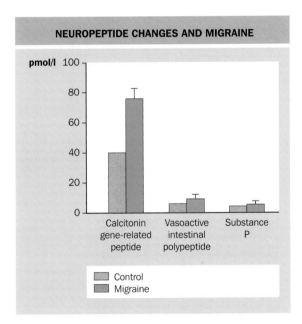

SENSITIZATION OF MENINGEAL AFFERENTS

NEUROPEPTIDE CHANGES AND MIGRAINE

• **Figure 5.7** *Sensitization of primary afferents to mechanical stimulation after application of an inflammatory 'soup'.[43]*

• **Figure 5.8** *Release of vasoactive peptides during migraine. Calcitonin gene-related peptide is a marker for activation of the trigeminovascular system and is elevated in primary headaches.[94]*

migraine attacks of substance P, neurokinin-1 receptor antagonists[82–85] casts some doubt upon the importance of peripherally released substance P in migraine. Furthermore, the potency of CP122 288 in neurogenically-induced PPE[86] must be viewed in the context of the fact that this compound at PPE blocking doses has no effect in acute migraine.[87] In addition, CP122 288 neither blocks fos expression in the trigeminocervical complex[88] nor

reduces CGRP release[89] after stimulation of the superior sagittal sinus in the cat. Similarly, the conformationally-restricted analogue of zolmitriptan 4991W93, a potent inhibitor of PPE,[90] is ineffective in animal models[91,92] and in the treatment of acute migraine.[93]

Neuropeptides and headache

Stimulation of the trigeminal ganglion in the cat leads to an increase in cranial levels of both substance P and CGRP. Similarly, stimulation of the trigeminal ganglion in humans undergoing thermocoagulation for trigeminal neuralgia leads to elevation in the cranial venous outflow of both peptides.[42] More specific stimulation of pain-producing intracranial structures, such as the superior sagittal sinus, also results in cranial venous release of CGRP and not substance P.[45] During migraine, in both adults and in adolescents CGRP is elevated in the external jugular vein blood, whereas substance P is not, (Figure 5.9).[94,95] These data clearly demonstrate activation of trigeminovascular neurons during migraine with or without aura. Similarly, CGRP but not substance P is elevated during acute attacks of cluster headache, both spontaneous[96] and provoked,[97] and during the pain of chronic paroxsymal hemicrania.[98] It is important to note in terms of understanding the pathophysiology of cluster headache that vasoactive intestinal polypeptide (VIP), a marker for cranial parasympathetic nerve activation, is also elevated in cluster headache and paroxysmal hemicrania.[96,98] Moreover, treatment with sumatriptan reduces CGRP levels in humans as their migraine subsides and in experimental animals during trigeminal ganglion stimulation.[99] Similarly, treatment with avitriptan, a potent clinically effective 5-HT$_{1B/1D}$ agonist[100,101] blocks CGRP release in experimental animals, while administration of the potent blocker of neurogenic PPE, CP122 288, is not effective at doses specific for PPE.[89] The fact that substance P, neurokinin-1 receptor antagonists, are ineffective in migraine is consistent with lack of release of substance P in migraineurs during headache[94,95] and with observations in our own model systems.[102] Since CGRP, but not substance P, is released in humans during migraine[103] it is likely that it is the CGRP-enriched innervation of the cerebral circulation[104,105] that plays the major role in the pain of migraine.

In cluster headache[96,97] and the closely related chronic paroxysmal hemicrania,[98] CGRP, but not substance P, is released. The latter syndromes may be lumped together under the pathophysiological rubric of trigeminal–autonomic cephalgias (TACs) and are associated with parasympathetic activation and release of VIP.[106] These data suggest that the animal models of trigeminovascular activation[81] can explain to the same extent the pain and some

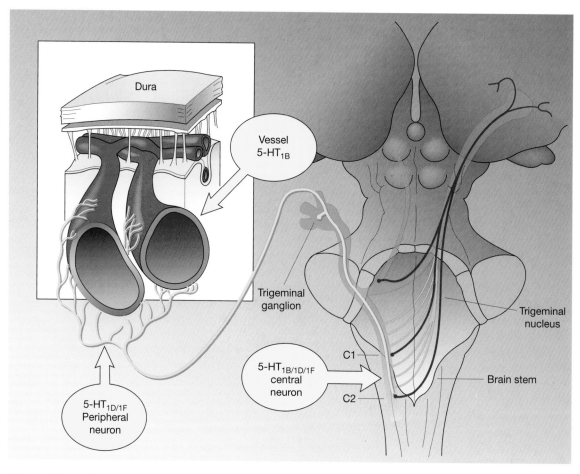

● **Figure 5.9** *Possible sites of action of triptans in the trigeminovascular system.*

of the associated symptoms of migraine and cluster headache.

To test the role of both CGRP and VIP in acute headache, specific antagonists will be required. A potent specific CGRP antagonist is now available,[107] so that the role of CGRP in acute migraine will soon be much clearer. Neurokinin-A is also elevated in migraine,[95] and can be released in experimental settings during trigeminal ganglion stimulation.[108] It is a potent vasodilator,[109,110] and provides a further avenue of exploration to understand the trigeminovascular system. Intriguing recent studies suggest that triptans may modulate CGRP release in terms of repressing the CGRP promoter in trigeminal ganglion cells,[111] offering a further avenue for migraine therapeutics. The release of these peptides offers the prospect of a marker for migraine that can be measured in a venous blood sample and seems highly predictive of antimigraine activity in humans. The development of specific nonpeptide

CGRP antagonists[107] offers the potential for an entirely non-vasconstrictor anti-migraine treatment, and the prospects for an entirely new approach to the management of analgesic, particularly opiate, overuse headaches.[112]

Central processing of trigeminovascular pain

The brainstem sites that are responsible for craniovascular pain have now begun to be mapped using fos-immunohistochemistry. After meningeal irritation with blood fos and offers a third site for the action of specific anti-migraine treatments (Figure 5.9) expression occurs in the trigeminal nucleus caudalis,[113] and after stimulation of the superior sagittal sinus, fos is expressed in cats[114] and monkeys[115] in the trigeminal nucleus caudalis and in the dorsal horn at the C_1 and C_2 levels (Figure 5.10). If metabolism is measured using 2-deoxyglucose, similar increases are seen in the brainstem following superior sagittal sinus stimulation.[116] These data contribute to the view that the trigemi-

FOS ACTIVATION IN THE TRIGEMINOCERVICAL COMPLEX OF THE MONKEY

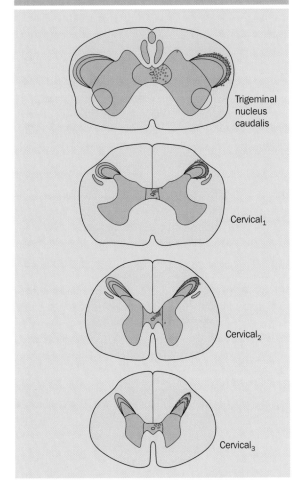

Trigeminal nucleus caudalis

Cervical$_1$

Cervical$_2$

Cervical$_3$

● **Figure 5.10** *Fos expression in the trigeminocervical complex of the monkey after stimulation of the superior sagittal sinus.[115]*

nal nucleus extends beyond the traditional nucleus caudalis to the dorsal horn of the high cervical region in a functional continuum that includes a cervical extension that could be regarded as a trigeminal nucleus cervicalis. The entire group of cells could usefully be labelled the trigeminocervical complex. A substantial portion of the trigeminovascular nociceptive information comes by way of the most caudal cells in the cervical spinal cord. Indeed, direct stimulation of the greater occipital nerve in the cat leads to increased metabolic activity in the entire trigeminocervical complex,[117] with neurons identifiable that receive input from both trigeminal meningeal and cutaneous cervical inputs.[118] It is most likely then that the trigeminocervical neurons are the site for referral of head

pain, and that this anatomical arrangement accounts for the distribution of pain in migraine and many other forms of headache. The rather diffuse activation of neurons in the trigeminal nucleus in visceral type pain, such as that arising from intracranial vessels, is to be contrasted with what is seen when pain stimuli are applied to discrete facial structures. Neuronal activation is more restricted[119] in line with the relatively good spatial localization of more superficial pain.

Experimental pharmacological evidence indicates that many of the abortive antimigraine drugs, such as ergots,[120,121] acetylsalicylic acid,[122] sumatriptan (after blood–brain barrier disruption),[123,124] zolmitriptan,[125] naratriptan,[126] eletriptan[88] and rizatriptan[127] act at second order trigeminal neurons to reduce cell activity, suggesting trigeminocervical complex neurons in the caudal brainstem as a possible target for antimigraine compounds. It is likely that this central action is largely mediated by the 5-HT$_{1B/1D}$ actions of the drugs because the effect of naratriptan can be antagonized by the 5-HT$_{1B/1D}$ antagonist GR127 935.[128] Similarly, and perhaps bringing the 5-HT argument full circle, 5-HT, when administered intravenously in experimental animals, will inhibit trigeminal neuron firing, an effect also blocked by GR127 935.[129] The results of autoradiographic studies indicate specific binding of DHE[120] and zolmitriptan[130] in the trigeminocervical complex neurons. Furthermore, inhibition of firing of trigeminal neuronal activity evoked by nociceptive trigeminovascular stimulation with microiontophoretic application of a range of 5-HT$_{1B/1D}$ receptor agonists locally,[91,131,132] as well as inhibitory effects of GABA-A[133] and opioid agonists,[134] indicate a substantial anatomic target for therapeutic intervention. Moreover, microiontophoretic studies allow us to conclude that there are both pre- and postsynaptic sites in the trigeminal nucleus,[135] offering the promise of ever more targeted treatments.

Following transmission in the caudal brainstem and high cervical spinal cord, information is relayed in a group of fibres (the quintothalamic tract) to the thalamus.[136,137] Processing of vascular pain in the thalamus occurs in the ventroposteromedial thalamus, the medial nucleus of the posterior complex, and the intralaminar thalamus.[138] If capsaicin, the active irritant found in chilli peppers, is applied to the superior sagittal sinus, trigeminal projections with a high degree of nociceptive input are processed in neurons, particularly in the ventroposteromedial thalamus and in its ventral periphery.[139] The properties and further higher centre connections of these neurons are the subject of ongoing studies that will allow us to build up a more complete picture of the trigeminovascular pain pathways (Table 5.1).

The future for acute treatments

There has been some effort to move away from drugs with a vasoconstrictor action, which all the 5-HT$_{1B/1D}$ agonist[140] compounds possess, to neurally active compounds. Initial attempts at such a strategy involved specific inhibitors of neurogenic plasma protein extravasation, such as CP122 288[86] and 4991W93.[90] Similarly, substance P (neurokinin-1) receptor antagonists, endothelin receptor antagonists, and a neurosteroid, have all been unsuccessful in clinical trials (see section on neurogenic plasma protein extravasation). Based on initial molecular biological studies, it has been suggested that the trigeminal ganglion may preferentially contain 5-HT$_{1D}$ receptors[141] and the blood vessels' 5-HT$_{1B}$ receptors.[142–146] Certainly, 5-HT$_{1B}$ receptors are found on human coronary vessels[147] (Table 5.4), which remains the Achilles' heel for triptans. The future demands that new purely neurally active drugs are

developed and tested to remove the small[148] but ever-present issue of safety. Two recent reports indicate that such a strategy will be effective. As mentioned above there is ample evidence for glutamatergic transmission in the trigeminal nucleus, and a preliminary study indicated that NMDA blockade with ketamine aborted migraine.[149] A further placebo-controlled study with an AMPA-kainate antagonist has also demonstrated efficacy in acute migraine.[150] Furthermore, an adenosine A$_1$ receptor agonist that is active with vascular effects in preclinical[151–153] and human[154] models is also effective in acute migraine.[155] Crucially, none of these compounds has any vasoconstrictor properties.

Stage 3. Central modulation – starting and stopping headache

The importance of brainstem mechanisms in the pathogenesis of migraine is underscored by the recent studies of Weiller et al[156] who reported brainstem activation in spontaneous migraine attacks. Using PET to measure regional CBF (rCBF), nine patients with right-sided migraine without aura were studied in the headache phase within hours of migraine onset. High rCBF values were found bilaterally in the cingulate, auditory association and visual association cortices, and on the left side only in the inferior anterocaudal cingulate cortex. There was increased rCBF in the left brainstem, anterior to the aqueduct and posterior to the corticospinal tract. Sumatriptan relieved the headache and its associated symptoms and reversed the cerebral, but

---

● **Table 5.4** *Location of triptan (5-HT$_{1B/1D}$) receptors in humans*

Site	5-HT$_{1B}$	5-HT$_{1D}$
Extracerebral cranial vessels	+++	±
Cerebral microvessels	–	+
Trigeminal ganglion	++	+++
Coronary vessels	+++	±

Note: + and – indicate relative strength of mRNA signal from tissues which is not quantitative nor does it indicate the relative contribution of the receptors to drug actions. Data are modified after Hamel.[143]

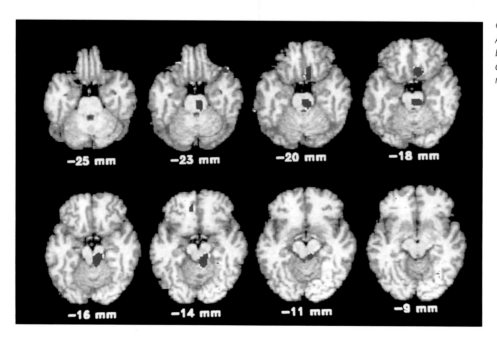

● **Figure 5.11**
Activation of the brainstem with PET during acute migraine.[156]

not the brainstem, increase in rCBF. Since the rCBF in the brainstem persisted despite headache resolution, it seems likely that the activation is owing to factors other than, or in addition to, increased activity of the endogenous antinociceptive system. Activation of the brainstem may be inherent in the migraine process itself. The brainstem center may integrate the migraine attack. Continued activation despite symptom resolution with sumatriptan may account for headache recurrence (Figure 5.11).

Central modulation of trigeminovascular pain

In the experimental animal, stimulation of the brainstem nucleus locus coeruleus (the main central noradrenergic nucleus) reduces CBF in a frequency-dependent manner[156] through an α_2 adrenoceptor-linked mechanism.[157] This reduction is maximal in the occipital cortex.[158] CBF is reduced up to 25% while extracerebral vasodilatation occurs in parallel.[159] Activating the main serotonin-containing nucleus in the brain stem, the midbrain dorsal raphe nucleus, can increase CBF.[160–163] These animal studies underpin the description in humans of activation of the periaqueductal grey matter (PAG) in the region of the dorsal raphe nucleus and in the dorsalateral pons near the locus coeruleus in PET studies during migraine without aura.[156] Moreover, these areas are active immediately after successful treatment of the headache but are not

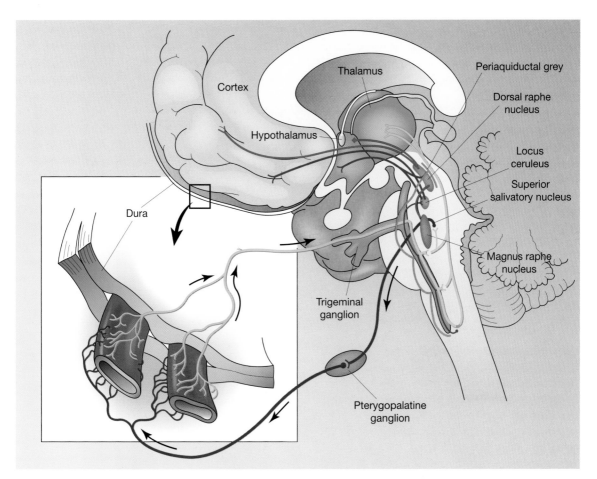

● **Figure 5.12** *Pathophysiology of migraine. Migraine involves dysfunction of brain-stem pathways that normally modulate sensory input. The key pathways for the pain are the trigeminovascular input from the meningeal vessels, which passes through the trigeminal ganglion and synapses on second-order neurons in the trigeminocervical complex. These neurons, in turn, project through the quintothalamic tract, and after decussating in the brain stem, form synapses with neurons in the thalamus. There is a reflex connection between neurons in the pons in the superior salivatory nucleus, which results in a cranial parasympathetic outflow that is mediated through the pterygopalatine, otic, and carotid ganglia. This trigeminal–autonomic reflex is present in normal persons[34] and is expressed most strongly in patients with trigeminal–autonomic cephalgias, such as cluster headache and paroxysmal hemicrania: it may be active in migraine. Brain imaging studies suggest that important modulation of the trigeminovascular nociceptive input comes from the dorsal raphe nucleus, locus ceruleus, and nucleus raphe magnus.*

active between headache attacks. Aura can exist in isolation from pain as a 'migraine equivalent'; it is thus possible that the aura originates in the central nervous system with the vascular changes being a secondary feature (Figure 5.12). How can changes in the brainstem seen in the PET studies occur contralateral to the pain? Are there crossed descending nociceptive control pathways from these regions? The contralateral changes may be owing to activation of ascending pain control systems that modulate thalamic transmission.[164] There are well-described connections from both ventrobasal and medial thalamus to the ipsilateral dorsal raphe nucleus.[165] Pain fibres from the trigeminal nucleus pass by way of the quintothalamic tract and decussate in the midbrain before synapsing on third order neurons in the ventrobasal thalamus and medial thalamic nuclei (see above section, Central processing of trigeminal pain). Alternatively, there is evidence for a descending inhibitory effect of PAG on trigeminal neurons after stimulation of the ventral–lateral region.[166]

Placement of an electrode into the region of the periaqueductal grey matter can evoke a migraine-like headache.[167] Cells in the same region can be activated after superior sagittal sinus stimulation.[168] Contingent negative variation (CNV), an event-related slow cerebral potential, is increased in amplitude and its habituation is lacking in patients with migraine without aura (Figure 5.13).[169–171] Furthermore, CNV is under aminergic control and normalizes after treatment with beta-blockers.[172] The visual evoked potential is augmented rather than habituated in migraine patients when studied between attacks.[173] These clinical observations taken together provide important components of the human data that argue that migraine is a disorder of the central nervous system.

Migraine and the blood–brain barrier

Some very compelling data from a clinical study of aura raises the possibility that the blood–brain barrier may not be normal in migraine. This is not a new suggestion,[174] although there has been little direct evidence for an altered barrier apart from a case report based on CT;[175] more recent MRI studies have been somewhat negative.[176] The era of more modern therapeutics, which has arguably started with sumatriptan, has provided interesting data. In a well-conducted study of patients with migraine with aura the effect of sumatriptan on the aura was examined. Sumatriptan did not shorten or lengthen the aura when compared to placebo. The most fascinating aspect of the study was that sumatriptan was not more effective than placebo for headache when it was given during the aura. Despite reliable delivery and a suitable drug level, with the

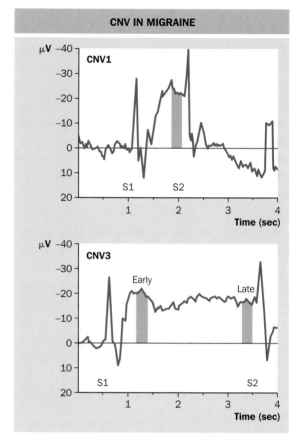

● *Figure 5.13* *Contingent negative variation (CNV) recorded with a 1 second (CNV1) and 3 second (CNV3) interstimulus interval. This method has been instrumental in examining some fundamental questions concerning migraine biology.*[169]

mean length of the aura being about 20 minutes, headache still occurred. Perhaps more remarkable is that the developed headache responded to a further sumatriptan injection.[177] These observations have been supported by analysis of the large Sumatriptan Clinical Trial Database that shows oral sumatriptan used during aura to be less likely to either produce a headache response or render the patient pain free.[178] In contrast triptans administered during mild headache are certainly effective.[179–181] Sumatriptan may not have access to a crucial receptor site during the aura that is made available by the pain process, which begs the question: what site does sumatriptan not normally have access to?

One obvious site would be behind the blood–brain barrier, which re-opens the very exciting possibility that the blood–brain barrier may not be normal in the headache phase of migraine. Better access, therefore, to sites within the central nervous system may be an advantage.

Blood–brain barrier change may be linked to observations of brainstem activation in migraine given that pontine activation has been documented.[156,182] Stimulation of the pontine cell group nucleus locus coeruleus, the main noradrenaline-containing nucleus in the central nervous system, can alter brain blood flow and blood–brain barrier permeability.[183] Modulation of central noradrenergic systems using tricylic antidepressants can alter blood–brain barrier permeability in experimental animals,[184] while central noradrenergic innervation is essential for maintaining blood–brain barrier integrity during some pathophysiological states.[185] Further imaging studies of brainstem changes during migraine and careful studies of the blood–brain barrier in migraine are warranted so that we can understand the implications of this altered physiology for therapeutics.

Observations on the pathophysiology of daily headache

A major cause of disability for patients, and consequently a substantial challenge for clinicians is the management of daily or near daily headache syndromes. An understanding of these conditions should be a primary goal of basic and clinical research.

The neurotrophins, a group of structurally related proteins, include nerve growth factor (NGF), brain derived nerve factor (BDNF), NT-3, NT-4, and NT-5, and have actions that are mediated by specific receptors.[186] A low-affinity (so-called P75) receptor binds all the neurotrophins. High-affinity receptors are now known to be the protein tyrosine kinases, TrkA, TrkB, and TrkC. NGF binds selectively to TrkA; BDNF and NT-5 to TrkB; and NT-3 to TrkC. In developing animals, NGF promotes the survival of sympathetic neurons and some sensory neurons. Evidence now links altered neurotrophin levels to the sensory disturbances (pain and hyperalgesia) associated with peripheral inflammatory states. One feature of the inflammatory response is a large upregulation of NGF production. The sensory neurons innervating the affected tissue show increased retrograde delivery of NGF and increased neuropeptide expression. Anti-NGF treatment can block hyperalgesia.[187] NGF may sensitize primary afferent nerve terminals, either directly through the high-affinity receptor on those terminals, or indirectly following the release of mediators from other local cells.[188] NGF degranulates mast cells, which express the high-affinity NGF receptor. Mast cells occur around the cerebral blood vessels and may be involved in neurogenic inflammation.[72] Increased NGF levels may also lead to a central neuronal sensitization.[189] NGF and inflammatory cytokines may change the behaviour of sensory neurons, making them more sensitive to

nociceptive stimuli. NGF increases the synthesis, transport, and neuronal content of substance P and CGRP. It also regulates two ion channels in sensory neurons: the capsaicin receptor ion channel[190] and the tetrodotoxin-resistant Na^+ channel.

Central sensitization and daily headache

The clinical evidence for sensitization in acute migraine is very compelling.[191] Sensitization of the trigeminal neurons would result in increased activation of the trigeminovascular system. Central sensitization is a well-described phenomenon in animal research.[192] It is manifested by increased spontaneous impulse discharges, increased responsiveness to noxious and non-noxious peripheral stimuli, and expanded receptive fields of nociceptive neurons. In animal models, conditioning stimuli that activate C (unmyelinated) fibres result in a marked and prolonged increase in the flexion withdrawal reflex in rats. In animal models of head pain there is good evidence for fos activation in the trigeminal nucleus caudalis and the dorsal horns at the C_1 and C_2 levels.[115] Fos is a marker for stimulation and may be one signal for the nervous system's adaptive responses to insult.[188,193] Fos and jun, two immediate early gene products that dimerize, can alter cell proteins, receptors, and other peptides, perhaps play a role in neuronal sensitization in headache. Repetitive C-fibre stimulation at constant intensity induces the phenomenon of wind-up, which is the increase in dorsal horn nociceptive neuron responsiveness in both magnitude and duration with each subsequent stimulus above a certain frequency.[194] Wind-up is sensitive to glutamate NMDA receptor antagonists. Neurons that exhibit wind-up are less sensitive to opioids than are neurons that do not exhibit this phenomenon. Wind-up is a short-lasting phenomenon that cannot alone explain the phenomenon of sensitization, which is of longer duration and may involve changes in neuronal plasticity.[188] Wind-up is mediated by NMDA and tachykinin receptors, is blocked by morphine pretreatment, and is accompanied by calcium entry via NMDA channels. It may be the trigger to long-lasting neuronal sensitization. The increased intracellular calcium induces translocation (from cytosolic to membrane-bound form) and activation of protein kinase C (PKC) and phosphorylation of the NMDA channel, which relieves the Mg^{2+} block on the ion channel. The increased calcium may also be responsible for the induction of the genes whose products are fos and jun[195] result in increased glutamate sensitivity. Local anaesthesia, non-NMDA and NMDA antagonists, and gangliosides (which prevent or reduce PKC translocation and activation) can interrupt this cascade. Nitric oxide (NO) is produced in response to NMDA receptor activation and contributes to fos activation in neurons of the trigeminocervical complex.[196]

Pain modulation in relationship to daily headache

The mammalian nervous system contains networks that modulate nociceptive transmission. In the rostroventromedial medulla are so-called 'off-cells' that inhibit and 'on-cells' that facilitate nociception. These cells are believed to modulate the activity of the trigeminal and dorsal horn neurons. Increased on-cell activity in the brainstem's pain modulation system could enhance the response to both painful and non-painful stimuli. Opiate withdrawal results in increased firing of the on-cells, decreased firing of the off-cells, and enhanced nociception.[197] A similar mechanism may occur during drug-induced headaches.[198] Some forms of chronic daily headache (see Chapter 8) may result, in part, from enhanced neuronal activity in the trigeminal nucleus caudalis as a result of enhanced on-cell or decreased off-cell activity. Other conditioned stimuli associated with pain and stress can also turn on the system and may account for some of the association between pain and stress. A tempting anatomical localization for neurons that seem to play a crucial role in frequent headache would be the mid-brain PAG. It has been shown that iron accumulates abnormally in the PAG of patients with both episodic and chronic migraine,[199] while a lesion in the same area can produce de novo a chronic migraine picture indistinguishable from that routinely seen in clinical practice[200] where no lesion can be demonstrated. Given the binding of ergot derivatives[120] and triptans to this area of the brain, it is tempting to consider these neurons as pivotal in the development of some daily headache syndromes.

Summary

Migraine should be viewed as a biologically determined, episodic syndrome of sensory sensitivity: certainly manifesting as head pain but not limited to head pain, with some mixture of sensitivity to light, sound, smell and movement, as well as changes in cutaneous sensation. It seems likely to involve intracranial structures, and is certainly associated with other neurological disturbances, such as might be seen in the aura phase. It is the syndromic nature of migraine, its ability to manifest as a collage of symptoms, that is its core characteristic. The brain and the connections that process and control head pain and other sensory information confer this attribute. The aminergic nuclei, whose usual role is to gate afferent pain information, modulate CBF and blood–brain barrier permeability, and control the signal-to-noise aspect of sensory inputs, are probably the crucial sites in migraine. Indeed, they are strong candidates for the physiological lesion in the classical neurological sense. When these modulatory controls are triggered or timed to dysfunction, the migrainous process is driven by the brain, releasing sensory inputs to create what Edward Liveing called a nerve storm.[201] At once, vessels pulsing normally can be felt to pulse, fluid in an otherwise satisfied stomach is perceived as nausea, normal lights, sounds, or smells are perceived as pungent or unpleasant, and normal movement is perceived to jar and disturb the head. The trigeminovascular system provides a therapeutic target for attack treatment as it arrests the final common pathway for expression of neurovascular head pain. The brain, however, provides the essential key to the disorder, the key to its genesis, and the key to its ultimate understanding and control.

References

1. Joutel A, Bausser MG, Biousee V. A gene for familial hemiplegic migraine maps to chromosome 19. Nat Genet 1993; 5: 40–5.
2. May A, Ophoff RA, Terwindt GM et al. Familial hemiplegic migraine locus on 19p13 is involved in the common forms of migraine with and without aura. Hum Genet 1995; 96: 604–8.
3. Terwindt GM, Ophoff RA, VanEijk R et al. Involvement of the CACNA1A gene containing region on 19p13 in migraine with and without aura. Neurology 2001; 56: 1028–32.
4. Ophoff RA, Terwindt GM, Vergouwe MN. Familial hemiplegic migraine and episodic ataxia type-2 are caused by mutations in the Ca^{2+} channel gene CACNLA4. Cell Tiss Res 1996; 87: 543–52.
5. Vahedi K, Joutel A, Van Bogaert P. A gene for hereditary paroxysmal cerebellar ataxia maps to chromosome 19p. Ann Neurol 1995; 37: 289–93.
6. Ramadan NM, Halvorson H, VandeLinde A et al. Low brain magnesium in migraine. Headache 1989; 29: 416–19.
7. Griggs RC, Nutt JG. Episodic ataxias as channelopathies. Ann Neurol 1995; 37: 285–7.
8. Ducros A, Joutel A, Vahedi K. Mapping of a second locus for familial hemiplegic migraine to 1q21–q23 and evidence of further heterogeneity. Ann Neurol 1997; 42: 885–90.
9. Gardner K, Barmada MM, Ptacek LJ, Hoffman EP. A new locus for hemiplegic migraine maps to chromosome 1q31. Neurology 1997; 49: 1231–8.
10. Ducros A, Deiner C, Joutel A et al. The clinical spectrum of familial hemiplegic migraine associated with mutations in a neuronal calcium channel. N Eng J Med 2001; 345: 17–24.
11. Somerville BW. The role of estradiol withdrawal in the etiology of menstrual migraine. Neurology 1972; 22: 355–65.

12. Nyholt DR, Dawkins JL, Brimage PJ et al. Evidence for an X-linked genetic component in familial typical migraine. Hum Mol Gen 1998; 7: 459–63.

13. Griffiths LR, Nyholt DR, Curtain RP et al. Migraine association and linkage studies of an endothelial nitric oxide synthase (NOS3) gene polymorphism. Neurology 1997; 49: 614–17.

14. Nyholt DR, Curtain RP, Gaffney PT et al. Migraine association and linkage analyses of the human 5-hydroxytryptamine (5HT$_{2A}$) receptor gene. Cephalalgia 1996; 16: 463–7.

15. Russell MB, Andersson PG, Thomsen LL, Iselius L. Cluster headache is an autosomal dominantly inherited disorder in some families: a complex segregation analysis. J Med Genet 1995; 32: 954–6.

16. Leone M, Russell MB, Rigamonti A et al. Increased familial risk of cluster headache. Neurology 2001; 56: 1233–6.

17. Russell MB, Andersson PG, Iselius L. Cluster headache is an inherited disorder in some families. Headache 1996; 36: 608–12.

18. Kupfermann I. Hypothalamus and limbic system II: motivation. In: Kandel ER, Schwartz JH, eds. Principles of neural science. Amsterdam: Elsevier Science Publishers, 1985: 626–35.

19. Swaab DF, Hofman MA, Lucassen PJ et al. Functional neuroanatomy and neuropathy of the human hypothalamus. Anat Embryol (Berlin) 1993; 187: 317–30.

20. Moore-Ede MC. The circadian timing system in mammals: two pacemakers preside over many secondary oscillators. Fed Proc 1983; 42: 2802–8.

21. Rasmussen BK, Olesen J. Migraine with aura and migraine without aura: an epidemiological study. Cephalalgia 1992; 12: 221–8.

22. Olesen J, Friberg L, Skyhoj-Olsen T. Timing and topography of cerebral blood flow, aura and headache during migraine attacks. Ann Neurol 1990; 28: 791–8.

23. Olesen J. Cerebral and extracranial circulatory disturbances in migraine: pathophysiological implications. Cerebrovasc Brain Metab Rev 1991; 3: 1–28.

24. Olesen J, Larsen B, Lauritzen M. Focal hyperemia followed by spreading oligemia and impaired activation of RCBF in classic migraine. Ann Neurol 1981; 9: 344–52.

25. Leao AAP. Spreading depression of activity in cerebral cortex. J Neurophysiol 1944; 7: 359–90.

26. Leao AAP. Pial circulation and spreading activity in the cerebral cortex. J Neurophysiol 1944; 7: 391–6.

27. Leao AAP. Further observations on the spreading depression of activity in the cerebral cortex. J Neurophysiol 1947; 10: 409–14.

28. Lauritzen M. Pathophysiology of the migraine aura. The spreading depression theory. Brain 1994; 117(Pt.1): 199–210.

29. Lauritzen M. Long-lasting reduction of cortical blood flow of the rat brain after spreading depression with preserved autoregulation and impaired CO2 response. J Cereb Blood Flow Metabol 1984; 4: 546–54.

30. Andersen AR, Friberg L, Skyhoj-Olsen T, Olesen J. SPECT demonstration of delayed hyperemia following hypoperfusion in classic migraine. Arch Neurol 1988; 45: 154–9.

31. Woods RP, Iacoboni M, Mazziotta JC. Bilateral spreading cerebral hypoperfusion during spontaneous migraine headaches. N Eng J Med 1994; 331: 1689–92.

32. Lashley KS. Patterns of cerebral integration indicated by the scotomas of migraine. Arch Neurol 1941; 46: 331–9.

33. Barkley GL, Tepley N, Nagel L et al. Magnetoencephalographic studies of migraine. Headache 1990; 30: 428–34.

34. Welch KMA, D'Andrea G, Tepley N et al. The concept of migraine as a state of central neuronal hyperexcitability. Neurol Clin 1990; 8: 817–28.

35. Welch KM, Ramadan NM. Mitochondria, magnesium and migraine. J Neurol Sci 1995; 134: 9–14.

36. Cutrer FM, Sorenson AG, Weisskoff RM et al. Perfusion-weighted imaging defects during spontaneous migrainous aura. Ann Neurol 1998; 43: 25–31.

37. Sanchez-del Rio M, Bakker D, Wu O et al. Perfusion weighted imaging during migraine: spontaneous visual aura and headache. Cephalalgia 1999; 19: 701–7.

38. Hadjikhani N, Sanchez del Rio M, Wu O et al. Mechanisms of migraine aura revealed by functional MRI in human visual cortex. Proc Nat Acad Sci 2001; 98: 4687–92.

39. Ruskell GL, Simons T. Trigeminal nerve pathways to the cerebral arteries in monkeys. J Anat 1987; 155: 23–37.

40. Liu-Chen LY, Mayberg MR, Moskowitz MA. Immunohistochemical evidence for a substance P containing trigeminovascular pathway to pial arteries in cats. Brain Res 1983; 268: 162–6.

41. Uddman R, Edvinsson L, Ekman R et al. Innervation of the feline cerebral vasculature by nerve fibers containing calcitonin gene-related peptide: trigeminal origin and co-existence with substance P. Neurosci Lett 1985; 62: 131–6.

42. Goadsby PJ, Edvinsson L, Ekman R. Release of vasoactive peptides in the extracerebral circulation of man. Ann Neurol 1988; 23: 193–6.

43. Feindel W, Penfield W, McNaughton F. The tentorial nerves and localization of intracranial pain in man. Neurology 1960; 10: 563.

44. Wolff HG. Headache and other head pain. 1963.

45. Zagami AS, Goadsby PJ, Edvinsson L. Stimulation of the superior sagittal sinus in the cat causes release of vasoactive peptides. Neuropeptides 1990; 16: 69–75.

46. Penfield W. A contribution to the mechanism of intracranial pain. Proc Assoc Res Nerv Men Dis 1934; 15: 399–415.

47. Penfield W, McNaughton FL. Dural headache and the innervation of the aura mater. Arch Neurol 1940; 44: 43–75.

48. Graham JR, Wolff HG. Mechanisms of migraine headache and action of ergotamine tartrate. Arch Neurol Psychiatry 1938; 39: 737–63.

49. Drummond PD, Lance JW. Extracranial vascular changes and the source of pain in migraine headache. Ann Neurol 1983; 13: 32–7.

50. Nichols FT, Mawad M, Mohr JP et al. Focal headache during balloon inflation in the vertebral and basilar arteries. Headache 1993; 33: 87–9.

51. Friberg L, Olesen J, Iversen HK, Sperling B. Migraine pain associated with middle cerebral artery dilatation – reversal by sumatriptan. Lancet 1991; 338: 13–17.

52. Olesen J, Thomsen LL, Iversen HK. Nitric oxide is a key molecule in migraine and other vascular headaches. Trends Pharmacol Sci 1994; 15: 149–53.

53. Thomsen LL, Kruuse C, Iversen HK, Olesen J. A nitric oxide donor (nitroglycerine) triggers genuine migraine attacks. Neurology 1994; 1: 73–80.

54. Sicuteri F. Vasoneuroactive substances and their implications in vascular pain. Res Clin Studies Headache 1967; 1: 6–45.

55. Curran DA, Hinterberger H, Lance JW. Total plasma serotonin, 5-hydroxyindoleacetic acid and p-hydroxy-m-methoxymandelic acid excretion in normal and migrainous subjects. Brain 1965; 88: 997–1010.

56. Anthony M, Hinterberger H, Lance JW. Plasma serotonin in migraine and stress. Arch Neurol 1967; 16: 544–92.

57. Kimball RW, Friedman AP, Vallejo E. Effect of serotonin in migraine patients. Neurology 1960; 10: 107–11.

58. Brewerton TD, Murphy DL, Mueller EA, Jimerson DC. Induction of migraine like headaches by the serotonin agonist m-chlorophenylpiperazine. Clin Pharmacol Ther 1988; 43: 605–9.

59. Brewerton TD, Murphy DL, Lesem MD et al. Headache responses following m-chlorophenylpiperazine in bulimics and controls. Headache 1992; 32: 217–22.

60. Feniuk W, Humphrey PP, Perren MJ. The selective carotid arterial vasoconstrictor action of GR43175 in anesthetized dogs. Br J Pharmacol 1989; 96: 83–90.

61. Humphrey PP, Feniuk W, Perren MJ et al. Serotonin and migraine. Ann NY Acad Sci 1990; 600: 587–98.

62. Hoyer D, Clarke DE, Fozard JR et al. VII International union of pharmacology classification of receptors for 5-hydroxytryptamine (serotonin). Pharmacol Reviews 1994; 46: 157–203.

63. Hartig PR, Hoyer D, Humphrey PPA, Martin GR. Alignment of receptor nomenclature with the human genome: classification of $5-HT_{1B}$ and $5-HT_{1D}$ receptor subtypes. Trends Pharmacol Sci 1996; 17: 103–5.

64. Pregenzer JF, Alberts GL, Im WB et al. Differential pharmacology between the guinea-pig and the gorilla $5-HT_{1D}$ receptor as probed with isochromas (5-HT_{1D}-selective ligands). Br J Pharmacol 1999; 127: 468–72.

65. Gomez-Mancilla B, Cutler NR, Leibowitz MT et al. Safety and efficacy of PNU-142633, a selective $5-HT_{1D}$ agonist, in patients with acute migraine. Cephalalgia 2001; 21: 727–32.

66. Fleishaker JC, Pearson LK, Knuth DW et al. Pharmacokinetics and tolerability of a novel $5-HT_{1D}$ agonist, PNU-142633F. Int J Clin Pharmacol Therap 1999; 37: 487–92.

67. Phebus LA, Johnson KW, Zgombick JM et al. Characterization of LY334370 as a pharmacological tool to study $5HT_{1F}$ receptors-binding affinities, brain penetration and activity in the neurogenic dural inflammation model of migraine. Life Sci 1997; 61: 2117–26.

68. Goldstein DJ, Roon KI, Offen WW et al. Selective serotonin 1F (5-HT(1F)) receptor agonist LY334370 for acute migraine: a randomised controlled trial. The Lancet 2001; 358: 1230–4.

69. Moskowitz MA, Cutrer FM. Sumatriptan: a receptor-targeted treatment for migraine. Ann Rev Med 1993; 44: 145–54.

70. Buzzi MG, Moskowitz MA, Shimizu T, Heath HH. Dihydroergotamine and sumatriptan attenuate levels of CGRP in plasma in rat superior sagittal sinus during electrical stimulation of the trigeminal ganglion. Neuropharmacol 1991; 30: 1193–200.

71. Markowitz S, Saito K, Moskowitz MA. Neurogenically mediated plasma extravasation in dura mater: effect of ergot alkaloids. A possible mechanism of action in vascular headache. Cephalalgia 1988; 8: 83–91.

72. Dimitriadou V, Buzzi MG, Theoharides TC, Moskowitz MA. Ultrastructural evidence for neurogenically mediated changes in blood vessels of the rat aura mater and tongue following antidromic trigeminal stimulation. Neuroscience 1992; 48: 187–203.

73. Strassman AM, Raymond SA, Burstein R. Sensitization of meningeal sensory neurons and the origin of headaches. Nature 1996; 384: 560–4.

74. Cutrer FM, Limroth V, Waeber C et al. New targets for antimigraine drug development. In: Goadsby PJ, Silberstein SD, eds. Headache. 17th edn. Boston: Butterworth-Heinemann, 1997: 58–74.

75. Buzzi MG, Sakas DE, Moskowitz MA. Indomethacin and acetyl salicylic acid block neurogenic plasma protein extravasation in rat dura mater. Eur J Pharmacol 1989; 165: 251–8.

76. Cutrer FM, Limmroth V, Ayata G, Moskowitz MA. Attenuation by valproate of c-fos immunoreactivity in trigeminal nucleus caudalis induced by intracisternal capsaicin. Br J Pharmacol 1995; 116: 3199–204.

77. Lee WK, Limmroth V, Ayata C et al. Peripheral GABA-A receptor mediated effects of sodium valproate on dural plasma protein extravasation to substance P and trigeminal stimulation. Br J Pharmacol 1995; 116: 1661–7.

78. Limmroth V, Lee WS, Cutrer FM, Moskowitz MA. $GABA_A$-receptor-mediated effects of progesterone, its ring-A-reduced metabolites and synthetic neuroactive steroids on neurogenic oedema in the rat meninges. Br J Pharmacol 1996; 117: 99–104.

79. Lee WS, Moussaoui SM, Moskowitz MA. Blockade by oral or parenteral RPR100893 (a nonpeptide NK1 receptor antagonist) of neurogenic plasma protein extravasation in guinea-pig dura mater and conjunctiva. Br J Pharmacol 1994; 112: 920–4.

80. May A, Gijsman HJ, Wallnoefer A et al. Endothelin antagonist bosentan blocks neurogenic inflammation, but is not effective in aborting migraine attacks. Pain 1996; 67: 375–8.

81. Edvinsson L. Experimental headache models in animals and man. 1st edn. London: Martin Dunitz, 1999.

82. Diener HC. Substance-P antagonist RPR100893–201 is not effective in human migraine attacks. In: Olesen J, Tfelt-Hansen P, eds. Proceedings of the VIth International Headache Seminar. New York: Lippincott-Raven, 1996.

83. Goldstein DJ, Wang O, Saper JR et al. Ineffectiveness of neurokinin-1 antagonist in acute migraine: a crossover study. Cephalalgia 1997; 17: 785–90.

84. Connor HE, Bertin L, Gillies S et al. Clinical evaluation of a novel, potent, CNS penetrating NK_1 receptor antagonist in the acute treatment of migraine. The GR205171 Clinical Study Group. Cephalalgia 1998; 18: 392.

85. Norman B, Panebianco D, Block GA. A placebo-controlled, in-clinic study to explore the preliminary safety and efficacy of intravenous L-758,298 (a prodrug of the NK1 receptor antagonist L-754,030) in the acute treatment of migraine. Cephalalgia 1998; 18: 407.

86. Lee WS, Moskowitz MA. Conformationally restricted sumatriptin analogues, CP-122,228 and CP-122,638, exhibit enhanced potency against neurogenic inflammation in aura mater. Brain Res 1993; 626: 303–5.

87. Roon KI, Olesen J, Diener HC et al. No acute antimigraine efficacy of CP-122,288, a highly potent inhibitor of neurogenic inflammation: results of two randomized double-blind, placebo-controlled clinical trials. Ann Neurol 2000; 47: 238–41.

88. Goadsby PJ, Hoskin KL. Differential effects of low dose CP122,288 and eletriptan on Fos expression due to stimulation of the superior sagittal sinus in the cat. Pain 1999; 82: 15–22.

89. Knight YE, Edvinsson L, Goadsby PJ. Blockade of CGRP release after superior sagittal sinus stimulation in cat: a comparison of avitriptan and CP122,288. Neuropeptides 1999; 33: 41–6.

90. Giles H, Honey A, Edvinsson L et al. Preclinical pharmacology of 4991W93, a potent inhibitor of neurogenic plasma protein extravasation. Cephalalgia 1999; 19: 402.

91. Storer RJ, Akerman S, Connor HE, Goadsby PJ. 4991W93, a potent blocker of neurogenic plasma protein extravasation, inhibits trigeminal neurons at 5-hydroxytryptamine (5-$HT_{1B/1D}$) agonist doses. Neuropharmacol 2001; 40: 911–17.

92. Knight YE, Edvinsson L, Goadsby PJ. 4991W93 inhibits release of calcitonin gene-related peptide in the cat but only at doses with $5HT_{1B/1D}$ receptor agonist activity. Neuropharmacol 2001; 40: 520–5.

93. Earl NL, McDonald SA, Lowry MT. Efficacy and tolerability of the neurogenic inflammation inhibitor, 4991W93, in the acute treatment of migraine. 4991W93 Investigator Group. Cephalalgia 1999; 19: 357.

94. Goadsby PJ, Edvinsson L, Ekman R. Vasoactive peptide release in the extracerebral circulation of humans during migraine headache. Ann Neurol 1990; 28: 183–7.

95. Gallai V, Sarchielli P, Floridi A. Vasoactive peptides levels in the plasma

of young migraine patients with and without aura assessed both interictally and ictally. Cephalalgia 1995; 15: 384–90.

96. Goadsby PJ, Edvinsson L. Human in vivo evidence for trigeminovascular activation in cluster headache. Brain 1994; 117: 427–34.

97. Fanciullacci M, Alessandri M, Figini M et al. Increases in plasma calcitonin gene-related peptide from extracerebral circulation during nitroglycerin-induced cluster headache attack. Pain 1995; 60: 119–23.

98. Goadsby PJ, Edvinsson L. Neuropeptide changes in a case of chronic paroxysmal hemicrania – evidence for trigeminoparasympathetic activation. Cephalalgia 1996; 16: 448–50.

99. Goadsby PJ, Edvinsson L. The trigeminovascular system in migraine: studies characterizing cerebrovascular and neuropeptide changes seen in humans and cats. Ann Neurol 1993; 33: 48–56.

100. Couch JR, Saper J, Meloche JP. Treatment of migraine with BMS180048: response at 2 hours. Headache 1996; 36: 523–30.

101. Ryan RE, Elkind A, Goldstein J. Twenty-four hour effectiveness of BMS 180048 in the acute treatment of migraine headaches. Headache 1997; 37: 245–8.

102. Goadsby PJ, Hoskin KL, Knight YE. Substance P blockade with the potent and centrally acting antagonist GR205171 does not effect central trigeminal activity with superior sagittal sinus stimulation. Neuroscience 1998; 86: 337–43.

103. Edvinsson L, Goadsby PJ. Neuropeptides in headache. Eur J Neurol 1998; 5: 329–41.

104. O'Connor TP, Van der Kooy D. Enrichment of vasoactive neuropeptide (calcitonin gene related peptide) in trigeminal sensory projection to the intracranial arteries. J Neurosci 1988; 8: 2468–76.

105. O'Connor TP, van der Kooy D. Pattern of intracranial and extracranial projections of trigeminal ganglion cells. J Neurosci 1986; 6: 2200–7.

106. Goadsby PJ, Lipton RB. A review of paroxysmal hemicranias, SUNCT syndrome and other short-lasting headaches with autonomic features, including new cases. Brain 1997; 120: 193–209.

107. Doods H, Hallermayer G, Wu D et al. Pharmacological profile of BIBN-4096BS, the first selective small molecule CGRP antagonist. Br J Pharmacol 2000; 129: 420–3.

108. Samsam M, Covenas R, Ahangari R et al. Simultaneous depletion of neurokinin A, substance P and calcitonin gene-related peptide from the caudal trigeminal nucleus of the rat during electrical stimulation of the trigeminal ganglion. Pain 2000; 84: 389–95.

109. Edvinsson L, Brodin E, Jansen I, Uddman R. Neurokinin A in cerebral vessels: characterization, localization and effects in vitro. Peptides 1988; 20: 181–97.

110. Jansen I, Alafaci C, McCulloch J et al. Tachykinins (substance P, neurokinin A, neuropeptide K, and neurokinin B) in the cerebral circulation: vasomotor responses in vitro and in situ. J Cerebral Blood Flow Metab 1991; 11: 567–75.

111. Durham PL, Sharma RV, Russo AF. Repression of the calcitonin gene-related peptide promoter by 5-HT1 receptor activation. J Neurosci 1997; 17: 9545–53.

112. Powell KJ, Ma W, Sutak M et al. Blockade and reversal of spinal morphine tolerance by peptide and non-peptide calcitonin gene-related peptide receptor antagonists. Br J Pharmacol 2000; 131: 875–84.

113. Nozaki K, Boccalini P, Moskowitz MA. Expression of c-fos-like immunoreactivity in brainstem after meningeal irritation by blood in the subarachnoid space. Neuroscience 1992; 49: 669–80.

114. Kaube H, Keay K, Hoskin KL et al. Expression of c-fos like immunoreactivity in the trigeminal nucleus caudalis and high cervical cord following stimulation of the sagittal sinus in the cat. Brain Res 1993; 629: 95–102.

115. Goadsby P, Hoskin KL. The distribution of trigeminovascular afferents in the non-human primate brain Macaca nemestrina: a c-fos immunocytochemical study. J Anat 1997; 190(Pt. 3): 367–75.

116. Goadsby PJ, Zagami AS. Stimulation of the superior sagittal sinus increases metabolic activity and blood flow in certain regions of the brainstem and upper cervical spinal cord of the cat. Brain 1991; 114: 1001–11.

117. Goadsby PJ, Hoskin KL, Knight YE. Stimulation of the greater occipital nerve increases metabolic activity in the trigeminal nucleus caudalis and cervical dorsal horn of the cat. Pain 1997; 73: 23–8.

118. Bartsch T, Goadsby PJ. Stimulation of the greater occipital nerve (GON) enhances responses of dural responsive convergent neurons in the trigeminocervical complex in the rat. Cephalalgia 2001; 21: 401–2.

119. Strassman AM, Vos BP, Mineta Y et al. Fos-like immunoreactivity in the superficial medullary dorsal horn induced by noxious and innocuous thermal stimulation of the facial skin in the rat. J Neurophysiol 1993; 70: 1811–21.

120. Goadsby PJ, Gundlach AL. Localization of [3H]-dihydroergotamine binding sites in the cat central nervous system: relevance to migraine. Ann Neurol 1991; 29: 91–4.

121. Hoskins KL, Kaube H, Goadsby PJ. Central activation of the trigeminovascular pathway in the cat is inhibited by dihydroergotamine: a c-Fos and electrophysiological study. Brain 1996; 119: 249–56.

122. Kaube H, Hoskin KL, Goadsby PJ. Intravenous acetylsalicylic acid inhibits central trigeminal neurons in the dorsal horn of the upper cervical spinal cord in the cat. Headache 1993; 33: 541–50.

123. Kaube H, Hoskin KL, Goadsby PJ. Sumatriptan inhibits central trigeminal neurons only after blood–brain barrier disruption. Br J Pharmacol 1993; 109: 788–92.

124. Shepheard SL, Williamson DJ, Williams J et al. Comparison of the effects of sumatriptan and the NKl antagonist CP-99,994 on plasma extravasation in the aura mater in c-fos mRNA expression in the trigeminal nucleus caudalis of rats. Neuropharmacol 1993; 34: 255–61.

125. Goadsby PJ, Hoskin KL. Inhibition of trigeminal neurons by intravenous administration of the serotonin (5HT)-1-D receptor agonist zolmitriptan (311C90): are brainstem sites a therapeutic target in migraine? Pain 1996; 67: 355–9.

126. Goadsby PJ, Knight YE. Naratriptan inhibits trigeminal neurons after intravenous administration through an action at the serotonin (5HT1B/1D) receptors. Br J Pharmacol 1997; 122: 918–22.

127. Cumberbatch MJ, Hill RG, Hargreaves RJ. Rizatriptan has central antinociceptive effects against durally evoked responses. Eur J Pharmacol 1997; 328: 37–40.

128. Clitherow JW, Scopes DI, Skingle M et al. Evolution of a novel series of [N,N-dimethylamino)propyl]- and piperazinylbenzanilides as the first selective 5-HT1D antagonists. J Med Chem 1994; 37: 2253–7.

129. Goadsby PJ, Hoskin KL. Serotonin inhibits trigeminal nucleus activity evoked by craniovascular stimulation through a 5-HT1B/1D receptor: a central action in migraine? Ann Neurol 1998; 43: 711–18.

130. Goadsby PJ, Knight YE. Direct evidence for central sites of action of zolmitriptan (311C90): an autoradiographic study in cat. Cephalalgia 1997; 17: 153–8.

131. Storer RJ, Goadsby PJ. Direct evidence using microiontophoresis that neurons of the caudal trigeminal nucleus contain 5HT1B/1D receptors. Cephalalgia 1997; 17: 241.

132. Boers P, Donaldson C, Zagami AS, Lambert GA. 5-HT1A and 5-HT1B/1D receptors are involved in the moculation of the trigeminovascular system of the cat: a microiontophoretic study. Neuropharmacol 2000; 39: 1833–47.

133. Storer RJ, Akerman S, Goadsby PJ. GABA receptors modulate trigeminovascular nociceptive neurotransmission in the trigeminocervical complex. Br J Pharmacol 2001; 134: 896–904.

134. Storer RJ, Akerman S, Goadsby PJ. Opioid receptors modulate nociceptive neurotransmission in the trigeminocervical complex. Cephalalgia 2001; 21: 354

135. Goadsby PJ, Akerman S, Storer RJ. Evidence for postjunctional serotonin (5HT1) receptors in the trigeminal nucleus caudalis. Ann Neurol 2002 (in Press)

136. May A, Bahra A, Buchel C et al. Hypothalamic activation in cluster headache attacks. Lancet 1998; 352: 275–8.

137. Bahra A, Matharu MS, Buchel C et al. Brainstem activation specific to migraine headache. Lancet 2001; 357: 1016–17.

138. Zagami AS, Lambert GA. Stimulation of cranial vessels excites nociceptive neurones in several thalarnic nuclei of the cat. Exp Brain Res 1990; 81: 552–66.

139. Zagami AS, Lambert GA. Craniovascular application of capsaicin activates nociceptive thalamic neurons in the cat. Neurosci Lett 1991; 121: 187–90.

140. Goadsby PJ. The pharmacology of headache. Prog Neurobiol 2000; 62: 509–25.

141. Rebeck GW, Maynard KI, Hyman BT, Moskowitz MA. Selective 5-HTID alpha serotonin receptor gene expression in trigeminal ganglia: implications for antimigraine drug development. Proc Natl Acad Sci USA 1994; 91: 3666–9.

142. Bouchelet I, Cohen Z, Yong W et al. Molecular basis for a possible role of 5-hydroxytryptamine (T-HT) 2B receptors in the aetiology of migraine headache. Proceedings from the International Business Communications Conference on serotonin receptors in the central nervous system: January 25–26, 1996.

143. Hamel E, Fan E, Linville D et al. Expression of mRNA for the serotonin 5-hydroxytryptamine ID beta receptor subtype in human bovine and cerebral arteries. Mol Pharmacol 1993; 44: 242–6.

144. Longmore J, Shaw D, Smith D et al. Differential distribution of 5HT(1D)- and 5HT(1B)-immunoreactivity within the human trigeminocerebrovascular system: implications for the discovery of new antimigraine drugs. Cephalalgia 1997; 17: 833–42.

145. Nilsson T, Longmore J, Shaw D et al. Contractile 5HT1B receptors in human cerebral arteries: pharmacologic characterization and localization with immunocytochemistry. Br J Pharmacol 1999; 128: 1133–40.

146. Razzaque Z, Heald MA, Pickard JD et al. Vasoconstriction in human isolated middle meningeal arteries: determining the contribution of 5-HT1B- and 5-HT1F-receptor activation. Br J Clin Pharmacol 1999; 47: 75–82.

147. Nilsson T, Longmore J, Shaw D et al. Characterization of 5HT receptors in human coronary arteries by molecular and pharmacological techniques. Eur J Pharmacol 1999; 372: 49–56.

148. Welch KM, Mathew NT, Stone P et al. Tolerability of sumatriptan: clinical trials and postmarketing experience. Cephalalgia 2000; 20: 687–94.

149. Nicolodi M, Sicuteri F. Relief of migraine attack with N-methyl-D-aspartic acid receptor antagonist ketamine: a double blind comparison with placebo-theoretic implications. Cephalalgia 1996; 16: 372.

150. Ramadan NM, Sang C, Chappell AS et al. IV LY293558, an AMPA/Kainate receptor antagonist, is effective in migraine. Cephalalgia 2001; 21: 267–8.

151. Bland-Ward PA, Feniuk W, Humphrey PP. The adenosine A1 receptor agonist GR79236 inhibits evoked firing of trigeminal nucleus caudalis (TNC) neurons in the rat. Cephalalgia 2000; 20: 271.

152. Honey AC, Bland-Ward PA, Connor HE et al. The adenosine A1 receptor agonist, GR79236, inhibits neurogenic vasodilation in the anesthetized rat. Cephalalgia 2000; 20: 419.

153. Goadsby PJ, Hoskin KL, Storer RJ, Edvinsson L, Connor HE. Adenosine (A1) receptor agonists inhibit trigeminovascular nociceptive transmission. Brain 2002: in press.

154. Giffin NJ, Kowacs F, Libri V, Williams P, Goadsby PJ, Kaube H. Effect of adenosine A_1 receptor agonist GR79236 on trigeminal nociception with blink reflex recordings in healthy human subjects. Cephalalgia 2002; 22: in press.

155. Humphrey PP, Bland-Ward PA, Carruthers AM et al. Inhibition of trigeminal nociceptive afferents by adenosine A1 receptor activation: a novel approach towards the design of new antimigraine compounds. Cephalalgia 2001; 21: 268–9.

156. Weiller C, May A, Limmroth V et al. Brainstem activation in spontaneous human migraine attacks. Nat Med 1995; 1: 658–60.

157. Goadsby PJ, Lambert GA, Lance JW. The mechanism of cerebrovascular vasoconstriction in response to locus coeruleus stimulation. Brain Res 1985; 326: 213–17.

158. Goadsby PJ, Duckworth JW. Low frequency stimulation of the locus coeruleus reduces regional cerebral blood flow in the spinalized cat. Brain Res. 1989; 476: 71–7.

159. Goadsby PJ, Lambert GA, Lance JW. Effects of locus coeruleus stimulation on carotid vascular resistance in the cat. Brain Res 1983; 278: 175–83.

160. Goadsby PJ, Piper RD, Lambert GA, Lance JW. The effect of activation of the nucleus rapine dorsalis (DRN) on carotid blood flow. I. The monkey. Am J Physiol 1985; 248: R257–62.

161. Goadsby PJ, Piper RD, Lambert GA, Lance JW. The effect of activation of the nucleus rapine dorsalis (DRN) on carotid blood flow. II. The cat. Am J Physiol 1985; 248: R263–9.

162. Underwood MD, Bakalian MJ, Arango V et al. Regulation of cortical blood flow by the dorsal rapine nucleus: topographic organization of cerebrovascular regulatory regions. Cereb Blood Flow Metabol 1992; 12: 664–73.

163. Underwood MD, Bakalian MJ, Arango V, Mann JJ. Effect of chemical-stimulation of the dorsal raphe nucleus on cerebral blood-flow in rat. Neurosci 1995; 199: 228–30.

164. Goadsby PJ, Fields HL. On the functional anatomy of migraine. Ann Neurol 1998; 43: 272.

165. Reichling DB, Basbaum AI. Collateralization of periaqueductal grey neurons to forebrain or diencephalon and to the medullary nucleus raphe magnus in the rat. Neurosci 1991; 42: 183–200.

166. Knight YE, Goadsby PJ. The periaqueductal grey matter modulates trigeminovascular input: a role of migraine? Neurosci 2001; 106: 793–800.

167. Raskin NH, Hosobuchi Y, Lamb S. Headache may arise from perturbation of brain. Headache 1987; 27: 416–20.

168. Hoskin KL, Bulmer DC, Lasalandra M et al. Fos expression in the midbrain periaqueductal gray after trigeminovascular stimulation. J Anat 2001; 197: 29–35.

169. Maertens de Noordhout A, Timsit-Berthier M, Timsit M, Schoenen J. Contingent negative variation and headache. Ann Neurol 1986; 19: 78–80.

170. Bocker KB, Timsit-Berthier M, Schoenen J, Brunia CH. Contingent negative variation and headache. Headache 1990; 30: 604–9.

171. Schoenen J, Timsit-Berthier M. Contingent negative variation: methods and potential interest in headache. Cephalalgia 1993; 13: 28–32.

172. De Noordhout AM, Berthier MT, Schoenen J. Contingent negative variation (CNV) in migraineurs before and during prophylactic treatment with beta-blockers. Cephalalgia 1985; 5: 34–5.

173. Schoenen J, Wang W, Albert A, Delwaide PJ. Potentiation instead of habituation characterizes visual evoked potentials in migraine patients between attacks. Eur J Neurol 1995; 2: 115–22.

174. Harper AM, MacKenzie ET, McCulloch J, Pickard JD. Migraine and the blood–brain barrier. Lancet 1977; 1: 1034–6.

175. Cermeno JA, Gobernado JM, Aimeno A. Transient blood–brain barrier (BBB) damage in migraine. Headache 1986; 26: 437

176. Nissila M, Parkkola R, Sonninen P, Salonen R. Intracerebral arteries and gadolinium enhancement in migraine without aura. Cephalalgia 1996; 16: 363

177. Bates D, Ashford E, Dawson R et al. Subcutaneous sumatriptan during the migraine aura. Neurology 1994; 44: 1587–92.

178. Goadsby PJ. The effect of migraine aura during an attack on treatment outcome: results from the sumatriptan naratriptan aggregated patient (SNAP). SNAP Database Study Group. Cephalalgia 2001; 21: 416.

179. Lipton RB, Stewart WF, Cady R et al. Sumatriptan for the range of headaches in migraine sufferers: results of the Spectrum Study. Headache 2000; 40: 783–91.

180. Cady RK, Lipton RB, Hall C et al. Treatment of mild headache in disabled migraine sufferers: results of the Spectrum Study. Headache 2000; 40: 792–7.

181. Cady RK, Sheftell F, Lipton RB et al. Effect of early intervention with sumatriptan on migraine pain: retrospective analyses of data from three clinical trials. Clin Therap 2000; 22: 1035–48.

182. Bahra A, Matharu MS, Buchel C, Frackowiak RSJ, Goadsby PJ. Brainstem activation specific to migraine headache. The Lancet 2001; 357: 1016–17.

183. Raichle ME, Hartman BK, Eichling JO, Sharpe LG. Central noradrenergic regulation of cerebral blood flow and vascular permeability. Proc Natl Acad Sci USA 1975; 72: 3726–30.

184. Preskorn SH, Hartman BK, Raichle ME, Clark HB. The effect of dibenzazepine (tricyclic antidepressants) on cerebral capillary permeability in the rat in vivo. J Pharmacol Exp Ther 1980; 213: 313–20.

185. Harik SI, McGunigal T. The protective influence of the locus ceruleus on the blood–brain barrier. Ann Neurol 1984; 15: 568–74.

186. Montalcini RL, Daltos R, Dellavalle F et al. Update of the NGF saga. J Neurol Sci 1995; 130: 119–27.

187. Dray A, Urban L, Dickenson A. Pharmacology of chronic pain. Trends Pharmacol Sci 1994; 15: 190–7.

188. Munglani R, Hunt SP. Molecular biology of pain. Br J Anaesth 1995; 75: 186–92.

189. Woolf CJ. Somatic pain: pathogenesis and prevention. Br J Anaesth 1995; 75: 169–76.

190. Caterina MJ, Schumacher MA, Tominaga M et al. The capsaicin receptor: a heat-activated ion channel in the pain pathway. Nature 1997; 389: 816–24.

191. Burstein R, Yarnitsky D, Aryeh IG et al. An association between migraine and cutaneous allodynia. Ann Neurol 2000; 47: 614–24.

192. Woolf CJ. Central sensitization: implications for the pathogenesis of headache. In: Rose FC, ed. Towards Migraine 2000. London: Elsevier, 1996, 173–81.

193. Hunt SP, Pini A, Evan G. Induction of c-fos like protein in spinal cord neurons following sensory stimulation. Nature 1987; 328: 1686–704.

194. Mendell LM. Physiologic properties of unmyelinated fibre projection to the spinal chord. Exp Neurol 1966; 16: 316–32.

195. Price DD, Mao J, Mayer DJ. Central neural mechanisms of normal and abnormal pain states. In: Fields HL, Liebeskind JC, eds. Progress in pain research and management. Washington: IASP Press, 1994, 61–84.

196. Hoskin KL, Bulmer DC, Goadsby PJ. Fos expression in the trigeminocervical complex of the cat after stimulation of the superior sagittal sinus is reduced by L-NAME. Neurosci 1999; 266: 173–6.

197. Fields HL, Heinricher MM, Mason P. Neurotransmitters as nociceptive modulatory circuits. Ann Rev Neurosci 1991; 219–45.

198. Scholz E, Diener HC, Geiselhart S, Wilkinson M. Drug-induced headache: does a critical dosage exist? In: Diener HC, ed. Drug-induced headache. Berlin: Springer-Verlag, 1988, 29–43.

199. Welch KM, Nagesh V, Aurora S, Gelman N. Periaqueductal gray matter dysfunction in migraine: cause or the burden of illness? Headache 2001; 41: 629–37.

200. Goadsby PJ. Neurovascular headache and a midbrain vascular malformation: evidence for a role of the brainstem in chronic migraine. Cephalalgia 2001; (In Press)

201. Liveing E. On megrim, sick headache, and some allied disorders: a contribution to the pathology of nerve-storms. Churchill, 1873.

202. Goadsby PJ, Lipton RB, Ferrari MD. Migraine: current understanding and management. N Eng J Med 2002; 346: 257–70.

section 2

Primary headache disorders

chapter 6

Migraine: diagnosis and treatment

Introduction

Many famous individuals from the worlds of arts and sciences have suffered from migraine headaches (Table 6.1).[1] Migraine is a primary episodic headache disorder characterized by various combinations of neurologic, gastrointestinal, and autonomic changes. In the United States, more than 17% of women, 6% of men, and 4% of children had had at least one migraine attack in the last year.[2–5] Migraine diagnosis is based on the retrospective reporting of headache characteristics and associated symptoms.[6] The physical and neurologic examinations, as well as laboratory studies, are usually normal and serve to exclude other, more ominous, causes of headache (see Chapters 2 and 4). Formal diagnostic criteria for migraine and other headache disorders were published by the International Headache Society (IHS) in 1988; however, these remain a guide and have a well-recognized group of false-negatives. The draft revised IHS system recognizes two major varieties of migraine: migraine without aura (formerly called common migraine) and migraine with aura (formerly called classic migraine).[7,8] The IHS system provides criteria for a total of seven subtypes of migraine (Table 6.2). In this chapter, we describe the migraine attack and its variants and their acute and preventive treatment based, in part, on the presence of any coexistent or comorbid disease.

Description of the migraine attack

Migraine has been recognized as a clinical entity for thousands of years. Aretaeus of Cappadocia, a Greek physician living in Rome in the first century AD, described migraine (heterocrania) and its associated mood changes and photophobia. 'There is much torpor, heaviness of head, anxiety, and weariness. For they flee the light; the darkness soothes their disease; nor can they bear readily to look upon or hear anything disagreeable.'

The migraine attack can be divided into four phases: the premonitory phase, which occurs hours or days before the headache; the aura phase, which immediately precedes the headache; the headache phase itself; and the headache resolution phase. Although most people experience more than one phase, no phase is obligatory for the diagnosis of migraine. A description of the four phases provides a convenient way of reviewing the protean manifestation of migraine (Figure 6.1).

Table 6.1 Some famous migraineurs

Julius Caesar	Thomas Jefferson	Ulysses S. Grant
Saint Paul	Friedrich Nietzsche	Peter Tchaikovsky
John Calvin	Immanuael Kant	Alfred Nobel
Queen Mary Tudor	Edgar Allan Poe	Leo Tolstoy
Blaise Pascal	Frédéric Chopin	Sigmund Freud
Carolus Linnaeus	Charles Darwin	Virginia Woolf
Lewis Carroll	Karl Marx	Princess Margaret

Adapted from Adler et al.[1]

Table 6.2 Proposed IHS migraine classification

1.	Migraine
1.1	Migraine without aura
1.2	Migraine with aura
1.2.1	Typical aura with migraine headache
1.2.2	Typical aura with nonmigraine headache
1.2.3	Typical aura without headache
1.2.4	Migraine with prolonged aura
1.2.5	Familial hemiplegic migraine
1.2.6	Sporadic hemiplegic migraine
1.2.7	Basilar-type migraine
1.2.8	Migraine with acute onset aura
1.3	Chronic migraine
1.3.1	Chronic migraine with medication misuse
1.3.2	Chronic migraine without medication misuse
1.4	Childhood periodic syndromes
1.5	Retinal migraine
1.6	Migrainous headache
1.7	Complications of migraine
1.7.1	Status migrainosus
1.7.1.1	Status migrainosus of migraine without aura
1.7.1.2	Status migrainosus of migraine with aura
1.7.2	Migrainous infarction
1.7.3	Persistent aura without infarction
1.7.4	Migraine triggered seizures

Premonitory phenomena (prodrome)

Premonitory phenomena occur in between 20% and 60% of migraineurs, often hours to days before headache onset. Usually patients describe a characteristic change in mood or behavior that may include psychological, neurologic, constitutional, or autonomic features (Table 6.3). Some people simply report a poorly characterized feeling that a migraine attack is coming. While the premonitory features are quite variable among individuals, they are often consistent within an individual (Figure 6.2). The fea-

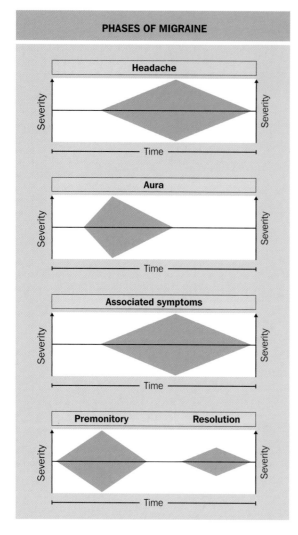

PHASES OF MIGRAINE

Figure 6.1 *Phases of migraine attack.*

tures of the premonitory phase, such as depression, cognitive dysfunction, and episodic bouts of food cravings, may be difficult to recognize as part of the migraine complex if a careful headache history is not taken or if these features occur in isolation or with a mild headache. A diary may be helpful to show the relationship of these periodic events to migraine (Table 6.3 and Figure 6.3).[9] These nonheadache symptoms can also occur during and after the headache.

Using a novel electronic diary system, Giffin and others (personal communication) showed that migraineurs who reported premonitory symptoms accurately predicted their full-blown headaches 72% of the time. A range of cognitive and physical symptoms was reported at a similar rate through all three phases of the migraine. The most common premonitory symptoms were feeling tired/weary (72% of attacks with warning features), difficulty concentrating (51%) and stiff neck (50%). Individuals who functioned poorly in the premonitory phase were the most likely to correctly predict their headaches.

Aura

The migraine aura is a complex of focal neurologic symptoms (positive or negative phenomena) that precedes, accompanies, or (rarely) follows an attack. Most aura symptoms develop over 5–20 minutes and usually last less than 60 minutes.[8] The aura can be characterized by visual, sensory, or motor phenomena, and may also involve language or brainstem disturbances (Table 6.4).

Headache usually occurs within 60 minutes from the end of the aura, but it may be delayed for several hours or entirely absent.[10,11] In one prospective study, headache followed the aura only 80% of the time.[10] Most patients do not feel normal during the gap between the aura offset and headache onset. Fears, somatic complaints, alter-

Table 6.3 *Premonitory symptoms (prodrome)*

Mental state	Neurological	General
Depressed	Photophobia	Stiff neck
Hyperactive	Difficulty concentrating	Food cravings
Euphoric	Phonophobia	Cold feeling
Talkative	Dysphasia	Anorexia
Irritable	Hyperosmia	Sluggishness
Drowsy	Yawning	Diarrhea or constipation
Restless		Thirst
		Urination
		Fluid retention

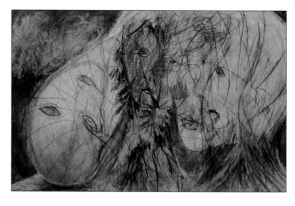

Figure 6.2 *'Mentally insufficient' by Angela Mark of Jamaica Plain, Massachusetts, USA. (© Sandoz Pharmaceuticals Corp.)*

EXAMPLE OF A MIGRAINE DIARY

	Date	Headache start time	Headache stop time	Severity (0-3 scale) 0=none 1=mild 2=moderate 3=severe	Associated symptoms (0-4 scale) 0=none 1=nausea 2=vomiting 3=photophobia 4=phonophobia	Disability (0-3 scale) 0=none 1=mild 2=moderate 3=severe	Medications taken to relieve headache	Any known triggers
Sunday								
Monday								
Tuesday								
Wednesday								
Thursday								
Friday								
Saturday								

● **Figure 6.3** *Example of a migraine diary.*

● **Table 6.4** *Characteristics of the visual aura*

Positive phenomena, negative phenomena, or both	Either may occur alone; positive phenomena often occur first and are followed by negative phenomena
Visual field	Scotoma often start centrally and migrate peripherally.
Shape	Fortification spectra often 'C'-shaped; scotoma bean shaped
Motion	Objects may rotate, oscillate, or boil
Flicker	Rate 10 cycles per second; may change during the course of the aura
Color	Gray, red, green, gold, yellow, blue, or purple; often have no specific color except excessively bright white
Clarity	May be blurry or fuzzy
Brightness	Often very bright.
Expansion	Buildup occurs in both fortification spectra and scotoma
Migration	Spectra may 'march' from the central area to periphery or sometimes vice versa

ations in mood, disturbances of speech or thought, or detachment from the environment or other people may occur. The headache may begin before or simultaneously with the aura, or the aura may occur alone. Patients can have more than one type of aura, with a progression from one symptom to another. Most patients with a sensory aura also have a visual aura.[12]

Auras may occur repeatedly, as frequently as many times an hour for as long as several months. These have been termed 'migraine aura status'.[9] Scotomata may occur repeatedly, even alternating sides; repetitive cycles of migrating sensory auras may occur for hours on end.[13] This presentation requires careful investigation before the diagnosis can be made.

Auras vary in their complexity. Elementary visual disturbances include scotomata, simple flashes (phosphenes), specks, or geometric forms. They may move across the visual field, sometimes crossing the midline. Shimmering or undulations in the visual field may also occur. These 'minor visual disorders' are more likely to occur during than before the headache.[14] Because they are bilateral, they are believed to arise from the occipital cortex. More complicated auras include teichopsia (Greek for 'town wall' and 'vision') or fortification spectrum, the most characteristic visual aura of migraine (Figure 6.4). An arc of scintillating lights, usually but not always beginning near the point of fixation, may form into a herringbone-like pattern that expands to encompass an increasing portion of a visual hemifield. It migrates across the visual field with a scintillating edge of often zigzag, flashing, or occasionally colored phenomena (Figure 6.5). Some characteristics of the aura are listed in Table 6.4. Migraine scotomata may occur simultaneously in both visual fields, but this is rare. They may even be synchronized to create an altitudinal, not a hemianoptic, pattern. The visions of Hildegard of Bingen, a 12th century mystic, have been attributed in part to her migrainous scintillating scotomas (Figure 6.6). Characteristic of the visions that she and other visionary prophets, including Ezekiel, saw were working, boiling, or fermenting lights.

Visual distortions and hallucinations can occur. These

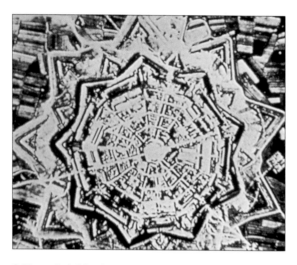

● **Figure 6.4** *Migraine with aura (aerial view of the fortified, walled city of Palmanova, Italy.)*

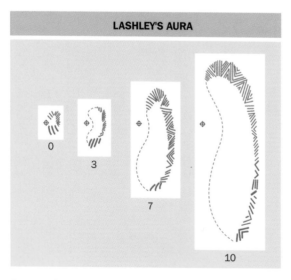

LASHLEY'S AURA

0

3

7

10

● **Figure 6.5** *Fortification spectra as depicted by Lashley.*

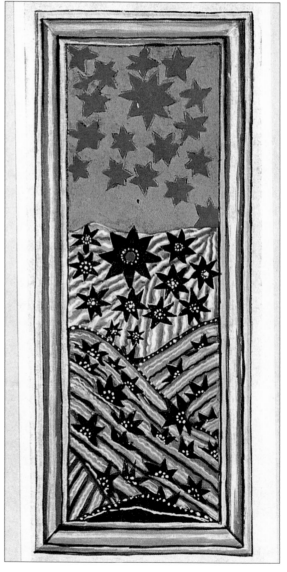

● **Figure 6.6** *'Vision of the fall of the angels' from a manuscript of Hildegard's Scivias, written in Bingen, AD 1180.*

attacks occur more commonly in children, are usually followed by a headache, and are characterized by a complex disorder of visual perception that may include metamorphopsia, micropsia, macropsia, zoom vision (opening up or closing down in the size of objects), or mosaic vision (fracturing of image into facets). In addition, nonvisual association cortex symptoms occur and include complex difficulties in perception and use of the body (apraxia and agnosia), speech and language disturbances, states of double or multiple consciousness associated with déjà vu or jamais vu, and elaborate dreamy, nightmarish, trance-like or delirious states.[9] Paresthesias, the second most common aura, are often cheiroaural, with numbness starting in the hand, migrating up the arm, and then jumping to involve the face, lips, and tongue. The leg is occasionally involved.[15] As with visual auras (with positive, followed by negative, symptoms), paresthesias may be followed by numbness and, in a few cases, loss of position sense. Paresthesias start or become bilateral in half of patients. Sensory auras rarely occur in isolation and usually follow a visual aura (Figure 6.7).[5–8,14–16] Motor symptoms can occur in as many as 18% of patients, most often in association with sensory symptoms;[10] however, true weakness is rare and is always unilateral.[15] Sensory ataxia is often reported as weakness;[15] hyperkinetic movement disorders, including chorea, have been reported.[9] Aphasic auras (speech abnormalities) including aphasia have been reported in 17% to 20% of patients.[10,15] However, since patients are rarely examined during an aura, many of these reported cases may be dysarthria, not aphasia.[15]

Headache phase

The typical headache of migraine is unilateral, throbbing, moderate to marked in severity, and aggravated by physical activity. Not all of these features are required to diagnose IHS migraine. Pain may be bilateral at onset (in 40% of cases) or start on one side and become generalized.[14] The headache of migraine can occur at any time of the day or night, but begins most frequently between 5 am and 12 noon.[14] The onset is usually gradual; the pain often peaks 2–12 hours into the attack and then gradually subsides. The median duration of an untreated migraine attack is 24 hours, with a usual range of 4–72 hours in adults and 1–48 hours in children (Figure 6.8).[8]

The head pain varies greatly in intensity, although the median pain intensity is 7–8 on a scale of 0–10, where 0 is no pain at all and 10 is pain as bad as it can be.[17] The pain is described as throbbing in 85% of cases, although throbbing pain is often described in other types of headache.[17] The pain is commonly aggravated by physical activity or simple head movement.[8]

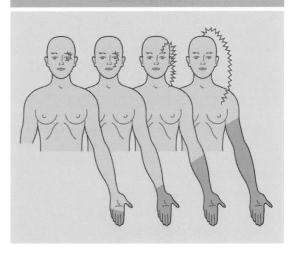

MIGRAINE AURA

● *Figure 6.7* *Paraesthesias, the second most common migraine aura. Adapted with permission.[18]*

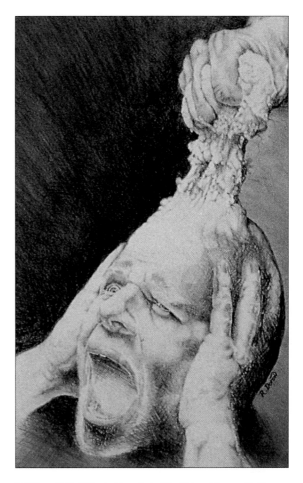

● *Figure 6.8* *'Gripping headache' by Richard Dorrow II of Athol, Massachusetts, USA. (© Sandoz Pharmaceuticals Corp.)*

The pain of migraine is invariably accompanied by other features. Anorexia is common, although food cravings can occur. Nausea occurs in almost 90% of patients, while vomiting occurs in about one-third of migraineurs (Figure 6.9).[18] Many patients experience marked sensory sensitivity, manifested by photophobia, phonophobia, and osmophobia, and seek a dark, quiet room (Figure 6.10).[7,18] Other systemic symptoms, including blurry vision, nasal stuffiness, anorexia, hunger, tenesmus, diarrhea, abdominal cramps, polyuria (followed by decreased urinary output after the attack), pallor (or, less commonly, redness) of the face, sensations of heat or cold, and sweating, may be noted during the headache phase. There may be localized edema of the scalp, the face, or under the eyes, tenderness of the scalp, unusual prominence of a vein or artery in the temple, or stiffness and tenderness of the neck. Impairment of concentration is common; less often there is memory impairment. Depression, fatigue, anxiety, nervousness, and irritability are common. Lightheadedness, rather than true vertigo, and a feeling of faintness may occur. The extremities tend to be cold and moist. As discussed below, the IHS selects particular associated features as cardinal manifestations for diagnosis.

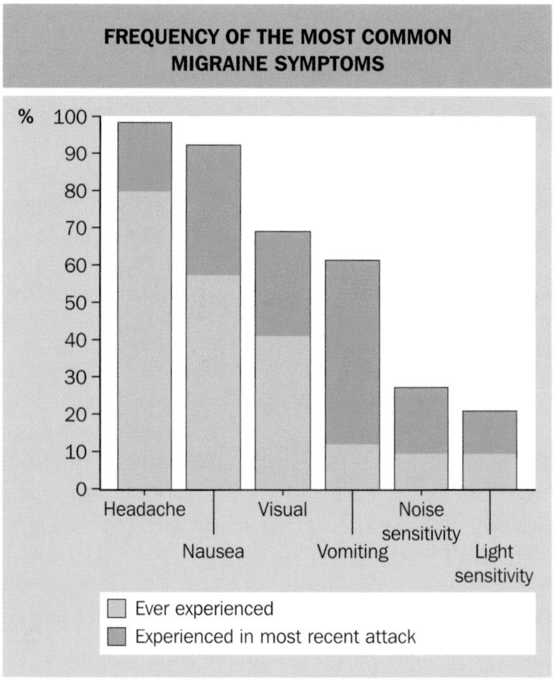

FREQUENCY OF THE MOST COMMON MIGRAINE SYMPTOMS

Ever experienced
Experienced in most recent attack

● **Figure 6.9** *Frequency of the most common migraine symptoms. Adapted with permission.*[18]

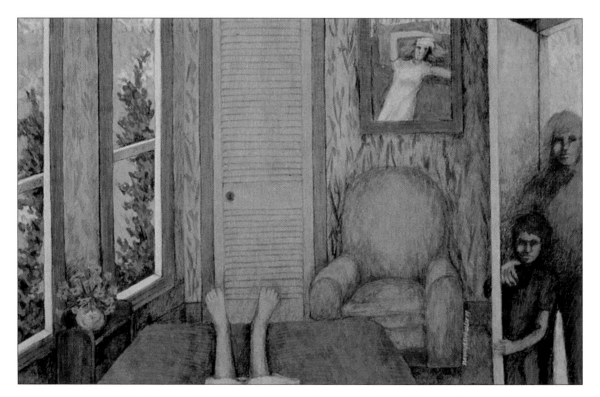

● **Figure 6.10** *'Serving time' by Nancy Ellen Wheeler of Scituate, Massachusetts, USA. (© Sandoz Pharmaceutical Corp.)*

Resolution phase

In the resolution phase, the pain wanes. Following the headache, the patient may feel tired, washed out, irritable, and listless and may have impaired concentration, scalp tenderness, or mood changes. Some people feel unusually refreshed or euphoric after an attack, while others experience depression and malaise.

Formal diagnostic criteria

Overview of the International Headache Society

To improve the classification of headache disorders both in clinical practice and in research, the IHS published diagnostic criteria for a broad range of headache disorders. These criteria, based on expert consensus, have had a major impact on clinical trials and on epidemiologic research, although they have not been widely employed in clinical practice.[19]

Despite its limitations,[6] the IHS system stands as a singular advance in headache classification. The criteria are being revised since significant empirical evidence and clinical experience have accumulated. The revision will provide the best available diagnostic 'gold standard' for clinicians and investigators (Table 6.2). Migraine continues to be subdivided into migraine with aura (1.1) and migraine without aura (1.2). In the new revision, chronic migraine will most likely be added to established categories including: childhood periodic symptoms (1.4); retinal migraine (1.5); migrainous headache (1.6); and complications of migraine (1.7).

Migraine without aura (common migraine) (Table 6.5)

To establish a diagnosis of IHS migraine without aura, five attacks are needed, each lasting 4–72 hours with at least two of four pain features and one of two associated characteristics. The four pain features include unilateral location, pulsating quality, moderate to severe intensity, and aggravation by routine physical activity. The attacks must have at least one of the following: nausea and/or vomiting or photophobia and phonophobia. Using these criteria, no single associated feature is mandatory for diagnosing migraine, although recurrent episodic attacks must be documented. The patient who has photophobia, phonophobia, and pulsatile pain aggravated by routine activity meets the criteria, as does the patient with typical unilateral throbbing pain and nausea. Other causes of migraine must be excluded.[8]

When migraine persists for more than 3 days, the term 'status migrainosus' is applied. Although migraine often begins in the morning, sometimes awakening the patient from sleep at dawn, it can begin at any time of the day or night. The frequency of attacks is extremely variable, from a few in a lifetime to several a week. The average migraineur experiences one or two headaches a month (Figure 6.11).[4,18] The requirement of at least five attacks is imposed because headaches simulating migraine may be caused by organic disease ranging from brain tumors to sinusitis to glaucoma.

The IHS also requires the exclusion of secondary headache disorders in one of several ways. Thus, migraine is both a diagnosis of inclusion, as specific combinations of features are required, and a diagnosis of exclusion, as alternative causes of headache must be systematically eliminated.

● **Table 6.5** *Migraine without aura (previously used terms: common migraine, hemicrania simplex). Diagnostic criteria*

A	At least five attacks fulfilling B–D.
B	Headache lasting 4–72 hours (untreated or unsuccessfully treated).
C	Headache has at least two of the following characteristics: 1 Unilateral location. 2 Pulsating quality. 3 Moderate or severe intensity. 4 Aggravation by routine physical activity (i.e. walking or climbing stairs).
D	During headache at least one of the following: 1 Nausea and/or vomiting. 2 Photophobia and phonophobia.
E	Not attributed to another disorder.

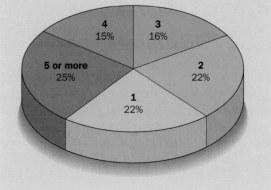

MIGRAINE ATTACKS PER MONTH

4 — 15%
3 — 16%
5 or more — 25%
2 — 22%
1 — 22%

● **Figure 6.11** *Frequency of migraine attacks experienced by migraineurs per month.*

Migraine with aura (classic migraine) (Table 6.6)

A diagnosis of migraine with aura (IHS migraine classification 1.2), the now-accepted term for classic migraine, requires at least two attacks with any three of the following four features: one or more fully reversible neurologic symptoms, aura developing over more than 4 minutes, aura lasting less than 60 minutes, and headache following aura with a symptom free interval of less than 60 minutes. Fewer attacks are required than for a diagnosis of migraine without aura, based on the assumption that the typical aura is highly specific for migraine. Once again, other causes of headache must be excluded.[8]

In the draft revision of the IHS criteria (Table 6.2), migraine with aura is subdivided into typical aura with migraine headache (1.2.1), typical aura with nonmigraine headache (1.2.2), typical aura without headache (1.2.3), migraine with prolonged aura (1.2.4), familial hemiplegic migraine (FHM) (1.2.5), sporadic hemiplegic migraine (1.2.6), basilar-type migraine (1.2.7), and migraine with acute onset aura (1.2.8).

The headache and associated symptoms of migraine with aura are similar to those of migraine without aura. Most sufferers who have migraine with aura also have attacks of migraine without aura. The aura usually lasts 20–30 minutes and typically precedes the headache, but it occasionally occurs only during the headache. In contrast to a transient ischemic attack (TIA), the aura of migraine evolves gradually and consists of both positive (e.g. scintillations, tingling) and negative (e.g. scotoma, numbness) features. If the aura is typical and stereotyped, the diagnosis of migraine with aura is warranted, even if the subsequent headache does not have the migrainous features described above. Indeed, typical migraine aura may be seen in association with other headache types, such as cluster headaches. Virtually any symptom or sign of brain dysfunction may be a feature of the aura, but most auras include visual features.

Focal symptoms and signs of the aura may persist beyond the headache phase. Formerly termed 'complicated migraine', the IHS classification has introduced two more specific labels: prolonged aura and migrainous infarction. If the aura lasts for more than 1 hour but less than 1 week, the term migraine with prolonged aura is applied. If the signs persist for more than 1 week but resolve, we use the term persistent aura; if a neuroimaging procedure demonstrates a stroke or the neurologic defect does not remit, a migrainous infarction has occurred. When the aura is not followed by the headache (particularly in mid- or late-life), it is considered a migraine equivalent.

Migraine variants

Basilar-type migraine

Basilar-type migraine has been called basilar artery migraine,[8] Bickerstaff's migraine,[20] and, recently, basilar migraine (Table 6.7). The term basilar migraine is misleading in that it implies a vascular mechanism, whereas the events are believed to be neural and not vascular. Although once viewed mainly as a disorder of adolescent girls, basilar-type migraine affects all age groups and both sexes, with the female predominance that typifies

---

● **Table 6.6** Migraine with aura (classic migraine)

Diagnostic criteria

A At least two attacks fulfilling B and C

B At least three of the following four characteristics:
1. Fully reversible aura symptoms explained by focal brain dysfunction
2. At least one aura symptom evolves gradually over at least 4 minutes or two or more symptoms evolve in succession
3. Each symptom lasts less than 60 minutes; if more than one aura symptom evolves in succession, overall duration may be proportionally increased
4. Headache begins during the aura or more frequently follows aura with a symptom-free interval of less than 60 minutes

C Not attributed to another disorder

● **Table 6.7** Basilar-type migraine

Description:
Migraine with aura where symptoms clearly originate from the brainstem or from simultaneous affection of both hemispheres

Diagnostic criteria:
A Fulfills IHS criteria for 1.2.

B Two or more aura symptoms of the following types:
Dysarthria
Vertigo
Tinnitus
Decreased hearing
Double vision
Ataxia
Decreased level of consciousness
Simultaneous bilateral visual symptoms in both the temporal and nasal field of both eyes
Simultaneous bilateral paresthesias
Simultaneous bilateral pareses

migraine. The aura often lasts less than 1 hour, is usually followed by a headache, and is nothing more than migraine with an aura clinically localized to the brainstem. In basilar-type migraine, a typical hemianoptic aura may involve both visual fields, leading at times to temporary blindness. This visual aura is usually followed by ataxia, vertigo, tinnitus, diplopia, nausea and vomiting, nystagmus, dysarthria, bilateral paresthesia, or a change in level of consciousness and cognition. Spells of basilar migraine can present a confusing picture. This disorder should be considered in patients with paroxysmal brainstem disturbances.

Confusional migraine

Confusional migraine[8,21] is characterized by a typical aura, a headache (which may be insignificant), and confusion, which may precede the headache or follow it. This again is nothing more than an aura that affects the centers that control consciousness. The confusion is characterized by inattention, distractability, and difficulty maintaining speech and other motor activities.

Ophthalmoplegic migraine

Ophthalmoplegic migraine is no longer considered migraine by the IHS and is being renamed. It is characterized by at least two attacks associated with ocular cranial nerve palsy (usually the third cranial nerve) with a dilated pupil and unilateral migrainous eye pain. Rarely, the fourth and sixth cranial nerves are involved. The duration of ophthalmoplegia varies from hours to months. Structural causes such as parasellar, retro-orbital, cavernous sinus or midcranial fossa lesion must be ruled out. The differential diagnosis also includes berry aneurysm, acute sphenoid sinusitis, and sphenoid mucocele. Ophthalmoplegic migraine is probably not a migraine variant but an idiopathic inflammatory neuritis. Mark et al[22] recently reported six patients with typical clinical features of ophthalmoplegic migraine who had enhancement of the cisternal segment of the oculomotor nerve during the acute phase. This was followed by resolution of the enhancement over several weeks as the symptoms resolved. Enhancement can occur in a variety of infectious[23–26] (Lyme disease, syphilis, coccidioidomycosis, HIV) and noninfectious (lymphoma, leukemia, sarcoid, Tolosa-Hunt, Fisher syndrome) inflammatory conditions. A lumbar puncture (LP) is needed to rule out infections and neoplastic causes. Ophthalmoplegic migraine may be due to a viral infection of the oculomotor nerve similar to Bell's palsy (a viral neuritis with nerve enhancement).[27] Contrast-enhanced magnetic resonance imaging (MRI) and magnetic resonance angiogram (MRA) is the procedure of choice in evaluating patients with oculomotor palsy. If MRI shows enhancement of the cisternal portion of the oculomotor nerve and lumbar puncture is negative, a presumptive diagnosis of ophthalmoplegic migraine can be made, but follow-up is necessary to be sure the symptoms resolve. If the MRI and LP are negative, conventional angiogram may still be necessary to rule out an aneurysm.[22] In addition, some cases of ophthalmoplegic migraine fit the criteria for the Tolosa-Hunt syndrome of painful ophthalmoplegia.[28]

Tolosa-Hunt syndrome (IHS 12.1.5)[8] is a rare, painful ophthalmoplegia owing to a granulomatous inflammation of the cavernous sinus. Diagnosis is based on the combination of one or more episodes of painful ophthalmoplegia with paralysis of the third, fourth, and/or sixth cranial nerves that lasts an average of 8 weeks untreated, pain relief with corticosteroids within 72 hours, and exclusion of other causes, including aneurysm, diabetes mellitus, paranasal mucocele, parasellar neoplasm, carotid cavernous fistula, sphenoid sinusitis, and other disorders of the cavernous sinus. de Arcaya et al[29] analysed computed tomography (CT) and MRI scans, with and without contrast enhancement, of the cranium and orbits of patients who fulfilled IHS criteria for the diagnosis of Tolosa-Hunt syndrome. CT scan, with and without contrast enhancement, showed an enlarged cavernous sinus in only one of five patients. MRI was abnormal in all four patients, showing a convex enlargement of the symptomatic cavernous sinus by an abnormal tissue isointense with gray matter on short TR/TE images and isohypointense on long TR/TE scans. It markedly enhanced after contrast injection and, in two patients, extended into the orbital apex and subtemporal fossa ipsilaterally. Three months after successful treatment with corticosteroids, the abnormal tissue, although diminished in size, was still visible on MRI. It only disappeared after 6 months of treatment. Painful ophthalmoplegia, cavernous sinus enlargement on MRI, and slow resolution with corticosteroid treatment are highly suggestive of Tolosa-Hunt syndrome.[29]

Hemiplegic migraine

The IHS[8] has subdivided hemiplegic migraine into two forms, sporadic and familial, both of which typically begin in childhood and often cease in adulthood. This separation may not be justified, and both forms may be part of the same syndrome.[16] The age of onset of hemiplegic migraine may be earlier than that of typical migraine. The attacks are frequently precipitated by minor head injury. Changes in consciousness ranging from confusion to coma are a feature of hemiplegic migraine, especially in childhood.[16] The hemiplegia may be part of the aura and last less than 1 hour (migraine with typical aura), or it may last for days or weeks. Headache may precede the hemiparesis or be absent. The onset of hemiparesis may be abrupt and simulate a stroke. The prevalence of hemiplegic migraine is uncertain and varies from 4% to 30% of cases of migraine.[14] The differential diagnosis of hemiplegic migraine includes stroke, homocystinuria, focal seizures, and MELAS syndrome.[21]

Familial hemiplegic migraine (FHM)

FHM (Table 6.8) has an autosomal dominant mode of inheritance with variable penetrance. The gene for 60% of affected families has been localized to the short arm of chromosome 19p13. A second locus is on chromosome 1. In some families linkage to both chromosome 1 and chromosome 19 has been excluded. Thus, clinical and genetic heterogeneity exists. A case has been made to classify FHM as a subtype of migraine because of:

- the paroxysmal occurrence of headache and the nausea, vomiting, and transient focal neuralgic symptoms, all of which are similar to migraine with aura;
- the fact that individuals with FHM and ordinary forms of migraine with and without aura coexist in the same families;
- the changes that occur in an affected individual over a lifetime.

● **Table 6.8** Familial Hemiplegic Migraine

Description:
Migraine with aura including any degree of paresis or hemiparesis and where at least one first- or second-degree relative has identical attacks.

Diagnostic criteria:

A At least two attacks fulfilling B–E

B Fully reversible symptoms including some degree of weakness plus at least one of the following: visual, sensory, or speech disturbance

C At least one symptom evolves over at least 5 minutes or symptoms occur in succession. Each symptom lasts less than 24 hours. If more symptoms are present, accepted duration is proportionally increased

D The aura is followed by headache

E At least one first- or second-degree relative has similar attacks

F Not attributed to another disorder

FHM is an autosomal dominant, genetically heterogenous form of migraine with aura with variable penetration. The aura is characterized by motor weakness of variable intensity. The syndrome includes attacks of migraine without aura, migraine with typical aura, and severe episodes with prolonged aura (up to several days or weeks), fever, meningismus, and impaired consciousness ranging from confusion to profound coma. Headache may precede the hemiparesis or be absent. The onset of the hemiparesis may be abrupt, and simulate a stroke.[30]

In 20% of unselected FHM families, patients can have fixed cerebellar symptoms and signs such as nystagmus and progressive ataxia. Cerebellar ataxia may occur before the first hemiplegic migraine attack and progress independently of the frequency or severity of hemiplegic migraine attacks. All these families have been shown to be linked to chromosome 19.[31] Episodic ataxia type 2 (EA2) is also an autosomal dominant disorder that is characterized by paroxysmal attacks of ataxia that last from 15 minutes to hours or days. It is provoked by emotional or physical stress, alcohol, or coffee, but not by startle, and is associated with interictal nystagmus and acetazolamide responsiveness. The gene for 60% of affected families has been localized to the short arm of chromosome 19p13, and has been cloned.[32] Mutations within CACNA1A, a gene encoding for the α1A subunit of a neuronal P/Q type calcium channel, cause both FHM and EA2. Another gene has been mapped to chromosome 1, CACNA1A.[33] All EA2 families have been linked to chromosome 19.[34,35]

This work demonstrates that at least one form of migraine is a calcium channelopathy, raising the possibility that other more common forms of migraine may also be channelopathies. This is discussed in detail in Chapter 5.

Cerebral autosomal dominant arteriopathy with subcortical infarcts and leukoencephalopathy

Cerebral autosomal dominant arteriopathy with subcortical infarcts and leukoencephalopathy (CADASIL) is an inherited arterial disease of the brain that has been mapped to chromosome 19 in two unrelated French families (Table 6.9).[36] Hutchinson et al[37] found four members of an Irish family with CADASIL who had a history and preceding diagnosis of FHM. The complete CADASIL syndrome consists of recurrent episodes of focal brain deficits (recurrent strokes) that start in mid-adult life and often lead to dementia, residual motor disability, and pseudobulbar palsy. Even before clinical symptoms or signs have developed, MRIs of at-risk individuals are often abnormal, with extensive areas of increased T2 signals in the white matter. FHM is distinguished from CADASIL by its earlier onset, benign prognosis, and normal MRI findings. It is

● **Table 6.9** Familial hemiplegic migraine (FHM) and cerebral autosomal dominant arteriopathy with subcortical infarcts and leukoencephalopathy (CADASIL)

	FHM	CADASIL	Migraine with WMA*
Genetics	AD	AD	AD
LOCUS	19*, 1	19	19 (?)
MRI	WNL	ABN	ABN
Migraine	Yes	Yes	Yes
Migraine with aura and hemiparesis	Yes	Yes	Yes
Stroke	No	Yes	No
Dementia	No	Yes	No

* White matter abnormalities; WNL when associated with cerebellar abnormalities

defined as migraine with aura with some hemiparesis, with at least one first-degree relative having identical attacks. Cases with associated cerebellar degeneration may be localized to chromosome 19. This suggests that a unique process, not typical of migraine, occurs in these families (Figures 6.13 and 6.14).

CADASIL can be diagnosed by the characteristic MRI abnormalities in a genetically at-risk family member.[37] MRI shows leukoencephalopathy of varying severity on T2-weighted images and multiple deep white matter infarcts on both T1- and T2-weighted images. Four of five members of the Irish family with the syndrome of FHM had the MRI findings of CADASIL (Figure 6.15).[37]

Chabriat et al[38] used MRI and genetic linkage analysis to study seven CADASIL families. The most frequent symptoms were recurrent subcortical ischemic events (84%), progressive or stepwise subcortical dementia with pseudobulbar palsy (31%), migraine with aura (22%), and mood disorders with severe depressive episodes (20%). All the symptomatic subjects had prominent signal abnormalities on MRI (these were also present in 19 asymptomatic subjects). The mean age at onset of symptoms was 45 years (SD 10.6 years), with attacks of migraine with aura occurring earlier in life (38.1 years; SD 8.03 years) than ischemic events (49.3 years; SD 10.7 years). The mean age at death was 64.5 (SD 10.6) years. On the basis of MRI data, the penetrance of the disease appears complete between 30 and 40 years of age.

The arteriopathy underlying CADASIL involves neither atherosclerosis nor amyloid deposition; rather, it involves pathology of the media of small cerebral arteries and to a lesser extent extracerebral arteries, including skin arterioles. Skin biopsy can be diagnostic. Ultrastructural examination reveals abnormal patches of agranular osmiophilic

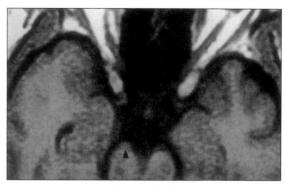

(A)

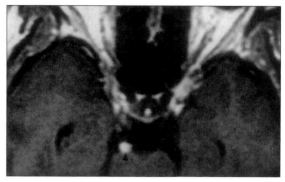

(B)

● **Figure 6.12** Case 1: 27-year-old woman with two prior episodes of headache and oculomotor nerve palsy. Axial noncontrast (A) and contrast-enhanced (B) T1-weighted images show focal nodular enhancement of the exit zone of the oculomotor nerve (arrowhead). Followup study showed virtually complete resolution of the enhancement.

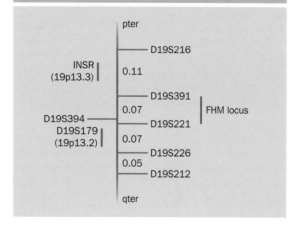

● **Figure 6.13** Genetic map of chromosome 19p region based on data from the Genome Data Base: distances are given in Morgans.

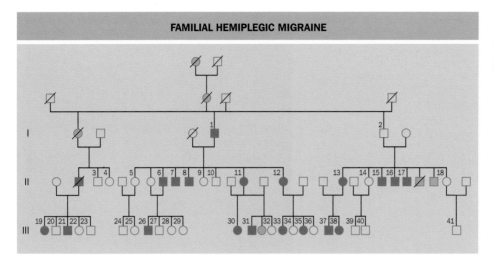

● Figure 6.14
Familial hemiplegic migraine: analysis of FHM genetic family pedigree.

material within the basal membranes of vascular smooth-muscle cells.[39]

In 1996, Joutel et al identified Notch3 as the defective gene in CADASIL.[40] Members of the Notch gene family encode evolutionarily conserved transmembrane receptors that are involved in cell fate specification during embryonic development. The Notch3 gene includes 33 exons encoding a protein of 2321 amino acids. Its extracellular domain contains 34 epidermal growth factor-like repeats that are involved in ligand-binding, whereas the intracellular domain carries the intrinsic signal-transducing activity. CADASIL gene identification has provided the information needed to set up a direct genotypic diagnostic test.[39]

Chabriat et al[41] also described one family with no evidence of migrainous infarct or prolonged aura, in which eight of the 12 examined members of the pedigree had throbbing headaches. The disorder was characterized by recurrent headache attacks with many features of migraine. The attacks usually lasted 2–48 hours (patients were asymptomatic between attacks) and were usually preceded by focal neurologic symptoms that developed gradually over 5–15 minutes and resolved in less than 60 minutes. Paresthesias and unilateral or bilateral blurring of vision were the most frequent of these symptoms. Six patients satisfied the IHS diagnostic criteria for migraine with typical aura, one for a migrainous disorder with aura, and one for migraine without aura. Some subjects had extremely unusual and severe attacks, including hyperthermia and stupor, that resolved in less than 24 hours (suggestive of subcortical brainstem involvement). Another had headache, coma, fever, and aseptic meningitis that resolved within 15 days. Most, but not all, of the subjects with migraine had striking MRI abnormalities. Numerous areas of decreased signal intensity on T1-weighted images and increased signal intensity were found in the basal ganglia and the subcortical white matter.

White matter abnormalities

White matter abnormalities (WMA) have been reported in migraine, particularly migraine with aura. Some believe this results from repeated ischemic insults that occur during the migrainous auras. However, they were also found in the family described by Chabriat et al[41] without evidence of stroke. Another explanation is that migraine with aura and WMA could be the consequence of the same underlying vascular disorder that is present in mitochondrial diseases or the antiphospholipid antibody syndrome. A mutation near the CADASIL locus could thus be a new cause of migraine associated with WMA on MRI (Table 6.9).

Aura without headache

Periodic neurologic dysfunction, which may be part of the migraine aura, can occur in isolation without the headache.[42] These phenomena (scintillating scotomata and recurrent sensory, motor, and mental phenomena) can be part of migraine, but they are accepted as migraine only after a full investigation and prolonged follow-up. Headaches occurring in association with aura symptoms help confirm the diagnosis.[7] Aura without headache often occurs at some time in patients with migraine with aura.[7]

Levy[43] found that 32% of Cornell neurologists had a history of transient neurologic loss, most commonly visual (field cuts, obscurations, scotomata), and less commonly nonvisual (hemiparesis, clumsiness, paresthesias, dysarthria). Migraine was reported in 29%, occurring in 44% of those reporting and 22% of those not reporting transient central nervous system (CNS) dysfunction. None

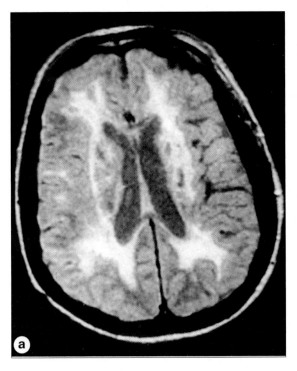

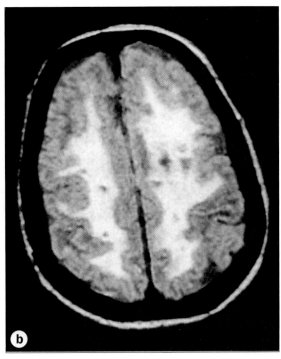

● **Figure 6.15** *MRI CADASIL. Brain MRI showing axial proton density sections at the level of the bodies of the lateral ventricles and centrum show confluent, severe, high-signal leukoencephalopathy, with discrete punctate low-signal lesions indicating cystic or necrotic lesions. Reproduced with permission.*[34]

● **Table 6.10** *Main criteria for the diagnosis of late-life migrainous accompaniments*

- Scintillations (or other visual display), paresthesias, aphasia, dysarthria and paralysis.
- Build-up of scintillations. Not seen in cerebrovascular disease.
- 'March' of paresthesias. Not seen in cerebrovascular disease.
- Progression from one accompaniment to another, often with a delay.
- Two or more similar attacks. Helps exclude embolism.
- Headache occurs in 50% of attacks.
- Episodes last 15–25 minutes.
- Characteristic mid-life 'flurry' of attacks.
- Generally benign course.
- Normal angiography: excludes thrombosis.
- Rule out: cerebral thrombosis, embolism and dissection, epilepsy, thrombocythemia, polycythemia, and thrombotic thrombocytopenia.

Adapted from Fisher.44

Fisher[44] described late-life migrainous accompaniments, which are transient neurologic phenomena frequently not associated with headache (Table 6.10). He reported on 188 patients over the age of 40 years; 60% were men and 57% had a history of recurrent headache. They had one or more attacks of episodic neurologic dysfunction, which lasted from 1 minute to 72 hours, with variable recurrence (one attack 27%, two to 10 attacks 45%, more than 10 attacks 28%). Fisher considered scintillating scotoma to be diagnostic of migraine even when it occurred in isolation, whereas other episodic neurologic symptoms (paresthesias, aphasia, and sensory and motor symptoms) needed more careful evaluation (Table 6.11).

Wijman et al[45] found that visual symptoms occurred in 186 subjects in the Framingham study. Visual symptoms typical of the visual aura of migraine were reported by 26 of 186 subjects (14%), with a prevalence of 1.23% overall (1.33% in women and 1.08% in men). The pattern of visual manifestations varied widely. The episodes were never accompanied by headaches in 58% of patients, and 42% had no headache history. Only in 19% of subjects did the migrainous visual episodes meet the IHS criteria for migraine aura, usually because one of the criteria ('at least one aura symptom develops gradually over more than 4

of the responders had developed any residual deficit or chronic neurologic disorder at 5-year follow-up, suggesting that these symptoms are benign migrainous accompaniments.

● **Table 6.11** *Migrainous accompaniments*

Visual-scintillating scotoma	Hemiplegia
Ophthalmoplegia	Cyclical vomiting
Paraesthesias	Brainstem symptoms
Oculosympathetic palsy	Seizures
Aphasia	Blindness
Mydriasis	Diplopia
Dysarthria	Blurring of vision
Confusion-stupor	Deafness
Dizziness	Hemianopia
Recurrence of old stroke deficit	

minutes') could not be reliably ascertained.

Three of 26 subjects (11.5%) had a stroke one or more years later; one had a subarachnoid hemorrhage 1 year later; one had a brainstem infarct 3 years later; and one had a cardioembolic stroke secondary to atrial fibrillation 27 years later. This stroke incidence rate of 11.5% was significantly lower than the stroke incidence rate of 33.3% in subjects with TIAs in the same cohort ($p = 0.030$) (these usually occurred within 6 months) and did not differ from the stroke incidence rate of 13.6% of those without migrainous phenomena or TIAs.

Visual migrainous phenomena are not rare, since they occur in 1.33% of women and in 1.08% of men in a general population sample and are usually benign. In addition, transient migrainous accompaniments – scintillating scotomata, numbness, aphasia, dysarthria, and motor weakness – may occur for the first time after the age of 45 years and be easily confused with TIAs of cerebrovascular origin (Table 6.11). In all but the most classic cases, the diagnostic method is still exclusion.[46] While many of these spells meet the IHS criteria for migraine aura without headache, others meet the diagnosis of acute-onset aura without headache, which is not recognized by the IHS.

Treatment

Effective migraine treatment begins with making an accurate diagnosis,[5] explaining it to the patient, and developing a treatment plan that considers the patient's diagnosis, symptoms, and any coincidental or comorbid conditions and deals with the most disturbing symptoms in the most appropriate way.[47] Comorbidity is defined as the co-occurrence of two disorders in the same individual at a greater frequency than mediated by chance. Conditions that occur in migraineurs with a higher prevalence than would be expected include stroke, epilepsy, mitral valve prolapse, Raynaud's syndrome, and psychological disorders, which include depression, mania, anxiety, and panic (Table 6.12). Co-occurring disease presents both therapeutic opportunities and therapeutic limitations. Migraine and epilepsy occur together; an antiepileptic drug may prevent both disorders and a tricyclic antidepressant (TCA) may prevent migraine and exacerbate epilepsy.

Symptom profiles should also be considered. For example, if nausea and vomiting are prominent, a nonoral route of drug administration is needed. Diagnosis must precede treatment, since a specific migraine medication may be useless or even dangerous if given to a patient with a migraine mimic. For example, a patient with an acute symptomatic headache due to meningitis or subarachnoid hemorrhage may respond to a triptan with relief of headache, lulling the physician into a false sense of diagnostic confidence.

After an initial clinical assessment (Chapter 4), we recommend asking patients to complete a headache calendar, recording the duration and severity of their headaches as well as their response to treatment (Figure 6.3). Non-pharmacologic treatment strategies include relaxation, biofeedback, and behavioural interventions, such as maintaining a regular schedule, getting adequate sleep and exercise, and giving up tobacco (Table 6.13).[6] Biofeedback is a useful treatment that serves to engage patients in cognitive behavioral therapy. It is especially useful for chil-

● **Table 6.12** *Migraine comorbid disease*

Cardiovascular	Psychiatric	Gastrointestinal	Neurologic	Other
Hypertension or hypotension	Depression	Irritable bowel syndrome	Epilepsy	Asthma
Raynaud's syndrome	Mania		Positional vertigo	Allergies
Mitral valve prolapse	Panic disorder		Essential tremor	
Angina/myocardial infarction	Anxiety disorder			
Stroke				

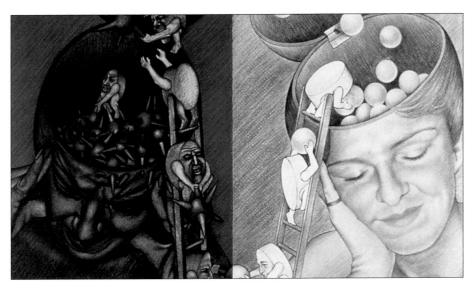

● **Figure 6.16** *'Relief'*
by Deborah Barrett of
Everett,
Massachusetts, USA.
(© Sandoz
Pharmaceuticals Corp.)

dren, pregnant women, and patients for whom stress is a trigger. Although behavioral interventions are important, drugs are the mainstay of treatment for most patients (Figure 6.16).

The pharmacologic treatment of migraine may be acute (abortive) or preventive (prophylactic).[6] Acute treatment attempts to reverse or stop the progression of a headache once it has started. Preventive therapy is given, even in the absence of a headache, to reduce the frequency and severity of anticipated attacks. Acute treatment is appropriate for most attacks, even for patients who are on preventive medication. It should not be used more than 2, or at most, 3 days a week, to prevent the development of rebound headaches. Preventive treatment is used more selectively, to decrease the occurrence of frequent attacks, for example.

In this chapter, we used, in part, the Technical Report created by Duke University and the American Academy of Neurology under contract to the Agency for Healthcare Policy and Research (AHCPR), in which evidence from controlled trials on the efficacy and tolerability of drug treatments for acute and preventive migraine headache was identified and summarized. These are the basis of the US Headache Consortium Guidelines.[48,49]

Treatment of the acute migraine headache

Many acute treatments are available for migraine. The choice depends on the severity and frequency of the headaches, the pattern of the associated symptoms, the presence of comorbid illnesses, and the patient's pattern of response to prior treatment (Table 6.14). Acute medication is indicated even if patients are using preventive medication. It is important to treat the headache as early as possible both to prevent its escalation and to increase the drug's effectiveness. Often migraine begins with pain of mild to moderate severity and is described as similar to a tension-type headache. As the headache increases in severity, it takes on more migraine-like features. Mild and severe migraine forms respond to triptans.[50,51]

Acute headache treatment medication can be specific or nonspecific (Table 6.15). Nonspecific medications are used to control the pain and associated symptoms of migraine or other pain disorders, while specific medications are effective for migraine (and cluster) headache but are not useful for nonheadache pain disorders. The migraine-specific medications include the ergots and triptans. Nonspecific medications include analgesics,

● **Table 6.13** Behavioral therapy

May help	Less likely to help
Regulate sleep	Avoid milk products
Regular exercise	Avoid citrus products
Regular meals	Avoid chocolate
Avoid monosodium glutamate	Avoid tyramine-
Avoid alcoholic beverages	containing food
Limit caffeine	
Limit medications	
Biofeedback, relaxation therapy, and stress management	

● **Table 6.14** *Acute medications: efficacy, side effects, relative contraindications, and indications*

Drug	*Efficacy	**AEs	Comorbid condition	
			Relative contraindications	Relative indications
Acetaminophen (APAP) (Paracetamol)	1+	1+	Liver disease	
Aspirin (Asa)	1+	1+	Kidney disease, ulcer disease, PUD, gastritis (age <15)	CAD, TIA
Butalbital, caffeine, and analgesics	2+	3+	Use of other sedative; history of medication overuse	
Caffeine (Asa and APAP)	2+	1+	Sensitivity to caffeine	
Isometheptene	2+	1+	Uncontrolled HTN, CAD, PVD	
Opioids	3+	4+	Drug or substance abuse, sedation	Pregnancy; rescue medication
NSAIDs	2+	2+	Kidney disease, PUD, gastritis	
Dihydroergotamine				
– IV	4+	2+	CAD, PVD, uncontrolled HTN	Orthostatic hypotension, prominent nausea or vomiting
– IM	3+	1+		
– IN	2+	1+		
Ergotamine				
– Tablets	2+	2+	Prominent nausea or vomiting, CAD, PVD, uncontrolled HTN	
– Suppositories	3+	3+		
Triptans				
Almotriptan				
– Tablets	3+	1+	CAD, PVD, uncontrolled HTN	
Frovatriptan				
– Tablets	2+	1+	CAD, PVD, uncontrolled HTN	
Naratriptan				
– Tablets	2+	1+	CAD, PVD, uncontrolled HTN	
Rizatriptan				
– Tablets	3+	1+	CAD, PVD, uncontrolled HTN	
Zolmitriptan				
– Tablets, intranasal	3+	1+	CAD, PVD, uncontrolled HTN	
Sumatriptan				
– SC injection	4+	1+	CAD, PVD, uncontrolled HTN	Prominent nausea or vomiting
– Intranasal	3+	1+	CAD, PVD, uncontrolled HTN	
– Tablets	3+	1+	CAD, PVD, uncontrolled HTN	

*Ratings are on a scale from 1+ (lowest) to 4+ (highest) based on response rates and consistency of response in double-blind placebo-controlled trails and our clinical experience.

**Ratings are from 1+ (fewest significant AEs) to 4+ (greatest significant Aes) in appropriate patients

AEs, adverse events; CAD, coronary artery disease; HTN, hypertension; NSAIDs, nonsteroidal antiinflammatory drugs; PUD, peptic ulcer disease; PVD, peripheral vascular disease; SC, subcutaneous;.TIA, transient ischemic attack.

antiemetics, anxiolytics, nonsteroidal anti-inflammatory drugs (NSAIDs), steroids, major tranquilizers, and opioids.[7] Preventive treatments include a selective group of medications from a broad range of drug classes, including notably β-blockers, calcium-channel blockers, antidepressants, serotonin antagonists, anticonvulsants, and NSAIDs. Optimizing therapy requires knowledge of alternative treatments and awareness of the patient's preferences. Some patients want to minimize their attack frequency and are willing to accept significant side-effects to achieve this goal. To others, tolerability is a higher priority than efficacy. Some patients are eager to try new therapies, while others

are afraid to change an established regimen. Some patients readily accept parenteral treatments, but others reject the idea of injections or suppositories.[6]

Acute treatment (Figure 6.17)

Treatment should be tailored to the attack and to the individual in whom it occurs. Determine the history of treatment, both prescription and over-the-counter, assessing both successes and failures. Be aware of all prescription and over-the-counter drugs that the patient is using, and assess the presence and risk for medication overuse. Acute headache medication overuse often causes treatment failure. Patient should be stratified primarily by severity and disability and treated with the medications most likely to be effective for that attack, taking into account the drug's efficacy, safety, and side-effects.

The formulation and route of administration are based on the attack severity, how rapidly it escalates, the patient's preference, the presence or absence of severe nausea or vomiting, and the need for rapid relief. Use a nonoral route and consider an antiemetic when there is significant early nausea or vomiting. Do not restrict antiemetics just to patients who are vomiting or likely to vomit. Nausea itself is one of the most disabling symptoms of migraine and should be treated appropriately.[52]

Individualize treatment. For patients with mild to moderate headaches, analgesics, NSAIDs, or a caffeine adjuvant compound can be useful. We often prescribe a triptan at the initial consultation as a first-line drug for severe attacks and as a backup medication for less severe attacks that do not adequately respond to simple or combination analgesics. Most patients prefer oral triptans. However, if rapid pain relief is required or if nausea or vomiting are prominent, nonoral treatment should be considered. If oral medication is ineffective or cannot be used due to gastrointestinal symptoms, we add an antiemetic or recommend suppositories, nasal spray, or injections, based on the patient's preferred route of administration. Suppositories include ergotamine, naproxen, indomethacin (indometacin), and prochlorperazine. Nasal sprays include transnasal butorphanol and dihydroergotamine (DHE), sumatriptan, and, soon, zolmitriptan. Injections include subcutaneous (SC) sumatriptan and intramuscular (IM) DHE, among others. We often prescribe more than one acute treatment at the time of the initial visit. For example, we may advise patients to use naproxen sodium for mild to moderate headaches and sumatriptan for more severe headaches.[6,7] It is important to get the treatment 'right' as soon as possible. Undertreatment leaves patients

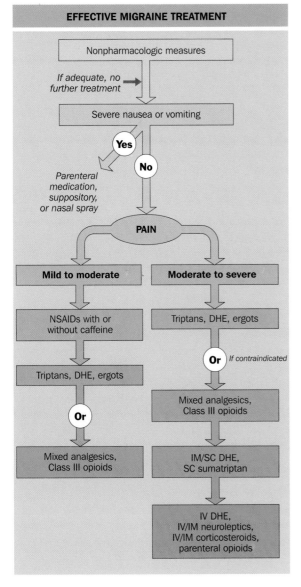

● *Figure 6.17 Effective migraine treatment begins with making an accurate diagnosis.*

with pain and disability, which often leads them to lapse from care.

Disability is a useful predictor of treatment need. In a randomized trial, high disability (MIDAS Grade IV) patients treated with aspirin plus metoclopramide (metoclopramide) failed treatment in 75% of cases. The study showed that patient outcomes improved using a stratified care approach – treating more disabled patients more aggressively as the first intention.[53] Disability can be defined by the amount of time a patient loses due to headache over a 3-month period and measured with the MIDAS Questionnaire. Backup medication is needed in the event that the initial treatment is inadequate. Triptans or DHE can be used if analgesics fail; neuroleptics or parenteral ketorolac or combination analgesics (with opioids or butalbital) can be used if triptans or ergots fail.

Acute headache medication is the best approach when attacks are infrequent or compliance is a problem. Treat at least two different attacks before deciding that a drug is ineffective. Be sure the dose is adequate and that no other factors interfere with its effect. It may be necessary to change formulation or route of administration or add an adjuvant. Consider changing the drug when the response is incomplete or too slow, the headache recurs, the results are inconsistent after an adequate trial at an adequate dose, or if the side-effects are bothersome. Guard against medication-overuse headache. In general, limit treatment with acute headache treatment to 2–3 days per week. Medication-overuse headache results from the too frequent use of acute headache medications, often resulting in more frequent headaches that are refractory to treatment. If medication overuse is suspected, keeping a diary can be very informative for both patient and physician.

Simple and combination analgesics and NSAIDs

We recommend simple analgesics for patients with mild to moderate headaches. Many individuals find headache relief with a simple analgesic, such as aspirin or acetaminophen (paracetamol), either alone or in combination with caffeine, a well established analgesic adjuvant. Butalbital combination products are useful where available, but medication overuse is an issue. We also use the combination of acetaminophen, isometheptene (a sympathomimetic), and dichloralphenazone (a chloral hydrate derivative). When patients are nauseated, we use antiemetics. Because of its lack of CNS problems, we recommend domperidone when it is available; metoclopramide is a good alternative. We often try naproxen sodium first, but we use a range of NSAIDs, often in combination with an antiemetic. Indomethacin, available as a 50 mg rectal suppository, and IM ketorolac are useful in

patients with severe nausea and vomiting.[7]

At least five different chemical classes of NSAIDs[54] have been used for headache treatment. The major mechanism of action of NSAIDs is the differential inhibition of one of the two subtypes of the enzyme cyclooxygenase (COX1, the constitutive, and COX2, the induced form) preventing prostaglandin synthesis.[55] COX1 is produced in normal quiescent conditions and is important when prostaglandins have a protective function, such as gastric mucus production and renal blood flow maintenance.[56]

NSAIDs are among the most commonly prescribed drugs in the world, but their use is limited by their gastrointestinal side-effects. These side-effects are primarily due to the suppression of prostaglandin synthesis (mainly through inhibition of COX1 activity), although several NSAIDs also have topical irritant properties.[57]

Nonselective COX inhibitors inhibit both COX1 and COX2 and include aspirin, naproxen, indomethacin, piroxicam, diclofenac, and ibuprofen. Some salicylates (sodium salicylate, salicylamide, and magnesium trisalicylate) can be used safely in patients with aspirin-induced asthma.[57] Marketed highly selective COX2 inhibitors include celecoxib and rofecoxib,[58] and many other compounds are in development.

The AHCPR analysed 33 controlled trials of NSAIDs and other nonopiate analgesics and found that aspirin, ibuprofen, tolfenamic acid, and naproxen sodium were superior to placebo in relieving the pain of migraine. Three trials showed that the combination of acetaminophen, aspirin, and caffeine (AAC; Excedrin®) was significantly more effective for headache relief than placebo in migraineurs.[59] Approximately 66% of patients treated migraine headache of moderate intensity, while 33% treated severe pain. Side-effects of NSAIDs include gastrointestinal upset, peptic ulcers and bleeding, abdominal pain, constipation, diarrhea, nausea, occasional paradoxical headache, lightheadedness, dizziness, somnolence, tinnitus, and fluid retention.

Acetaminophen's efficacy in acute migraine treatment has now been established.[60] The danger of Reye's syndrome makes acetaminophen preferable to aspirin for children who have headaches and are younger than 15 years.[61] Acetaminophen is an alternative to aspirin or the other NSAIDs for patients who have gastritis or bleeding disorder. Ibuprofen in over-the-counter doses has also been shown to be effective,[62] although AAC has been shown to be more effective than ibuprofen.[63]

Barbiturate hypnotics

No randomized, placebo-controlled studies have established the efficacy of butalbital-containing agents in the treatment of acute migraine headaches.[64] Because of concerns about overuse, medication-overuse headache, and withdrawal, the use of butalbital-containing analgesics should be limited and carefully monitored. Their use should be limited to situations wherein a more specific or less potentially problematic agent cannot be used or is ineffective. They may be very effective as back-up medications when other migraine medications have failed. For an individual attack, patients should take one or two tablets or capsules, with a maximum of six per attack. The most frequent adverse reactions are drowsiness and dizziness. Drug use should be limited to no more than 2–3 treatment days per week.

Ergotamine and dihydroergotamine (DHE) (Figure 6.18)

We sometimes use ergotamine[65] to treat moderate to severe migraine if analgesics do not provide satisfactory headache relief or if they produce significant side-effects and cost is a factor. However, with time and experience, the triptans are preferred to ergots for most patients. Some patients still respond preferentially to rectal ergotamine. Patients who cannot tolerate ergotamine because of nausea are pretreated with an antiemetic. Ergotamine tartrate, originally derived from a rye fungus (Claviceps purpurea), is an ergopeptide, which consists of a natural D-lysergic acid linked to a tricyclic peptide moiety by a peptide bond. Ergotamine tartrate is still available as a sublingual preparation and, in combination with caffeine, as an oral tablet and a suppository. The evidence to support ergotamine's efficacy for migraine treatment is inconsistent. For individual attacks, patients can take up to six 1 mg tablets or two suppositories over 24 hours. Use should not exceed 2 dosage days per week.[66,67] In certain circumstances, these limits may be liberalized (e.g. cluster headache, intractable menstrual migraine).

DHE has fewer side-effects than ergotamine and can be administered intramuscularly, subcutaneously, or intravenously (IV). DHE is given in doses up to 1 mg IM or IV per treatment, with a maximum of 3 mg/day. A nasal spray (NS) is available at 2 mg/treatment. The best evidence exists for DHE NS. No placebo-controlled trials in migraine patients have demonstrated the efficacy and safety of DHE SC, IM, or IV as monotherapy. We limit monthly use to 18 ampoules or 12 events. DHE remains useful because it is effective in most patients, is associated with a low headache recurrence rate (<20%), and is less likely than ergotamine to exacerbate nausea or produce rebound headache. Repetitive IV DHE is a mainstay of acute symptomatic treatment for intractable headache.[68–70]

Women who are attempting to become pregnant and patients with uncontrolled hypertension, sepsis, renal or hepatic failure, and coronary, cerebral, or peripheral vascular disease should avoid ergotamine and DHE. Nausea is a common side-effect of ergotamine, but it is less common with DHE (unless it is given intravenously). Other side-effects include dizziness, paresthesias, abdominal cramps, and chest tightness; rare idiosyncratic arterial and coronary vasospasm can occur. We recommend an electrocardiogram for all patients before their first dose of DHE, particularly if there are any cardiac risk factors (including age >40 years).

Selective 5-HT₁ agonists (triptans)

Sumatriptan (Figure 6.19)

The first marketed selective $5\text{-HT}_{1B/1D}$ agonist (triptan) was sumatriptan, followed by zolmitriptan, naratriptan, rizatriptan, and almotriptan. As of this writing frovatriptan and eletriptan are available in some countries. Sumatriptan is the most extensively studied agent in the history of migraine, with over 9 000 000 individual patients and over 400 000 000 attacks treated as of December 2001. Sumatriptan is extensively metabolized in the liver by MAO-A; therefore its use as an oral or nasal spray formulation is relatively contraindicated in patients who are on monoamine oxidase (MAO) inhibitors (MAOIs).

Sumatriptan is available in an injectable preparation (6 mg SC), a nasal spray (20 mg), tablets (25, 50, or 100 mg), and, in a few countries, a suppository (25 mg). SC sumatriptan has a very rapid onset of action. Placebo-controlled trials consistently showed that SC sumatriptan (6 mg), oral sumatriptan, and sumatriptan nasal spray are effective.[71,72] Sumatriptan relieves headache pain, nausea, photophobia, and phonophobia and restores the patient's ability to function normally.

ERGOTAMINE AND DIHYDROERGOTAMINE

Ergotamine

Dihydroergotamine

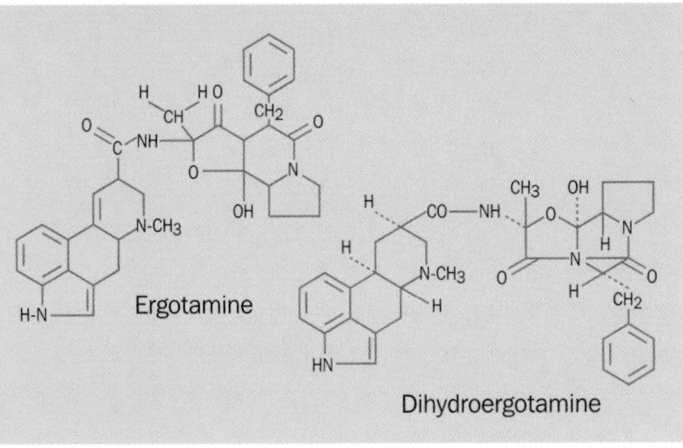

● **Figure 6.18** *Molecular structure of ergotamine and dihydroergotamine.*

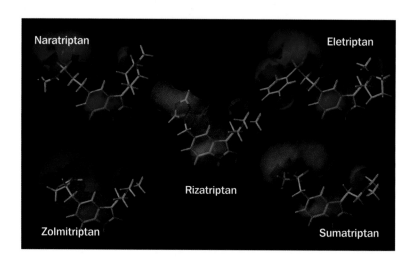

● **Figure 6.19** *Structure of triptans.*

Although 80% of patients get pain relief from an initial SC dose of sumatriptan and approximately 60% of patients get relief with oral sumatriptan, headache recurs in about one-third of patients. Recurrences are most likely in patients with long-duration headaches. Recurrences respond well to a second dose of sumatriptan or to simple and combination analgesics.[73,74]

None of the triptans should be used by patients with ischemic heart disease, Prinzmetal's angina, uncontrolled hypertension, vertebrobasilar migraine, or by patients who are at high risk for these conditions. Sumatriptan's common side-effects include pain at the injection site, tingling, flushing, burning, and warm or hot sensations. Dizziness, heaviness, neck pain, and dysphoria also can occur. These side-effects generally abate within 45 minutes. Sumatriptan causes noncardiac chest pressure in approximately 4% of patients. We obtain an electrocardiogram on patients over the age of 40 years and those with risk factors for heart disease before using sumatriptan. Adverse events – most commonly malaise/fatigue, dizziness/vertigo, asthenia, and nausea – were generally more frequent (and in some cases significantly more frequent) with the oral triptans than with placebo. We sometimes give the first dose of sumatriptan in the office at a time the patient does not have a headache.[75]

New triptans (Table 6.16)

Following the introduction of sumatriptan, a number of new compounds with $5HT_{B/D}$ agonist activity were developed. Those include: almotriptan, eletriptan, frovatriptan, naratriptan, rizatriptan, and zolmitriptan. All can penetrate the CNS to some extent. Each compound has been shown in experimental settings to constrict extracerebral intracranial vessels, inhibit activity in peripheral trigeminal neurons, and, since each can penetrate the CNS to some extent, block transmission in the trigeminal nucleus. Each compound can constrict the human coronary artery. All were initially developed as oral tablets (Table 6.16).[76]

Zolmitriptan is the second triptan to be marketed in both the UK and USA. Zolmitriptan displays high affinity at human recombinant $5\text{-}HT_{1B/1D}$ receptors and modest affinity for $5\text{-}HT_{1A}$ and $5\text{-}HT_{1F}$ receptors; it lacks significant affinity for other 5-HT receptors and a wide variety of monoamine receptors.[83–88] It is more lipophilic than sumatriptan.[84] It is available as 2.5 and 5-mg tablets and as 2.5 and 5-mg orally disintegrating tablets. A nasal spray formulation will soon be available.

Zolmitriptan has a high oral bioavailability (40%), a T-max of about 2.5 hours, and is metabolized by the cytochrome P450 system to an active metabolite that is degraded by MAO-A. Zolmitriptan (2.5 or 5 mg) is signific-

● **Table 6.15** *Migraine treatment*

Acute (symptomatic)	Specific:	for only migraine
	Non-specific:	for any pain disorder or associated symptoms
Preventive (prophylactic)	Episodic:	immediately prior to triggering event
	Subacute:	for limited time
	Chronic:	continuous

● **Table 6.16** *Selective serotonin (5HT$_1$) agonists*

	Almotriptan	Eletriptan	Frovatriptan	Naratriptan	Rizatriptan	Sumatriptan	Zolmitriptan
5HT$_{1B/1D}$ affinity	✓	✓	✓	✓	✓	✓	✓
Agonist activity	F	P	F	F	F	F	F
Cranial vasoconstrictor	✓	✓	✓	✓	✓	✓	✓
Coronary vasoconstrictor	✓	✓	✓	✓	✓	✓	✓
Inhibitor NI	✓	✓	✓	✓	✓	✓	✓
CNS penetration	✓	✓	✓	✓	✓	✓	✓

CNS, central nervous system; F, full Agonist; P, partial agonist.

antly more effective than placebo for headache relief and complete relief at 2 and 4 hours.[83,89,90] Zolmitriptan demonstrated a headache response of 64% with a therapeutic gain of 34% for the 2.5-mg dose and a headache response of 65% and a 37% therapeutic gain for the 5-mg dose.[89] The recommended starting dose of 2.5 mg provides the best balance of benefit and side-effects, although some patients may benefit from the higher 5-mg dose. A randomized, controlled, parallel trial that compared sumatriptan 25 and 50 mg with zolmitriptan 2.5 and 5 mg over the course of a series of headaches showed that both doses of zolmitriptan were either comparable or statistically superior to both doses of sumatriptan for headache relief, consistency of response, and 24-hour headache relief rates.[91] One small study did not support the use of zolmitriptan during the aura phase for the short-term prevention of migraine.[92]

A metaanalysis of the phase II/III placebo-controlled studies of zolmitriptan demonstrated a headache response at 2 hours of 64% (95% confidence interval (CI) 59–69%), with a therapeutic gain (which refers to the difference in response between active drug and placebo) of 34% (95% CI: 27–41%) for 2.5 mg, and a headache response of 66% (95% CI: 62–70%), with a corresponding therapeutic gain of 37% (95% CI: 30–44%) for the 5-mg dose.[93] The headache-free endpoint at 2 hours for 2.5 mg was 25% (95% CI: 21–29%), with a therapeutic gain of 19% (95% CI: 14–24%), and for 5 mg was 34% (95% CI: 30–38%), with a therapeutic gain of 28% (95% CI: 23–33%). Increasing the dose increased adverse events; the therapeutic penalty rates were 17% (95% CI: 11–23%) and 29% (95% CI: 23–35%) for 2.5 mg and 5 mg, respectively. Therefore, the recommended starting dose of 2.5 mg provides the best balance of benefit and side-effects, although some patients may benefit from the higher 5-mg dose. In all studies, zolmitriptan reduced the incidence of photophobia,

phonophobia, and nausea compared with placebo.

Oral eletriptan, with a 50% bioavailability and a half-life of 5 hours, is rapidly absorbed.[77] Eletriptan has interactions with drugs that are metabolized by cytochrome p450 (including C4P3A4). Eletriptan 40 mg was at least as good as sumatriptan 100 mg at 2 hours, and eletriptan 80 mg was superior to sumatriptan 100 mg in a parallel-group controlled study. Headache improvement was evident at 1 hour, with a response rate of 43% in patients who received eletriptan 40 mg and 40% in patients who received eletriptan 80 mg (currently registered in Switzerland; this dosage is not registered in the USA), compared with only 21% and 19% for those who received sumatriptan and placebo, respectively. Treatment-related adverse events were reported by 23% of patients on placebo, 18% of patients on eletriptan 20 mg, 25% of patients on eletriptan 40 mg, 36% of patients on eletriptan 80 mg, and 37% of patients on sumatriptan 100 mg.[78]

Oral eletriptan was more effective than Cafergot[T].[79] At 2 hours after treatment, more patients in the eletriptan 40 and 80-mg groups had a headache response than those in the Cafergot[T] group (54–68% vs 33%; $p < 0.0001$), and more eletriptan patients were completely pain-free (28–38% vs 10%; $p < 0.00001$).

Oral naratriptan differs from sumatriptan primarily in its longer half-life, longer T-max (3–5 hours), higher oral bioavailability (70%), and lipophilicity. It has a mean response of 48% at 2 hours after administration, but therapeutic gains are comparatively modest (21%). Relief rates with naratriptan were lower than with the other oral triptans.[49,72] The rate of recurrence was lowest for the 2.5-mg dose (25%) when compared with a recurrence rate of 38% for sumatriptan in the comparative studies done in the development programme. Tolerability for the 2.5-mg dose of naratriptan is very good, with a rate of adverse events for naratriptan (2.5 mg) equal to that of placebo.[80,81]

Rizatriptan has rapid oral absorption and high oral bioavailability at 45% for the 10-mg dose. Rizatriptan was significantly better than placebo for headache relief and complete relief at 2 hours. Rizatriptan (5 and 10 mg) has high consistency from attack to attack in formal blinded consistency studies and a wafer (Melt) formulation that many patients, particularly those with nausea as a prominent feature, find convenient, as it dissolves on the tongue and requires no water, although absorption is gastrointestinal, not transbuccal.[49] Rizatriptan has a significant interaction with propranolol, which requires that the dose be halved to 5 mg, and its use is contraindicated with MAOIs because of its route of metabolism. Rizatriptan was significantly better than placebo at relieving recurrent headache pain.[82]

The newly-developed 5-$HT_{1B/1D}$ agonist, almotriptan, has shown significant headache relief for the acute treatment of migraine. A single oral dose of 6.25 mg or 12.5 mg of almotriptan or placebo was administered during three different migraine attacks.[94,95] The overall percentages of attacks were 38.4%, 59.9% and 70.3% for placebo, 6.25 mg and 12.5 mg respectively. Pain-free values at two hours were 15.5%, 29.9% and 38.8% for placebo, 6.25 mg and 12.5 mg respectively.

Frovatriptan is a 5$HT_{1B/1D}$ receptor agonist with a high affinity for the 5$HT_{1B/1D}$ receptors. A randomized, double-blind, placebo-controlled, parallel-group, outpatient study of placebo and 2.5, 5, 10, 20, or 40 mg of frovatriptan allocated in a 1 : 1 : 1 : 2 : 2 : 2 ratio was performed in 38 USA centers. At 2 hours there was a two-fold significant difference in response rates between all doses of frovatriptan (40–48%) and placebo (22%) ($p \leq 0.012$). More patients in each of the frovatriptan groups had relief of associated migraine symptoms and functional improve-ment than did those in the placebo group. Low recurrence rates were observed: 9–14% for frovatriptan and 18% for placebo, although in direct comparison with sumatriptan, the rates were comparable.[96]

The triptans are safe and effective for the acute treatment of migraine headaches. To date, no evidence supports their use during the aura phase of a migraine attack given that injectable sumatriptan is ineffective in aura.[97] The triptans are appropriate first-line treatment choices and may be considered for patients with moderate to severe migraine who have no contraindications to these agents. Because of their inability to take oral medications, patients with nausea and vomiting may be given intranasal or SC sumatriptan. Initial treatment with any triptan is a reasonable choice when the headache is moderate to severe or an adequate trial of NSAIDs or other nonopiate analgesics (including combination NSAIDs such as AAC) has failed to provide adequate relief in the past.

Opioids

If nonopioid medications do not provide adequate pain relief, we use codeine in combination with simple analgesics and sometimes butalbital or caffeine in the USA. We also use, in restrictive circumstances, more potent narcotic analgesics, such as propoxyphene, butorphanol, meperidine (pethidine), morphine, hydromorphone, and oxycodone, alone and in combination with simple analgesics.[6,7] Because medication overuse and rebound headache pose a threat with narcotic use, these agents are most appropriate for patients whose severe headaches are relatively infrequent. Although butorphanol is a mixed agonist–antagonist, it clearly causes rebound headache and medication overuse syndromes. Transnasal butorphanol tartrate (1 mg followed by 1 mg 1 hour later) is an

● **Table 6.17** Doses of opioids equivalent to 10 mg parenteral morphine

Drug	Oral dose (mg)	Oral-to-parenteral dose ratio	Parenteral dose (mg)
Butorphanol	NA	NA	2
Codeine	200	1.5 : 1	130
Hydromorphone	7.5	5 : 1	1.5
Meperidine	300	4 : 1	75
Methadone	20	2 : 1	10
Morphine			
Single dose	60	6 : 1	10
Repeated dose	30	3 : 1	10
Oxycodone	15	2 : 1	30

NA, not applicable

effective acute outpatient treatment that not only rapidly relieves the pain of migraine, but circumvents problems with oral absorption. Opioids should not be used more than 2 days a week on average (Table 6.17). In women with intractable menstrual migraine, we sometimes use narcotics on a more regular basis. These drugs are also especially helpful to patients who either do not respond to simple analgesics or cannot take ergots or sumatriptan. Pregnant women can use codeine or meperidine (pethidine) with caution.[98] Opioids are also useful for patients who awaken in the middle of the night with a headache. Sedation, which is sometimes an undesirable side-effect, may help the patient go back to sleep and awaken headache-free in the morning.

Adjunctive treatment

Nausea and vomiting can be as disabling as the headache itself. Gastric stasis and delayed gastric emptying decrease the effectiveness of oral medication.[7] We use metoclopramide or domperidone as an antiemetic and a prokinetic to enhance the absorption of oral medications. Promethazine intravenously (0.15 mg/kg diluted in 50 ml of 5% dextrose or normal saline) or ondansetron (a selective 5-HT_3-receptor antagonist) orally (8-mg tablet) or intravenously (4–8 mg) can be used by patients who cannot tolerate metoclopramide because of side-effects. We use the neuroleptics, chlorpromazine, droperidol, and prochlorperazine, intravenously, intramuscularly, and by suppository, for nausea, vomiting, and pain. Prochlorperazine suppositories (25 mg) are used as a primary treatment for headache and nausea and also as a rescue medication.

Sixteen trials (AHCPR Technical Report) compared the efficacy of rectally (PR) and parenterally administered antiemetics. Prochlorperazine IM, IV, or PR was relatively safe and effective for the treatment of migraine headache and associated nausea and vomiting. Prochlorperazine IV, IM, and PR may be a therapeutic choice for migraine in the appropriate setting. Prochlorperazine PR may be considered an adjunct in the treatment of acute migraine with nausea and vomiting. Prochlorperazine (Compazine[T]) can be administered IV 7.5–15 mg over 5–10 minutes via a saline drip or 'slow push.'[99,100]

Chlorpromazine (Thorazine[T]) can be administered IV (10–25 mg three to four times per day) diluted in 20–30 ml of saline by rapid drip or 'slow push' over several minutes. Chlorpromazine can also be administered intramuscularly or parenterally. It is important to be sure that a patient is adequately hydrated before chlorpromazine is administered or hypotension may result.

Droperidol is a parenteral neuroleptic. IV droperidol was effective in a pilot study of 35 patients with status migrainosus or refractory migraine in an ambulatory infusion center. Droperidol (2.5 mg) was given IV every 30 minutes until either three doses were given or the patient was completely or almost headache-free.[101] The success rate (headache-free or mild headache) was 88% in patients with status migrainosus and 100% in patients with refractory migraine.

Silberstein et al[102] evaluated the efficacy and tolerability of four different doses (0.1, 2.75, 5.5 or 8.25 mg) of IM droperidol vs. placebo for the acute treatment of migraine with or without aura in a double blind, placebo-controlled, randomized, parallel-group, 22-center study. More patients in the 2.75, 5.5 and 8.25-mg treatment groups experienced a significant reduction in headache by 2 hours (moderate or severe to none or mild; 87%, 81%, and 84%, respectively) compared with placebo (57%). Headache improvement ≥2 grade levels, less headache recurrence, less rescue medication use, and fewer non-headache-associated symptoms were significantly associated with droperidol doses ≥2.75 mg. Adverse effects (AEs) occurring in more than 5% of patients receiving droperidol included asthenia, anxiety, akathisia, somnolence, and injection site reactions. Most AEs were mild to moderate.

Droperidol is safe and effective in treating status migrainosus and refractory migraine. Patients should be warned of sedation and akathisia,[101] which can be treated with diphenhydramine or benzotropine.[102]

Corticosteroids

Studies have suggested that corticosteroids are effective in the treatment of headache. The mechanism by which the corticosteroids exert their effect in migraine is uncertain. Hydrocortisone or Solu-Medrol[T] (methyl prednisolone sodium succinate) can be given IV in the following manner: 100 mg via a saline drip over 10 minutes every 6 hours for 24 hours; every 8 hours for 24 hours; every 12 hours for 24 hours; and then a final dose. Dexamethasone (Decadron[T]) can be administered IV or IM, starting at a dose of 8–20 mg per day in divided doses, rapidly tapering over 2–3 days. Oral dexamethasone 1.5–4 mg twice daily for 2 days with a taper over 3 more days has also proven useful for less disabled migraineurs with prolonged migraine headache.

Preventive treatment

Preventive medications are usually taken, whether or not headache is present, to reduce attack frequency, duration, or severity. Preventive treatment can be either preemptive, short-term, or long-term. Preemptive treatment is used when there is a known headache trigger, such as exercise or sexual activity, or a clear premonitory feature indicative of impending headache; patients are instructed to treat before the headache begins with a single dose of a pre-emptive agent. For example, single doses of indomethacin 25 or 50 mg can be given 1–2 hours prior to exercise to prevent exercise-induced migraine. Short-term prevention is used when a patient undergoes a time-limited exposure to a provoking factor, such as menstruation or ascent to a high altitude. The patient is instructed to treat for several days during a period of increased headache risk; examples of this include using NSAIDs or naratriptan for menstrual migraine. Long-term preventive medication is taken on a daily basis, usually over months, to decrease the frequency of migraine attacks.[7,52]

Recommendations for long-term migraine prevention often focus on the number of attacks that occur each month. The clinician, however, must take into account the patient's response to acute medication, his or her needs or preferences, and the characteristics of the attack. Circumstances that might warrant chronic preventive treatment include:

- Recurring migraine that significantly interferes with the patient's daily routine despite acute treatment. (e.g. two or more attacks a month that produce disability that lasts 3 or more days or headache attacks that are infrequent but produce profound disability);
- Failure of, contraindication to, or troublesome side-effects from acute medications;
- Overuse of acute medications;
- Special circumstances, such as hemiplegic migraine or attacks with a risk of permanent neurologic injury;
- Very frequent headaches (more than two per week) with the risk of rebound headache development; or
- Patient preference, that is, the desire to have as few acute attacks as possible.

During pregnancy, preventive medications should be avoided unless severe pain or disability create benefits from medication that overshadow the risks.[77] The major medication groups for preventive migraine treatment include β-adrenergic blockers, antidepressants, calcium channel antagonists, serotonin antagonists, anticonvulsants, and NSAIDs. If preventive medication is indicated, the agent should be chosen from one of the major categories, based on side-effect profiles and coexistent comorbid conditions (Table 6.18).[6]

Preventive medications should be started at a low dose and increased slowly until therapeutic effects develop, side-effects develop, or the ceiling dose for the agent in question is reached. Migraineurs frequently require a lower dose of a preventive medication than is needed for other indications. TCAs such as amitriptyline, are used in doses of 100–200 mg/day for depression, while 10–20 mg/day is often effective for migraine. In addition, migraineurs may be more sensitive to the side-effects of medication. A starting dose of 25–50 mg/day of amitriptyline is common in patients with depression, whereas this dose can produce intolerable side-effects in migraineurs. Divalproex or valproate is often effective at a dose of 500–1000 mg/day for migraine, while higher doses may be necessary to effectively treat epilepsy or mania.[104] It is important to remember that some patients may respond to lower doses of preventive medications, but it may be necessary to increase the dose to tolerance before assuming the agent is ineffective.

A full therapeutic trial may take 2–6 months. In controlled clinical trials, efficacy is often first noted after 4 weeks of treatment; benefits may continue to increase over 3 months of therapy. It is not uncommon for a patient to be treated with a new preventive medication for 1–2 weeks without effect and then prematurely discontinue it, based on the mistaken belief that it was not effective.

To obtain maximal benefit from preventive medication, the patient should not overuse analgesics or ergot derivatives. In addition, oral contraceptives, hormonal replacement therapy, or vasodilating drugs, such as nifedipine or nitroglycerine, may interfere with preventive drugs.

Migraine headaches may improve with time independent of treatment; if the headaches are well controlled, a drug holiday can be undertaken following a slow taper programme. Many patients experience continued relief after discontinuing the medication or may not need the same dose. Dose reduction may provide a better risk-to-benefit ratio. A woman of childbearing potential should be on adequate contraception before starting migraine medication. However, some women who are pregnant or who are attempting to become pregnant may still require preventive medications. If this is absolutely necessary, inform the patient and her partner of any potential risks and pick the medication with the least adverse effects on the fetus.

Medication

β-Blockers

The AHCPR Technical Report analysed 74 controlled trials of β-blockers for migraine prevention.[76] Propranolol, nadolol, atenolol, metoprolol, and timolol have been shown to be effective. The β-blockers that are partial agonists and have intrinsic sympathomimetic activity have not

● **Table 6.18** *Choices of preventive treatment in migraine: influence of comorbid conditions*

Drug	*Efficacy	*Adverse events	Comorbid condition	
			Relative contraindication	**Relative indication**
β-blockers	4+	2+	Asthma, depression, CHF, Raynaud's disease, diabetes	HTN, angina
Antiserotonin				
Pizotifen	3+	2+	Obesity	
Methysergide	4+	4+	Angina, PVD	Orthostatic hypotension
Calcium channel blockers				
Verapamil	2+	1+	Constipation, hypotension	Migraine with aura, HTN, angina, asthma
Flunarizine	4+	2+	Parkinson's	Hypertension, FHM
Antidepressants				
TCAs	4+	2+	Mania, urinary retention, heart block	Other pain disorders, depression, anxiety disorders, insomnia
SSRIs	2+	1+	Mania	Depression, OCD
MAOIs	4+	4+	Unreliable patient	Refractory depression
Anticonvulsants				
Divalproex/valproate	4+	2+	Liver disease, bleeding disorders	Mania, epilepsy, anxiety disorders
Gabapentin	2+	2+	Liver disease, bleeding disorders	Mania, epilepsy, anxiety disorders
Topiramate	3+	2+	Kidney stones	Mania, epilepsy, anxiety disorders
NSAIDs				
Naproxen	2+	2+	Ulcer disease, gastritis	Arthritis, other pain disorders

*Ratings are on a scale from 1+ (lowest) to 4+ (highest) based on magnitude of effect and strength of evidence
CHF, congestive heart failure; HTN, hypertension; MAOIs, monoamine oxidase inhibitors; NSAIDs, nonsteroidal anti-inflammatory drugs; OCD, obsessive–compulsive disorder; PVD, peripheral vascular disease; SSRI, serotonin specific reuptake inhibitor; TCA, tricyclic antidepressants.

been found to be effective for the prevention of migraine.

Since the relative efficacy of the different β-blockers (propranolol, metoprolol, timolol, nadolol, and atenolol) has not been clearly established, choose a β-blocker based on β-selectivity, convenience of drug formulation, side-effects, and the patient's individual reaction.[6,7] We often use nadolol and atenolol because of their long half-life and favorable side-effect profile, although propranolol remains a very useful drug. Since β-blockers can produce behavioral side-effects such as drowsiness, fatigue, lethargy, sleep disorders, nightmares, depression, memory disturbance, and hallucinations, we avoid them when patients have depression or low energy. Decreased exer-

cise tolerance limits their use by athletes. Less common side-effects include impotence, orthostatic hypotension, significant bradycardia, and aggravation of intrinsic muscle disease. We find β-blockers especially useful for patients with comorbid angina or hypertension. They are relatively contraindicated for patients with congestive heart failure, asthma, Raynaud's disease, and insulin-dependent diabetes.

Antidepressants

The currently available antidepressants consist of a number of different classes of drugs with different mechanisms of action:

(1) MAOIs: (a) selective and reversible; (b) nonselective and irreversible;
(2) monoamine reuptake inhibitors: (a) nonselective TCAs; (b) selective serotonin reuptake inhibitors (SSRIs); (c) selective serotonin and norepinephrine reuptake inhibitors (SNRIs);
(3) monoamine receptor targeted drugs: (a) serotonin (trazadone, trazodone); (b) norepinephrine α_2 NE antagonist (mirtazepine, mirtazapine); (c) dopamine (bupropion).

Future antidepressant drugs may be based on substance P antagonism.

A total of 16 controlled trials investigated the efficacy of the TCAs amitriptyline and clomipramine and the SSRIs fluoxetine and fluvoxamine. The TCAs most commonly used for migraine (and tension-type) headache prophylaxis include amitriptyline, nortriptyline, doxepin and protriptyline. Amitriptyline is the only antidepressant with fairly consistent support for its efficacy in migraine prevention. Other agents have not been rigorously evaluated; their use is based largely on clinical experience and uncontrolled reports. Fluoxetine was significantly better than placebo in a small study, but not in a second substantial migraine prevention trial.

We often use TCAs for patients who have a sleep disturbance. We use SSRIs, such as fluoxetine, paroxetine, and sertraline, to treat coexistent depression, based on their favorable side-effect profiles and not their established efficacy. Fluoxetine is of proven value in chronic daily headache.[105] Anecdotally, venlafaxine, the first specific SNRI, may be effective, but no studies have been performed. The dose ranges from 75 to 275 mg/day in divided doses or as a long-acting preparation.

Side-effects from TCAs are common. Most involve antimuscarinic effects, such as dry mouth and sedation. The drugs also cause increased appetite and weight gain; cardiac toxicity and orthostatic hypotension occur occasionally. Sexual dysfunction is not uncommon with SSRIs and can be treated with amantadine.[106] Antidepressants are especially useful in patients with comorbid depression and anxiety disorders.

Calcium-channel blockers

Calcium channels can be divided into two broad categories: calcium entry channels, which allow extracellular calcium to enter the cell, and calcium release channels, which allow intracellular calcium (in storage sites in organelles) to enter the cytoplasm. Calcium entry channels can be subdivided into the voltage-gated (opened by depolarization), ligand-gated (opened by chemical messengers, such as glutamate), and capacitative (activated by deple-

tion of intracellular calcium stores) subtypes. There are six functional subclasses of voltage-gated calcium (Ca^{2+}) channels that are named T, L, N, P, Q, and R. They fall into two major categories: high-voltage activated channels and the unique low-voltage activated T-type, which is activated at negative potentials.[107] The three major classes of L-type Ca^{2+} channel blockers are the dihydropyridines (e.g. nifedipine), benzothiazepines (e.g. diltiazem), and phenylalkylamines (e.g. verapamil). Regions of the α_1 subunit contain the binding sites for all these drugs.[107]

The AHCPR Technical Report identified 45 controlled trials of calcium antagonists.[76] A metaanalysis was statistically significant in favor of flunarizine (not available in the USA). Nimodipine had mixed results in placebo-controlled trials. The evidence for nifedipine was difficult to interpret. Verapamil was more effective than placebo in two of three trials, but both positive trials had high dropout rates, rendering the interpretation of the findings uncertain. Of the calcium-channel blockers available in the USA, verapamil is the most widely used, despite the limited evidence base.[6,7] Verapamil is especially useful for patients with comorbid hypertension or with contraindications, such as asthma and Raynaud's disease, to β-blockers. We also use verapamil for patients who have migraine with prolonged aura or migrainous infarction, although flunarizine, when available, is a much better option. Because verapamil has an especially favorable side-effect profile, we use it preferentially on patients unlikely to tolerate cognitive side-effects. Constipation is verapamil's most common side-effect. Although flunarizine is the most effective drug of this class, it is not universally available. In addition, its antidopaminergic activity sometimes produces symptoms of parkinsonism. Although these side-effects may limit dose, they are not a major problem in practice. Flunarizine can worsen depression and should be used with care when patients have a history of significant depression.

Antiepileptic drugs

Antiepileptic drugs (AEDs) are increasingly recommended for migraine prevention because of placebo-controlled, double-blind trials that prove them effective. Nine controlled trials of five different anticonvulsants were included in the AHCPR Technical Report. Five studies provided strong, consistent support for the efficacy of divalproex sodium and sodium valproate. An extended release form of divalproex sodium demonstrated comparable efficacy to the tablet formulation with an adverse event profile almost identical to placebo. In a long-term safety study of divalproex sodium,[108] reasons for premature discontinuation (67%) included administrative problems (31%), drug intolerance (21%), and treatment ineffectiveness (15%). The most frequently reported adverse events were nausea (42%), infection (39%), alopecia (31%), tremor (28%), asthenia (25%), dyspepsia (25%), and somnolence (25%). Divalproex was found to be safe and initial improvements were maintained for periods in excess of 1080 days. No unexpected adverse events or safety concerns unique to the use of divalproex in the prophylactic treatment of migraine were found.

Many patients find divalproex sodium to be effective at a low dose (500–1000 mg/day). It can now be given as an extended release preparation at bedtime. Side-effects include sedation, hair loss, tremor, and changes in cognitive performance. Nausea, vomiting, and indigestion can occur, but these are self-limited side-effects. Hepatotoxicity is the most serious side-effect, but irreversible hepatic dysfunction is extremely rare in adults. Pancreatitis has also been reported. Baseline liver function studies should be obtained, but routine follow-up studies are probably not routinely needed in adults on monotherapy. Follow-up is necessary to adjust the dose and monitor side-effects.

Silberstein[109] published practical recommendations and clinical guidelines for using valproate for headache prophylaxis:

(1) Before initiating divalproex sodium, perform a physical examination and take a thorough medical history, with special attention to hepatic, hematologic, and bleeding abnormalities. Obtain screening baseline laboratory studies to help identify risk factors that could influence drug selection.
(2) To minimize gastrointestinal side-effects, use the delayed extended release formulation. Begin with a dose of 500 mg at bedtime. Increase the dose to 1000 mg a day.
(3) Obtain follow-up divalproex levels to test for compliance, toxicity, and drug reactions.
(4) See the patient on a regular basis (every 1–2 months) during the first 6–9 months of therapy.
(5) It is not necessary to monitor blood and urine in otherwise healthy and asymptomatic patients on monotherapy.
(6) If mild hepatic transaminase elevation occurs, continue divalproex sodium at the same dose or a lower dose until the enzymes normalize.
(7) Tremor may occur in 10% of treated patients. If this is bothersome, decrease the dose of divalproex sodium or use propranolol.

Gabapentin (1800–2400 mg), in a randomized, placebo-controlled, double-blind trial, was superior to placebo in reducing the frequency of migraine attacks. The responder rate was 36% for gabapentin and 14% for placebo.[110] The most common adverse events were dizziness or giddiness and drowsiness. Relatively high patient withdrawal rates due to adverse events were reported in some trials.[76]

Topiramate is a structurally unique anticonvulsant that was discovered by serendipity. Topiramate is a derivative of the naturally occurring monosaccharide D-fructose and contains a sulfamate functionality. Topiramate is rapidly and almost completely absorbed. The average elimination half-life is approximately 21 hours. Topiramate has been tested for inhibitory activity on six isozymes of carbonic anhydrase CA. The relevance of the carbonic anhydrase inhibitory activity to the anticonvulsant activity of topiramate is not known.

Topiramate has been associated with weight loss, not weight gain (a common reason to discontinue preventive medication) with chronic use. Shuaib et al[111] studied 37 patients with frequent migraines (more than 10 headaches a month) who were treated with topiramate (25–100 mg a day). In addition to migraine, most had chronic daily headache and all had failed treatment on a number of preventive drugs. Patients maintained a daily diary to record the frequency and severity of headaches and the amount and type of rescue medication used. Over a 3–9-month follow-up, 11 patients (30%) had a significant improvement in headache frequency.

Edwards et al[112] enrolled 30 migraineurs in a placebo-controlled, double-blind prevention trial of topiramate. Percent responders (patients with ≥50% reduction in 28-day migraine headache frequency) during the 18-week double-blind phase was topiramate 46.7% and placebo 6.7% (statistically significant ($p = 0.035$)). Potter et al[113] evaluated the efficacy and safety of topiramate in migraine prophylaxis. The median percent reduction in monthly headache rate was 33% (topiramate) versus 8% (placebo); $p - 0.0061$). Topiramate should be started at a dose of 15–25 mg/day at bedtime and increased weekly to 100–200 mg/day in divided doses. Adverse events include weight loss, paresthesias, and cognitive dysfunction (which can often be controlled by slow titration). Topirimate should be used with caution in patients who have a history of renal calculi.

Divalproex sodium and topiramate are especially useful when migraine occurs in patients with comorbid epilepsy, anxiety disorder, or manic-depressive illness. It can be safely administered to patients with depression, Raynaud's disease, asthma, and diabetes, circumventing the contraindications to β-blockers. With the exception of valproic acid and phenobarbital, many AEDs interfere with the efficacy of oral contraceptives.[114,115] Caution is therefore advised in women on AEDs and oral contraceptives.

Serotonin antagonists

Methysergide is an effective migraine prophylactic drug.

Side-effects include transient muscle aching, claudication, abdominal distress, nausea, weight gain, and hallucinations. Frightening hallucinations after the first dose are not uncommon.[116] The major complication of methysergide is the rare (1/2500) development of retroperitoneal, pulmonary, or endocardial fibrosis, the unreasonable fear of which prevents its more widespread use.[116] To prevent this complication, a medication-free interval of 4 weeks following each 6-month course of continuous treatment is recommended. We find methysergide to be a very effective drug with minimal side-effects, but we reserve its use because of the need for a drug holiday.[7]

Pizotifen

Pizotifen is a benzocycloheptathiophene derivative that is structurally similar to cyproheptadine and the TCAs. It has a long elimination half-life (about 23 hours) and can be given as a single evening dose. Pizotifen is a $5-HT_2$ and histamine-1 antagonist with the side-effects of drowsiness and increased appetite with associated weight gain. Pizotifen has proven effective in controlled[117] and placebo-controlled[118-120] trials. In an open trial, it was less effective than methysergide[121] but more effective than placebo. In another placebo-controlled trial, it was as effective as naproxen sodium, and both were more effective than placebo. Pizotifen (2–3 mg) daily was as effective as flunarazine 10 mg daily. Pizotifen is often used for adolescent migraineurs at doses of 0.5–1.5 mg daily. Adults, in contrast, may require up to 3 mg daily. Pizotifen has no interaction with specific antimigraine compounds, such as ergotamine or the triptans. Pizotifen is not available in the USA.

Natural products

Feverfew (Tanacetum parthenium) is a medicinal herb used by some patients to self-treat migraine. The clinical effectiveness of feverfew for migraine prevention has not been established beyond reasonable doubt. More clinical trials are needed, both on a larger scale and with various feverfew extracts, including parthenolide-free sesquiterpene lactone chemotypes.[122]

Riboflavin

Schoenen et al[123] (1988c) compared riboflavin (400 mg) with placebo in migraineurs in a randomized trial of 3 months' duration. Riboflavin was significantly superior to placebo in reducing the attack frequency ($p = 0.005$), headache days ($p = 0.012$), and migraine index (0.012). The proportion of patients improved by at least 50% in headache days, i.e. 'responders', was 15% for placebo, 59% for riboflavin ($p = 0.002$).

Newer treatments

Silberstein et al[124] evaluated the safety and efficacy of pericranial Botulinum toxin type A (Botox[R]): injections as prophylactic treatment of chronic moderate to severe migraine. One hundred twenty-three patients who had two to eight moderate to severe IHS-defined migraine attacks during a 1-month baseline were randomized to treatment with either 0, 25, or 75 U of Botulinum toxin type A injected symmetrically into glabellar, frontalis, and temporalis muscles. The 25 U Botulinum toxin type A treatment group fared significantly better than the placebo group by the following measures: reduction in mean frequency of moderate to severe migraines during days 31–60; incidence of 50% reduction and a decrease in at least two mild to severe migraines at days 61–90; reduction in mild to severe migraine during days 61–90; reduction of days with phonophobia during days 31–90; and improvement by patient global assessment for days 31–60 postinjection. Further studies of this agent are indicated before it is used routinely in clinical practice.

Setting treatment priorities

The goals of treatment are to relieve or prevent the pain and associated symptoms of migraine and to optimize the patient's ability to function normally. The medications used to treat migraine can be divided into five major categories (Table 6.19):

(1) Drugs with documented high efficacy and mild to moderate AEs, which include ß-blockers, amitriptyline, and divalproex;
(2) Drugs with lower documented efficacy and mild to moderate AEs, which include SSRIs, calcium channel antagonists, gabapentin, riboflavin, and NSAIDs;
(3) Drug use based on opinion (a) mild to moderate AEs and (b) major AEs or complex management;
(4) Drugs with documented high efficacy that have significant AEs (or are difficult to use), which include methysergide and MAOIs; and
(5) Drugs with proven limited or no efficacy, which include cyproheptadine, lithium, and phenytoin.

Choose a drug based on its proven efficacy, the patient's preferences and headache profile, the drug's side-effects, and the presence or absence of coexisting or comorbid disease (Table 6.18). Use the drug with the best risk-to-benefit ratio for the individual patient and take advantage of the drug's side-effect profile. An underweight patient would be a candidate for one of the medications that commonly produce weight gain, such as a TCA; in contrast, one would try to avoid these drugs in the overweight patient. Tertiary TCAs that have a sedating effect would be useful at bedtime for patients with insomnia. The older

● Table 6.19 *Preventive drugs*

Efficacy	AEs	Drugs
High	Low to moderate	Propranolol, timolol, amitriptyline, divalproex
High	Prominent	Methysergide
Low	Low to moderate	NSAIDs – aspirin, flurbiprofen, ketoprofen, naproxen sodium β-Blockers—atenolol, metoprolol, nadolol Calcium Channel Blockers—verapamil Anticonvulsants—gabapentin, topirimate Other—fenoprofen, feverfew, vitamin B2 Pizotifen
Unproven	Low to moderate	Antidepressants—doxepin, nortriptyline, imipramine, protriptyline venlafaxine, fluvoxamine, mirtazepine, paroxetine, protriptyline, sertraline, trazodone
	Major or complex management	Methergine, MAOIs
Proven not effective or low		Acebutolol, carbamazepine, clomipramine, clonazepam, indomethacin (indometacin), lamotrigine, nabumetone, nicardipine, nifedipine, pindolol

AEs, adverse effects; NSAID, nonsteroidal antiinflammatory drug; MAOI, monoamine oxidase inhibitor

patient with cardiac disease or patients with significant hypotension may not be able to use TCAs or calcium channel or ß-blockers but could easily use divalproex. In the athletic patient, ß-blockers should be used with caution. Medication that can impair cognitive functioning should be avoided in patients who are dependent on their wits.[52]

Comorbid and coexistent diseases have important implications for treatment. In some instances, two or more conditions may be treated with a single drug. When migraine and hypertension and/or angina occur together, β-blockers or calcium-channel blockers may be effective for all conditions.[6,7] For the patient with migraine and depression, TCAs or SSRIs may be especially useful.[125] For the patient with migraine and epilepsy[80] or migraine and manic depressive illness,[80] divalproex sodium, gabapentin, and topiramate are the drugs of choice. The pregnant migraineur who has a comorbid condition that needs treatment should be given a medication that is effective for both conditions and has the lowest potential for adverse effects on the fetus. If an individual has more than one disease, certain categories of treatment may be relatively contraindicated. For example, β-blockers should be used with caution in the depressed migraineur, while TCAs, neuroleptics, or sumatriptan may lower the seizure threshold and should be used with caution in the epileptic migraineur.

Drug combinations are commonly used for patients with refractory headache disorders. Some combinations, such as antidepressants and β-blockers, are suggested; others, such as β-blockers and calcium-channel blockers, should be used with caution; and some, such as MAOIs and SSRIs, are contraindicated because of potentially lethal interactions (Table 6.20). Many clinicians find that an antidepressant/β-blocker combination acts synergistically. Divalproex or topiramate, used in combination with antidepressants, is a logical choice to treat refractory migraine that is complicated by depression or bipolar disease. Some clinicians cautiously use the combination of phenelzine and amitriptyline in refractory headache patients.

Use of acute medication in patients on preventive treatment

Preventive medication is considered effective if it decreases the attack frequency more than 50%. Thus, patients treated with preventive medication may continue to have attacks of episodic migraine and tension-type headache. Menstrual migraine attacks often persist to a greater extent than nonmenstrual attacks. Preventive medication may also decrease the intensity and duration of the attacks, and in some cases may make acute medications more effective. The use of preventive and abortive medication in concert presents a new set of complexities. First, the amount of acute medication must be limited to prevent the development of drug-induced daily rebound headache and loss of efficacy of the preventive medication. This is one of the causes of secondary failure of

Table 6.20 Drug Combinations

Suggested	
Antidepressants	Beta-blocker
	calcium channel blocker
	divalproex, gabapentin, topiramate
	methysergide
Methysergide	calcium channel blocker
SSRI	TCAs
Caution	
β-blocker	calcium channel blocker
	methysergide
MAOIs	amitriptyline or nortriptyline
Contraindications	
MAOIs	SSRIs
	most TCAs (except amitriptyline or
	nortriptyline)
	doxepin and trazadone
	carbamazepine
NSAIDs	lithium

MAOIs, monoamine oxidase inhibitors; NSAIDs, nonsteroidal antiinflammatory drugs; SSRIs, selective serotonin reuptake inhibitors; TCAs, tricyclic antidepressants

preventive medication. Second, certain abortive medications should be used with caution in the presence of some preventive medications (Table 6.21). Ergotamine, DHE, and sumatriptan could potentially enhance vasospastic properties in the presence of methysergide. However, many authorities have found that the ergots are more effective when patients are treated with methysergide, and we have used the combination in selected patients without any problem. MAOIs increase the half-life and the area under the curve of oral sumatriptan. Therefore, the dose of oral sumatriptan should be reduced and used cautiously, if at all, in patients taking MAOIs. Meperidine and sympathomimetics are a potentially lethal addition to MAOIs and may result in serotonin syndrome or hypertensive crisis.

Status migrainosus

Status migrainosus is an attack of migraine, the headache phase of which lasts more than 72 hours whether it is treated or not.[8] It is characterized by the severe, persistent headache often associated with intractable nausea and vomiting. Factors responsible for triggering status migrainosus include emotional stress, depression, abuse of medications, anxiety, diet, hormonal factors, and multiple nonspecific factors.[126] Status migrainosus may be secondary to an acute neurologic disorder. Prior to instituting treatment, serious organic causes of headache must be excluded.[126] Patients with status migrainosus need aggressive treatment. They usually present in the emergency department, but can be treated in outpatient infusion centers. The principles of treatment for status migrainosus include:

(1) Fluid and electrolyte replacement (if indicated);
(2) Drug detoxification;
(3) Intravenous pharmacotherapy to control pain;
(4) Treatment of associated symptoms of nausea and vomiting; and
(5) Concurrent implementation of migraine prophylaxis (if indicated).

Table 6.21 Cautions in acute medication use

	Caution	Contraindicated
Methysergide	Ergotamine, DHE, 5-HT$_1$ agonists	
Monoamine oxidase inhibitors	Sumatriptan (SC), naratriptan, zolmitriptan, and frovatriptan	Meperidine, sympatho-mimetics (Midrin), rizatriptan, sumatriptan (PO, IN), eletriptan
NSAIDs	Other NSAIDs or aspirin containing compounds	
Divalproex	Overuse of short-acting barbiturates	

NSAIDs, nonsteroidal anti-inflammatory drugs; DHE, dihydroergotamine; PO, orally; IN, intranasally; SC, subcutaneously

We start treatment by rehydrating the patient with intravenous fluids and using one of the treatment options in Table 6.22). If the headache persists and is associated with intractable nausea and vomiting, hospital admission may be required. Some indications for admission are listed in Table 6.23. Various treatment options have been explored for treating this type of headache. IV chlorpromazine and prochlorperazine are effective in controlling intractable headache.[6,7,99,127] Chlorpromazine was found to be more effective than the combination of meperidine and dimenhydrinate, and prochlorperazine was more effective than placebo in treating emergency department

---

● Table 6.22 *Treatment of status migrainosus*

- Start IV
- Pretreat with prochlorperazine 5–10 mg IV or metoclopramide 10 mg IV
- Treat with DHE 0.5–1 mg IV
- If headache persists after 1 hour give additional 0.5 mg DHE IV
- Additions – dexamethasone 4 mg IV; diazepam 5–10 mg IV
- Alternatives: ketorolac 30–60 mg IM
    opioids
    chlorpromazine .1 mg/kg
    droperidol 1–2.5 mg IV or IM

DHE, dihydroergotamine; IM, intramuscular; IV, intravenous

● Table 6.23 *Indications for admission to hospital*

A Emergency or urgent admission

Diagnosis itself warrants admission
- Migraine variants such as hemiplegic migraine.
- Suspected CNS infection.
- Acute vascular disorder.
- Drug toxicity.
- Status migrainosus.
- Failed outpatient treatment of severe headache.

B Nonemergent admission

- Headache causing interruption and compromise of the ability to carry out activities of daily living.
- Chronic daily refractory headache or cluster headache that does not respond to aggressive outpatient treatment.
- Headache complicated by significant depression or psychiatric disturbance.
- Headache accompanied by significant medical or surgical problem.
- Headache treatment requiring polypharmacy with potentially dangerous drug interactions or requiring close observation during initiation (monoamine oxidase inhibitors).
- Headache complicated by drug overuse that could not be safely or effectively treated overnight.

---

patients.[100] Neuroleptics are locally irritating when given intravenously; they are more effective than when given intramuscularly or by suppository. We have found that haloperidol (5 mg), droperidol (1–2.5 mg), and thiothixene (5 mg) given intramuscularly are effective as adjunct or primary treatment for the severe migraine headache.[69] IV haloperidol and IV droperidol have recently been used successfully. We now use repetive intravenous droperidol (1–2.5 mg q6hr) in combination with diphenhydramine suppositories as needed.

IV prochlorperazine 5 mg, followed by IV DHE, is a safe and effective means of terminating a migraine attack.[105] The combination of IV metoclopramide and IV DHE is more effective in treating an acute migraine attack than is IM meperidine.[6,7] Prochlorperazine (10 mg, 2 ml) and DHE (1 mg, 1 ml) can be mixed in a syringe and 2 cc of the mixture can be injected intravenously. If the headache is not relieved in 15–30 minutes, the remainder of the dose can be injected. The addition of 5–10 mg of IV diazepam may help terminate the headache attack.

Repetitive intravenous dihydroergotamine (DHE)

Patients who have truly intractable headaches should be admitted to the hospital and treated with repeated doses of repetitive IV DHE.[9] The patient should be pretreated with metoclopramide 10 mg IV and then given DHE 0.5 mg (Figure 6.20). If the patient has no nausea and the headache persists, another 0.5 mg DHE is given. If the patient's headache is gone, 0.5–1 mg DHE is continued every 8 hours. If nausea develops, the dose of DHE is decreased and the metoclopramide increased. Both drugs are continued as needed, the DHE every 8 hours until the patient is headache-free, at which time it is tapered and discontinued.

Repetitive IV DHE was effective in eliminating chronic intractable headache in 89% of patients within 48 hours in one series. IV diazepam was only partially effective in eliminating such headaches (13% within 3–6 days). We have found that repetitive IV DHE is effective in eliminating prolonged migraine, providing a break from attacks to patients with cluster headache, and is helpful in the management of chronic daily headache of the chronic migraine type, with or without rebound.

By breaking the headache cycle and making the patient's headaches more manageable, IV DHE seems to have a prolonged effect on the patient's well-being. It is uncertain whether this is a result of DHE, the active metabolite 8-hydroxydihydroergotamine, the cessation of overused drugs, or the removal of the patient from a stressful environment, but patients frequently do well after hospital discharge.[125]

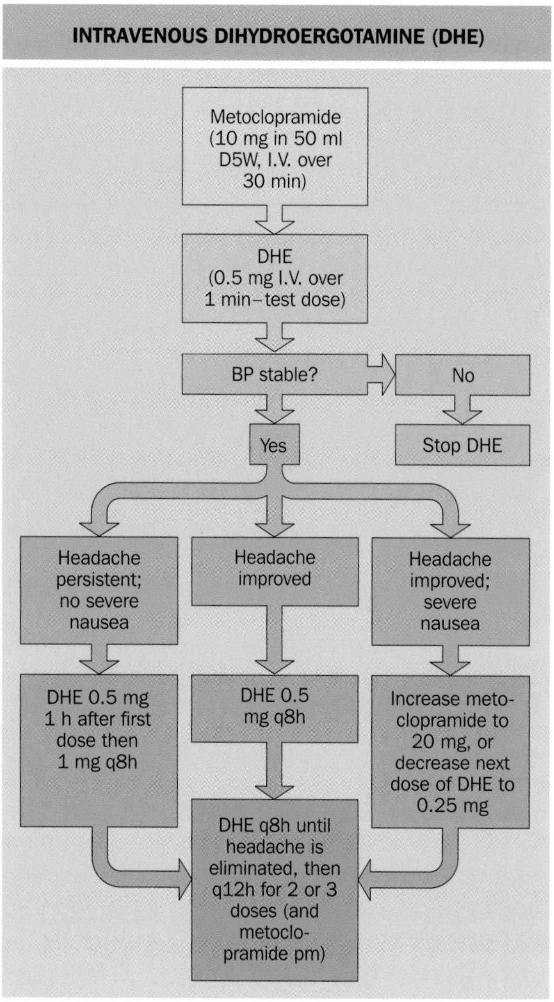

INTRAVENOUS DIHYDROERGOTAMINE (DHE)

● **Figure 6.20** *Treatment protocol of repetitive intravenous dihydroergotamine (DHE).*

Some clinicians advocate the use of parenteral corticosteroids, either alone or in combination with other symptomatic medications, to treat the severe resistant headache. Controlled studies have shown corticosteroids to be effective in the treatment of headache associated with altitude sickness.[6,7] Dexamethasone 4 mg IV following pretreatment with IV metoclopramide may be effective in the treatment of acute migraine headache.[6,7] The addition of dexamethasone to a narcotic regimen seems to provide additional relief.[6,7] Clinical experiences also support the view that steroids, such as a rapidly-tapering short course of prednisone (starting with 80–100 mg/day) or dexamethasone (Decadron[T], starting with 8–20 mg/day), will assist in terminating an otherwise refractory migraine

headache. Inpatients can be treated with high-dose IV corticosteroids, alone or in conjunction with neuroleptics or DHE, to help terminate a headache cycle.

Some advocate using naproxen or indomethacin rectal suppositories or IM ketorolac, especially in situations where neuroleptics, narcotics, and DHE are relatively contraindicated.

A maximum of two doses of sumatriptan (6 mg SC) separated by 1 hour can be given within 24 hours. However, sumatriptan should not be given for at least 24 hours following ergotamine or DHE. A repeat injection is not effective if injection fails. Headache recurrence, which occurs in about 40% of patients, may limit sumatriptan's use in status migrainosus and chronic daily headache.

After acute treatment is completed, most patients with status migrainosus require continuing care. This should include a preventive treatment program using standard migraine preventive drugs.

Menstrual migraine

Migraine can occur before, during, or after menstruation, or at the time of ovulation.[129] When migraine occurs before menstruation (premenstrual migraine) it may be associated with other features of premenstrual syndrome (PMS) (Table 6.24). Migraine that occurs during menstruation is often associated with dysmenorrhea and may be more difficult to treat. It is important to differentiate between the two conditions, because medications that may be useful in treating headache related to dysmenorrhea may not help headache associated with PMS.[127]

The prevalence of menstrual migraine depends upon the definition used and the population studies; in clinical-based series, the frequency of menstrual migraine has been reported to be as high as 60–70%. Based on retrospective analysis, prevalence ranges from 26% to 60% in headache clinic patients. The prevalence is lower in non-headache clinic patients. The relative frequency of menstrual migraine depends on the means of ascertainment.[130] Women with migraine are more likely to have

● **Table 6.24** *Premenstrual syndrome*

Depression	Backache
Anxiety	Breast tenderness
Crying spells	Swelling
Difficulty in thinking	Nausea
Lethargy	

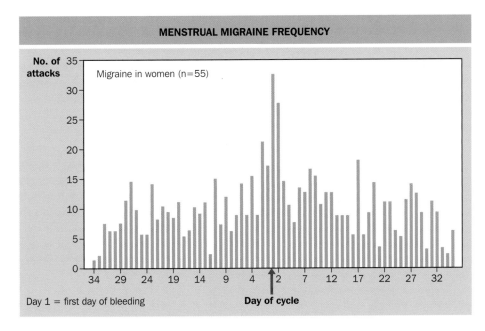

migraine headaches at the time of menses (Figure 6.21). Women with PMS have more headaches prior to the onset of menses, but most women have more headaches just before or with menstruation. Some women have migraine (usually without aura) only with menses. Menstrual migraine can be defined by looking at attacks triggered by menstruation on a regular basis (Table 6.25). Attacks that occur only with menstruation, even if infrequent, have been called 'true menstrual migraine'. Attacks that occur both at menstruation and at other times of the month are termed 'menstrually triggered migraine'. A frequency indicator (e.g. frequent >70%, common 35–70%, and infrequent <35%) would look at the tightness of this association. The quality of these attacks, their response to treatment, and the hormonal changes in such patients could then be analysed based on this association. Migraine attacks occurring 2–7 days before the onset of menses would be called 'premenstrual'; those occurring from −1 to +4 days, 'menstrual'. These cut-offs are arbitrary.[129] In our view, the hormonal events surrounding menstruation trigger migraines in biologically vulnerable individuals; menstrual migraine is not a different type of migraine.

Menstrual migraine occurs at the time of the greatest fluctuation in estrogen levels (Figure 6.22). Attempts to find consistent differences in ovarian hormone levels between women with menstrual migraine and controls have not yielded consistent results. Some authors have reported higher estrogen and progestin levels, but others have not;[129] most find that testosterone, follicle-stimulating hormone, and luteinizing hormone (LH) levels are similar to controls. In Beckham et al's[131] study, headache activity correlated with high progesterone during the luteal phase. Since progesterone is the marker for the luteal phase, it tells us nothing regarding any causal association between luteal headaches and progesterone.[129]

● **Table 6.25** *Menstrual migraine definition*

Premenstrual migraine	Menstrual migraine
Attacks occur −7 to −2 days*	Attacks occur −1 to +4 days*
* Day 0 onset of menses	

● **Table 6.26** *Treatment of menstrual migraine*

Standard preventive treatment
Short-term perimenstrual preventive treatment<BI>
  Nonsteroidal anti-inflammatory drugs (NSAIDs)
  Ergotamine and its derivatives
  Triptans
  Magnesium
Hormonal therapy
  Estrogens (with or without androgens or progestin)
  Combined oral contraceptives
  Synthetic androgens (danazol)
  Antiestrogen (tamoxifen)
  Medical oophorectomy (GnRH analogs)
Dopamine agonists (bromocriptine)

GnRH, gonadotrophin-releasing hormone

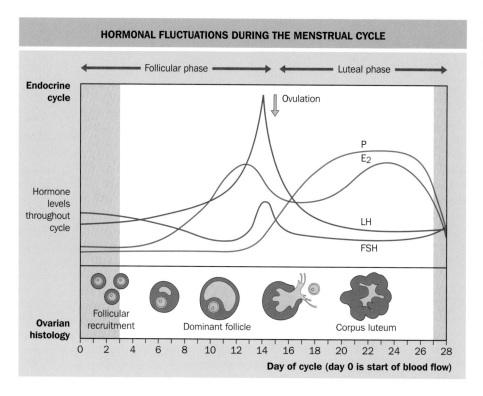

HORMONAL FLUCTUATIONS DURING THE MENSTRUAL CYCLE

● *Figure 6.22*
Hormonal fluctuations during the menstrual cycle.

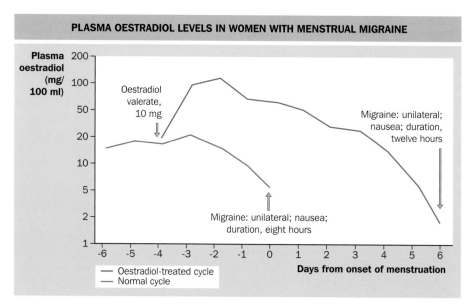

PLASMA OESTRADIOL LEVELS IN WOMEN WITH MENSTRUAL MIGRAINE

● *Figure 6.23*
Plasma oestradiol levels in women with menstrual migraine (adapted from ref. 132).

Somerville[132] reported that menstrual migraine headache occurs during or after the simultaneous fall of estrogens and progesterone. Estrogens given premenstrually delay the onset of migraine but not menstruation.[129] In contrast, progesterone administration delays menstruation but does not prevent migraine.[129] Somerville concluded that estrogen withdrawal may trigger migraine attacks in susceptible women (Figure 6.23). Estrogen-withdrawal migraine requires several days of exposure to high levels of estrogen. When Somerville used an erratic delivery system of long-acting estrogen implants to suppress migraine, his patients developed irregular bleeding and headaches associated with fluctuating estrogen levels.

The initial treatment of women who have migraine

throughout their menstrual cycle should include general measures, such as reassurance, identification and elimination of triggers, use of abortive and prophylactic medications, psychological modalities, and sleep hygiene.[129] These measures may eliminate all headaches except those associated with the menses.[129] Menstrually-related migraine typically occurs at the same time of month or in association with symptoms that herald its occurrence, allowing the timed use of medications (Table 6.26).[129] Menstrual migraine may differ from nonmenstrual migraine in that menstrual migraine is not associated with an aura, is of longer duration, and may be more subject to headache recurrence after treatment. Drugs that have proven effective or are commonly used for the acute treatment of menstrual migraine include NSAIDs, DHE, the triptans, and AAC.

Prostaglandin production may be enhanced in menstrual migraine. The effectiveness of the NSAIDs[129] may be a result of blocking prostaglandin synthesis by inhibiting the enzyme COX. The meclofenamates, in addition, are prostaglandin receptor antagonists. One NSAID, ketoprofen, inhibits the formation of leukotrienes by inhibiting 5-lipooxygenase. NSAIDs in adequate doses can be used abortively or prophylactically 1–2 days before the expected onset of headache and continued for the duration of vul-

nerability. If the first NSAID is ineffective, other classes of NSAIDs should be tried (Figure 6.24).[129]

DHE is effective for the treatment of menstrual migraine.[69,133,134] Sumatriptan, zolmitriptan, and rizatriptan are as effective for menstrually associated migraine[135] as for nonmenstrually associated migraine and, in addition, control the nausea and vomiting associated with attacks.[136,137] If severe menstrual migraine cannot be controlled with NSAIDs, ergots, DHE, or selective $5HT_1$ agonists (triptans), then analgesics combined with opioids, opioids alone,[7] high dose corticosteroids, major tranquilizers (chlorpromazine, haloperidol, thiothixene, droperidol), or a course of IV DHE can be tried.[7,69] Women with frequent, severe menstrual migraine are candidates for preventive therapy (either continuous or short-term) and often respond better to acute therapy when on preventive treatment.

Women who are using preventive medication but continue to have menstrual migraine can increase the medication dose prior to their menses. Women who do not use preventive medicine or have migraine exclusively with their menses can just be treated perimenstrually with short-term prophylaxis.[138–140] Regular periods and a predictable relationship between the attacks and the menses are essential for this strategy to succeed. Treating coexistent PMS may help control premenstrual headache. Drugs that have been used perimenstrually for short-term prophylaxis include NSAIDs, ergotamine, DHE, methysergide, methergine, the triptans, and magnesium. NSAIDs in adequate doses can be used preventively 1–2 days before the expected onset of headache and continued for the duration of vulnerability. If the first NSAID fails, a different NSAID from another chemical class should be tried.

Ergotamine and DHE can be used prophylactically at the time of menses without significant risk of developing ergot dependence. Ergotamine tartrate, at bedtime or twice a day, is an effective prophylactic agent. Ergotamine in combination with belladonna and phenobarbital (Bellergal[T]) may be useful in treating other PMS symptoms in addition to headache.[129]

DHE NS, given every 8 hours for 6 days beginning 3 days before the expected onset of headache, was used in a placebo-controlled, double-blind, short-term trial for the treatment of menstrual migraine. The mean pain severity rating for DHE NS was lower than placebo for 67.5% of the 40 evaluable patients.[141]

Oral sumatriptan (25 mg tid) was used 2–3 days before the expected headache onset and continued for a total of 5 days in an open-label study of 20 women with menstrual migraine.[142] In 126 sumatriptan-treated cycles, headache was absent in 52.4% of subjects and reduced in severity

PROSTAGLANDINS AND THE MECHANISM OF ACTION OF NSAID

Cell → Cell lysis → Arachidonic acid → COX 1 / COX 2 → Endoperoxides → Prostacyclins (PGE$_1$), Prostaglandins PGE$_1$, PGE$_2$, Thromboxane A$_2$ (Thromboxane B$_2$)

NSAIDs ← COX 1, COX 2
Selective COX 2 Inhibitors ← COX 2

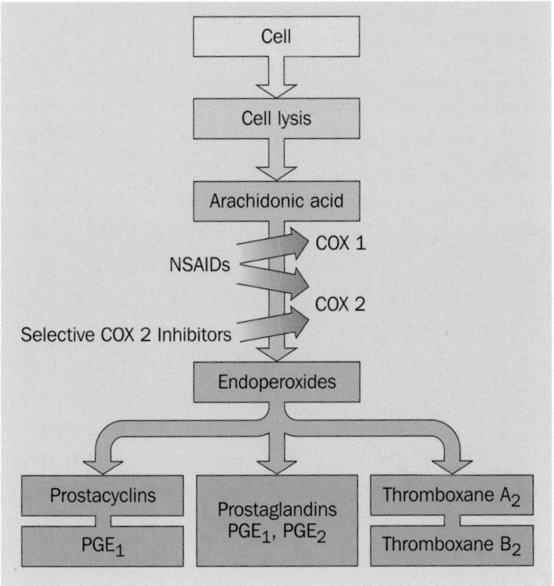

● *Figure 6.24* *Prostaglandins and the mechanism of action of NSAID.*

by 50% or greater in 42%. Breakthrough headaches were rare and significantly reduced in severity compared with the baseline headaches. Naratriptan, which has a longer half-life than sumatriptan, is currently in placebo-controlled, double-blind trials for short-term perimenstrual prophylaxis of menstrual migraine.[142]

Popular but ineffective treatments for menstrual migraine include diuretics and vitamins. Diuretics help with fluid retention but not with menstrual migraine.[143,144] The efficacy of pyridoxine to treat both PMS and menstrual migraine has not been proven in double-blind studies.[145,146]

If severe menstrual migraine cannot be controlled with these measures, a trial of hormonal therapy may be indicated.[129] Successful hormonal therapy of menstrual migraine has been reported with estrogens,[136] estrogen antagonists, prolactin-release inhibitors, and estrogens in combination with progesterone or testosterone. Progesterone is not effective in the treatment of headache or other symptoms of PMS despite many favorable anecdotal reports.[129]

The decrease in estrogen levels during the late luteal phase of the menstrual cycle is a trigger for migraine,[99] and estrogen replacement prior to menstruation has been used to prevent migraine. In two double-blind crossover studies, percutaneous estradiol gel used perimenstrually significantly reduced headache.[129] Magos et al, in both an open and a double-blind study, found estradiol implants (available investigationally in the USA) and cyclic progesterones to be effective in menstrual migraine.[147] The estradiol cutaneous patch provides a relatively stable plasma-estrogen level over the time of application.[148] Levels are less stable with higher dose patches. Serum estrogen levels rise within 4 hours of applying the transdermal patch and are proportional to the dose (patch TTS 25, serum level of 23 pg/ml; TTS 50, serum level 39 ng/ml; TTS 100 serum level 74 pg/ml).[149]

The TTS 25 patch used from 4 days before to 4 days after menstruation was not as effective as the TTS 100 patch.[150] It may be necessary to maintain the serum estradiol level between 60 and 80 pg/ml during the crucial week to prevent menstrual migraine.[129] TTS 50 patches (TTS = 39 pg/ml) were not significantly different from placebo in one placebo-controlled double-blind trial[150] and in another placebo-controlled trial, except for patients who had abnormal CNV and normal ES2.[151]

A combination of estrogens and progestogens or progestogens alone in the form of oral contraceptives (discussed below) is a reasonable approach for some patients with intractable menstrual migraine, particularly if it is associated with severe dysmenorrhea.[129] We now use continuous oral contraceptives with breaks every 3–4 months

as a first-line therapy.

Danazol, an androgen derivative, may be effective in the prophylaxis of menstrual migraine at a dose of 200–600 mg/day, starting before the expected onset of the headache and continuing through the menses.[129] Tamoxifen, an anti-estrogen, in doses of 5–15 mg/day for days 7–14 of the luteal cycle has provided significant relief of menstrual headache without side-effects.[129] Both these treatments should be reserved for very severe menstrual migraine that is refractory to other modalities.

Hysterectomy and oophorectomy have not been shown to be effective migraine treatment; we do not recommend this approach. However, medical ovariectomy using gonadotrophin-releasing hormone (GnRH) analogs to suppress ovulation are effective in refractory PMS. Since GnRH analogs induce menopause, treatment is usually limited to 6 months unless replacement estrogens are used.[129]

Premenstrual migraine sufferers who have had a hysterectomy without an oophorectomy continue to have cyclic mental and physical symptoms during the late luteal phase of the menstrual cycle, demonstrating that neither the presence of the uterus nor the occurrence of menstruation is necessary for the maintenance of PMS.[129]

Some physicians are again advocating the use of hysterectomy and oophorectomy for women with severe intractable PMS or menstrual migraine who respond to medical ovariectomy.[152,153] There are no long-term follow-up or controlled studies to suggest the effectiveness of this radical procedure.

The effects of ovariectomy and hysterectomy on PMS and headache are contaminated by the postoperative use of daily estrogen. No study is placebo-controlled, and women with PMS are very sensitive to placebo. The use of continuous estrogen alone could account for the positive results.[153]

Another strategy is a dopamine receptor agonist, either short-term or continuously. Bromocriptine (Parlodel[T]),[154–157] a dopamine D2 receptor agonist, is an inhibitor of PRL release. A dose of 2.5–5 mg a day during the luteal phase of the menstrual cycle may decrease the premenstrual symptoms of breast engorgement, irritability, and headache. In an open trial,[158] 24 women with severe, disabling menstrual migraine (occurring within 3 days of menstruation) were treated with continuous bromocriptine, 2.5 mg three times daily. Seventy-five per cent of the women had at least a 25% reduction in headache compared to baseline. Overall headache frequency decreased 72%. None of the patients had less than a 10% increase in headache; three could not tolerate bromocriptine, and three did not benefit.

Migraine in the menopause

Menopause is the permanent cessation of menstruation. In postmenopausal women, steroid sex hormone levels are low and gonadotropin levels are elevated. The menopause is associated with both early and late symptoms. Hot flushes, a vasomotor change, correlate with bursts of activity in hypothalamic pacemaker neurons leading to pulses of GnRH and, thus, LH. Hormonal replacement with estrogens (estrogen replacement therapy), alone or in combination with progestins (hormone replacement therapy), is often used to treat symptoms and prevent steoporosis.

Although migraine prevalence peaks in the early 40s, either exacerbations or improvement may occur at menopause. Neri et al[159] investigated 556 consecutive postmenopausal women attending an outpatient clinic and found that headache was present in 13.7%. Most had headache prior to the onset of menopause. Many (62%) had migraine without aura; the remainder had tension-type headache. None had migraine with aura or cluster headache. Two-thirds of women with prior migraine improved with physiological menopause. In contrast, two-thirds of women who had surgical menopause had worsening of migraine. Other studies have shown that hysterectomy or oophorectomy is not an effective treatment for migraine at any age,[160] despite recent suggestions to the contrary.[149,161] Estrogen replacement therapy can exacerbate migraine or, alone or with testosterone, relieve it.[129] This has been confirmed in one, but not another, double-blind study. The use of drugs for treatment of migraine in menopausal women who do not need replacement estrogens should be guided by their cardiac and renal status. Refractory cases may be treated with hormonal replacement.[129,135]

Headache management can be difficult in women who require estrogen replacement therapy for menopausal symptoms but develop headaches as a result of the therapy. Several empirical strategies may be utilized (Table 6.27). Reducing the dose of estrogen or changing the type of estrogen from a conjugated estrogen to pure estradiol, to synthetic ethinyl estradiol, or to a pure estrone may significantly reduce headache. Changing from interrupted to continuous administration may be very effective if the headaches are associated with estrogen withdrawal. Parenteral estrogens, with or without adjunct hormones, can be effective. The estradiol cutaneous patch, which provides a physiological ratio of estradiol to estrone and a steady-state concentration of estrogen, has been associated anecdotally with fewer headache side-effects; however, this has not been proven in any controlled study.

● **Table 6.27** *Treatment of oestrogen replacement headache*

- Reduce oestrogen dose
- Change oestrogen type from conjugated oestrogen to pure oestradiol to synthetic oestrogen to pure oestrone
- Convert from interrupted to continuous dosing
- Convert from oral to parenteral dosing
- Add androgens

Migraine associated with oral contraceptive use

Hormonal contraceptive steroids are available as oral preparations (oral contraceptives, OCs), SC implants, depo-injections, and, in some countries, vaginal preparations.[160,162] The transdermal estrogen patch has been advocated for contraception by some.[148,153] There are three major types of OC formulations: two are combined oral contraceptives (fixed-dose and phasic combinations) and one is progestin only. The OCs most commonly used in the USA contain combinations of synthetic estrogen (ethinyl estradiol or mestranol) and synthetic progestin. In an attempt to minimize the associated androgenic side-effects, the type of synthetic progestin has been changed. The sequential formulations use fixed amounts of estrogen and progestin; these are taken 21 days each month and followed by a steroid-free period of 7 days.[163,164] There has been a progressive decrease in the ethinyl estradiol content in COCs; most now contain 35 mg or less. Formulations with 50 μg or more of estrogen are now called first-generation OCs. Those with less than 50 μg of estrogen are called second generation OCs. Formulations with the new progestins, desogestrel, norgestimate, and gestodene, are called third-generation OCs.

The new formulation of OCs, containing 35 mg of ethinyl estradiol and one of the new progestins, are comparable in efficacy with each other and with established agents (Table 6.28).[165–169] In addition, they may be associated with stronger suppression of ovarian activity. These properties have allowed a further reduction in the estrogenic content of OCs to 20 μg; no data show that further decreases in the estrogen dose confer any added benefit.[170] Absolute contraindications to OC use include a history of vascular disease, including thromboembolism, thrombophlebitis, atherosclerosis, and stroke, and systemic disease that may affect the vascular system, such as lupus erythematosus or diabetes with retinopathy or nephropathy. Uncontrolled hypertension and cigarette smoking by OC users over age 35 are also contraindications.

● **Table 6.28** *Oral contraceptives*

Progestin	Dose (mg)	Oestrogen	Dose (μg)
Monophasic			
Desogestrel	0.15	Ethinyloestradiol	30, 35
Ethynodiol diacetate	1.0	Ethinyloestradiol	35, 50
Levonorgestrel	0.15	Ethinyloestradiol	30
Norethindrone	0.4, 0.5, 1.0	Ethinyloestradiol	30, 35, 50
Norethindrone acetate	1.0, 1.5	Ethinyloestradiol	20, 30, 50
Norgestimateol	0.25	Mestranol	50
Norgestrel	0.5	Ethinyloestradiol	50
Multiphasic			
Norethindrone	0.5 (7), 1.0 (14)	Ethinyloestradiol	35
Norethindrone	0.5 (7), 0.75 (7), 1.0 (7)	Ethinyloestradiol	35
Norgestamate	0.180 (7), 0.215 (7), 0.290 (7)	Ethinyloestradiol	30

● **Table 6.29** *Oral contraceptives and stroke risk*

Factor		Odds ratio
Oestrogen dose (μg)	>50	8–10
	50	2–4
	30–40	1.5–2.5
Progestogen alone		1
Smoking		1.5–1.6

Adapted from Lidegaard.[171]

Persistent controversy exists concerning OCs and the risk of stroke in migraineurs. During the last two decades, at least 15 retrospective studies have looked at the influence of OCs on the risk of cerebral thromboembolic events. Most (11/15) were conducted during a period when high-dose estrogen pills were widely used. These data suggest that OCs that contain more than 50 μg, 50 μg, and 30–40 μg of estrogen are associated with odds ratios for cerebral thromboembolic attacks of about 8–10, 2–4, and 1.5–2.5, respectively, whereas those containing only a progestin are not associated with any increased risk (Table 6.29).[171]

Bousser and Kittner[172] reviewed the relationship between OCs and stroke. Since 1962, more than 25 studies devoted to the relationship between OCs and stroke have been performed. They are all case–control or cohort epidemiologic studies and thus contain the difficulties and biases that are inherent in these types of studies. The following conclusions can be drawn from these studies: high estrogen content (≥50 μg) increases the risk of stroke, all stroke subtypes, and stroke death; low estrogen content (<50 μg) carries a very low or no risk of stroke; there are no data on progestogen-only OCs; stroke risk is greatly increased if associated risk factors are present, in particular, hypertension, cigarette smoking, and migraine; OCs, even at low doses, significantly increase the risk of cerebral venous thrombosis, which is further enhanced if congenital thrombophilia is present; and the attributable risk of stroke in young women using OCs is about one per 200 000 woman-years. The contra-

ceptive and noncontraceptive benefits of low-dose OCs vastly outweigh their risks, provided other risk factors are absent or well controlled.

The older combined OCs can induce, change, or alleviate headache. OCs can trigger the first migraine attack, most often in women with a family history of migraine. Existing migraine may exacerbate and headaches may occur on the days off the OC. The headache pattern may become more severe and frequent and may be associated with neurologic symptoms. In most women, however, the headache pattern does not change, and some women may have a distinct improvement in their headaches.[129]

New onset of migraine usually occurs in the early cycles of OC use, but it can occur after prolonged OC usage. Stopping the OCs may not bring immediate headache relief, or there may be a delay of 6–12 months or no improvement. Studies from neurologic or migraine clinics show increased incidence and severity of migraine in users of the older OCs. While headaches frequently occur on the days off the OC, many women have relief with OCs. Studies from contraceptive clinics and general practitioners are more favorable towards OCs. Four double-blind, placebo-controlled studies showed no difference in headache incidence between OC and placebo. Both groups had a decreasing incidence of headache with continued observation. Some uncontrolled studies show an increase in headache frequency in women on OCs. A new OC containing 35 mg of the new, third-generation progestin, norgestimate (Ortho-Cyclen[T]), was associated with a low incidence of headaches over three cycle intervals.

Contraception with progestins alone is a hormonal alternative to the use of the combined OCs. Progestins have no effect on blood clotting or platelet aggregation and are the contraceptive of choice for hypertensive women.

Norplant[T], a system of subdermal implants that release a steady dose of levonorgestrel (a progestin), is an effective contraceptive that lasts 5 years. The primary side-effects are irregular menstrual bleeding and headaches.

Headache, which was the primary reason cited for removal other than menstrual disturbance, occurs in about 5–20% of patients. Recently, Depo-Provera[T] (medroxyprogesterone acetate suspension), a long-acting parenteral progestin, has been approved as a contraceptive agent. The exact frequency of headache with use of this drug is uncertain.

The IHS Task Force concluded that there is no contraindication to the use of OCs in women with migraine in the absence of migraine aura or other risk factors.[173] We use them with caution in women with migraine with typical aura in the absence of other risk factors. Women should be counseled and regularly assessed for additional risk factors. There is a potentially increased risk of ischemic stroke in women with migraine who are using combined oral contraceptives and have additional risk factors. Risk factors should be identified and evaluated; migraine type, particularly migraine with aura, should be diagnosed; women who have migraine and smoke should stop smoking before starting combined oral contraceptives; other risk factors, such as hypertension and hyperlipidemia, should be treated; and nonethinylestradiol methods should be considered for women who are at increased risk of ischemic stroke, particularly those with multiple risk factors. Progestogen-only hormonal contraceptive use is probably not associated with an increased risk of ischemic stroke. No specific tests need to be undertaken other than those routinely performed or indicated by the patient's history or the presence of specific symptoms, e.g. a patient with a relative who experienced arterial disease when aged 45 years or less. Migraine-related symptoms that may necessitate further evaluation and/or cessation of combined oral contraceptives include a new persisting headache, new onset of migraine aura, increased headache frequency or intensity, or the development of unusual aura symptoms, particularly prolonged aura.

OCs may generate new headaches or aggravate or ameliorate pre-existing headaches. This variability is also noted with pregnancy and menopause and may be a consequence of a variation in intrinsic estrogen neuronal response. Women with intractable menstrual migraine or a history of headache relief with oral contraceptives may be candidates for a trial of OCs. They must be followed for headache aggravation or the development of neurologic symptoms. Progestins can be used for contraception when estrogens have caused increased headaches or are contraindicated.

References

1. Adler CS, Adler SM, Friedman AP. A historic perspective on psychiatric thinking about headache. In: Adler CS, Adler SM, Packard RC, eds. Psychiatric Aspects of Headache. Baltimore: Williams and Wilkins, 1987, 3–21.

2. Lipton RB, Diamond S, Reed M et al. Migraine diagnosis and treatment: results from the American Migraine Study II. Headache 2001; 41: 638–45.

3. Lipton RB, Stewart WF, Diamond S et al. Prevalence and burden of migraine in the United States: data from the American Migraine Study II. Headache 2001; 41: 646–57.

4. Stewart WF, Lipton RB, Celentano DD, Reed ML. Prevalence of migraine in the United States. Relation to age, income, race, and other sociodemographic factors. JAMA 1992; 267: 64–9.

5. Lipton RB, Stewart WF. Migraine in the United States: epidemiology and healthcare utilization. Neurology 1993; 43: 6–10.

6. Silberstein SD, Lipton RB. Overview of diagnosis and treatment of migraine. Neurology 1994; 44: 6–16.

7. Silberstein SD, Saper JR, Freitag F. Migraine: diagnosis and treatment. In: Silberstein SD, Lipton RB, Dalessio DJ, eds. Wolff's Headache and other Head Pain. 7th ed. New York: Oxford University Press, 2001, 121–237.

8. Headache Classification Committee of the International Headache Society. Classification and diagnostic criteria for headache disorders, cranial neuralgia, and facial pain. Cephalalgia 1988; 8: 1–96.

9. Silberstein SD, Young WB. Migraine aura and prodrome. Sem Neurol 1995; 45: 175–82.

10. Jensen K, Tfelt-Hansen P, Lauritzen M, Olesen J. Classic migraine, a prospective recording of symptoms. Acta Neurol Scand 1986; 73: 359–62.

11. Blau JN. Classical migraine: symptoms between visual aura and headache onset. Lancet 1992; 340: 355–6.

12. Olesen J. Some clinical features of the acute migraine attack. An analysis of 750 patients. Headache 1978; 18: 268–71.

13. Sacks O. Migraine: understanding a common disorder. Berkeley: University of California Press, 1985.

14. Selby G, Lance JW. Observation on 500 cases of migraine and allied vascular headaches. J Neurol Neurosurg Psychiatry 1960; 23: 23–32.

15. Manzoni G, Farina S, Lanfranchi M, Solari A. Classic migraine–clinical findings in 164 patients. Eur Neurol 1985; 24: 163–9.

16. Bradshaw P, Parsons M. Hemiplegic migraine, a clinical study. Q J Med 1965; 133: 65–85.

17. Stewart WF, Schechter A, Lipton RB. Migraine heterogeneity: disability, pain intensity, attack frequency, and duration. Neurology 1994; 44: S24-S39.

18. Silberstein SD. Migraine symptoms: results of a survey of self-reported migraineurs. Headache 1995; 35: 387–96.

19. Lipton RB, Silberstein SD, Stewart WF. An update on the epidemiology of migraine. Headache 1994; 34: 319–28.

20. Bickerstaff ER. Migraine variants and complications. In: Blau JN, ed. Migraine: Clinical and Research Aspects. Baltimore: Johns Hopkins University Press, 1987, 55–75.

21. Hosking G. Special forms: variants of migraine in childhood. In: Hockaday JM, ed. Migraine in childhood. Boston: Butterworths, 1988, 35–53.

22. Mark AS, Casselman J, Brown D et al. Ophthalmoplegic migraine: reversible enhancement and thickening of the

cisternal segment of the oculomotor nerve on contrast-enhanced MR images. Am J Neuroradiol 1998; 19: 1887–91.

23. Nelson JA, Wolfe MD, Yuh WT, Peeples ME. Cranial nerve involvement with Lyme borreliosis demonstrated by magnetic resonance imaging. Neurology 1992; 42 (suppl 3, part 1): 673.

24. Pachner AR, Duray P, Steere AC. Central nervous system manifestations of Lyme disease. Arch Neurol 1989; 46: 790–5.

25. Blake PY, Mark AS, Kattah J, Kolsky M. MR of oculomotor nerve palsy. Am J Neuroradiol 1995; 16: 241–51.

26. Schmitt T, Erbguth F, Taghavy A. Oculomotor paralysis as the leading symptom of meningovascular syphilis: report of two patients and review of the literature. Nervemarzt 1993; 64: 668–72.

27. May M. Idiopathic (Bell's) palsy, herpes zoster and other facial nerve disorders of viral origin. In: May M, ed. The Facial Nerve. New York: Thieme Medical, 1986, 365–99.

28. Hansen SL, Borelli-Miller L, Strange P et al. Opthalmoplegic migraine: diagnostic criteria, incidence of hospitalization and possible etiology. Acta Neurol Scand 1990; 81: 54–60.

29. de Arcaya AA, Cerezal L, Canga A et al. Neuroimaging diagnosis of Tolosa-Hunt syndrome: MRI contribution. Headache 1999; 39: 321–5.

30. Whitty CWM. Familial hemiplegic migraine. In: Rose FC, ed. Handbook of Clinical Neurology. New York: Elsevier, 1986, 141–53.

31. Tournier-Lasserve E. Hemiplegic migraine, episodic ataxia type 2, and the others. Neurology 1999; 53: 3–4.

32. Ophoff RA, Terwindt GM, Vergouwe MN. Familial hemiplegic migraine and episodic ataxia type-2 are caused by mutations in the Ca2+ channel gene CACNLA4. Cell Tiss Res 1996; 87: 543–52.

33. Gardner K, Barmada MM, Ptacek LJ, Hoffman EP. A new locus for hemiplegic migraine maps to chromosome 1q31. Neurology 1997; 49: 1231–8.

34. Ducros A, Joutel A, Vahedi K. Mapping of a second locus for familial hemiplegic migraine to 1q21–q23 and evidence of further heterogeneity. Ann Neurol 1997; 42: 885–90.

35. Ducros A, Deiner C, Joutel A et al. The clinical spectrum of familial hemiplegic migraine associated with mutations in a neuronal calcium channel. N Eng J Med 2001; 345: 17–24.

36. Tournier-Lasserve E, Joutel A, Melki J. Cerebral autosomal arteriopathy with subcortical infarcts and leukoencephalopathy maps to chromosomes. Nat Genet 1993; 3: 256–9.

37. Hutchinson M, O'Riordan J, Javed M et al. Familial hemiplegic migraine and autosomal dominant arteriopathy with leukoencephalopathy. Ann Neurol 1995; 38: 817–24.

38. Chabriat H, Vahedi K, Iba-Zizen MT et al. Clinical spectrum of CADASIL: a study of seven families. Lancet 1995; 346: 934–9.

39. Joutel A, Vahedi K, Corpechot C et al. Strong clustering and stereotyped nature of Notch3 mutations in CADASIL patients. Lancet 1997; 350: 1511–15.

40. Joutel A, Corpechot C, Ducros A et al. Notch3 mutations in CADASIL, a hereditary adult-onset condition causing stroke and dementia. Nature 1996; 383: 707–10.

41. Chabriat H, Tournier-Lasserve E, Vahedi K et al. Autosomal dominant migraine with MRI white-matter abnormalities mapping to the CADASIL locus. Neurology 1995; 45: 1086–91.

42. Whitty CWM. Migraine without headache. Lancet 1967; ii: 283–5.

43. Levy DE. Transient CNS deficits: a common, benign syndrome in young adults. Neurology 1988; 38: 831–6.

44. Fisher CM. Late life migraine accompaniments as a cause of unexplained transient ischemic attacks. Can J Neurol Sci 1980; 7: 9–17.

45. Wijman C, Wolf PA, Kase CS et al. Migrainous visual accompaniments are not rare in late life: the Framingham Study. Stroke 1998; 29: 1539–43.

46. Fisher CM. Late-life migraine accompaniments – further experience. Stroke 1986; 17: 1033–42.

47. Lipton RB, Silberstein SD. Why study the comorbidity of migraine? Neurology 1994; 44: 4–5.

48. Ramadan NM, Silberstein SD, Freitag FG et al. Evidence-based guidelines of the pharmacological management for prevention of migraine for the primary care provider. Neurology 1999. Available at: http:/www.neurology.org

49. Matchar DB, Young WB, Rosenberg JA et al. Evidence-based guidelines for migraine headache in the primary care setting: pharmacological management of acute attacks. http: //www aan com 2000;

50. Cady RK, Lipton RB, Hall C et al. Treatment of mild headache in disabled migraine sufferers: results of the Spectrum Study. Headache 2000; 40: 792–7.

51. Lipton RB, Stewart WF, Hall CB et al. Sumatriptan (50 mg) treats the full spectrum of headaches in disabling migraine: Results of a randomized, double-blind, placebo-controlled trial.

Headache 2000; (In Press)

52. Silberstein SD. Preventive treatment of migraine: an overview. Cephalalgia 1997; 17: 67–72.

53. Lipton RB, Stewart WF, Stone AM et al. Stratified care vs. step care strategies for migraine. The Disability in Strategies of Care (DISC) study, a randomized trial. JAMA 2000; 284: 2499–505.

54. Pradalier A, Clapin A, Dry J. Treatment review: nonsteroid antiinflammatory drugs in the treatment and long-term prevention of migraine attacks. Headache 1988; 28: 550–7.

55. Campbell WB. Lipid-derived autocoids: eicosanoids and platelet-activating factor. In: Gilman AG, Rall TW, Taylor P, eds. The Pharmacological Basis of Therapeutics 8th ed. New York: Pergamon Press, 1990, 600–17.

56. Cashman J, McAnulty G. Nonsteroidal antiinflammatory drugs in perisurgical pain management: mechanisms of action and rationale for optimum use. Drugs 1995; 49: 51–70.

57. Wallace JL, Cirino G. The development of gastrointestinal-sparing nonsteroidal antiinflammatory drugs. Trends Pharmacol Sci 1994; 15: 405–6.

58. Frölich JC. A classification of NSAIDs according to the relative inhibition of cyclooxygenase isoenzymes. Trends Pharmacol Sci 1997; 18: 30–4.

59. Lipton RB, Stewart WF, Ryan RE et al. Efficacy and safety of the nonprescription combination of acetaminophen, aspirin, and caffeine in alleviating headache pain of an acute migraine attack: three double-blind, randomized, placebo-controlled trials. Arch Neurol 1998; 55: 210–17.

60. Lipton RB, Baggish JS, Stewart WF, Codispoti M. Efficacy and safety of acetaminophen in the treatment of migraine: results of a randomized, double-blind, placebo-controlled, population-based study. Arch Intern Med 2000; 160: 3486–92.

61. Silberstein SD. Twenty questions about headaches in children and adolescents. Headache 1990; 30: 716–27.

62. Kellstein DE, Lipton RB, Geetha R et al. Evaluation of a novel solubilized formulation of ibuprofen in the treatment of migraine headache: a randomized, double-blind, placebo-controlled, dose-ranging study. Cephalalgia 2000; 20: 233–43.

63. Goldstein JL, Silverstein FE, Agrawal NM et al. Reduced risk of upper gastrointestinal ulcer complications with celecoxib, a novel COX-2 inhibitor. Am J Gastroenterol 2000; 95: 1681–90.

64. Silberstein SD, McCrory DC. Butalbital in the treatment of headache: history,

pharmacology, and efficacy. Headache 2001; 41: 953–67.

65. Silberstein SD, Young WB. Safety and efficacy of ergotamine tartrate and DHE in the treatment of migraine and status migrainosus. For the working panel of the headache and facial pain section of the American Academy of Neurology. Neurology 1995; 45: 577–84.

66. Saper JR. Changing perspectives of chronic headache. Clin J Pain 1986; 2: 19–28.

67. Tfelt-Hansen P, Saxena PR, Dahlof C et al. Ergotamine in the acute treatment of migraine: a review and European consensus. Brain 2000; 123: 9–18.

68. Raskin NH. Repetitive intravenous dihydroergotamine as therapy for intractable migraine. Neurology 1986; 36: 995–7.

69. Silberstein SD, Schulman EA, Hopkins MM. Repetitive intravenous DHE in the treatment of refractory headache. Headache 1990; 30: 334–9.

70. Edmeads J. Emergency management of headache. Headache 1988; 28: 675–9.

71. Silberstein SD. Practice parameter – evidence-based guidelines for migraine headache (an evidence-based review): report of the Quality Standards Subcommittee of the American Academy of Neurology for the United States Headache Consortium. Neurology 2000; 55: 754–62.

72. Ferrari MD, Roon KI, Lipton RB, Goadsby PJ. Oral triptans (serotonin 5-HT$_{1B/1D}$ agonists) in acute migraine treatment: a metaanalysis of 53 trials. Lancet 2001; 358: 1668–75.

73. Pilgrim AJ, Blakeborough P. The clinical efficacy of sumatriptan in the acute treatment of migraine. Rev Contemp Pharmacother 1994; 5: 295–310.

74. Edmeads J. Advances in migraine therapy: focus on oral sumatriptan. Neurology 1995; 45: 3–4.

75. Goadsby PJ, Lipton RB, Ferrari MD. Migraine – current understanding and treatment. N Engl J Med 2002; 346: 257–70.

76. Gray RN, Goslin RE, McCrory DC et al. Drug treatments for the prevention of migraine headache. Prepared for the Agency for Health Care Policy and Research, Contract No. 290–94–2025 (Technical Review 2.3, February). Available from the National Technical Information Service, Accession No. 127953. 1999.

77. Färkkilä M. A dose-finding study of eletriptan (UK-116,044) (5–30 mg) for the acute treatment of migraine. Cephalalgia 1996; 16: 387–8.

78. Goadsby PJ, Ferrari MD, Olesen J et al. Eletriptan in acute migraine: a double-blind, placebo-controlled comparison to sumatriptan. Eletriptan Steering

Committee. Neurology 2000; 54: 156–63.

79. Reches A. Comparison of the efficacy, safety and tolerability of oral eletriptan and Cafergot® for the acute treatment of migraine. On behalf of the Eletriptan Steering Committee. Cephalalgia 1999; 19: 355 (Abstract).

80. Kempsford RD, Baille P, Fuseau E. Oral naratriptan tablets (2.5 mg–10 mg) exhibit dose-proportional pharmacokinetics. Neurology 1997; 48: A66 (Abstract).

81. Klassen A, Elkind A, Asgharnjad M et al. Naratriptan tablets are effective and well-tolerated in the acute treatment of migraine: results of a double-blind, placebo-controlled, parallel group trial. Headache 1997; 37: 640–5.

82. Teall J, Tuchman M, Cutler N et al. Rizatriptan (MAXALT) for the acute treatment of migraine and migraine recurrence. A placebo-controlled, outpatient study (Rizatriptan 022 Study Group). Headache 1998; 38: 281–7.

83. Visser WH, Klein KB, Cox RC et al. 311C90, a new central and peripherally acting 5-HT$_{1D}$ receptor agonist in the acute oral treatment of migraine: a double-blind, placebo-controlled, dose-range finding study. Neurology 1996; 46: 522–6.

84. Goadsby PJ, Edvinsson L. Peripheral and central trigeminovascular activation in cat is blocked by serotonin (5HT)-1D receptor agonist 311C90. Headache 1994; 34: 394–9.

85. Goadsby PJ, Hoskin KL. Inhibition of trigeminal neurons by intravenous administration of the serotonin (5HT1B/D receptor agonist zolmitriptan (311C90): are brainstem sites a therapeutic target in migraine? Pain 1996; 67: 355–9.

86. Goadsby PJ, Knight YE. Direct evidence for central sites of action of zolmitriptan (311C90): an autoradiographic study in cat. Cephalalgia 1997; 17: 153–8.

87. Thomsen LL, Dixon R, Lassen LH et al. 311C90 (zolmitriptan), a novel centrally and peripheral acting oral 5-nydroxytryptamine-1D agonist: a comparison of its absorption during a migraine attack and in a migraine-free period. Cephalalgia 1996; 16: 270–5.

88. Palmer KG, Spencer CM. Zolmitriptan. CNS Drugs 1997; 7: 468–78.

89. Rapoport AM, Ramadan NM, Adelman JU et al. Optimizing the dose of zolmitriptan (Zomig, 311C90) for the acute treatment of migraine: a multicenter, double-blind, placebo-controlled, dose range-finding study. 017 Clinical Trial Study Group. Neurology 1997; 49: 1210–18.

90. Solomon GD, Cady RK, Klapper JA et al. Clinical efficacy and tolerability of

2.5 mg zolmitriptan for the acute treatment of migraine. Neurology 1997; 49: 1219–25.

91. Gallagher RM, Dennish G, Spierings EL, Chitra R. A comparative trial of zolmitriptan and sumatriptan for the acute oral treatment of migraine. Headache 2000; 40: 119–28.

92. Dowson A. Can oral 311C90, a novel 5-HT1D agonist, prevent migraine headache when taken during an aura? Eur Neurol 1996; 36(suppl 2): 28–31.

93. Goadsby PJ. A triptan too far? J Neurol Neurosurg Psychiatry 1998; 64: 143–7.

94. Robert M, Cabarrocas X, Zayas JM et al. Overall response of oral almotriptan in the treatment of three migraine attacks. On behalf of the Almotriptan Multiple Attacks Study Group. Cephalalgia 1999; 19: 363 (Abstract).

95. Pascual J, Falk RM, Piessens F et al. Consistent efficacy and tolerability of almotriptan in the acute treatment of multiple migraine attacks: results of a large, randomized, double-blind, placebo-controlled study. Cephalalgia 2000; 20: 488–96.

96. Easthope S, Goa KL. Frovatriptan. CNS Drugs 2001; 15: 1–7.

97. Bates D, Ashford E, Dawson R et al. Subcutaneous sumatriptan during the migraine aura. Neurology 1994; 44: 1587–92.

98. Silberstein SD. Migraine and pregnancy. Neurol Clin 1997; 15: 209–31.

99. Callaham M, Raskin N. A controlled study of dihydroergotamine in the treatment of acute migraine headache. Headache 1986; 26: 168–71.

100. Jones J, Sklar D, Dougherty J, White W. Randomized double-blind trial of intravenous prochlorperazine for the treatment of acute headache. JAMA 1989; 261: 1174–85.

101. Wang SJ, Silberstein SD, Young WB. Droperidol treatment of status migrainosus and refractory migraine. Headache 1997; 37: 377–82.

102. Silberstein SD, Young WB, Mendizabal J et al. Efficacy of intramuscular droperidol for migraine treatment: a dose response study. Neurology 2001; 56: A64 (Abstract).

103. Silberstein SD, Young WB, Mendizabal JE et al. Acute migraine treatment with the dopamine receptor antagonist, droperidol: results of a randomized, double-blind, placebo-controlled, multicenter trial. Submitted for publication 2001;

104. Silberstein SD, Willmore LJ. Divalproex sodium: migraine treatment and monitoring. Headache 1996; 36: 239–42.

105. Saper JR, Silberstein SD, Lake AE, Winters ME. Double-blind trial of

fluoxetine: chronic daily headache and migraine. Headache 1994; 34: 497–502.

106. Stein DJ, Hollander E. Sexual dysfunction associated with the drug treatment of psychiatric disorders: incidence and treatment. CNS Drugs 1994; 2: 78–86.

107. Varadi G, Mori Y, Mikala G, Schwartz A. Molecular determinants of Ca2+ channel function and drug action. Trends Pharmacol Sci 1995; 2: 43–9.

108. Silberstein SD, Collins SD. Safety of divalproex sodium in migraine prophylaxis: an open-label, long-term study (for the long-term safety of depakote in headache prophylaxis study group). Headache 1999; 39: 633–43.

109. Silberstein SD. Divalproex sodium in headache – literature review and clinical guidelines. Headache 1996; 36: 547–55.

110. Mathew NT, Rapoport A, Saper J et al. Efficacy of gabapentin in migraine prophylaxis. Headache 2001; 41: 119–28.

111. Shuaib A, Ahmed F, Muratoglu M, Kochanski P. Topiramate in migraine prophylaxis: a pilot study. Cephalalgia 1999; 19: 379 (Abstract).

112. Edwards KR, Glantz MJ, Shea P et al. A double-blind, randomized trial of topiramate versus placebo in the prophylactic treatment of migraine headache with and without aura. Cephalalgia 2000; 20: 316 (Abstract).

113. Potter DL, Hart DE, Calder CS, Storey JR. A double-blind, randomized, placebo-controlled, parallel study to determine the efficacy of topiramate in the prophylactic treatment of migraine. Neurology 2000; 54: A15 (Abstract).

114. Coulam CB, Annagers JR. New anticonvulsants reduce the efficacy of oral contraception. Epilepsia 1979; 20: 519–25.

115. Hanston PP, Horn JR. Drug interaction. Newsletter 1985; 5: 7–10.

116. Silberstein SD. Methysergide. Cephalalgia 1998; 18: 421–35.

117. Speight TM, Avery GS. Pizotifen (BC-105): a review of its pharmacological properties and its therapeutic efficacy in vascular headaches. Am J Med Sci 1972; 240: 327–31.

118. Arthur GP, Hornabrook RW. The treatment of migraine with BC105 (pizotifen): a double-blind trial. N Z Med J 1971; 73: 5–9.

119. Lawrence ER, Hossain M, Littlestone W. Sanomigran for migraine prophylaxis: controlled multicenter trial in general practice. Headache 1977; 17: 109–12.

120. Capildeo R, Rose FC. Single-dose pizotifen, 1.5 mg nocte: a new approach in the prophylaxis of

migraine. Headache 1982; 22: 272–5.

121. Curran DA, Lance JW. Clinical trial of methysergide and other preparations in the management of migraine. J Neurol Neurosurg Psychiatry 1964; 27: 463–9.

122. Vogler BK, Pittler MH, Ernst E. Feverfew as a preventive treatment for migraine: a systematic review. Cephalalgia 1998; 18: 704–8.

123. Schoenen et al. 1998.

124. Silberstein SD, Mathew N, Saper J, Jenkins S. Botulinum toxin type A as a migraine preventive treatment. Headache 2000; 40: 445–50.

125. Silberstein SD, Lipton RB, Breslau N. Migraine: association with personality characteristics and psychopathology. Cephalalgia 1995; 15: 337–69.

126. Couch JR, Diamond S. Status migrainosus: causative and therapeutic aspects. Headache 1983; 23: 94–101.

127. Silberstein SD. Status migrainosus. La Jolla: Arbor, 1995.

128. Bell R, Montoya D, Snualb A, Lee MA. A comparative trial of three agents in the treatment of acute migraine headache. Ann Emerg Med 1990; 19: 1079–82.

129. Silberstein SD, Merriam GR. Sex hormones and headache. In: Goadsby PJ, Silberstein SD, eds. Headache. Newton: Butterworth–Heinemann, 1997,143–73.

130. Johannes CB. Hormonal factors in the relationship to migraine headache attacks in young women. A dissertation submitted to The Johns Hopkins University in conformity with the requirements for the degree of Doctor of Philosophy. 1989: (UnPub)

131. Beckham et al.

132. Somerville BW. The role of estradiol withdrawal in the etiology of menstrual migraine. Neurology 1972; 22: 355–65.

133. D'Alessandro R, Gamberini G, Lozito A, Sacquegna T. Menstrual migraine, intermittent prophylaxis with a timed-release pharmacological formulation of dihydroergotamine. Cephalalgia 1983; 3: 156–8.

134. Diamond S, Freitag FG, Diamond ML, Urban GJ. Subcutaneous dihydroergotamine mesylate (DHE) in the treatment of menstrual migraine. Headache Q1996; 7: 145–7.

135. Solbach MP, Waymer RS. Treatment of menstruation-associated migraine headache with subcutaneous sumatriptan. Obstet Gynecol 1993; 82: 769–72.

136. de Lignières B, Vincens M, Mauvais-Jarvis P et al. Prevention of menstrual migraine by percutaneous oestradiol. Br Med J (Clin Res Ed) 1986; 293: 1540.

137. Sheftel F, Silberstein SD, Rapoport A. Pharmacological treatment of chronic headache. Drug Therapy 1992; 22: 47–59.

138. Silberstein SD, Merriam GR. Estrogens, progestins, and headache. Neurology 1991; 41: 775–93.

139. Raskin NH. Headache 2nd ed. New York: Churchill–Livingstone, 1988.

140. Silberstein SD, Saper JR. Migraine: diagnosis and treatment. In: Dalessio DJ, Silberstein SD, eds. Wolff's Headache and other Head Pain. 6th ed. New York: Oxford University Press, 1993, 96–170.

141. Silberstein SD. DHE-45 in the prophylaxis of menstrually related migraine. Cephalalgia 1996; 16: 371.

142. Newman LC, Lipton RB, Lay CL, Solomon S. A pilot study of oral sumatriptan as intermittent prophylaxis of menstruation-related migraine. Neurology 1998; 51: 307–9.

143. Lundberg PO. Endocrine headaches. In: Rose FC, ed. Handbook of Clinical Neurology. Volume 48 ed. New York: Elsevier, 1986, 431–40.

144. Reid RL, Yen SSC. Premenstrual syndrome. Am J Obstet Gynecol 1981; 139: 85–104.

145. Williams MJ, Harris RI, Dean BC. Controlled trial of pyridoxine in the premenstrual syndrome. J Int Med Res 1985; 1: 174–9.

146. Hagen I, Nesheim B, Tuntland T. No effect of vitamin B-6 against premenstrual tension: a controlled clinical study. Acta Obstet Gynecol Scand 1985; 64: 667–70.

147. Magos AL, Brincat M, Studd JWW. Treatment of the premenstrual syndrome by subcutaneous estradiol implants and cyclical oral norethisterone: placebo controlled study. Br Med J (Clin Res Ed) 1986; 292: 1629–33.

148. Stumpf PG. Pharmacokinetics of estrogen. Obstet Gynecol 1990; 75: 9–17.

149. Schwartz J, Freeman R, Frishman W. Clinical pharmacology of estrogens: cardiovascular actions and cardioprotective benefits of replacement therapy in postmenopausal women. J Clin Pharmacol 1995; 35: 1–16.

150. Pfaffenrath V. Efficacy and safety of percutaneous estradiol vs. placebo in menstrual migraine. Cephalalgia 1993; 13: 168 (Abstract).

151. Smits MG, VanderMeer YG, Pfeil JP et al. Perimenstrual migraine: effect of estraderm TTS and the value of contingent negative variation and exteroceptive temporalis muscle suppression test. Headache 1993; 34: 103–6.

152. Casson P, Hahn PM, VanVugt DA, Reid

RL. Lasting response to ovariectomy in severe intractable premenstrual syndrome. Obstet Gynecol 1990; 162: 99–105.

153. Watson NR, Studd JW, Savvas M et al. Treatment of severe premenstrual syndrome with estradiol patches and cyclical oral norethisterone. Lancet 1989; 2: 730–2.

154. Wentz AC. Management of the menopause. In: Jones HW, Wentz AC, Burnett LS, eds. Novak's Textbook of Gynecology 11th ed. Baltimore: Williams and Wilkins, 1985, 397–442.

155. Andersch B, Hahn L, Wendestam C et al. Treatment of premenstrual syndrome with bromocriptine. Acta Endocrinol 1978; 88: 165–74.

156. Ylostalo P, Kauppila A, Puolakka J et al. Bromocriptine and noresthisterone in the treatment of premenstrual syndrome. Obstet Gynecol 1982; 58: 292–8.

157. Andersen AN, Larsen JF, Steenstrup OR et al. Effect of bromocriptine on the premenstrual syndrome: a double-blind clinical trial. Br J Obstet Gynecol 1977; 84: 370–4.

158. Herzog AG. Continuous bromocriptine therapy in menstrual migraine. Neurology 1995; 48: 101–2.

159. Neri I, Granella F, Nappi RMGC et al. Characteristics of headache at menopause: a clinico-epidemiologic study. Maturitas 1993; 17: 31–7.

160. Baird DT, Glasier AF. Hormonal contraception. N Eng J Med 1993; 328: 1543–9.

161. Pradalier A, Vincent D, Beaulieu PH et al. Correlation between estradiol plasma level and therapeutic effect on menstrual migraine. In: Rose FC, ed. New advances in Headache Research 4th ed. London: Smith-Gordon, 1994, 129–32.

162. MacGregor EA, DeLignieres B. The place of combined oral contraceptives in contraception. Cephalalgia 2000; 20: 157–63.

163. Wentz AC. Contraception and family planning. In: Jones HW, Wentz AC, Burnett LS, eds. Novak's Textbook of Gynecology 11th ed. Baltimore: Williams and Wilkins, 1985, 204–39.

164. Derman R. Oral contraceptives: a reassessment. Obstet Gyn Survey 1989; 44: 662–8.

165. Speroff L, DeCherney A, The Advisory Board for the New Progestins. Evaluation of a new generation of oral contraceptives. Obstet Gynecol 1993; 81: 1034–47.

166. Corson SL. Contraceptive efficacy of a monophasic oral contraceptive containing desogestrel. Am J Obstet Gynecol 1993; 168: 1017–20.

167. Huber J. Clinical experience with a new norgestimate-containing oral contraceptive. Int J Fertil 1992; 32: 47–53.

168. Dunson TR, McLaurin VL, Israngkura B et al. A comparative study of two low-dose combined oral contraceptives: results from a multicenter trial. Contraception 1993; 48: 109–19.

169. Shoupe D. Effects of desogestrel on carbohydrate metabolism. Am J Obstet Gynecol 1993; 168: 1041–7.

170. Mishell DR. Family planning: contraception, sterilization, and pregnancy termination. In: Mishell DR, Stenchever MA, Droegemueller W, Herbst AL, eds. Comprehensive Gynecology 3rd ed. St. Louis: Mosby, 1997; 283–52.

171. Lidegaard Ø. Oral contraception and risk of a cerebral thromboembolic attack: results of a case–control study. Br Med J Clin Res 1993; 306: 956–63.

172. Bousser MG, Kittner SJ. Oral contraceptives and stroke. Cephalalgia 2000; 20: 183–9.

173. Bousser MG, Conard J, Kittner S et al. Recommendations on the risk of ischemic stroke associated with use of combined oral contraceptives and hormone replacement therapy in women with migraine (the International Headache Society Task Force on Combined Oral Contraceptives and Hormone Replacement therapy). Cephalalgia 2000; 20: 155–6.

chapter 7

Tension-type headache: diagnosis and treatment

A primary headache disorder requires exclusion of other disorders. Patients with secondary organic headache types often have symptoms that mimic tension-type headache (TTH). Pericranial tenderness can also be found in other primary headaches, as well as asymptomatic headaches, e.g. intracerebral lesions, such as tumour or haemorrhage and therefore, one must be alert for atypical symptoms or any abnormalities on neurologic examination.

This vague, ambiguous description is not operational. It not only includes clinical features, triggers, and a proposed mechanism (contraction of skeletal muscles), but suggests that the headache has a psychological basis, which is a prejudiced and unproven allegation.[3,4] The IHS definition[1] attempts to define this type of headache more precisely and to distinguish between patients with episodic tension-type headache (ETTH) and those with chronic tension-type headache (CTTH). CTTH is used by the IHS[1] instead of 'chronic daily headache' (CDH), which they state was the previously used term. CDH and CTTH are not identical and the substitution has created confusion.[4] TTH of both the episodic and chronic type are now subclassified into those associated with or unassociated with disorder of the pericranial muscles. These subclassifications are based on the presence or absence of tenderness or increased electromyographic (EMG) activity. TTH is no longer presumed to be caused by chronic muscle contraction, but it may be associated with muscle tenderness and increased EMG activity. We will review the new IHS classification of TTH and discuss the pathogenesis and treatment of TTH as well as its relationship to migraine. The IHS system remains imperfect; the degree to which TTH should ever have features of nausea, photophobia, or phonophobia needs to be considered, and will be in the current revision process. CDH will be considered in Chapter 8.

Episodic tension-type headache

Definition and clinical characteristics

ETTH is defined[1] as recurrent episodes of headache that meet the IHS diagnostic criteria (Table 7.1). TTH is the most common headache type there is. The lifetime prevalence (in Denmark) is 69% in men and 88% in women and the 1-year prevalence is 63% in men and 86% in women.[5] In Israel, the prevalence of non-migrainous headaches in Jewish immigrants is 65% in men and 66% in women.[6] In the United States, the 1-year prevalence of TTH is about 40%, with a slight female preponderance (Figure 7.1) (See Chapter 3).[7]

TTH varies in frequency as well as in severity, from rare, brief episodes to frequent, often continuous, disabling headaches. In Denmark, 59% of the population had 1 day or less each month of TTH, and 3% had more than 15 days a month.[8] In the United States, 0.5% of the population have daily severe headache.[9] The 1-year prevalence of frequent (> 1 per month) TTH is 20–30%. TTH is more prevalent in women than in men; the prevalence declines with age in both sexes. TTH prevalence does not differ significantly with socioeconomic background.[10,11] Among Danish TTH sufferers, only 16% had ever consulted a doctor because of their headache.[10]

TTH classically has no premonitory symptoms or aura, although the headache that follows a migraine aura may be featureless.[1] The pain is a dull, achy, non-pulsatile feeling of tightness, pressure, or constriction (vice-like or hatband-like), and is usually mild to moderate in severity, in contrast to the moderate to severe pain of migraine. The pain intensity increases with the headache attack frequency.[12] Most patients have bilateral pain, but the location varies considerably within and between patients, and can involve the frontal, temporal, occipital, or parietal regions, alone or in combination; it commonly changes location during the attack.[8] Occipital location is less common than frontal or temporal location. Some patients have neck or jaw discomfort or have frank problems with their temporomandibular joint.[13] The presence of reciprocal clicking of the temporomandibular joint or pain with maximum jaw opening and pain upon palpation are said to be sensitive clinical signs of oromandibular dysfunction.[14] Unilateral headache occurs in 10–20% of patients.[11,12] Whether these patients had CDH of the chronic migraine type, hemicrania continua, or true ETTH is not clear. Scalp tenderness is more frequent and more severe in migraine or TTH patients during a headache than in non-headache controls, is greatest at the site of the headache, and may persist for several days after the headache subsides.[15] TTH does not usually interfere with daily activities[13] and physical activity normally has no influence on headache intensity.[16]

Some patients may have tender spots and sharply

● **Table 7.1** *Tension-type headache (IHS)*

2.1	**Episodic tension-type headache**

Diagnostic criteria:

A At least 10 previous headache episodes fulfilling criteria (B–D) listed below. Number of days with such headache <180/year (<15/month).

B Headache lasting from 30 minutes to 7 days.

C At least two of the following pain characteristics:
1 Pressing/tightening (non-pulsating) quality.
2 Mild or moderate intensity (may inhibit, but does not prohibit activities).
3 Bilateral location.
4 No aggravation by walking stairs or similar routine physical activity.

D Both of the following:
1 No nausea or vomiting (anorexia may occur).
2 Photophobia and phonophobia are absent, or one but not the other is present.

2.1.1 Episodic tension-type headache associated with disorder of pericranial muscles

Diagnostic criteria:

A Fulfills criteria for 2.1.

B At least one of the following:
1 Increased tenderness of pericranial muscles.
2 Increased EMG level of pericranial muscles.

2.1.2 Episodic tension-type headache unassociated with disorder of pericranial muscles

Diagnostic criteria:

A Fulfills criteria for 2.1.

B No increased tenderness or EMG activity of pericranial muscles.

2.2 Chronic tension-type headache

Diagnostic criteria:

A Average headache frequency >15 days/month (180 days/year) for >6 months fulfilling criteria (B–D).

B At least two of the following pain characteristics:
1 Pressing/tightening quality.
2 Mild or moderate severity (may inhibit but does not prohibit activities).
3 Bilateral location.
4 No aggravation by walking stairs or similar routine physical activity.

C Both of the following:
1 No vomiting.
2 No more than one of the following: nausea, photophobia or phonophobia.

2.2.1 Chronic tension-type headache associated with disorder of pericranial muscles

2.2.2 Chronic tension-type headache unassociated with disorder of pericranial muscles

DIAGNOSIS OF EPISODIC TENSION-TYPE HEADACHE

Headache pain accompanied by two of the following symptoms:

• Pressing/tightening (nonpulsating) quality
• Bilateral location
• Not aggravated by routine physical activity

Headache pain accompanied by both of the following symptoms:

• No nausea or vomiting
• Photophobia and phonophobia absent or only one present

Fewer than 15 days per month with headache

No evidence of organic disease

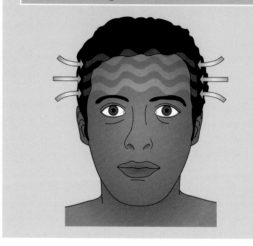

● **Figure 7.1** *Diagnosis of episodic tension-type headache.*

localized nodules in the pericranial or cervical muscles that can be detected by manual palpation of the pericranial and neck muscles. In general, ETTH sufferers, whether or not they are having a headache, have more muscle tenderness than do headache-free controls.[17] Most patients have no associated symptoms, but some report slight photophobia, phonophobia, or nausea.[8] Lack of sleep is a common precipitating factor, with TTH occurring in 39% of healthy volunteers after sleep deprivation.[18] TTH subjects have more problems sleeping than do migraineurs or non-headache controls.[19,20] TTH is subdivided by the IHS up to the fourth digit code to indicate possible causative factors. This empiric subdivision is useful mainly for research purposes. For example, coexistence of oromandibular dysfunction and headache is frequent but could be due to chance. The prevalence of oromandibular dysfunction does not differ between subjects with frequent TTH, migraineurs, and headache-free persons.[21] Psychological and psychiatric causative factors, defined according to the DSM-IV criteria, could be the result, rather than the cause, of recurrent pain. In fact, a prospective population-based study showed that moderate to severe nonmigrainous headache is a risk factor for depression.[22]

A primary headache disorder requires exclusion of other organic disorders. TTH is the most frequent but the least distinct of the primary headache disorders. Its clinical diagnosis is based chiefly on the absence of symptoms that characterize migraine (unilaterality, pulsatility, aggravation by physical activity, associated symptoms, etc.). There is no diagnostic test for TTH. Patients with secondary organic headache types often have symptoms that mimic TTH.[23] Pericranial tenderness can also be found in other primary headaches, as well as asymptomatic headaches, e.g. in intracerebral lesions, such as tumour or haemorrhage; therefore, one must be alert for atypical symptoms or any abnormalities on neurologic examination.

The prognosis and clinical course of TTH are variable. Patients with frequent ETTH may be at increased risk of developing CTTH over a period of many years.[14] Whether patients with more severe TTH are at increased risk for developing migraine or whether migraineurs are more likely to develop more severe and frequent TTH is still controversial.

Differential diagnosis

Tension-type headache is the most frequent but the least distinct of the primary headache disorders. Its diagnosis is based chiefly on the absence of symptoms that characterize migraine (unilaterality, pulsatility, aggravation by physical activity, and associated symptoms). Patients with secondary organic headache types often have symptoms that mimic TTH.[23] Pericranial tenderness occurs in both migraine and in symptomatic headaches due to meningitis and subarachnoid haemorrhage. Since there is no laboratory test that will confirm the diagnosis of TTH (or any of the other primary headaches), one must always consider an underlying structural or metabolic disease when evaluating a patient who fulfills the diagnostic criteria of TTH. This is especially true if the headaches are of recent onset, if the headache changes, if there are important symptoms other than those associated with the primary headaches, and if there are positive neurological signs.

TTH may be misdiagnosed as a 'sinus headache' if the headache is bifrontal (anterior to the frontal sinuses) or if a postnasal drip or thickening of the sinus mucosa is present, or as a 'cervicogenic headache' if neck stiffness or cervical spondylosis is present. However, one should not be reassured that a patient has TTH just because routine physical and neurologic examinations are normal. Daily headaches can be due to a chronic subdural haematoma or to increased intracranial pressure secondary to idiopathic intracranial hypertension. The headaches are easily diagnosed when papilloedema is present. If the patient does not have papilloedema, it can be difficult to differentiate the headache from CTTH. Metabolic changes such as those associated with subtle carbon monoxide poisoning can also mimic a TTH.[24]

The pain of oromandibular or temporomandibular joint dysfunction or disease may radiate to the temple and beyond and may be misdiagnosed as TTH. Pain arising from disease or dysfunction of the cervical structures may radiate to the occipital areas and sometimes to other parts of the head, but neck movement almost invariably is a trigger that distinguishes dental disease from ETTH. Head and neck disease may trigger a TTH. Dental disease and sinusitis, as well as less common disorders, should be looked for if a patient complains of this type of pain.

Migraine and ETTH have traditionally been considered distinct entities. The IHS continues this distinction, although patients can be classified as having both migraine and TTH. However, some clinicians and epidemiologists believe that migraine and TTH are related entities that differ more in severity than in kind.[25–31] Both migraine and TTH may be 'benign recurring headaches which occur in the headache-prone'. The majority of migraineurs (62%) also have TTH, and 25% of TTH patients also have migraine. A migraine headache may begin as a TTH that develops migrainous features when it increases in severity.[29]

Iversen et al[8] examined the clinical characteristics of migraine and ETTH in relation to the old ad hoc and the new IHS diagnostic criteria. Eighty-one patients diagnosed as having migraine, TTH, or both, according to previous criteria,[1] were re-analysed using the new IHS diagnostic criteria. Use of the new IHS criteria did not radically change the headache diagnosis.

Sixty-three percent of patients with only ETTH, 17% of patients with only migraine, and 41% of patients with both disorders had pericranial and neck muscle tenderness. ETTH pain was usually mild to moderate in severity and changed location in half the attacks. Almost 20% of the ETTHs were unilateral and 10% were pulsating and throbbing. ETTH was more variable and often shorter in duration than migraine.

Routine physical activity typically aggravates pain in migraine but not in TTH. However, physical activity exacerbates TTH in patients who also have migraine. Photophobia, phonophobia, and nausea are less frequent in patients who have only TTH than in patients who also have migraine. Iversen[8] has speculated that patients with both migraine and TTH may differ from patients with pure TTH. What we call 'TTH' may be two distinct disorders. The first disorder may be attacks of mild migraine. The second may be a pure TTH that is not associated with other features of migraine (sensitivity to movement, nausea, or photophobia) or with attacks of severe migraine. The fact that sumatriptan is effective for TTH that occurs in migraineurs but not for TTH that occurs in nonmigraineurs supports this concept.[32]

CTTH (Table 7.1) requires head pain for 15 days a month for at least 6 months; many patients have daily headaches. Although the pain criteria are identical to ETTH, the IHS allows nausea but not vomiting, or either photophobia or phonophobia occurring alone, while the presence of nausea is consistent with the IHS diagnosis of CTTH but not ETTH.[1] This anomaly is likely to be corrected in the revision of the IHS classification, with nausea being eliminated from the criteria for TTH. These headaches are often diffuse or bilateral and frequently involve the posterior aspect of the head and neck. Patients with CTTH, in contrast to those with chronic migraine, do not have prior or coexistent episodic migraine, and most features of migraine are absent, as well. We proposed several modifications to the 1988 IHS classification of CTTH.[33,34] The need to include any migrainous features in the IHS definition of CTTH may be a result of the practice of including chronic migraine under the rubric of CTTH. If chronic migraine is classified separately, there may be no need to include migrainous features in the diagnostic criteria for CTTH; indeed, it is desirable to define CTTH so it can be studied. Coexistent migraine and CTTH might exist with the caveat that the nonmigrainous headaches have no migrainous features. Guitera et al have suggested, based on population-based epidemiological data, that CTTH and migraine can coexist if and only if the current headache has no migrainous features and there is a remote history of migraine.[35]

CTTH that has evolved from ETTH presupposes prior evidence of ETTH. Diagnostic confidence increases if ETTH frequency increases to meet the criteria of CTTH. Although there is no explicit headache duration in the IHS definition of CTTH, available evidence does not support a critical value. (We arbitrarily chose 4 hours to separate out cluster headache and the other shorter-duration daily headaches.) It is likely that CTTH is itself aetiologically and biologically heterogeneous. We also distinguish between CTTH associated with medication overuse (2.2.01) and CTTH not associated with medication overuse (2.2.0.2.).

Mechanisms of tension-type headache

The previous belief that TTH arose from the sustained contraction of pericranial muscles, perhaps as a consequence of emotion or tension or a reaction to head pain, led to this headache being called 'muscle contraction headache'. Tonic muscle contraction could then lead to tissue ischaemia and a 'vascular' headache. Migraineurs have as much if not more muscle contraction than patients with TTH,[23,36–38] and, in fact, we now know that no correlation exists between muscle contraction, tenderness, and the presence of headache.[39] Biofeedback using EMG is as effective in TTH as in migraine.[40] There is no evidence of muscle ischaemia in TTH. Temporal muscle blood flow is normal in CTTH at rest and during teeth clenching,[41] and amyl nitrite (a vasodilator) worsens TTH.[42,43]

During an attack, most migraine and TTH patients have more muscle tenderness than do nonheadache controls.[44] While the total amount of muscle tenderness correlates to headache intensity, there is no pattern to the tenderness or correlation to the headache site. In addition, some nonheadache controls have tender spots.[45] TTH patients frequently have normal pericranial EMG levels when recordings are performed at rest and in one muscle. Abnormal findings increase with multiple recording sites and under stressful conditions.[46] Pericranial tenderness and EMG levels are not correlated, and patients with abnormal EMG levels or increased tenderness do not differ clinically from those without such an abnormality.[47] Patients with ETTH, CTTH, and migraine may have increased EMG activity in some muscles when multiple muscles are sampled under different conditions.[45,48] No increase in neck-muscle EMG activity was found during continuous monitoring by ambulatory EMG during a headache attack.[49]

Exteroceptive suppression (ES) is the inhibition of voluntary EMG activity of the temporalis muscle induced by trigeminal nerve stimulation.[50] Two successive ES (ES1 and ES2) silent periods can be seen (Figure 7.2). ES2, a multisynaptic reflex subject to limbic and other modulation, was originally reported to be absent in 40% of patients with CTTH and reduced in duration in 87%, whereas ES1, an oligosynaptic reflex, was normal. More recent studies have not confirmed these findings. Zwart and Sand found normal ES2 values in a small, blinded study of 11 patients with CTTH.[51] Bendtsen et al[52] and Lipchik et al[53,54] did not find abnormalities in ES2 in blinded studies of patients with CTTH. Measures of ES2's duration depend on difficult to control methodological variables, level of arousal, anxiety, and drug use. It is unclear why the results differ in CTTH. Could ES2 be abnormal in a subset of CTTH patients?[55]

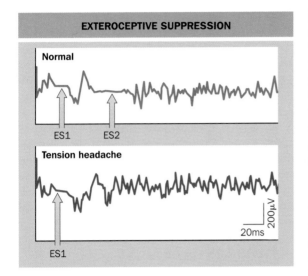

EXTEROCEPTIVE SUPPRESSION

Normal

ES1   ES2

Tension headache

200μV

20ms

ES1

● **Figure 7.2** _Exteroceptive suppression of temporalis muscle. Note absence of ES2 in tension-type headache._[50]

Schoenen et al[46] measured the ES2, pain threshold, EMG activity, anxiety scores, and response to biofeedback in 32 women with CTTH, and found an abnormal EMG in 62.5% of the patients when three different muscles and three states were tested. ES2 duration was reduced in 87% of patients. Reduced Achilles tendon pain thresholds were found in half of CTTH patients when compared with headache-free controls.[44] Biofeedback moderately but significantly increased the pain threshold, perhaps by normalizing limbic input to the brainstem pain modulating system. Increased EMG activity or decreased pain thresholds were found in 72% of the patients,[44] consistent with a diagnosis of CTTH 'associated with disorder of pericranial muscles', but these findings were not present in the remaining 28% of patients, consistent with a diagnosis of CTTH 'unassociated with such disorder'. Headache severity, anxiety, ES2, and response to biofeedback did not differ between these two groups, suggesting that their separation may be artificial or a consequence of the headache. Nitric oxide may play a role in the pathophysiology of TTH. A nitric oxide (NO) synthetase inhibitor reduced headache and muscle hardness, whereas the NO donor glyceryl trinitrate caused more headache in patients with CTTH than in healthy controls.[56–58] In a placebo-controlled study, a NO synthesis inhibitor significantly reduced the pain of CTTH, again suggesting a role for NO generation in the pain.[59]

Fibromyalgia, myofascial pain syndrome, tension myalgia, and tension-type headache

Fibromyalgia is a chronic disorder of widespread pain and musculoskeletal tenderness throughout the body[60] that mainly affects women (90%). Associated symptoms include sleep disturbance (75%), morning stiffness (77%), fatigue (81%), paraesthesias, headache (52.8%), and anxiety (47.8%) or depression (31.5%). Because it is associated with a decreased pain threshold, pain from other disorders may be exacerbated.[61]

Motor dysfunction (loss of the reciprocal innervation of muscles during voluntary activity),[62] tender spots, relief with trigger point injection, and, when chronic, associated anxiety and depression may be present in both fibromyalgia and TTH. The myofascial pain syndrome[63] is distinguished from fibromyalgia by being a focal, self-limited disorder associated with trigger points. Decreased pain threshold and involvement of the pain control systems may also be present, suggesting that TTH may overlap with localized fibromyalgia of the pericranial structures.

Biochemical changes in tension-type headache

Platelets, the major source of serotonin in the blood and plasma, account for 98% of the circulating blood level. Some have found that patients with CTTH have significantly lower platelet serotonin content than do normal controls,[64–67] while others have found normal values or elevated platelet serotonin in CTTH patients.[68–72] Patients who have ETTHs have lower mean levels of circulating plasma epinephrine, norepinephrine, and dopamine during a headache, suggesting decreased sympathetic activity.[65] Some ETTH patients have higher plasma serotonin levels, while others have lower plasma serotonin levels, during a headache.[73,74] Patients with severe headache show abnormalities of cerebrospinal beta-endorphin and release of luteinizing hormone induced by naloxone.[75]

Platelet gamma-aminobutyric acid (GABA) levels in patients with CTTH (43.1 ± 11.8 pmol/1012 platelets) are significantly higher than in migraineurs (30.9 ± 11.7) and healthy controls (34.7 ± 8.1). The platelet, a model of monamine neurons, may have elevated GABA levels to counter the state of neuronal hyperexcitability seen during an attack of migraine and continually during CTTH.[76] Elevated GABA levels are found in the CSF during migraine attacks.[77] Valproic acid, which among other actions is a GABA-mimetic agent, is effective in the treatment of migraine, CDH, and cluster headache, suggesting that the increased GABA levels are a reaction to, not a cause of, head pain.

Relationship to depression

Many have attempted to portray TTH as a primary psychological disorder.[78] This conclusion, based on studies of patients with CDH frequently complicated by medication overuse, does not address ETTH. Merikangas et al,[79] following a cohort of ETTH patients from Zurich, have found no evidence of associated anxiety or depression, in contrast to the frequent association of anxiety and depression with migraine and the psychological distress of patients with CDH. This did not address the specificity issue, because the difference in the rates of depression between the two headache conditions might have been explained by differences in severity.

In a recent study, Breslau et al examined the migraine/depression comorbidity in a large scale epidemiologic study, the Detroit Area Study of Headache.[22] Three groups (persons with migraine ($n = 536$), persons with other severe headaches of comparable pain severity and disability ($n = 162$), and matched controls with no history of severe headache ($n = 586$)) were identified by a random-digit dialing telephone survey of 4765 persons aged 25–55 years. The lifetime prevalence of major depression in persons with migraine was 40.7%; in those with other severe headaches it was 35.8%; and in controls it was 16.0%. Sex-adjusted odds ratios in the two headache groups, relative to controls, were approximately the same magnitude, 3.5 and 3.2. However, examination of the bidirectional relationship between major depression and each headache type yielded different results. With respect to migraine, a bidirectional relationship was observed: migraine signalled an increased risk for the first onset of major depression and major depression signalled an increased risk for the first time occurrence of migraine; sex-adjusted hazard ratios were 2.4 and 2.8, respectively (both statistically significant). In contrast, severe nonmigraine headache signalled an increased risk for major depression, but there was no evidence of a significant influence in the reverse direction; i.e. from major depression to severe headache; sex-adjusted hazard ratios were 3.6 and 1.6, respectively (only the first statistically significant).[80]

Some believe that CTTH can mask depression or other serious emotional disorders. A persistent, vague headache for which no organic cause can be determined (as is true for migraine) is frequently blamed on underlying psychic distress.[78] The psychological problems these patients have could be the result, not the cause, of their chronic pain. The relationship between headache and depression is complicated. 'Depression headache' has been described in detail.[81,82] In one series, 84% of depressed patients complained of headache. The source of this population is

not clear, nor is it clear whether the headache preceded the depression, followed the depression, or was a comorbid condition. Patients with depression headache frequently suffer from chronic migraine[82] (see Chapter 8).

Depression may be a result, not a cause, of chronic pain. Additionally, depression, anxiety, and chronic headache may be comorbid conditions with a common biological basis, as is true for the conditions of migraine, depression, and anxiety. Prior to the onset of either migraine or CTTH, patients show an increase in perceived stressful life events, whereas headache-free controls do not. This may be a result of an idiosyncratic, biologically-determined overreaction to significant life events in these patients.[83] Serotonin has been implicated in the genesis of migraine, depression, and anxiety disorders, and may be the biological basis for their comorbidity.[3,84]

Summary

TTH is probably a clinical manifestation of abnormal neuronal sensitivity and pain facilitation, not abnormal muscle contraction: pain sensitivity is increased; tenderness is increased in some pericranial muscles; EMG is increased in some pericranial muscles, under some conditions independent of headache; and tenderness and increased EMG activity vary independently. Thus, headache is not directly related to muscle contraction and focal tenderness. ES2 may be abnormal in some subtypes; this suggests abnormal modulation of the interneurons that connect the trigeminal nerve to the motor neurons. This abnormality may be a consequence of abnormal modulation from the basal ganglia, the limbic system, or the serotonergic neurons from the nucleus raphe dorsalis. The trigeminal nucleus caudalis, which is the major relay nucleus for head and face pain, receives nociceptive input from cephalic blood vessels and pericranial muscles, and it receives dual supraspinal input, both inhibitory and facilitory.[85] Recent evidence suggests the presence of central pain facilitory neurons (on-cells) in the ventromedial medulla.[86] In addition, the trigeminal nucleus caudalis can be sensitized as a result of intense neuronal activation (Figure 7.3).

In CTTH, there may be hypersensitivity of neurons in the trigeminal nucleus caudalis neurons as a result of supraspinal facilitation. If the vascular nociceptor is hypersensitive in migraine, then perhaps in CTTH associated with a disorder of the pericranial muscles, the myofascial nociceptor is hypersensitive. In CTTH not associated with a disorder of the pericranial muscles, there may be less myofascial nociceptor hypersensitivity and a general increase in nociception. CTTH may be the result of an interaction between endogenous nociceptive brainstem activity and peripheral input (Figure 7.2). Acute ETTH can

HEADACHE PAIN PATHWAYS

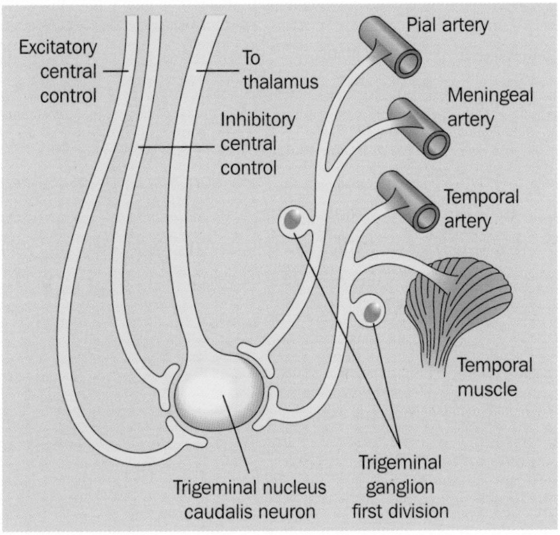

● **Figure 7.3** *Headache pain pathways: vascular supraspinal myogenic model. Trigeminal nucleus caudalis has excitatory and inhibitory central control. It receives input from both arteries and muscle.*[42]

be brought on by physical or psychological stress or by nonphysiological working positions. Increased nociception from strained muscles trigger the attack in an individual with altered pain modulation. Emotional mechanisms may also reduce endogenous antinociception. Long-term potentiation of nociceptive neurons and decreased activity in the antinociceptive system could cause CTTH. Sensitization of the trigeminal nucleus caudalis neurons can result in normal nonpainful stimuli becoming painful, producing trigger spots, an overlap in the symptoms of migraine and TTH, and activation of the trigeminal vascular system.

The pain from intense stimulation or injury usually diminishes as healing progresses and disappears when healing is complete. However, another type of pain occurs when the peripheral or central nervous system malfunctions. Three spatiotemporal characteristics of pain can be seen during both normal and pathophysiological pain:[87]

- as pain intensity increases, the area in which the pain is experienced often enlarges (radiation),
- the pain often outlasts the evoking stimulus, and
- repeated nociceptive stimulation may slowly increase the perceived intensity of pain, even without an increase in the peripheral input (sensitization).

Jensen and Olesen[88] used 30 minutes of sustained teeth-clenching (10% of maximal EMG signal) to trigger TTH in 58 patients who had frequent, but not daily, CTTH or ETTH and

58 matched controls. Within 24 hours, 69% of patients (more than would be expected) and 17% of controls developed TTH. Shortly after clenching, EMG amplitude was significantly increased in the trapezius but not in the temporal muscle, and tenderness (which was increased at baseline in the headache patients) further increased only in the patients who subsequently developed headache. Mechanical pain thresholds remained unchanged in the group that developed headache but increased in the group that did not develop headache. Pain tolerance decreased in the patients who developed headache, was unchanged in the remaining patients, and increased in controls, suggesting that headache patients do not effectively activate their antinociceptive system. This study clearly shows that peripheral mechanisms alone cannot explain TTH, but they could act as a trigger for a central process. Tenderness, not muscle contraction, correlates to headache development. Tenderness may have a central cause or result from muscle contraction causing activation and chemical sensitization on myofascial mechanoreceptors, or their afferent fibres, or both. Therapeutic approaches should consider the relative importance of peripheral and central mechanisms, since they may vary, producing complex interactions.

Genetics

The high prevalence of ETTH in the population results in a positive family history simply by chance in 99% of probands with four first-degree relatives. Thus a positive family history does not imply a genetic disorder.[89] Russell et al evaluated CTTH in a family study of 122 probands and 377 first-degree relatives.[90] Sensitivity, specificity, predictive values, and chance-corrected agreement rate for the diagnosis of CTTH were 68%, 86%, 53% (PVpos), 92% (PVneg), and 0.48, respectively. The low sensitivity of CTTH assessed by proband report indicates that a clinical interview of family members is necessary. Clinically interviewed parents, siblings, and children had a 2.1- to 3.9-fold increased risk of CTTH compared with the general population. The proband's gender did not influence the risk of CTTH among first-degree relatives. The significantly increased familial risk, with no increased risk found in spouses, suggests that a genetic factor is involved in CTTH. Russell believes that CTTH may have genetic heterogeneity.[89]

Treatment of tension-type headache

Episodic TTH is the most common headache type, and most sufferers self-medicate with simple analgesics or do not take medication at all or consult a health care professional. People may seek help if ETTHs occur with unusual frequency or intensity.[91] The main categories of treatment for TTH consists of psychophysiological therapy, physical therapy, and pharmacotherapy.

Psychophysiological therapy involves reassurance, counselling, stress management, relaxation therapy, and biofeedback. The use of traditional acupuncture is controversial and was not more effective than placebo in one study.[92] A metaanalysis,[93] while suggesting that acupuncture had a role in the treatment of headache, found the evidence unconvincing. Two recent studies showed no efficacy.[94,95] Physical therapy consists of: modality treatments (heat, cold packs, ultrasound, and electrical stimulation); improvement of posture through stretching, exercise and traction; trigger point injections or occipital nerve blocks; and a programme of regular exercise, stretching, balanced meals, and adequate sleep.[96]

Pharmacotherapy

Acute therapy, to stop or reduce the severity of the individual attack, consists of the structured use of simple analgesics alone or in combination with caffeine, anxiolytics, or codeine, and nonsteroidal antiinflammatory drugs (NSAIDs). Because of the potential of drug-induced headache, these drugs must be limited (Table 7.2). Optimizing therapy requires knowledge of alternative treatments and awareness of the patient's preferences. Many acute treatments are available. The choice depends on the severity and frequency of the headaches, the associated symptoms, the presence of coexistent illness, and the patient's treatment profile. Oral medications, such as analgesics, NSAIDs, or a caffeine adjuvant compound are useful for patients with mild-to-moderate headaches not complicated by nausea. We begin with simple analgesics for patients with mild-to-moderate headaches. Many individuals find headache relief with over-the-counter analgesics such as naproxen sodium, ibuprofen, aspirin, or acetaminophen (paracetamol), alone or in combination with caffeine. When we use prescription drugs, we add butalbital or use the combination of acetaminophen, isometheptene, and dichloralphenazone. Although this combination may be more effective than simple analgesics or NSAIDs, one must be cautious when prescribing butalbital-containing components since the addiction potential is so high. Because of the risk of dependency, abuse, and CDH, analgesic overuse must be avoided.

Simple analgesics and NSAIDs are effective for the acute treatment of TTH. Aspirin, the most commonly used analgesic, is more effective than placebo and comparable to acetaminophen. Dose-response curves for aspirin have

● **Table 7.2** *Acute medications for tension-type headache**

Drug		Efficacy	Side effects
Analgesics	Aspirin	2+	2
	Acetaminophen**	2+	1
Non-steroidal anti-inflammatory drugs	Indomethacin	3	2
	Ibuprofen	2+	2
	Naproxen	3+	2
	Fenoprofen	2	2
	Ketoprofen	2	2
	Ketorolac	3	3
Combination	Aspirin and/or acetaminophen plus caffeine	3+	2
	Aspirin or acetaminophen plus butalbital with caffeine	3+	3
Muscle relaxants	Orphenadrine	0 (?)	3
	Carisoprodol	0 (?)	3
	Methocarbamal	0 (?)	3
	Diazepam	0 (?)	3
	Cyclobenzaprine	0 (?)	3
	Chlorphenesin	0 (?)	3
	Chloroxazone	0 (?)	3

* Rated on a 1–3 scale.
** Paracetamol.

been established for headache.[97,98] Acetaminophen (650 and 1000 mg) had greater efficacy than placebo and its effect was indistinguishable from that of similar doses of aspirin, but had fewer side effects.[99] The NSAIDs have antiinflammatory, analgesic, and antipyretic properties and are quickly absorbed when taken orally, with a time to peak plasma concentration (max) of less than 2 hours.[100] Ibuprofen and naproxen are significantly more effective than placebo and may be more effective than aspirin or acetaminophen.[101,102] In a controlled, double-blind, crossover trial of ibuprofen, aspirin, and placebo conducted with 50 TTH outpatients, ibuprofen was as effective as aspirin in the relief of pain. No statistical data were reported, nor was there any mention of the details of the scoring system for headache.[102] Two recent studies using the IHS guidelines found 400 or 800 mg of ibuprofen to be significantly more effective than placebo or 1000 mg of acetaminophen.[103] A low dose of ibuprofen (200 mg) was superior to 500 mg of aspirin.[101]

Naproxen sodium, in a multicentre, randomized, double-blind, three-way parallel study,[104] provided a significantly greater percentage change in mean pain intensity compared with acetaminophen ($p < 0.01$) or placebo ($p < 0.001$). Sevelius et al found that naproxen sodium provided earlier and better pain relief than aspirin in various pain states, including headache, and its effect was consistent over time.[98] Other NSAIDs, such as ketoprofen, ketorolac, or indomethacin (indometacin), are also effective, but are less well studied. Five comparative trials of ketoprofen have been published.[105–109] Ketoprofen 50 mg was more effective than ibuprofen 200 mg or acetaminophen 1000 mg.[110] The efficacy of ketoprofen 12.5 mg did not significantly exceed that of placebo in one study, nor did acetaminophen.[107] Ketoprofen 25 mg was more effective than 12.5 mg, and both were more effective than 1000 mg of acetaminophen and significantly more effective than placebo in a study of 703 subjects with TTH.[111] Fifty milligrams of ketoprofen, but not acetaminophen, was more effective than placebo.[105]

The major side effects of NSAIDs are gastrointestinal symptoms (bleeding, nausea, vomiting, constipation, ulcers, epigastric pain, and diarrhoea). Dermatological (rash, pruritus) and central nervous system (CNS) side-effects (headache, lethargy, confusion) are less common, and even rarer are oedema, leukopenia, thrombocytopenia, and liver-function abnormalities. Contraindications include hypersensitivity to aspirin or any NSAID, peptic ulcers, treatment with anticoagulants, bleeding tendency, and severe renal, cardiac, or liver impairment within the last three months.

There is no evidence that muscle relaxants, such as the mephenesin-like compounds, baclofen, diazepam, tizanidine, cyclobenzaprine or dantrolene sodium, are effective in the treatment of ETTH.

Combination analgesics, sedatives, and tranquillizer/ analgesic combinations have been used in the treatment of acute TTH.[112] A single-dose, placebo-controlled study found that adding a muscle relaxant to a compound analgesic was complementary.[113] A comparison of meprobamate and aspirin with a butalbital-aspirin-phenacetin combination found them to be equally effective, but the later had significantly more CNS adverse events. A multicentre, double-blind, randomized clinical study found that a meprobamate/acetylsalicylic acid combination was significantly more effective than aspirin alone. The combination of analgesics with caffeine, sedatives, or tranquillizers may be more effective than simple analgesics or NSAIDs. Caffeine (130 or 200 mg) as an adjunct significantly increases the efficacy of simple analgesics and ibuprofen.[114–115] Eight publications reported on ten separate controlled trials of butalbital-containing combination drugs to treat TTH.[97,116–122] The butalbital-containing compounds have been shown to be efficacious in placebo-controlled trials among patients with ETTHs. Short-term adverse events appeared to be infrequent and mild.

Patients can overuse the medications they take for acute headache attacks. When an acute medication for episodic headache is taken more often than 2 days a week, daily or almost-daily headaches may develop.[123] The overused medication may transiently relieve the pain, but when the effect wears off and some degree of headache returns, the natural tendency is to take more medication. This is a common reason that ETTH or migraine evolves to CTTH or chronic migraine.[24,123] Acute medication should be taken no more than 2 days a week. If TTH consistently occurs more than 2 days a week, preventive therapy is warranted.

Preventive treatment is designed to reduce the frequency and severity of headache attacks and should be considered if the frequency (more than two per week), duration (> 3–4 hours), and severity might lead to significant disability or to the overuse of abortive medication. We prefer to begin treatment with the tricyclic antidepressants or serotonin-specific reuptake inhibitors (SSRIs), but any of the migraine preventive drugs can be used empirically. If preventive medication is indicated, the agent should be chosen from one of the major categories, based on side-effect profiles and coexistent comorbid conditions (Chapter 6).

Tricyclic antidepressants are the drugs that are most commonly used for TTH. Amitriptyline is the most frequently used tricyclic antidepressant. Lance and Curran conducted a placebo-controlled, crossover trial of amitriptyline (10–25 mg three times a day) in 27 CTTH patients.[124] Twelve responded to amitriptyline, 12 had no improvement with either amitriptyline or placebo, and three responded to both treatments (significantly favouring amitriptyline). Diamond and Baltes tested two different dosage ranges of amitriptyline (10–60 mg daily and 25 and 150 mg daily) versus placebo.[125] The lower dose range was more effective than placebo, but no significant effect of the higher dose range was found. Gobel et al compared amitriptyline (75 mg daily) to placebo.[126] Headache duration was reduced significantly in the amitriptyline group in the last week of the 6-week study; analgesic intake was unaltered. A large, multicentre, parallel-group trial by Pfaffenrath et al compared amitriptyline (50–75 mg daily) to amitriptyline oxide (60–90 mg daily), and to placebo.[127] No significant difference was found between the active treatments and placebo. In a three-way crossover study, Bendsten et al compared amitriptyline 75 mg daily, citalopram (an SSRI) 20 mg daily, and placebo in nondepressed patients who were resistant to previous treatments.[128] Amitriptyline reduced the AUC (headache duration times headache intensity) by 30% compared with placebo (highly significant), whereas citalopram had only a slight, insignificant effect

(12%). These placebo-controlled studies suggest that amitriptyline has a statistically significant and clinically relevant effect in the treatment of CTTH.[129] Holroyd et al[130] conducted a randomized, placebo-controlled trial on the management of CTTH with tricyclic antidepressant medication alone, stress management alone, and both treatments in combination. Participants were randomly assigned to receive tricyclic antidepressant (amitriptyline hydrochloride, up to 100 mg a day or nortriptyline hydrochloride up to 75 mg a day) medication (n = 53), placebo (n = 48), stress management (e.g. relaxation, cognitive coping) therapy (three sessions and two telephone contacts) plus placebo (n = 49), or stress management therapy plus antidepressant medication (n = 53). Combined therapy was more likely to produce clinically significant (≥ 50%) reductions in headache index scores (64% of participants) than antidepressant medication (38% of participants; p = 0.006), stress management therapy (35%; p = 0.003), or placebo (29%; p = 0.001). On other measures the combined therapy and its two component therapies produced similar outcomes.

Other antidepressants, such as doxepin, nortriptyline, or protriptyline, have been used. The SSRIs have fewer side-effects than the tricyclic antidepressants and are often preferred by patients. In one controlled trial, fluoxetine (20–40 mg) was more effective than placebo for patients with chronic daily headache.[131] Langemark and Olesen compared paroxetine (20–30 mg daily) with sulpiride, a dopamine antagonist used as a neuroleptic.[132] Patients improved with both treatments, although a tendency to better efficacy was found for sulpiride.

Muscle relaxants may be effective in the preventive treatment of CTTH. Tizanidine was compared with placebo in a randomized, double-blind, crossover study in 37 women who were 20–59 years of age and had CTTH.[76] The treatment periods were 6 weeks with an intervening 2-week washout period. Treatment began with 2 mg three times a day and the daily dose could be increased to 6 mg three times a day. The effect of the treatment was measured by visual analogue scale, verbal rating scale, number of headache-free days, number of analgesics needed, and the dose of trial medication needed. Tizanidine was statistically significantly more effective than placebo in all these measurements.[129]

Other agents have been used in the treatment of chronic headaches, usually the mixed variety of migraine and CTTH. In an open trial, significant success was reported with propranolol or a combination of propranolol plus amitriptyline.[133] An open trial of 30 subjects found that valproic acid, in doses of 1000–2500 mg, was effective in treating mixed migraine and CTTH.[134] However, these were probably cases of chronic migraine.

Preventive medications should be started at a low dose and increased slowly until therapeutic effects develop or until the ceiling dose for the agent in question is reached. Tricyclic antidepressants, such as amitriptyline, are often used in doses of 100–200 mg/day for depression, while 10–20 mg/day is often effective for TTH. (A starting dose of 25–50 mg/day of amitriptyline is common in patients with depression, whereas it can produce intolerable side-effects in migraineurs.) With fluoxetine, for example, we begin with 10 mg and slowly increase the dose. While some patients respond to lower doses of preventive medications, it may be necessary to increase the dose to tolerance before assuming the agent is ineffective. A full therapeutic trial may take 2–6 months. Patients may be treated with a new preventive medication for 1–2 weeks without effect and then prematurely discontinue it, causing both patient and physician to believe it was not effective. To obtain maximal benefit from preventive medication, the patient should not overuse analgesics. Headaches may improve with time independent of treatment; if the headaches are well controlled, a drug holiday can be undertaken following a slow taper programme. Many patients experience continued relief after discontinuing the medication or may not need the same dose. Dose reduction may provide a better risk-to-benefit ratio. The other medications used to treat migraine and depression have been used to treat ETTH and CTTH (see Chapter 6).

Nonpharmacologic treatments

Nonpharmacologic treatment modalities should be considered in primary headache management. Patients should be taught healthy habits, such as obtaining adequate sleep, eating balanced meals, and getting regular exercise, and told to eliminate unhealthy habits, such as smoking and excess drinking. Since patients may be concerned about an underlying brain tumour or other serious disease, the diagnosis should be discussed and the patient reassured. Psychological factors should be addressed. Depression, anxiety, or both may coexist with, or aggravate, TTH, and these conditions, which are likely to be consequences rather than causes of the headache, need to be treated appropriately if they are present.[81,83]

Psychophysiological therapy involves reassurance, counselling, stress management, relaxation therapy, and biofeedback. EMG biofeedback enables patients to control muscle tension by providing continuous information pertaining to the state of tension of one or more muscles, with the frontalis muscle being the most common site. Feedback can be auditory (for example, clicks that vary in rate) or visual (such as bars that vary in length). Sessions last about 1 hour and include an adaptation phase, a baseline phase, a training phase, and a self-control phase.[135] Efficacy improves when patients learn to either increase or decrease their pericranial EMG activity.[136]

The most commonly used forms of relaxation training are progressive relaxation training and autogenic training. The goal of progressive relaxation training is to help patients recognize tension and relaxation in everyday life. Patients learn to sequentially tense and then release or relax various groups of muscles throughout the body. They are told to practice relaxation training daily at home, and audiotapes are usually provided for assistance.[135] Autogenic training, developed by Schultz and Luthe, is based on autosuggestion.[137] It seeks to simultaneously regulate mental and somatic functions by passively concentrating on a formula, such as 'my forehead is cool'.

Two main variations of cognitive–behavioural therapy have been developed. In the original formulation, Holroyd and colleagues focused on altering maladaptive cognitive responses that were assumed to mediate the occurrence of headaches.[138,139] In contrast, Bakal et al developed a treatment approach that emphasized modifying the stress reactions that are associated with headaches (feelings of helplessness, anxiety, and fear) rather than modifying stress reactions to environmental and interpersonal events.[140] The goal of cognitive therapy is to teach patients to identify and challenge dysfunctional thoughts and subsequently the underlying maladaptive assumptions and beliefs.[135,141,142]

Metaanalytical and narrative reviews have concluded that EMG biofeedback training, relaxation training, and cognitive–behavioural therapy effectively reduce TTH.[143] EMG biofeedback training, either alone or with relaxation training, and cognitive–behavioural therapy each yield at least a 50% reduction in TTH activity. Improvements reported with these treatments, as well as with relaxation training alone, are significantly more pronounced than improvements reported with placebo–control treatments or observed in untreated patients.[144] Improvement is often maintained for long periods without contact with the therapist. Improvements achieved with psychological treatments have generally been maintained for 3–9 months.

Cognitive–behavioural interventions, such as stress management programmes, may effectively reduce TTH activity when used alone, but these modalities may be more useful in conjunction with biofeedback or relaxation therapies, particularly for patients who have a high level of daily stress. Physical therapy may be warranted for patients who have TTH associated with pericranial muscle disorders.[145] Physical therapy techniques include modality treatments (heat, cold packs, and ultrasound), stretching, exercise, trigger point injections or occipital nerve blocks,

acupuncture, ergonomic instruction, massage, and manipulations.[96] A systematic review of randomized control trials on complementary/alternative therapies in the treatment of TTH and cervicogenic headache has been published by Vernon et al.[146] The evidence is inconsistent for most therapeutic modalities. The use of traditional acupuncture is controversial and was not more effective than placebo in one study but was as effective as massage in another.[92,147]

Massage may be useful for acute episodes of TTH, but the long-term benefit is uncertain. Most studies have found only a moderate effect on pain intensity and frequency.[146,148]

Bove and Nilsson conducted a randomized, controlled trial lasting 19 weeks at an outpatient facility of a National Health Service-funded chiropractic research institution in Denmark.[149] Subjects included 26 men and 49 women who were 20–59 years of age and had IHS ETTH. One group received soft tissue therapy and spinal manipulation (the manipulation group), and the other group received soft tissue therapy and a placebo laser treatment (the control group). All participants received eight treatments over 4 weeks performed by the same chiropractor. Daily hours of headache, pain intensity per episode, and daily analgesic use were recorded in diaries. Based on intent-to-treat analysis, no significant differences between the manipulation and control groups were observed in any of the three outcome measures. However, by week 7, each group experienced significant reductions in mean daily headache hours (manipulation group, reduction from 2.8 to 1.5 hours); control group, reduction from 3.4 to 1.9 hours). As an isolated intervention, spinal manipulation did not seem to have a positive effect on ETTH in this trial. However, one small trial suggested that manipulation might be effective[150] and another trial suggested that it may be as effective as amitriptyline.[151]

Oromandibular treatment may be helpful for some TTH patients. Most studies that claim efficacy of treatments, such as occlusal splints, therapeutic exercises for masticatory muscles, or occlusal adjustment, are uncontrolled. Many headache-free individuals have signs and symptoms of oromandibular dysfunction;[20,152] therefore, irreversible dental treatments should not be recommended for treating TTH.[20] Patients rarely benefit from oromandibular treatment.

Other treatments

Botulinum toxin injected into pericranial muscles was effective for TTH in one open trial and in two of five placebo-controlled, double-blind trials. In a randomized, single-blind trial, Porta[153] studied the safety and efficacy of botulinum toxin A (BTX-A) injections in pericranial muscles for the treatment of TTH. Patients randomly received either BTX-A (20) or the steroid methylprednisolone (20). The drug was injected in the tender points of cranial muscles, which were determined using pressure pain threshold measurements using an electronic algometer. At 60 days postinjection, the reduction in pain score was statistically significantly greater in patients who received BTX-A compared with those who received steroid.

Smuts et al conducted a double-blind, placebo-controlled, randomized study involving 40 CTTH patients who received intramuscular injections of either BTX-A (Botox® 100 units in 2 ml saline) or placebo (2 ml saline) at predefined areas in the neck and temporal muscles.[154] The number of headache-free days was significantly increased in the BTX-A group three months after treatment compared with controls (238 versus 56 days; $p = 0.001$). These patients may have had chronic migraine.

Gobel et al did not find any difference in ten CTTH patients who were treated on a double-blind basis with either 10 i.u.[155] of Botox® injected into the frontal muscle and the auricular muscle on each side and 20 i.u. injected into the splenius capitis muscle on each side, or the corresponding quantity of saline as placebo. Relja and Korsic reported a significant and long-lasting decrease in headache intensity in 16 CTTH patients in a double-blind, placebo-controlled study.[156] Botox® and/or placebo (saline)

were injected into the most tender pericranial muscle. BTX-A treatment resulted in a significant decrease of the total tenderness score, obtained by the palpation method, 2 weeks, 4 weeks, and 8 weeks after injections. Placebo had no effect. According to patients' diaries, the severity and the duration of the attacks decreased significantly during the BTX-A treatment period.[156]

Schmitt et al,[157] in a placebo-controlled, double-blind trial, compared 20 units of BTX-A with saline, injecting into fixed sites. No difference was noted. Rollnik et al[158] compared 200 units of Dysport® (a type of botulinum toxin type A) with saline in a placebo-controlled double-blind trial. Sites were fixed and no differences were noted. Most studies chose a standarized design with defined injection sites. There was no individual selection of trigger points, and patients with a long therapy-resistant case history were typically included in the studies.

One lesson from the experience to date with BTX-A in therapy of tension-type headache is that the injection should be performed at the site of the pain or the trigger points and not on a standardized basis. Injection is made specifically into the affected muscle in the treatment of patients with dystonia, and this must also be done in the treatment of pain. BTX-A would fail to have a therapeutic effect on spasmodic torticollis under a bilateral standardized injection regime, and the same applies to the treatment of TTH.[159]

References

1. Headache Classification Committee of the International Headache Society. Classification and diagnostic criteria for headache disorders, cranial neuralgia, and facial pain. Cephalalgia 1988; 8: 1–96.
2. Ad Hoc Committee on Classification of Headache. Classification of headache. Arch Neurol 1962; 6: 13–16.
3. Silberstein SD. Advances in understanding the pathophysiology of headache. Neurology 1992; 42: 6–11.
4. Silberstein SD. Chronic daily headache and tension-type headache. Neurology 1993; 43: 1644–9.
5. Rasmussen BK, Jensen R, Schroll M, Olesen J. Epidemiology of headache in a general population – a prevalence study. J Clin Epidemiol 1991; 44: 1147–57.
6. Abramson JH, Hopp C, Epstein LM. Migraine and nonmigrainous headaches. A community survey in Jerusalem. J Epidemiol Community Health 1980; 34: 188–93.
7. Schwartz BS, Stewart WF, Simon D, Lipton RB. Epidemiology of tension-type

headache. JAMA 1998; 279: 381–3.
8. Iversen HK, Langemark M, Andersson PG et al. Clinical characteristics of migraine and episodic tension-type headache in relation to old and new diagnostic criteria. Headache 1990; 30: 514–19.
9. Newman LC, Lipton RB, Solomon S, Stewart WF. Daily headache in a population sample: results from the American Migraine Study. Headache 1994; 34: 295
10. Waters WE. Migraine: intelligence, social class, and familial prevalence. Br Med J 1971; 2: 77–81.
11. Rasmussen BK. Migraine and tension-type headache in a general population: psychosocial factors. Int J Epidemiol 1992; 21: 1138–43.
12. Drummond PD. Scalp tenderness and sensitivity to pain in migraine and tension headache. Headache 1987; 27: 45–50.
13. Langemark M, Olesen J, Poulsen DL, Bech P. Clinical characterization of patients with chronic tension headache.

Headache 1988; 28: 590–6.
14. Schiffman E, Haley D, Backer C, Lindgren B. Diagnostic criteria for screening headache patients for temporomandibular disorders. Headache 1995; 35: 121–4.
15. Silberstein SD. Twenty questions about headaches in children and adolescents. Headache 1990; 30: 716–27.
16. Rasmussen BK, Jensen R, Olesen J. A population-based analysis of the diagnostic criteria of the international headache society. Cephalalgia 1991; 11: 129–34.
17. Hatch JP, Moore PJ, Cyr-Provost M et al. The use of electromyography and muscle palpation in the diagnosis of tension-type headache with and without pericranial muscle involvement. Pain 1992; 49: 175–8.
18. Blau JN. Sleep deprivation headache. Cephalalgia 1990; 10: 157–60.
19. Rasmussen BK. Migraine and tension-type headache in a general population: precipitating factors, female hormones, sleep pattern, and relation to lifestyle.

Pain 1993; 53: 65–72.

20. Paiva T, Batista A, Martins P, Martins A. The relationship between headaches and sleep disturbances. Headache 1995; 35: 590–6.

21. Jensen R, Rassmussen BK, Pedersen B et al. Prevalence of oromandibular disorders in a general population. J Orofac Pain 1993; 7: 175–82.

22. Breslau N, Schultz LR, Stewart WF et al. Headache and major depression: is the association specific to migraine? Neurology 2000; 54: 308–13.

23. Forsyth PA, Posner JB. Intracranial neoplasms. In: Olesen J, Tfelt-Hansen P, Welch KMA, eds. The Headaches. 2nd edn. New York: Raven Press, 2000, 849–61.

24. Solomon S, Newman LC. Episodic tension-type headaches. In: Silberstein SD, Lipton RB, Dalessio DJ, eds. Wolff's Headache and other Head Pain. 7th edn. New York: Oxford University Press, 2001, 238–46.

25. Bakal DA. The Psychobiology of Chronic Headache. New York: Springer, 1982.

26. Waters WE. Series in Clinical Epidemiology: Headache. Littleton: PSG, 1986.

27. Featherstone HJ. Migraine and muscle contraction headaches: a continuum. Headache 1985; 25: 194–8.

28. Raskin NH. Headache. 2nd edn. New York: Churchill-Livingstone, 1988.

29. Saper JR. Changing perspectives of chronic headache. Clin J Pain 1986; 2: 19–28.

30. Marcus DA. Migraine and tension-type headaches: the questionable validity of current classification systems. Clin J Pain 1992; 8: 28–36.

31. Ziegler DK, Hassanein RS. Specific headache phenomena: their frequency and coincidence. Headache 1990; 30: 152–6.

32. Lipton RB, Stewart WF, Cady R et al. Sumatriptan for the range of headaches in migraine sufferers: results of the spectrum study. Headache 2000; 40: 783–91.

33. Pfaffenrath V, Isler H. Evaluation of the nosology of chronic tension-type headache. Cephalalgia 1993; 13: 60–2.

34. Mathew NT, Stubits E, Nigam MR. Transformation of episodic migraine into daily headache: analysis of factors. Headache 1982; 22: 66–8.

35. Guitera V, Munoz P, Castillo J, Pascual J. Transformed migraine: a proposal for the modification of its diagnostic criteria based on recent epidemiological data. Cephalalgia 1999; 19: 847–50.

36. Ziegler DK, Hassanein R, Hassanein K. Headache syndromes suggested by factor analysis of symptom variables in a headache prone population. J Chronic Dis 1972; 25: 353–63.

37. Lichstein KL, Fischer SM, Eakin TL et al. Psychophysiological parameters of migraine and muscle-contraction headaches. Headache 1991; 31: 27–34.

38. Sutton EP, Belar CD. Tension headache patients versus controls: a study of EMG parameters. Headache 1982; 22: 133–6.

39. Arena JG, Hannah SL, Bruno GM et al. Effect of movement and position of muscle activity in tension headache sufferers during and between headaches. J Psychosom Res 1991; 35: 187–95.

40. Ziegler DK. The headache symptom: how many entities. Arch Neurol 1985; 42: 273–7.

41. Langemark M, Jensen K, Olesen J. Temporal muscle blood flow in chronic tension -type headache. Arch Neurol 1990; 47: 654–8.

42. Silberstein SD, Lipton RB, Solomon S, Mathew NT. Classification of daily and near daily headaches: proposed revisions to the IHS classification. Headache 1994; 34: 1–7.

43. Martin PR, Mathews AM. Tension headaches: psychophysiological investigation and treatment. J Psychosom Res 1978; 22: 389–99.

44. Olesen J. Clinical and pathophysiological observations in migraine and tension-type headache explained by integration of vascular, supraspinal and myofascial inputs. Pain 1991; 46: 125–32.

45. Langemark M, Olesen J. Pericranial tenderness in tension headache: a blind, controlled study. Cephalalgia 1987; 7: 249–55.

46. Schoenen J, Bottin D, Hardy F, Gerard P. Cephalic and extracephalic pressure pain threshold in chronic tension-type headache. Pain 1991; 47: 145–9.

47. Schoenen J, Gerard P, De Pasqua V, Sianard-Gainko J. Multiple clinical and paraclinical analyses of chronic tension-type headache associated or unassociated with disorder of pericranial muscles. Cephalalgia 1991; 11: 135–9.

48. Pritchard DW. EWG cranial muscle levels in headache sufferers before and during headache. Headache 1989; 29: 103–8.

49. Hatch JP, Prihoda TJ, Moore PJ. A naturalistic study of the relationships among electromyographic, psychological stress, and pain in ambulatory tension-type headache patients and headache-free controls. Neurology 1991; 37: 1834–6.

50. Schoenen J, Jamart B, Gerard P et al. Exteroceptive suppression of temporalis muscle activity in chronic headache. Neurology 1987; 37: 1834–6.

51. Zwart JA, Sand T. Exteroceptive suppression of temporalis muscle activity: a blind study of tension-type headache, migraine, and cervicogenic headache. Headache 1995; 35: 338–43.

52. Bendtsen L, Jensen R, Brennum J et al. Exteroceptive suppression of temporal muscle activity is normal in patients with chronic tension-type headache and not related to actual headache state. Cephalalgia 1996; 16: 251–6.

53. Lipchik GL, Holroyd KA, France CR et al. Central and peripheral mechanisms in chronic tension-type headache. Pain 1996; 64: 475

54. Lipchik GL, Holroyd KA, Talbot F, Greer M. Pericranial muscle tenderness and exteroceptive suppression of temporalis muscle activity: a blind study of chronic tension-type headache. Headache 1997; 37: 368–76.

55. Schoenen J, Bendtsen L. Neurophysiology of tension-type headache. In: Olesen J, Tfelt-Hansen P, Welch KMA, eds. The Headaches. 2nd edn. Philadelphia: Lippincott Williams & Wilkins, 2000: 579–87.

56. Ashina M, Bendtsen L, Jensen R et al. Possible mechanisms of action of nitric oxide synthase inhibitors in chronic tension-type headache. Brain 1999; 122: 1629–35.

57. Ashina M, Lassen LH, Bendtsen L et al. Effect of inhibition of nitric oxide synthase on chronic tension-type headache: a randomized crossover trial. Lancet 1999; 353: 287–9.

58. Lassen LH, Ashina M, Christiansen I et al. Nitric oxide synthase inhibition in migraine. Lancet 1997; 349: 401–2.

59. Ashina M, Bendtsen L, Jensen R, Olesen J. Nitric oxide-induced headache in patients with chronic tension-type headache. Brain 2000; 123: 1830–7.

60. Wolfe F, Smythe HA, Yanus MB. The American College of Rheumatology 1990 criteria for the classification of fibromyalgia: report of the Multicenter Criteria Committee. Arthritis Rheum 1990; 33: 160–72.

61. Wolfe F. Two muscle pain syndromes: fibromyalgia and the myofascial pain syndrome. Pain Mgt 1990; 3: 153–64.

62. Makashima K, Takahashi K. Exteroceptive suppression of the masseter, temporalis and trapezius muscles produced by mental nerve stimulation in patients with chronic headaches. Cephalalgia 1991; 11: 23–8.

63. Travell J, Simons DG. Myofascial pain and dysfunction: the trigger point manual. Baltimore: Williams & Wilkins, 1983.

64. Rolf LH, Wiele G, Bruno GG. 5-Hydroxytryptamine in platelets of patients with muscle contraction headache. Headache 1991; 21: 10–11.

65. Anthony M, Lance JW. Plasma serotonin in patients with chronic tension headaches. J Neurol Neurosurg Psychiatry 1989; 52: 182–4.

66. Nakano T, Shimomura T, Takahashi K, Ikawa S. Platelet substance P and 5-hydroxytryptamine in migraine and tension-type headache. Headache 1993; 33: 528–32.

67. Shimomura T, Takahashi K. Alteration of platelet serotonin in patients with chronic tension-type headache during cold pressor test. Headache 1990; 30: 581–3.

68. Bendtsen L, Jensen R, Hindberg I et al. Serotonin metabolism in chronic tension-type headache. Cephalalgia 1997; 17: 843–8.

69. Ferrari MD, Odink J, Frolich M et al. Release of platelet metenkephalin, but not serotonin, in migraine. A platelet response unique to migraine patients? J Neurol Sci 1989; 93: 51–60.

70. Shukla R, Shanker K, Nag D et al. Serotonin in tension headache. J Neurol Neurosurg Psychiatr 1987; 50: 1682–4.

71. D'Andrea G, Hasselmark L, Cananzi AR et al. Metabolism and menstrual cycle rhythmicity of serotonin in primary headaches. Headache 1995; 35: 216–21.

72. Leira R, Castillo J, Martinez F et al. Platelet-rich plasma serotonin levels in tension-type headache and depression. Cephalalgia 1993; 13: 346–8.

73. Castillo J, Martinez F, Leira R. Plasma monoamines in tension-type headache. Headache 1994; 34: 531–5.

74. Kitano A, Shimomura T, Takeshima T. Increased 11-dehydrothromboxane B2 in migraine: platelet hyperfunction in patients with migraine during headache-free period. Headache 1994; 34: 515–18.

75. Silberstein SD, Merriam GR. Estrogens, progestins, and headache. Neurology 1991; 41: 775–93.

76. Kowa H, Shimomura T, Takahashi K. Platelet gamma-aminobutyric acid levels in migraine and tension-type headache. Headache 1992; 32: 229–32.

77. Welch KMA, Chabi E, Bartosh K et al. Cerebrospinal fluid gamma aminobutyric acid levels in migraine. Br Med J 1975; 3: 516–17.

78. Martin MJ, Rome HP, Swenson WM. Muscle contraction headache. A psychiatric review. Res Clin Stud Headache 1967; 1: 184.

79. Merikangas KR, Angst J. Migraine and psychopathology: epidemiologic and genetic aspects. Clin Neuropharmacol 1992; 15: 275A.

80. Silberstein SD, Lipton RB, Breslau N. Neuropsychiatric aspects of primary headache disorders. In: Yudofssky SC, Hales RE, eds. Textbook of Neuropsychiatry. 4th edn. Washington: American Psychiatric Press, Inc., 2000.

81. Diamond S. Muscle contraction in headache. In: Dalessio DJ, ed. Wolff's headache and Other Head Pain. New York: Oxford University Press, 1987, 172–89.

82. Diamond S. Depression and headache. Headache 1983; 23: 122–6.

83. DeBenedittis G, Lorenzetti A, Pieri A. The role of stressful life events in the onset of chronic primary headache. Pain 1990; 40: 65–75.

84. Peatfield RC. Pain, headache, and depression: a discussion. New York: Oxford University Press, 1990.

85. Basbaum AI, Fields HL. Endogenous pain control mechanisms: reviews and hypothesis. Ann Neurol 1978; 4: 451–62.

86. Fields HL, Heinricher M. Brainstem modulation of nociceptor-driven withdrawal reflexes. Ann NY Acad Sci 1989; 563: 34–44.

87. Scholz E, Diener HC, Geiselhart S, Wilkinson M. Drug-induced headache: does a critical dosage exist? In: Diener HC, ed. Drug-induced Headache. Berlin: Springer-Verlag, 1988, 29–43.

88. Jensen R, Olesen J. Initiating mechanisms of experimentally induced tension-type headache. Cephalalgia 1996; 16: 175–82.

89. Russell MB, Olesen J. Genetics of tension-type headache. In: Olesen J, Tfelt-Hansen P, Welch KMA, eds. The Headaches. 2nd edn. Philadelphia: Lippincott Williams & Wilkins, 2000, 561–3.

90. Russell MB, Stergaard S, Endtsen L, Olesen J. Familial occurrence of chronic tension-type headache. Cephalalgia 1999; 19: 207–10.

91. Solomon S. OTC analgesics in treating common primary headaches: a review of safety and efficacy. Headache 1994; 34: 13–21.

92. Tavola T, Gala C, Conte G, Invernizzi G. Traditional Chinese acupuncture in tension-type headache: a controlled study. Pain 1992; 48: 325–9.

93. Melchart D, Linde K, Fischer P et al. Acupuncture for recurrent headaches: a systematic review of randomized controlled trials. Cephalalgia 1999; 19: 779–86.

94. Karst M, Reinhard M, Thum P et al. Needle acupuncture in tension-type headache: a randomized, placebo-controlled study. Cephalalgia 2001; 21: 637–42.

95. White AR, Resch KL, Chan JC et al. Acupuncture for episodic tension-type headache: a multicenter randomized controlled trial. Cephalalgia 2000; 20: 632–7.

96. Silberstein SD, Lipton RB. Overview of diagnosis and treatment of migraine.

Neurology 1994; 44: 6–16.

97. Glassman JM, Soyka JP. Muscle contraction (tension) headache; a double blind study comparing the efficacy and safety of meprobamate-aspirin with butalbital-aspirin-phenacetin-caffeine. Curr Ther Res 1980; 28: 904–9.

98. Sevelius H, Segre M, Bursick R. Comparative analgesic effects of naproxen sodium, aspirin, placebo. J Clin Pharm 1980; 20: 480–8.

99. Peters BH, Fraim CJ, Masel BE. Comparison of 650 mg aspirin and 1000 mg acetaminophen with each other, and with placebo in moderately severe headache. Am J Med 1983; 76: 36–42.

100. Tfelt-Hansen P, McEwen J. Nonsteroidal antiinflammatory drugs in the treatment of the acute migraine attack. In: Olesen J, Tfelt-Hansen P, Welch KMA, eds. The Headaches. 2nd edn. New York: Raven Press, 2000, 391–9.

101. Nebe J, Heier M, Diener HC. Low-dose ibuprofen in self-medication of mild to moderate headache: a comparison with acetylsalicylic acid and placebo. Cephalalgia 1995; 15: 531–5.

102. Ryan RE. Motrin – a new agent for symptomatic treatment of muscle contraction headache. Headache 1977; 16: 280–3.

103. Schachtel BP, Furey SA, Thoden WR. Nonprescription ibuprofen and acetaminophen in the treatment of tension-type headache. J Clin Pharmacol 1996; 36: 1120–5.

104. Miller DS, Talbot CA, Simpson W, Korey A. A comparison of naproxen sodium, acetaminophen and placebo in the treatment of muscle contraction headache. Headache 1987; 27: 392–6.

105. Dahlof CG, Jacobs LD. Ketoprofen, paracetamol and placebo in the treatment of episodic tension-type headache. Cephalalgia 1996; 16: 117–23.

106. Lange R, Lentz R. Comparison of ketoprofen, ibuprofen and naproxen sodium in the treatment of tension-type headache. Drugs Exp Clin Res 1995; 21: 89–96.

107. Mehlisch DR, Weaver M, Fladung B. Ketoprofen 12.5 and 25 mg, extra-strength Tylenol 1000 mg and placebo for the treatment of patients with episodic tension-type headache. Cephalalgia 1997; 17: 274

108. Steiner TJ, Lange R. Ketoprofen (25mg) in the symptomatic treatment of episodic tension-type headache: double-blind placebo-controlled comparison with acetaminophen (1000 mg). Cephalalgia 1998; 18: 38–43.

109. Vangerven JM, Schoemaker RC, Jacobs

LD et al. Self-medication of a single headache episode with ketoprofen, ibuprofen or placebo, home-monitored with an electronic patient diary. Br J Clin Pharmacol 1996; 42: 475–81.

110. Autret A, Unger PH, Euraxi Group, Lesaichot JL. Naproxen sodium versus ibuprofen in episodic tension headache. Cephalalgia 1997; 17: 446

111. Mehlisch DR, Weaver M, Fladung B. Ketoprofen, acetaminophen and placebo in the treatment of tension headache. Headache 1998; 38: 579–89.

112. Mathew NT, Schoenen J. Acute pharmacotherapy of tension-type headache. In: Olesen J, Tfelt-Hansen P, Welch KMA, eds. The Headaches. Philadelphia: Lippincott Williams & Wilkins, 2000, 661–6.

113. Atkinson D. A single dose placebo-controlled study to assess the effectiveness of adding a muscle relaxant to a compound analgesic in the treatment of tension headaches. J Intern Med 1979; 7: 560–5.

114. Migliardi JR, Armellino JJ, Friedman M et al. Caffeine as an analgesic adjuvant in tension headache. Clin Pharmacol Ther 1994; 56: 576–86.

115. Diamond S, Freitag FG, Balm TK, Berry DA. The use of a combination agent of ibuprofen and caffeine in the treatment of episodic tension-type headache. Cephalalgia 1997; 17: 446

116. Friedman AP. Assessment of Fiorinal with codeine in the treatment of tension headache. Clin Ther 1986; 8: 703–21.

117. Friedman AP, Boyles WF, Elkind AH et al. Fiorinal with codeine in the treatment of tension headache – the contribution of components to the combination drug. Clin Ther 1988; 10: 303–15.

118. Friedman AP, Diserio FJ. Symptomatic treatment of chronically recurring tension headache: a placebo-controlled, multicenter investigation of Fioricet and acetaminophen with codeine. Clin Ther 1987; 10: 69–81.

119. Hwang DS, Mietlowski MJ, Friedman AP. Fiorinal with codeine in the management of tension headache: impact of placebo response. Clin Ther 1987; 9: 201–22.

120. Thorpe P. Controlled and uncontrolled studies on 'Fiorinal-PA' for symptomatic relief in tension headache. Med J Aust 1970; 2: 180–1.

121. von Graffenried B, Hill RC, Nuesch E. Headache as a model for assessing mild analgesic drugs. J Clin Pharmacol 1980; 20: 131–44.

122. von Graffenried B, Nuesch E. Nonmigrainous headache for the evaluation of oral analgesics. J Clin Pharmacol 1980; 10: 225–31.

123. Mathew NT, Kurman R, Perez F. Drug induced refractory headache – clinical features and management. Headache 1990; 30: 634–8.

124. Lance JW, Curran DA. Treatment of chronic tension headache. Lancet 1964; 1: 1236–9.

125. Diamond S, Baltes B. Chronic tension headache treated with amitriptyline: a double blind study. Headache 1971; 11: 110–16.

126. Gobel H, Hamouz V, Hansen C et al. Chronic tension-type headache: amitriptyline reduces clinical headache-duration and experimental pain sensitivity but does not alter pericranial muscle activity readings. Pain 1994; 59: 241–9.

127. Pfaffenrath V, Diener HC, Isler H et al. Efficacy and tolerability of amitriptylinoxide in the treatment of chronic tension-type headache: a multicentre controlled study. Cephalalgia 1994; 14: 149–55.

128. Bendtsen L, Jensen R, Olesen J. A nonselective (amitriptyline), but not a selective (citalopram), serotonin reuptake inhibitor is effective in the prophylactic treatment of chronic tension-type headache. J Neurol Neurosurg Psychiatr 1996; 61: 285–90.

129. Mathew NT, Bendtsen L. Prophylactic pharmacotherapy of tension-type headache. In: Olesen J, Tfelt-Hansen P, Welch KMA, eds. The Headaches. 2nd edn. Philadelphia: Lippincott Williams & Wilkins, 2000, 667–73.

130. Holroyd KA, O'Donnell FJ, Stensland M et al. Management of chronic tension-type headache with tricyclic antidepressant medication, stress management therapy, and their combination: a randomized controlled trial. JAMA 2001; 285: 2208–16.

131. Saper JR, Silberstein SD, Lake AE, Winters ME. Double-blind trial of fluoxetine: Chronic daily headache and migraine. Headache 1994; 34: 497–502.

132. Langemark M, Olesen J. Sulpiride and paroxetine in the treatment of chronic tension-type headache. An exploratory double-blind trial. Headache 1994; 34: 20–4.

133. Mathew NT. Prophylaxis of migraine and mixed headache. A randomized controlled study. Headache 1981; 21: 105–9.

134. Mathew NT, Ali S. Valproate in the treatment of persistent chronic daily headache. An open label study. Headache 1991; 31: 71–4.

135. Holroyd KA, Martin PR. Psychological treatments of tension-type headache. In: Olesen J, Tfelt-Hansen P, Welch KMA, eds. The Headaches. 2nd edn. New York: Raven Press, 2000: 643–51.

136. Philips C, Hunter M. The treatment of tension headache. I. Muscular abnormality and biofeedback. Behav Res Ther 1981; 19: 485–98.

137. Schultz J, Luthe W. Autogenic training: a psychophysiologic approach in psychotherapy. New York: Grune & Stratton, 1959.

138. Holroyd KA, Andrasik FA. A cognitive-behavioral approach to recurrent tension and migraine headache. In: Kendall PE, ed. Advances in Cognitive-Behavioral Research and Therapy. New York: Academic Press, 1982; 275–320.

139. Holroyd KA, Andrasik F, Westbrook T. Cognitive control of tension headache. Cogn Ther Res 1977; 1: 121–33.

140. Bakal DA, Demjen S, Kaganov JA. Cognitive behavioral treatment of chronic headache. Headache 1981; 21: 81–6.

141. Beck AT. Cognitive Therapy and the Motional Disorders. New York: International Universities Press, 1976.

142. Meichenbaum DA. Cognitive Behavior Modification: an Integrative Approach. New York: Plenum, 1977.

143. Bogaards MC, ter Kuile MM. Treatment of recurrent tension headache: a meta-analytic review. Clin J Pain 1994; 10: 174–90.

144. Holroyd KA, Penzien DB. Client variables and behavioral treatment of recurrent tension headaches: a meta-analytic review. J Behav Med 1986; 9: 515–36.

145. Hammill JM, Cook TM, Rosecrance JC. Effectiveness of a physical therapy regimen in the treatment of tension-type headache. Headache 1996; 36: 149–53.

146. Vernon H, McDermaid CS, Hagino C. Systematic review of randomized clinical trials of complementary/alternative therapies in the treatment of tension-type and cervicogenic headache. Complement Ther Med 1999; 7: 142–55.

147. Ahonen E, Mahlmaki S, Partenen J et al. Effectiveness of acupuncture and physiotherapy on myogenic headache: a comparative study. Acupunct Electrother Res 1984; 9: 141–50.

148. Carlsson JY, Jensen R. Physiotherapy of tension-type headache. In: Olesen J, Tfelt-Hansen P, Welch KMA, eds. The Headaches. 2nd edn. Philadelphia: Lippincott Williams & Wilkins, 2000, 651–6.

149. Bove G, Nilsson N. Spinal manipulation in the treatment of episodic tension-type headache: a randomized controlled trial. JAMA 1998; 280: 1576–9.

150. Hoyt WH, Shaffer F, Bard DA et al. Osteopathic manipulation in the treatment of muscle contraction headache. J Amer Osteopath Assoc 1979; 78: 322–5.

151. Boline PD, Kassak K, Bronfort G et al. Spinal manipulation vs amitriptyline for the treatment of chronic tension-type

headache: randomized clinical trial. J Manipulative Physiol Therap 1995; 18: 148–54.

152. Reik L. Unnecessary dental treatment of headache patients for temporomandibular joint disorders. Headache 1985; 25: 246–8.

153. Porta M. A comparative trial of botulinum toxin Type A and methylprednisolone for the treatment of tension-type headache. Cur Rev Pain 2000; 4: 31–5.

154. Smuts JA, Baker MK, Smuts HM et al. Botulinum toxin type A as prophylactic treatment in chronic tension-type headache. Cephalalgia 1999; 19: 454 (Abstract).

155. Gobel H, Lindner V, Krack P et al. Treatment of chronic tension-type headache with botulinum toxin. Cephalalgia 1999; 19: 455 (Abstract).

156. Relja MA, Korsic M. Treatment of tension-type headache by injections of botulinum toxin type A: double-blind placebo-controlled study. Neurology 1999; 52: A203 (Abstract).

157. Schmitt WJ, Slowey E, Fravi N et al. Effect of Botulinum toxin A injections in the treatment of chronic tension-type headache: a double-blind, placebo-controlled trial. Headache 2001; 41: 658–64.

158. Rollnik JD, Tanneberger O, Schubert M et al. Treatment of tension-type headache with botulinum toxin type A: a double-blind, placebo-controlled study. Headache 2000; 40: 300–5.

159. Gobel H, Heinze A, Kuhn KH, Austermann K. Botulinum toxin A in the treatment of headache syndromes and pericranial pain syndromes. Pain 2001; 91: 195–9.

chapter 8

Chronic daily headache: diagnosis and treatment

Introduction

The classification of very frequent primary headache disorders and the appropriate use of the term 'chronic daily headache' (CDH) are still controversial. Some authors use CDH to refer to 'transformed migraine', a distinct clinical syndrome described below. Others use the term for any headache disorder that occurs on a daily or near-daily basis, regardless of etiology. The International Headache Society (IHS) has now begun to address the classification of very frequent primary headache disorders. In this chapter, we use the term 'CDH' to refer to the broad group of headache disorders that occur more frequently than 15 days a month and we discuss those that have an average duration of 4 hours or longer. Headaches lasting less than four hours a day are discussed primarily in Chapters 9 and 10.

When a patient has frequent headaches (>15 days/month) that are not related to a structural or systemic illness, the physician faces a substantial diagnostic and therapeutic challenge. Although only 0.5% of the population have severe headaches on a daily basis,[1] and only 2–3% meet IHS criteria for chronic tension-type headache (CTTH),[2,3] these groups account for the majority of consultations in headache subspecialty practices.[3] Often these patients are overusing medication, and this may play a role in initiating or sustaining the pattern of frequent headaches. Anxiety, depression, and other psychological disturbances may accompany CDH and require treatment.[4]

Patients with CDH are difficult to classify using the current IHS classification system.[5–8] Many individuals with CDH are placed in the CTTH group or are given two diagnoses. If there are superimposed attacks of severe headache, a second diagnosis of migraine is often assigned. Several lines of evidence (outlined below) suggest that at least some patients with CDH evolving from migraine have the biology of the migraineur. Therefore, it seems inappropriate to classify their headaches as a form of tension-type headache (TTH). An approach to classifying CDH is presented in Table 8.1. We classify CDH into primary and secondary varieties and subclassify primary CDH on the basis of average daily headache duration into long-duration (≥ 4 hours) and short-duration (< 4 hours) subgroups. Causes of long-duration CDH include chronic (transformed) migraine (CM), CTTH, new daily persistent headache (NDPH), and hemicrania continua (HC).

Causes of short-duration CDH include chronic cluster headache, paroxysmal hemicrania (PH), short-lasting unilateral neuralgiform headache attacks with conjunctival injection and tearing (SUNCT), hypnic headache, idiopathic stabbing headache, and the cranial neuralgias. Both short- and long-duration primary and secondary CDH disorders can be associated with analgesic, ergotamine, or triptan overuse. Cervicogenic headache[9] is a unilateral pain disorder that does not switch sides,[10] occurs mainly in women, and may be associated with ipsilateral blurred vision, tinnitus, lacrimation, tingling, difficulty swallowing, photophobia, arm pain, and, when more severe, nausea and anorexia. 'Neck triggers' and reduced cervical range of motion are characteristic of the disorder. It is uncertain whether cervicogenic headache is an independent entity, or migraine, or TTH with a cervical trigger.[11]

Headache is a common accompaniment of cervical disc lesions.[12,13] High cervical bony defects and root damage (such as that caused by Paget's disease) that involves the bones of the base of the skull and the upper cervical spine are associated with headache. Since most of the population over the age of 40 years has radiological changes of cervical spondylosis but few have symptoms, it is

● **Table 8.1** Chronic daily headache

Primary variety
Headache duration >4 hours Chronic migraine Chronic tension-type headache New daily persistent headache Hemicrania continua
Headache duration <4 hours Cluster headache Chronic paroxysmal hemicrania SUNCT Hypnic headache Idiopathic stabbing headache
Secondary variety
Post-traumatic headache
Cervical spine disorders
Headache associated with vascular disorders: arteriovenous malformation; arteritis, including giant cell arteritis; dissection; subdural hematoma
Headache associated with nonvascular intracranial disorders (intracranial hypertension, infection (Epstein–Barr virus, HIV), neoplasm)
Other (temporomandibular joint disorder; sinus infection)

important not to attribute headache to X-ray abnormalities simply because these radiographic abnormalities are present. However, 40% of patients with spondylosis or symptomatic cervical disc disease, such as radiculopathy or myelopathy, have headache as a major complaint.[14] Even in the absence of uniform terminology, a systematic approach to these difficult patients is needed.

Secondary CDH may be caused by a range of structural, metabolic, and systemic disorders. CDH may be a presentation of idiopathic intracranial hypertension; in the majority of cases the diagnosis is easily made when papilledema is present. Some patients do not have papilledema; this condition can mimic primary CDH (see Chapter 8). Mosek et al[15] prospectively measured the cerebrospinal fluid opening pressure of 24 patients who had CDH without papilledema. The average cerebrospinal fluid opening pressure was 170 ± 41 mm cerebrospinal fluid, and five patients (21%) had an opening pressure of greater than 200 mm. The mean cerebrospinal fluid opening pressure of CDH patients was 13 mm higher than that of nonheadache patients ($p = 0.05$) after adjusting for body mass index, age, sex, and various nonheadache disorders. The odds of having a cerebrospinal fluid opening pressure greater than 200 mm cerebrospinal fluid was five times greater for CDH patients than nonheadache patients.

Several authors have examined the relative frequency of some of these conditions in clinic patients with CDH. Most had CDH evolving from migraine, some began de novo, and a few had CDH that had evolved from episodic tension-type headache (ETTH). Many, if not most, patients had CDH associated with medication overuse.[16] In population studies, CM and CTTH are the most frequent causes of primary CDH of long duration, followed by NDPH and HC.[17]

In this chapter, we discuss the classification and treatment of primary CDH of long duration, highlighting the four categories above. We discuss our proposed revisions to the IHS system and offer criteria for CM, CTTH, NDPH and HC (Table 8.2).[4] The new IHS classification will provide criteria for each of these disorders.

Chronic migraine

Patients with CM often have a past history of episodic migraine beginning in their teens or twenties.[18] In subspecialty clinics, most of these patients are women, 90% of whom have a history of migraine without aura. The headaches grow more frequent (over months to years) and the associated symptoms of photophobia, phonopho-

● **Table 8.2** Headache classification for chronic daily headache (CDH)

Daily or near daily headache lasting >4 hours/day for >15 days/month

1.8 Chronic migraine	
	1.8.1 with medication overuse
	1.8.2 without medication overuse
2.2 Chronic tension-type headache (CTTH)	
	2.2.1 with medication overuse
	2.2.2 without medication overuse
4.7 New daily persistent headache (NDPH)	
	4.7.1 with medication overuse
	4.7.2 without medication overuse
4.8 Hemicrania continua (HC)	
	4.8.1 with medication overuse
	4.8.2 without medication overuse

Adapted from Silberstein et al.[4]

bia, and nausea become less severe and less frequent than during typical migraine (Figure 8.1).[19,20] Patients often develop a pattern of daily or nearly-daily headaches that phenomenologically resemble CTTH. That is, the pain is mild to moderate and not associated with photophobia, phonophobia, or gastrointestinal features. Other features of migraine, including unilaterality, gastrointestinal symptoms, and aggravation by menstruation and other trigger factors, may persist. Many patients have attacks of full-blown migraine superimposed on a background of less severe headaches.

In clinic-based studies, about 80% of patients who have CM overuse symptomatic medication.[19,21–24] Their headache frequency may have increased during a period of increasing medication use (Figure 8.1). Stopping the overused medication frequently results in headache improvement, although this may take days or weeks to occur (Figure 8.2). Many patients have significant long-term improvement after detoxification. In population studies, less than one-third of CDH sufferers overuse medication.[25] Thus, medication overuse is not necessary for the development of CDH.

Eighty percent of patients with CM have depression.[19,23] The depression often lifts when the pattern of medication overuse and daily headache is interrupted. Although CM is widely recognized as a clinical entity, widely accepted formal diagnostic criteria are still lacking. We proposed and then revised criteria for what was then called transformed migraine (Table 8.3). We believed that transformed migraine was a form of migraine and that its diagnosis depended upon a past history of IHS migraine with a

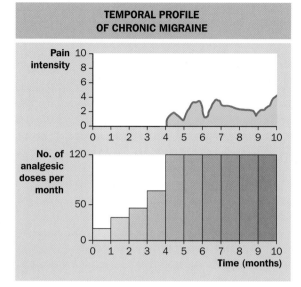

**TEMPORAL PROFILE
OF CHRONIC MIGRAINE**

● **Figure 8.1** *Temporal profile of transformed migraine provided by a 30-year-old woman who has a ten year history of headache. For many years she had bouts of episodic migraine without aura but with some nausea lasting 6–8 hours which she treated with a caffeine/analgesic mixture. About one year ago her headaches became more frequent and she started to increase her use of analgesics. After four months she experienced daily, bilateral headaches which were mild to moderate in intensity and associated with periodic migraine exacerbations.*

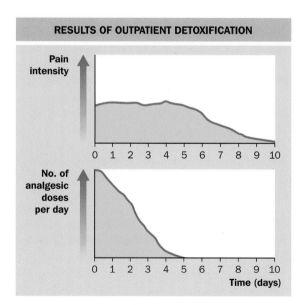

RESULTS OF OUTPATIENT DETOXIFICATION

● **Figure 8.2** *Results of outpatient detoxification. An improvement in CDH occurred within days of stopping the overuse of analgesics. Breakthrough headaches were treated with intramuscular dihydroergotamine administration.*

● **Table 8.3** *Proposed '1995' criteria for transformed (now chronic) migraine.*

1.8 Transformed migraine
A Daily or almost daily (>15 days/month) head pain for >1 month
B Average headache duration of >4 hours/day (if untreated)
C At least one of the following: • History of episodic migraine meeting any IHS criteria 1.1 to 1.6 • History of increasing headache frequency with decreasing severity of migrainous features over at least 3 months • Headache at some time meets IHS criteria for migraine 1.1 to 1.6 other than duration
D Does not meet criteria for new daily persistent headache (4.7) or hemicrania continua (4.8)
E At least one of the following: • There is no suggestion of one of the disorders listed in groups 5–11 • Such a disorder is suggested, but it is ruled out by appropriate investigations • Such disorder is present, but first migraine attacks do not occur in close temporal relation to the disorder

Adapted from Silberstein et al.[4]

process of transformation leading to CDH. The period of transformation was characterized by increasing headache frequency and decreasing prominence of associated migrainous features.

Our criteria provide three alternative diagnostic links to migraine:

- a prior history of IHS migraine;
- a clear period of escalating headache frequency with decreasing severity of migrainous features (which were both required in the 1994 criteria); or
- current superimposed attacks of headaches that meet all the IHS criteria for migraine except duration.

To avoid undue diagnostic overlap, we proposed hierarchical rules. If a patient meets the criteria for two disorders, the rules establish which diagnosis should be used. Thus, the diagnosis of CM precludes a diagnosis of either episodic migraine (IHS 1.11.7) or CTTH.

Although migraine transformation most often develops with medication overuse, transformation may occur without overuse.[21,26] Using the IHS criteria, a firm diagnosis of 'headache induced by substance use or exposure' requires that the headaches remit after the overused medication is discontinued. Figure 8.2 illustrates a patient whose daily headache remitted but whose episodic migraine continued when medication overuse was eliminated. In such a patient, the diagnosis changes from episodic migraine to transformed migraine with medication overuse, back to episodic migraine. This criterion is difficult to apply reliably, and diagnosis is impossible until the overused medication is discontinued. As an alternative, we provide definitions for medication overuse based on a review of published reports and clinical experience (see below).[4,27]

Chronic tension-type headache (Table 8.4)

Patients who have a history of ETTH may develop daily headaches. These headaches are usually diffuse or bilateral and frequently involve the posterior aspect of the head and neck. In CTTH, in contrast to CM, most features of migraine are absent, as is prior or coexistent episodic migraine.

● **Table 8.4** *Proposed diagnostic criteria for chronic tension-type headache (CTTH)*

2.2 Chronic tension-type headache

A Average headache frequency >15 days/month (180 days/year) with average duration of >4 hours/day (if untreated) for 6 months fulfilling criteria (B–D) listed below

B At least two of the following pain characteristics:
1 Pressing/tightening quality
2 Mild or moderate severity (may inhibit, but does not prohibit activities)
3 Bilateral location
4 No aggravation by walking stairs or similar routine physical activity

C History of episodic tension-type headache in the past (needs to be tested)

D History of evolutive headaches which gradually increased in frequency over at least a 3 month period (needs to be tested)

E Both of the following:
1 No vomiting
2 No more than one of nausea, photophobia, or phonophobia (needs to be tested).

F Does not meet criteria for hemicrania continua (4.8), new daily persistent headache (4.7) or transformed migraine (1.8).

G At least one of the following:
1 There is no suggestion of one of the disorders listed in groups 5–11
2 Such a disorder is suggested, but it is ruled out by appropriate investigations.
3 Such disorder is present, but first headache attacks do not occur in close temporal relation to the disorder.

Adapted from Silberstein et al.[4]

We propose several modifications to the current criteria for CTTH. The current criteria for CTTH (IHS 2.2) require head pain on at least 15 days a month for at least 6 months. Although the pain criteria are identical to ETTH, the IHS classification allows nausea, but not vomiting. Operational rules are needed regarding nausea, photophobia, and phonophobia, and for the decision regarding the prominence of these features.[8] Mild nausea or mild photophobia and phonophobia may prove to be compatible with the diagnosis of CTTH if better measures of symptom severity are developed.[8,27] However, the need to include any of these migrainous features in the IHS definition of CTTH may be a result of including cases of CM under the rubric of CTTH.

CTTH evolving from ETTH requires a prior diagnosis of ETTH. Diagnostic confidence increases if ETTH increases in frequency until the criteria of CTTH are met. No explicit time durations of headache are specified in the IHS definition of CTTH. Although CTTH usually has an average headache duration of >4 hours (Table 8.4), we believe that the broad range of durations included in the IHS criteria are compatible with the diagnosis. CTTH can exist in two varieties: headaches associated with (2.2.0.1) and not associated with (2.2.0.2) medication overuse. One could argue that CTTH could begin without preceding ETTH, analogous to the situation that exists in chronic cluster (i.e. unrelenting from onset). However, cluster headache involves a series of episodic attacks, not a constant headache.

Russell et al[28] evaluated CTTH via a family study of 122 probands and 377 first-degree relatives. Sensitivity, specificity, predictive values, and chance-corrected agreement rates for the diagnosis of CTTH were 68%, 86%, 53% (PVpos), 92% (PVneg), and 0.48, respectively. The low sensitivity of CTTH assessed by proband report indicates that a clinical interview of family members is necessary. Clinically-interviewed parents, siblings, and children had a 2.1- to 3.9-fold increased risk of CTTH compared with the general population. The proband's gender did not influence the risk of CTTH among first-degree relatives. The significantly increased familial risk, with no increased risk found in spouses, suggest that a genetic factor is involved in CTTH.

New daily persistent headache (Table 8.5)

NDPH is the abrupt development (over <3 days) of a headache that does not remit.[29] NDPH is likely to be a heterogeneous disorder. Some cases may reflect a postviral syndrome.[29] Patients with NDPH are generally younger than those with CM.[29]

● **Table 8.5** *Proposed criteria for new daily persistent headache (NDPH)*

4.7 New daily persistent headache
A Average headache frequency >15 days/month for >1 month
B Average headache duration >4 hours/day (if untreated). Frequently constant without medication but may fluctuate
C No history of tension-type headache or migraine which increases in frequency and decreases in severity in association with the onset of NDPH (over 3 months)
D Acute onset (developing over <3 days) of constant unremitting headache
E Headache is constant in location? (Needs to be tested)
F Does not meet criteria for hemicrania continua (4.8)
G At least one of the following: 1 There is no suggestion of one of the disorders listed in groups 5–11. 2 Such a disorder is suggested, but it is ruled out by appropriate investigations. 3 Such disorder is present, but first headache attacks do not occur in close temporal relation to the disorder.

Adapted from Silberstein et al.[4]

● **Table 8.6** *Proposed criteria for hemicrania continua*

4.8 Hemicrania continua (HC)*
A Headache present for at least 1 month
B Strictly unilateral headache
C Pain has all of the following present: 1 Continuous but fluctuating 2 Moderate severity, at least some of the time 3 Lack of precipitating mechanisms
D 1 Absolute response to indomethacin, or 2 One of the following autonomic features with severe pain exacerbation: • Conjunctival injection • Lacrimation • Nasal congestion • Rhinorrhoea • Ptosis • Eyelid edema
E At least one of the following: 1 There is no suggestion of one of the disorders listed in groups 5–11. 2 Such a disorder is suggested, but it is ruled out by appropriate investigations. 3 Such disorder is present, but first headache attacks do not occur in close temporal relation to the disorder.
F May have associated idiopathic stabbing headache

Adapted from Goadsby and Lipton.[31]
* HC is usually non-remitting, but rare cases of remission have been reported.

We elected not to classify NDPH as a type of de novo CTTH, for it is not clear whether or not this condition is etiologically related to TTH. Since NDPH and CTTH have similar characteristics, the disorders are distinguished by the presence or absence of a past history of headache. NDPH requires the absence of a history of evolution from migraine or ETTH. Excluding all patients with a history of ETTH is problematic, as almost 70% of men and 90% of women have had a TTH at some time in the past. We allow a diagnosis of NDPH in patients with migraine or ETTH if these disorders do not increase in frequency to give rise to NDPH. The constancy of location is uncertain and needs to be field-tested. NDPH may or may not be associated with medication overuse (4.7.1, 4.7.2). A diagnosis of NDPH takes precedence over CM and CTTH.

Hemicrania continua (Table 8.6)

HC is a relatively rare,[30] indomethacin (indometacin)-responsive headache disorder characterized by a continuous, unilateral headache that varies in intensity, waxing and waning without disappearing completely. The continuous unilateral headache is frequently associated with exacerbations of more severe pain. These painful exacerbations are often associated with autonomic disturbances such as ptosis, miosis, tearing, and sweating.[31] It may (rarely) alternate sides.[32] It is frequently associated with jabs and

jolts (idiopathic stabbing headache). HC is not reliably triggered by neck movements, but tender spots in the neck may be present. Patients may have photophobia, phonophobia, and nausea.

We present a patient history to illustrate the important features of this disorder.[31] A 45-year-old woman presented with a 10-year history of daily unilateral headache. In the remote past, she had had occasional periods of left-sided headache lasting from 1 month to 1 year. At the time of presentation, she had a constant, widely distributed, left-sided hemicranial headache that waxed and waned in severity. The pain was usually mild to moderate, but eight to 20 times a month she experienced exacerbations that lasted as long as 12 hours, characterized by more severe left periorbital and hemicranial pain accompanied by left-side miosis, ptosis and nasal congestion. The exacerbations were also associated with nausea and sensitivity to sensory stimuli. Her past medical history was unremarkable. General medical and neurologic examinations and routine laboratory studies were unremarkable. Magnetic resonance imaging (MRI) of the head was normal.

The patient had been treated with several beta-blockers, calcium-channel blockers, tricyclic antidepressants, selective serotonin reuptake inhibitors (SSRIs), methysergide, and divalproex sodium without substantial relief. Inpatient treatment with dihydroergotamine did not improve her headaches. Acute treatment with several non-steroidal anti-inflammatory drugs (NSAIDs) and transnasal butorphanol and butalbital combination products was not helpful. Subcutaneous sumatriptan produced short-term relief during painful exacerbations. Following a tentative diagnosis of HC, she was started on indomethacin 50 mg t.i.d. Her headache resolved following each dose of indomethacin but recurred at the end of the dosing interval. Her regimen was gradually increased to a final dose of 75 mg t.i.d. with ranitidine (150 mg b.i.d.). Her other medications have been tapered and she is headache-free unless she skips a dose of indomethacin.

This patient illustrates the prompt and enduring response to indomethacin that typifies the disorder. Requiring a therapeutic response as a diagnostic criterion is problematic. It effectively excludes the diagnosis of HC in patients who were never treated with indomethacin (perhaps because of ulcer disease) and patients who failed to respond to indomethacin. Treatment response is generally not part of IHS case definitions of headache disorders. Cases have been described that did not respond to indomethacin but otherwise meet the phenotype. For this reason, we have provided an alternate means of diagnosis (Table 8.6), which is controversial.[33]

HC exists in both continuous and remitting forms. In the continuous form, which must be differentiated from CM, headaches occur on a daily basis, sometimes for years. Many patients with this disorder overuse acute medication. In the remitting form, periods of daily headache alternate with pain-free remissions. Both forms meet the criteria outlined in Table 8.6. HC takes precedence over the diagnosis of other types of primary CDH.

Clinical features

HC, a unilateral, continuous, indomethacin-responsive headache with periodic exacerbations, was believed to be a rare disorder. Peres et al recently reported 34 new cases and suggested that HC may be more common than has been appreciated.[34] The number of patients with unilateral CDH who respond to indomethacin is unknown.

Sixty-three of the 93 previously reported patients were typical indomethacin-responsive cases. Of these, 53 (84%) were continuous (approximately two-thirds continuous from onset), and 10 (16%) were remitting. Peres' patients were similar: 30 patients (88.2%) had the continuous form, 18 (52.9%) from onset and 12 (35.3%) transformed from remitting; four (11.8%) were remitting.

Thirty patients had atypical features, including headaches that alternated sides,[35] bilateral pain,[36] unresponsiveness to indomethacin,[37,38] posttraumatic,[39] association with hemiplegic migraine,[20] and evolution from cluster headache.[40] Two secondary cases have been reported, one with a mesenchymal tumor[41] and another with HIV.[42] The four bilateral reported cases were either remitting (two patients) or had transformed from remitting (two patients).

A preponderance of women (5:1) was present in the first 18 reported cases;[32] the gender ratio has decreased as more cases were reported (1.8:1).[43] Summarizing all the cases where gender data is available, there are 61 women and 22 men, with a 2.8:1 woman:man ratio. The sex ratio in our patients (2.4:1) was similar.[34]

Exacerbations are a common feature of HC, occurring in 74% of reported cases and in all of Peres' patients. Nocturnal exacerbations occur and could result in a mistaken diagnosis of cluster or hypnic headache. Thirty percent of the reported cases had nocturnal exacerbations that usually lasted 1–2 hours; 29.4% of Peres' patients had nocturnal exacerbations.

The associated symptoms of HC can be divided into three main categories: autonomic symptoms, idiopathic stabbing headache and migrainous features. Autonomic symptoms (conjunctival injection, tearing, rhinorrhea, nasal stuffiness, eyelid edema, and forehead sweatiness) are not as prominent in HC as in cluster headache or PH and can be absent. They occurred in 63% of 41 cases with available descriptions and in 73.5% of Peres' patients during painful exacerbations, but not with baseline headache. The most common symptom in both our series and the literature was tearing; conjunctival injection and ptosis were slightly more frequent in the literature than we observed.

Idiopathic stabbing headache syndrome is defined as a sharp pain that lasts less than 1 minute. It occurs in headache-free individuals and in patients with tension-type, migraine, and cluster headache. It often responds to indomethacin. It occurs in patients with HC more frequently in the exacerbation periods. Idiopathic stabbing headache syndrome was described in 26% of the cases in the literature and in 41% of Peres' patients. Its prevalence in the general population is reported to be 30%.[44] Because of its low sensitivity and specificity, it should be not be part of the diagnostic criteria for HC.

Migrainous features were common. Twenty-four (70.6%) of Peres' patients met IHS criteria for migraine in the exacerbation period, but none did in the baseline period. IHS diagnostic criteria for migraine could not be applied to previously reported cases because of lack of information. Nevertheless, 23 patients (50%) had at least one migrainous feature: either nausea, vomiting, photophobia, or phonophobia.

HC is one of the indomethacin-responsive headaches; others are chronic and episodic paroxysmal hemicrania (Chapter 10), exertional headaches, and some cases of migraine and cluster headache (Chapter 9). The reported effective dose of indomethacin for HC ranged from 50 to 300 mg a day. We found the most common effective dose to be 150 mg a day (range 25–225 mg). Drugs other than indomethacin that are reported to be effective in HC include ibuprofen (800 mg t.i.d.),[45] piroxicam beta-cyclodextrin (20–40 mg a day),[46] and rofecoxib.[47] Other classes of drugs have not been successful in controlling HC, including sumatriptan.[48] Injectable indomethacin 50 mg intramuscularly ('indotest') has been used as a diagnostic test for HC.[34] Complete pain relief was reported to occur within 2 hours. Six patients who met the HC phenotype but were not responsive to indomethacin were reported.[37,38] Whether these patients truly have HC is uncertain.

The long-term outcome of indomethacin response was investigated in eight patients.[49] Indomethacin was discontinued after 3, 7, and 15 months and patients remained pain-free. Three patients discontinued treatment because of side-effects and had headache recurrence; two had relief with aspirin. Two other patients continue to take indomethacin and had partial relief. Symptomatic cases of HC with loss of response to indomethacin have also been reported.[41] These cases suggest that escalating doses or loss of indomethacin's efficacy should be treated with suspicion and the patient reevaluated.

Pathophysiological studies

The relative rarity of HC has made it difficult to study its pathophysiology. Pain pressure thresholds are reduced in patients with HC, as they are in PH patients.[50] In contrast, orbital phlebography is relatively normal compared with patients with PH,[50] although it should be observed that this area is controversial. Pupillometric studies have shown no clear abnormality in HC, and studies of facial sweating have shown modest changes, similar to those seen in PH.[50]

Drug overuse and rebound headache

Patients with frequent headaches of all kinds may overuse opioids, simple analgesics, ergotamine, and triptans (Figure 8.3).[51] Medication overuse by headache-prone patients frequently produces CDH (drug-induced 'rebound headache') accompanied by dependence on symptomatic medication. In addition, medication overuse can make headaches refractory to preventive medication.[26,52–55]

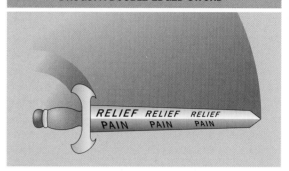

DRUGS: A DOUBLE-EDGED SWORD

● **Figure 8.3** *Overuse of medication by headache-prone patients frequently produces drug-induced CDH accompanied by dependence on symptomatic medication.*

Although stopping the symptomatic medication may result in withdrawal symptoms and a period of increased headache initially, the general rule is subsequent headache improvement.[55–59] Many CDH patients who were withdrawn from ergotamine and analgesics and given no further therapy stopped having daily headaches, although they often still had episodic migraine attacks.[60,61]

In subspecialty centers, most patients with drug-induced headache have a history of episodic migraine that has been converted into CM as a result of medication overuse.[22,26,52,55,61–64] Patients with CTTH, HC, and NDPH may also overuse symptomatic medications. Drug-induced CDH, or, as Isler[65] has termed it, 'painkiller headache', has been reported since the 17th century, with occurrences reaching epidemic proportions in Switzerland after World War II.

The epidemiology of chronic drug-induced headache is uncertain since some headaches are drug-induced and some are just associated with drug overuse. In some European headache centers, 5–10% of the patients have drug-induced headache. One series of 3000 consecutive headache patients reported that 4.3% had drug-induced headaches.[66] Experience in the United Kingdom suggests that drug-associated headache is more common in Europe than the literature suggests. In American specialty headache clinics, as many as 50–80% of patients who presented with CDH used analgesics on a daily or near-daily basis.[58] These differences may reflect the genuine influence of patterns of healthcare use. In the United States, over-the-counter analgesics are readily available and patients often consult multiple physicians who may not be aware of other analgesics that the patient is taking. In population studies, only 20–30% of patients with CDH overuse medications (A Scher, personal communication).[25]

Clinical features of rebound headache

Analgesic rebound headache has not been demonstrated in placebo-controlled trials. However, stopping daily low-dose caffeine frequently results in withdrawal headache.[67] In a controlled study of caffeine withdrawal, 64 normal adults (71% women) with low to moderate caffeine intake (the equivalent of about 2.5 cups of coffee a day) were given a 2-day caffeine-free diet and either placebo or replacement caffeine. Under double-blind conditions, 50% of the patients who were given placebo had a headache by day 2, compared with 6% of those given caffeine. Nausea, depression, and flu-like symptoms were very common in the placebo group. This study is relevant since caffeine is frequently used by headache sufferers for pain relief, often in combination with analgesics or ergotamine. The study is a model for short-term caffeine withdrawal, but does not demonstrate the long-term consequences of detoxification. In a community-based telephone survey of 11 112 subjects in Lincoln and Omaha, Nebraska, USA, 61% reported daily caffeine consumption, and 11% of the caffeine consumers reported symptoms upon stopping coffee.[68] A group of those who reported withdrawal symptoms was assigned to one of three regimes: abrupt caffeine withdrawal, gradual withdrawal, and no change. One third of the abrupt-withdrawal group and an occasional member of the gradual-withdrawal group had symptoms that included headache and tiredness.

The actual dose limits and time needed to develop rebound headaches have not been defined in rigorous studies. In addition, the relationship of drug half-life to the development of rebound is unknown. Our clinical knowledge is derived from observing patterns of medication use in patients who have rebound headaches. Because there may be large individual differences in susceptibility to rebound headaches, anecdotal data must be generalized cautiously. Overuse is believed to occur when patients take opioids or ergotamine tartrate more often than 2 days a week, three or more simple analgesics a day more often than 5 days a week, or triptans or combination analgesics containing barbiturates or sedatives more often than 3 days a week (Figure 8.4).[26,52–54,69]

Specific limits are necessary to prevent analgesic, ergotamine, and triptan overuse. The frequency of days of ergotamine use (treatment days, events) is as important as, if not more important than, the total monthly dose.[23,56] Rebound can develop when patients take as little as 0.5–1 mg of ergotamine three times a week.[54,59,69,70] Sumatriptan and the other triptans, which are effective in acute migraine treatment, have been reported to induce rebound headache.[71] We recommend limiting the use of triptans to two or at most three days a week.[51] Careful

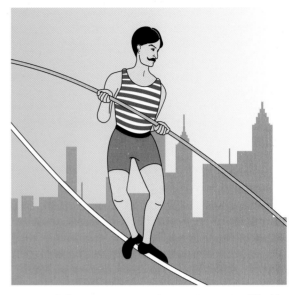

● **Figure 8.4** *Responsible use of analgesics can be difficult!*

monitoring is required when the headache frequency reaches two or more days a week.

Most daily headache patients overuse symptomatic medication[72] and may develop psychological dependence, tolerance, and abstinence syndromes. Medication overuse may be responsible, in part, for the transformation of episodic migraine or ETTH into daily headache and for the perpetuation of the syndrome. However, medication overuse is not the sine qua non of CM or CTTH. Some patients develop CM or CTTH without overusing medication, and others continue to have daily headaches long after the overused medication is discontinued. Medication overuse is usually motivated by a patient's desire to treat the headaches. However, some headache patients may overuse combination analgesics to treat their mood disturbance. Medication overuse rarely represents primary substance abuse.

In addition to exacerbating the headache disorder, drug overuse has other serious effects. The overuse of symptomatic drugs may interfere with the effectiveness of preventive headache medications. The extended use of large amounts of medication may cause renal or hepatic toxicity in addition to tolerance, habituation, or dependence. ('Tolerance' refers to the decreased effectiveness of the same dose of an analgesic, often leading to the use of higher doses to achieve the same degree of effectiveness. 'Habituation' and 'dependence' are, respectively, the psychological and physical need to repeatedly use drugs).

Psychiatric comorbidity

Anxiety, depression, and bipolar disease are more frequent in migraine patients than in non-migraine control subjects.[73,74] Since CM evolves from migraine, one would also expect psychiatric comorbidity in CM. In a clinic-based study of 630 patients with CDH, including patients with CM, CTTH, NDPH and posttraumatic headache, the Minnesota Multiphasic Personality Inventory (MMPI) was abnormal in 61%, compared with 12.2% of patients with episodic migraine. Zung and Beck Depression Scale scores were significantly higher in the CDH patients than in migraine controls.[52] In several subspecialty center-based studies, depression occurred in about 80% of CM patients.[26,52,54] Clinical experience suggests that comorbid depression often improves when the cycle of daily head pain is broken.[75] The biological relationship of migraine vulnerability to rebound headache and psychiatric comorbidity remains to be clarified. Mitsikostas and Thomas[76] found more anxiety and depression in headache sufferers than in healthy controls. High headache attack frequency, a long history of headaches, and female gender correlated to more anxiety and depression. Verri et al[77] found current psychiatric comorbidity in 90% of primary CDH patients, 81% of migraineurs, and 83% of chronic low back pain patients. Generalized anxiety disorders were the most common in each group.

Psychiatric comorbidity is a predictor of intractability. The MMPI was abnormal in 100% of patients with primary CDH who failed to respond to aggressive management (31% of the primary CDH group), compared with 48% of the responders. Physical, emotional, or sexual abuse, parental alcohol abuse, and a positive dexamethasone suppression test also correlated highly with a poor response to aggressive management. Curioso et al[78] found that 31 of 69 (45%) primary CDH patients had an adjustment disorder, 16 (23%) had major depression, 12 (17%) were dysthymic, six (9%) had generalized anxiety disorder, one (2%) was bipolar, and three (4%) were normal. The risk of a bad outcome after treatment was significantly greater for patients with major depression compared with those without. Primary CDH patients who have major depression or have abnormal Beck Depression Inventory scores have worse outcomes at 3–6 months compared with patients who are not depressed.

Epidemiology

In population-based surveys, primary CDH occurs in 4.1% of Americans, 4.35% of Greeks, 3.9% of elderly Chinese, and 4.7% of Spaniards.[17,79–82] Population-based estimates for the 1-year period prevalence of CTTH are 1.7% in Ethiopia,[79] 3% in Denmark,[80] 2.2% in Spain,[25] 2.7% in China,[81] and 2.2% in the United States.[17]

Scher et al[17] ascertained the prevalence of CDH in Baltimore County, Maryland. The overall prevalence of primary CDH was 4.1% (5.0% women, 2.8% men; 1.8 : 1 women to men ratio). In both men and women, prevalence was highest in the lowest educational category. More than half (52% women, 56% men) met criteria for CTTH (2.2%), almost one-third (33% women, 25% men) met criteria for CM (1.3%), and the remainder (15% women, 19% men) were unclassified (0.6%). Overall, 30% of women and 25% of men who were frequent headache sufferers met IHS criteria for migraine (with or without aura). On the basis of chance, migraine and CTTH would co-occur in 0.22% of the population; CM occurring in 1.3% of this population would suggest that their co-occurrence is more than random.

Castillo et al[25] found that 4.7% of the population of Cantalucia, Spain had CDH. None had HC, 0.1% had NDPH, 2.2% had CTTH, and 2.4% had CM. Overuse of symptomatic medication occurred in 19% of CTTH patients and 31.1% of CM patients.

Wang et al[81] looked at the characteristics of primary CDH in a population of elderly Chinese (over 65 years of age) in two townships on Kinmen Island in August 1993. Sixty patients (3.9%) had CDH. Significantly more women than men had primary CDH (5.6% and 1.8%, $p < 0.001$). Of the primary CDH patients, 42 (70%) had CTTH (2.7%), 15 (25%) had CM (1%), and three (5%) had other CDH. The significant risk factors of primary CDH included analgesic overuse (OR = 79), a history of migraine (OR = 6.6), and a Geriatric Depression Scale-Short Form score of 8 or above (OR = 2.6). At follow-up in 1995 and 1997, approximately two-thirds of patients still had CDH. Compared with the patients in remission, the patients with persistent primary CDH in 1997 had a significantly higher frequency of analgesic overuse (33% vs. 0%, $p = 0.03$) and major depression (38% vs. 0%, $p = 0.04$).

Pathophysiology

The source of pain in CDH is unknown. Chronic continuous pain is often because of ongoing peripheral activation of nociceptors (e.g. chronic inflammation), although at times chronic pain may occur in the absence of painful stimuli. Peripheral sensitization owing to tissue damage or inflammation reduces the threshold of nociceptive afferent input at the injury site, resulting in local pain and tenderness. Central sensitization results from increased excitability of spinal neurons, producing an exaggerated response, so that non-painful stimuli feel painful even outside the injured site. Although the pathophysiology of CDH is unknown, recent work suggests several mechanisms that could contribute to the process. CDH may be due to:

- abnormal excitation of peripheral nociceptive afferent fibers with peripheral sensitization (perhaps due to chronic neurogenic inflammation);
- enhanced responsiveness of the nucleus caudalis neurons (central sensitization);
- defective pain modulation;
- spontaneous central pain;
- continuous activity of the 'migraine brainstem generator'; or
- a combination of these (see Chapter 5).

Drug-induced headache mechanisms

Overuse of analgesics, barbiturates, or ergotamine-containing compounds may contribute to the transformation of episodic migraine into CM. Some believe that drug-induced CDH is owing to a rebound effect wherein medication withdrawal triggers the next headache, which, in turn, leads to the consumption of more drugs. This may produce a vicious cycle resulting in more frequent drug use and drug-induced CDH. Formulations of drugs that maintain sustained, non-fluctuating levels might avoid the development of drug-induced headache.[82] The consequences of drug discontinuation depend on the type of therapeutic response it engenders. Discontinuation might be associated with relapse for several reasons. These include:

- loss of therapeutic drug effects;
- rebound changes caused by drug withdrawal; or
- re-induction of the primary pathophysiological process with the occurrence of a new episode.[82,83]

Increased activity of the on-cells in the pain modulation system of the brainstem could enhance the response to any painful or non-painful stimuli and result in sensitization. The activity of this system is enhanced during opioid withdrawal. A similar mechanism may occur during drug-induced headaches. CM not associated with drug overuse may result from sensitization of nociceptors in the nucleus caudalis as a result of enhanced on-cell activity, which could be, in part, a problem of the network that modulates pain from the head and face. Continued high fluctuating doses of ergots, analgesics, or opioids could result in resetting of the pain control mechanisms in susceptible individuals, perhaps by enhancing on-cell activity, enhancing central sensitization through N-methyl-D-aspartate receptors, or blocking adaptive antinociceptive changes. Compensatory adaptive changes associated with frequent headaches (if they occur) may not be enough to allow continued drug effectiveness. If tolerance has decreased drug effectiveness, a drug holiday could renew the response.[82] Drug overuse may, in part, prevent the occurrence of antinociceptive adaptive changes.

The transformation of episodic to chronic headache or the development of de novo CDH probably is a result of sensitization in the pathways of the trigeminal system. This could result from a painful peripheral receptor stimulus (other painful disorders in the trigeminal or cervical territory), from stressful events that could enhance pain perception, or from neurochemical or hormonal changes. Increased on-cell activity, decreased central pain inhibition, and activation of the peripheral nociceptor may act together to produce CDH. Whether increased kindling and N-methyl-D-aspartate receptor activity or nerve growth factor (NGF) and NGF mast cell activation occur is not known for certain, but these theoretical possibilities suggest potential therapy. In addition, the phenomenon of contingent tolerance (see Chapter 5) may be at work. Clinical strategies based on these concepts might be used to reverse tolerance in the long-term treatment of migraine or transformed migraine. Changing the patient's drug to one that has a different mechanism of action and does not show cross-tolerance or discontinuing the ineffective drug and re-introducing it later may be effective in some CM patients.

Treatment

Overview (Figures 8.5–8.7)

It can be difficult to treat patients who are suffering from CDH, especially those who have the complications of medication overuse and comorbid depression.[22,54] We recommend the following steps. First, exclude secondary headache disorders; second, diagnose the specific long-duration primary CDH disorder (i.e. CM, CTTH, NDPH, or HC); and third, identify comorbid medical and psychiatric conditions and exacerbating factors, especially medication overuse. Limit all symptomatic medications (with the possible exception of the long-acting NSAIDs). For out-

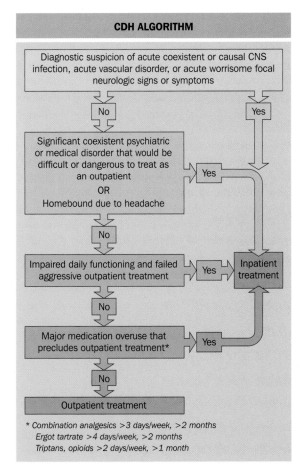

● **Figure 8.5** *CDH treatment algorithm.*

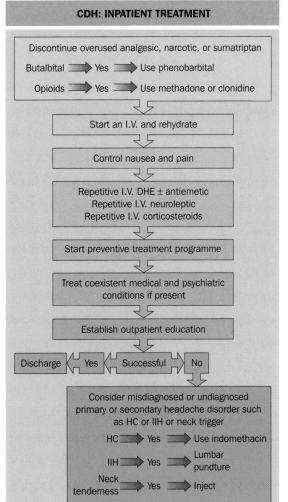

● **Figure 8.6** *CDH inpatient treatment algorithm.*

patients, gradually taper the overused medications, at a rate of 10% a week, often replacing them with NSAIDs. Patients should be started on a programme of preventive medication (to decrease reliance on symptomatic medication), with the explicit understanding that the drugs may not become fully effective until medication overuse has been eliminated and the washout period completed.[84] Patients need education and continuous support during the detoxification period, which may require several months. If outpatient detoxification proves difficult or is dangerous, hospitalization may be required. The detoxification process can last from 2–10 weeks after medication overuse is eliminated. Withdrawal symptoms include severely exacerbated headaches accompanied by nausea, vomiting, agitation, restlessness, sleep disorder, and (rarely) seizures. Barbiturates and benzodiazepines must be tapered gradually to avoid a serious withdrawal syndrome. The washout period may last 3–8 weeks; once it is

over, there is frequently considerable headache improvement.[16,22,59,85]

Inpatient and outpatient (ambulatory infusion unit or at-home) detoxification options are available. A consensus paper by the German Migraine Society recommends outpatient withdrawal for highly motivated patients who do not take barbiturates or tranquilizers with their analgesics. Inpatient treatment is recommended for patients who fail outpatient treatment, have high depression scores, or take tranquilizers, codeine, or barbiturates.[86]

Hospitalization may be necessary for severe dehydration, for which parenteral therapy may be necessary; diagnostic suspicion (confirmed by appropriate diagnostic testing) of organic etiology; prolonged, unrelenting headache with associated symptoms, such as nausea and

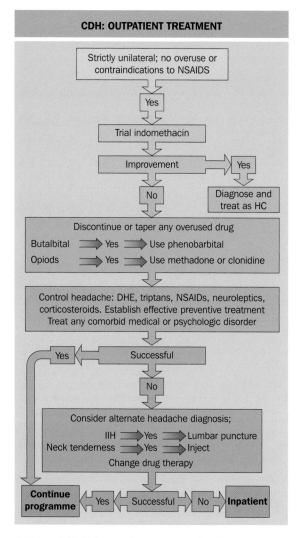

CDH: OUTPATIENT TREATMENT

Strictly unilateral; no overuse or contraindications to NSAIDS

Yes

Trial indomethacin

Improvement → Yes

No

Diagnose and treat as HC

Discontinue or taper any overused drug

Butalbital → Yes → Use phenobarbital

Opioids → Yes → Use methadone or clonidine

Control headache: DHE, triptans, NSAIDs, neuroleptics, corticosteroids. Establish effective preventive treatment Treat any comorbid medical or psychologic disorder

Yes ← Successful

No

Consider alternate headache diagnosis;

IIH → Yes → Lumbar puncture

Neck tenderness → Yes → Inject

Change drug therapy

Continue programme ← Yes ← Successful → No → **Inpatient**

● *Figure 8.7* *CDH outpatient treatment algorithm.*

vomiting, which, if allowed to continue, would pose a further threat to the patient's welfare; status migraine; dependence on analgesics, ergots, opioids, barbiturates, or tranquilizers; pain that is accompanied by serious adverse reactions or complications from therapy wherein continued use of such therapy aggravates or induces further illness; pain that occurs in the presence of significant medical disease but appropriate treatment of headache symptom aggravates or induces further illness; failed outpatient detoxification, for which inpatient pain and psychiatric management may be necessary; or treatment requiring co-pharmacy with drugs that may cause a drug interaction, thus necessitating careful observation (monoamine oxidase inhibitors and beta-blockers).

Disturbances in mood and function are common and require management with behavioral methods of pain management and supportive psychotherapy (including biofeedback, stress management, and cognitive behavioral therapy). Treatment of the comorbid psychiatric illness is often necessary before the CDH comes under control. Psychophysiological therapy involves reassurance, counselling, stress management, relaxation therapy, and biofeedback. The use of traditional acupuncture is controversial, and has not proven more effective than placebo.[87] Physical therapy consists of modality treatments (heat, cold packs, ultrasound, and electrical stimulation); improvement of posture through stretching, exercise, and traction; trigger point injections; occipital nerve blocks; and a programme of regular exercise, stretching, balanced meals, and adequate sleep.[88] It has been our experience that treating painful trigger areas in the neck can result in the improvement of intractable CDH.

Acute pharmacotherapy

Choosing the acute medication depends upon the diagnosis. CM patients who do not overuse symptomatic medication can treat acute severe headache exacerbations with antimigraine drugs, including triptans, dihydroergotamine, and ergotamine, as well as opioids. These drugs must be strictly limited to prevent the development of superimposed rebound headache that will complicate treatment and require detoxification. The risk of rebound is much lower for dihydroergotamine and triptans than for analgesics, opioids, and ergotamine. In our experience, rebound hardly, if ever, occurs with dihydroergotamine, but can occur with daily triptan use. CTTH and NDPH can be treated with nonspecific headache medication and HC can be treated with supplemental doses of indomethacin.

Preventive pharmacotherapy

Patients with daily headaches should be treated primarily with preventive medications, with the explicit understanding that medications may not become fully effective until the overused medication has been eliminated. It may take 3–6 weeks for treatment effects to develop.

The following principles guide the use of preventive treatment:[89]

- from among the first-line drugs, choose preventive agents based on their side-effect profiles, comorbid conditions, and specific indications (e.g. indomethacin for HC);
- start at a low dose;
- increase the dose gradually until efficacy is achieved, the patient develops side-effects, or the ceiling dose for the drug in question is reached;

- explain to the patient that treatment effects develop over weeks and treatment may not become fully effective until rebound is eliminated;
- if one agent fails and if all other things are equal, choose an agent from another therapeutic class;
- monotherapy is preferred, but be willing to use combination therapy;
- communicate realistic expectations.

Most preventive agents used for CDH have not been examined in well-designed double-blind studies. Table 8.7 summarizes an assessment of the efficacy, safety, and evidence for a number of agents.[84] Antidepressants are attractive agents for use in CDH (CM, CTTH, NDPH), since many patients have comorbid depression and anxiety. The most widely used antidepressants are the tricyclic antidepressants, which include nortriptyline (Aventyl[T], Pamelor[T]), amitriptyline (Elavil[T]),[89–99] and doxepin[84] (Sinequan[T]) (start at 10–25 mg at bedtime and gradually increase). Fluoxetine (Prozac[T]), a SSRI, is coming into wider use for daily headaches; evidence from a double-blind study demonstrates its efficacy in CDH.[90,100] Fluvoxamine appears to be effective[101] and may have analgesic properties.[102] Other SSRIs, the new selective norepinephrine- and serotonin-re-uptake inhibitors, such as venlafaxine, and the monoamine oxidase inhibitors may have a therapeutic role, but this has not been proven.[103]

Beta-blockers (propranolol, nadolol) remain a mainstay of therapy for migraine[84] and are used for CM. Their value in true CTTH is uncertain.[96,104] Since clinicians fear that beta-blockers may exacerbate depression;[105] they are often used in combination with antidepressants. Beta-blockers are relatively contraindicated in patients with asthma and Raynaud's disease.

Calcium-channel blockers are well tolerated;[84] however, the only evidence that supports their use for CM is anecdotal. Verapamil (Calan[T]) is the most widely prescribed agent in this family. Diltiazem (Cardizem[T]) and nifedipine (Procardia[T]) are of unproven efficacy. Flunarizine (flunarazine)[75,84] is effective and widely used in Canada, Europe, and Southeast Asia, but is not available in the United States.

The anticonvulsant, divalproex sodium (Depakote[T]),[106] is an important drug for use in CDH, even for patients who have not obtained relief from other agents. Four double-blind, placebo-controlled studies demonstrate its efficacy in migraine.[106–109] Smaller open studies support its utility in CM.[110] Doses lower than those used in epilepsy (250 mg two to three times a day) may be sufficient. Divalproex sodium is an especially useful agent for patients who have comorbid epilepsy and manic-depressive illness and, possibly, anxiety disorders.

Table 8.7 Summary of prophylactic drugs for use in chronic daily headache

Drug	Clinical efficacy	Side effects	Clinical evidence*
Antidepressants			
Amitriptyline	+++	++	+++
Doxepin	+++	++	++
Fluoxetine	++	+	+++
Anticonvulsants			
Divalproex	+++	++	++
Beta-blockers			
Propranolol, nadolol, etc.	++	+	+
Calcium-channel blockers			
Verapamil	++	+	+
Miscellaneous			
Methysergide	+++	+++	+

Modified from Tfelt-Hansen and Welch[84]
All categories are rated from + to ++++ based on a combination of published literature and clinical experience.
*Ratings of +++ for clinical evidence indicate at least one double-blind, placebo-controlled study. A rating of ++ indicates open well-designed studies and + indicates ratings based on clinical experience. A rating of ++++ requires at least two double-blind placebo-controlled trials.

Topiramate is a newer antiepileptic agent that has a range of pharmacological actions. It has few side-effects when used in low doses, although as doses escalate cognition impairment is common. Its chronic use has been associated with weight loss, not weight gain. Shuaib et al[111] found it to be effective in an open label study in which most patients had CDH in addition to migraine and all had failed previous preventive treatment. This uncontrolled study suggests that topiramate may be useful for CM.

The ergot derivative, methysergide,[84] is the first US Food and Drug Administration Agency-approved migraine preventive drug, and one that is sometimes unreasonably feared. It is an effective migraine preventive agent and can be safely combined with tricyclic antidepressants, SSRIs, or calcium-channel blockers. The usual initial dose of methysergide is 2 mg twice a day. It can be increased to a maximum of 8 mg/day (2 mg four times a day); higher doses, although not recommended by the Physicians' Desk Reference, are sometimes useful.

NSAIDs can be used for both symptomatic and preventive headache treatment. Naproxen sodium is effective in prevention at a dose of one or two 275-mg tablets twice a day.[112] Other effective NSAIDs include tolfenamic acid, ketoprofen, mefenamic acid, fenoprofen, and ibuprofen.[113,114] Aspirin was found to be effective in one study[115] and equal to placebo in another.[116] The short-acting NSAIDs, such as ibuprofen and aspirin, may cause rebound, and their use should be limited. It is uncertain whether or not the other NSAIDs cause rebound. CM, CTTH, NDPH, and HC may all be unilateral. The only feature that separates HC is indomethacin responsiveness, which is not unique to HC. We used absolute responsiveness to indomethacin to define the presence of the disorder. It is uncertain if nonresponsive patients have the same biology as indomethacin-responsive patients do. HC is not a rare disorder. All cases of chronic unilateral daily headaches should receive an indomethacin trial early in treatment. We give indomethacin a therapeutic trial (up to 150–225 mg/day for 2 weeks) to rule out HC, but otherwise limit the use of other NSAIDs.

Although monotherapy is preferred, it is sometimes necessary to combine preventive medications. Antidepressants are often used with beta-blockers or calcium-channel blockers, and divalproex sodium may be used in combination with any of these medications.

Other Treatments

Open and small placebo-controlled trials have suggested that CTTH may improve following injection with botulinum toxin A (Botox® (BTX-A)); whether this is due to paralysis of muscles or to unknown mechanisms is uncertain. There is limited evidence that botulinum toxin decreases the frequency of migraine attacks.[117,118] This treatment needs further controlled studies.

Detoxification

Outpatient

Two general outpatient strategies can be followed. One approach is to taper the overused medication, gradually substituting a long-acting NSAID as effective preventive therapy is established. The alternative strategy is to abruptly discontinue the overused drug, substitute a transitional medication to replace the overused drug, and subsequently taper the transitional drug. Drugs used for this purpose include NSAIDs, dihydroergotamine, corticosteroids, and triptans. Serious withdrawal syndromes that can be produced by the overused drug must be prevented. For example, if high doses of a butalbital-containing analgesic combination are abruptly discontinued, phenobarbital should be used to prevent barbiturate withdrawal. Similarly, benzodiazepines must be gradually tapered. Outpatient treatment, while preferable for motivated patients, is not always safe or effective.

Patients who do not need hospital-level care but cannot be safely or adequately treated as outpatients can be considered for ambulatory infusion treatment. Out-

patient ambulatory infusion treatment is effective for migraine status and uncomplicated primary CDH with and without rebound. It must be done in a hospital or a supervised medical setting where the patient can be monitored frequently (every 15 minutes). Under these circumstances, repetitive intravenous (i.v.) treatment can be given twice a day for several consecutive days. Although ambulatory infusion treatment is better than outpatient treatment for many patients, major concerns still exist. No long-term observation is available in an outpatient setting, and many problems manifest themselves in an intensely-monitored interactive environment. Contraindications to outpatient ambulatory infusion treatment include the possibility of withdrawal symptoms occurring at night when patients are withdrawn from long-acting or potent drugs; psychiatric disorders that interfere with treatment (these patients cannot be treated aggressively as outpatients); and comorbid medical illnesses that require prolonged monitoring.

Inpatient

If outpatient treatment fails or is not safe, or if significant medical or psychiatric comorbidity is present, inpatient treatment may be needed.[84] The goals of inpatient treatment include:

- detoxification and rehydration;
- pain control with parenteral therapy;
- establishment of effective prophylaxis;
- interruption of the cycle of pain;
- patient education; and
- establishment of outpatient methods of pain control.[84]

The detoxification process can be enhanced and shortened and the patient's symptoms made more tolerable by coadministering repetitive i.v. dihydroergotamine and metoclopramide or domperidone (Figure 8.8),[85] which helps control nausea. Following 10 mg i.v. metoclopramide or a domperidone suppository, dihydroergotamine 0.25 or 0.5 mg is administered intravenously. Subsequent doses are adjusted based on pain relief and side-effects. Patients who are not candidates for dihydroergotamine or are truly intolerant of the drug may require repetitive i.v. neuroleptics, such as chlorpromazine, prochlorperazine, droperidol and/or corticosteroids. These agents may also supplement repetitive i.v. dihydroergotamine in refractory patients.[16] Hospitalization can also be used for patient education, for introducing behavioral methods of pain control, and for adjusting an outpatient programme of preventive and acute therapy. In our experience,[16] repetitive i.v. dihydroergotamine is a safe and effective means of rapidly controlling intractable headache.

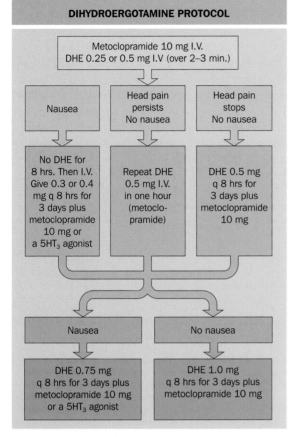

DIHYDROERGOTAMINE PROTOCOL

Metoclopramide 10 mg I.V.
DHE 0.25 or 0.5 mg I.V (over 2–3 min.)

Nausea

Head pain persists
No nausea

Head pain stops
No nausea

No DHE for 8 hrs. Then I.V. Give 0.3 or 0.4 mg q 8 hrs for 3 days plus metoclopramide 10 mg or a 5HT$_3$ agonist

Repeat DHE 0.5 mg I.V. in one hour (metoclopramide)

DHE 0.5 mg q 8 hrs for 3 days plus metoclopramide 10 mg

Nausea

No nausea

DHE 0.75 mg q 8 hrs for 3 days plus metoclopramide 10 mg or a 5HT$_3$ agonist

DHE 1.0 mg q 8 hrs for 3 days plus metoclopramide 10 mg

● **Figure 8.8** *Dihydroergotamine treatment protocol. After Raskin.*[85]

Prognosis

The 'natural history' of CDH disorders, and of rebound headache in particular, have never been studied and probably never will be for ethical and technical reasons. Recognition of the rebound process probably is itself therapeutic and could affect the patient's behavior or the physician's approach. Retrospective analysis suggests that there may be periods of stable drug consumption and phases of accelerated medication use. Patients who are treated aggressively generally improve. No studies report spontaneous improvement of rebound headache, although this may happen. We performed follow-up evaluations on 50 hospitalized CDH drug overuse patients who were treated with repetitive i.v. dihydroergotamine and became headache-free.[119] Once detoxified, treated, and discharged, most patients did not resume daily analgesic or ergotamine use. Seventy-two percent continued to show significant improvement at 3 months, and 87% continued to show significant improvement after 2 years. Patients

with drug-induced CDH, while difficult to treat, often return to a state of intermittent episodic headache after detoxification and treatment with a preventive medication. Our 2-year success rate of 87% is consistent with the long-term success rates reported in the literature.[119]

Why treatment fails (Table 8.8)

When patients fail to respond to therapy or announce at the first consultation that they have already tried everything and nothing will work, it is important to try to identify the reason or reasons that treatment has failed. The cause of treatment failure may be an incomplete or incorrect diagnosis. For example:

- an undiagnosed secondary headache disorder is the major source of the head pain;
- a misdiagnosed primary headache disorder is present (i.e. HC is mistaken for CM, episodic paroxysmal hemicrania or hypnic headache is mistaken for cluster); and
- two or more different headache disorders are present. In addition, important exacerbating factors, such as medication overuse, may have been missed or pharmacotherapy may have been inadequate. Other factors may also be present.

● **Table 8.8** *Why treatment fails*

The diagnosis is incomplete or incorrect
An undiagnosed secondary headache disorder is present
A primary headache disorder is misdiagnosed
Two or more different headache disorders are present
Important exacerbating factors may have been missed
Medication overuse (including OTCs)
Caffeine overuse
Dietary or lifestyle triggers
Hormonal triggers
Psychosocial factors
Other medications which trigger headaches
Pharmacotherapy has been inadequate
Ineffective drug
Excessive initial doses
Inadequate final doses
Inadequate duration of treatment
Other factors
Unrealistic expectations
Comorbid conditions complicate therapy
Inpatient treatment required

Prevention

Headache sufferers often do not realize that excessive or frequent self-treatment may perpetuate or exacerbate their headaches. Since most headache sufferers do not seek medical advice until and unless the pain becomes frequent or intense, the opportunity for diagnosis and physician intervention to halt the cycle is often missed. Physicians need to screen CDH patients for analgesic overuse. Headache patients must be informed about the risks of analgesic overuse and rebound headache. Yet, even when patients are aware of the risks, they may still overmedicate. This requires continued vigilance on the part of the treating physician.

Patients who overuse medication may feel ashamed and out of control. They may be unable to provide an accurate history of drug use. To facilitate this process, the condition of medication overuse rebound should be explained as a part of the natural history of migraine. Even if the patient is not overusing acute medication at the time, all symptomatic headache medications, with the possible exception of the long-acting NSAIDs, need to be limited.

References

1. Newman LC, Lipton RB, Solomon S, Stewart WF. Daily headache in a population sample: results from the American Migraine Study. Headache 1994; 34: 295.
2. Rasmussen BK. Migraine and tension-type headache in a general population: psychosocial factors. Int J Epidemiol 1992; 21: 1138–43.
3. Schwartz BS, Stewart WF, Simon D, Lipton RB. Epidemiology of tension-type headache. JAMA 1998; 279: 381–3.
4. Silberstein SD, Lipton RB, Solomon S, Mathew NT. Classification of daily and near daily headaches: proposed revisions to the IHS classification. Headache 1994; 34: 1–7.
5. Solomon S, Lipton RB, Newman LC. Evaluation of chronic daily headache – comparison to criteria for chronic tension-type headache. Cephalalgia 1992; 12: 365–8.
6. Sanin LC, Mathew NT, Bellmyer LR, Ali S. The International Headache Society (IHS) headache classification as applied to a headache clinic population. Cephalalgia 1994; 14: 443–6.
7. Messinger HB, Spierings ELH, Vincent AJP. Overlap of migraine and tension-type headache in the International Headache Society classification. Cephalalgia 1991; 11: 233–7.
8. Pfaffenrath V, Isler H. Evaluation of the nosology of chronic tension-type headache. Cephalalgia 1993; 13: 60–2.
9. Sjaastad O, Saumte C, Hovdahl H. Cervicogenic headache, a hypothesis. Cephalalgia 1983; 3: 249–56.
10. Sjaastad O. The headache challenge in our time: cervicogenic headache. Funct Neurol 1990; 5: 155–8.
11. Pfaffenrath V, Kaube H. Diagnostics of cervicogenic headache. Funct Neurol 1990; 5: 159–64.
12. Edmeads J. The cervical spine and headache. Neurology 1988; 38: 1874–8.
13. Brain WR. Some unsolved problems of cervical spondylosis. Br Med J 1963; 1: 771–7.
14. Edmeads JG. Disorders of the neck: cervicogenic headache. In: Silberstein SD, Lipton RB, Dalessio DJ, eds. Wolff's headache and other head pain. 7th edn., New York: Oxford University Press, 2001, 447–58.
15. Mosek A, Swanson JW, O'Fallon WM et al. CSF opening pressure in patients with chronic daily headache. Cephalalgia 1999; 19: 323 (Abstract).
16. Silberstein SD, Schulman EA, Hopkins MM. Repetitive intravenous DHE in the treatment of refractory headache. Headache 1990; 30: 334–9.
17. Scher AI, Stewart WF, Liberman J, Lipton RB. Prevalence of frequent headache in a population sample. Headache 1998; 38: 497–506.
18. Silberstein SD, Lipton RB, Sliwinski M. Classification of daily and near-daily headaches: field trial of revised IHS criteria. Neurology 1996; 47: 871–5.
19. Mathew NT. Transformed migraine. Cephalalgia 1993; 13: 78–83.
20. Saper JR, Silberstein SD, Gordon CD et al. Handbook of Headache Management: A Practical Guide to Diagnosis and Treatment of Head, Neck, and Facial Pain. 2nd edn. Baltimore: Lippincott Williams & Wilkins, Inc., 1999.
21. Mathew NT, Stubits E, Nigam MR. Transformation of episodic migraine into daily headache: analysis of factors. Headache 1982; 22: 66–8.
22. Mathew NT, Reuveni U, Perez F. Transformed or evolutive migraine. Headache 1987; 27: 102–6.
23. Saper JR. Headache Disorders: Current Concepts in Treatment Strategies. Littleton: Wright-PSG, 1983.
24. Saper JR, Silberstein SD, Gordon CD, Hamel RL. Handbook of Headache Management. Baltimore: Williams & Wilkins, 1993.
25. Castillo J, Munoz P, Guitera V, Pascual J. Epidemiology of chronic daily headache in the general population. Headache 1999; 39: 190–6.
26. Mathew NT, Kurman R, Perez F. Drug induced refractory headache – clinical features and management. Headache 1990; 30: 634–8.
27. Silberstein SD, Lipton RB. Chronic daily headache including transformed migraine, chronic tension-type headache, and medication overuse. In: Silberstein SD, Lipton RB, Dalessio DJ, eds. Wolff's headache and other head pain. 7th edn. New York: Oxford University Press, 2001, 247–82.
28. Russell MB, Stergaard S, Endtsen L, Olesen J. Familial occurrence of chronic tension-type headache. Cephalalgia 1999; 19: 207–10.
29. Vanast WJ. New daily persistent headaches: definition of a benign syndrome. Headache 1986; 26: 317.
30. Newman LC, Lipton RB, Solomon S. Hemicrania continua: 7 new cases and a literature review. Headache 1993; 32: 267.
31. Goadsby PJ, Lipton RB. A review of paroxysmal hemicranias, SUNCT syndrome and other short-lasting headaches with autonomic features, including new cases. Brain 1997; 120: 193–209.
32. Bordini C, Antonaci F, Stovner LJ et al. 'Hemicrania Continua' – a clinical review. Headache 1991; 31: 20–6.
33. Pareja JA, Antonaci F, Vincent M. The hemicrania continua diagnosis. Cephalalgia 2001; 21: 940–6.
34. Peres MF, Silberstein SD, Nahmias A et al. Hemicrania continua is not that rare. Neurology 2001; 57: 948–51.
35. Marano E, Giampiero V, Gennaro DR et al. Hemicrania continua: a possible case with alternating sides. Cephalalgia 1994; 14: 307–8.
36. Pasquier F, Leys D, Petit H. Hemicrania

continua: the first bilateral case. Cephalalgia 1987; 7: 169–70.

37. Kuritzky A. Indomethacin-resistant hemicrania continua. Cephalalgia 1992; 12: 57–9.

38. Pascual J. Hemicrania continua. Neurology 1995; 45: 2302–3.

39. Lay CL, Newman LC. Posttraumatic hemicrania continua. Headache 1999; 39: 275–9.

40. Centonze V, Bassi A, Causarano V et al. Simultaneous occurrence of ipsilateral cluster headache and chronic paroxysmal hemicrania: a case report. Headache 2000; 40: 54–6.

41. Antonaci F, Sjaastad O. Hemicrania continua: a possible symptomatic case due to mesenchymal tumor. Funct Neurol 1992; 7: 471–4.

42. Brilla R, Evers S, Soros P, Husstedt IW. Hemicrania continua in an HIV-infected outpatient. Cephalalgia 1998; 18: 287–8.

43. Wheeler SD. Clinical spectrum of hemicrania continua. The American Academy of Neurology Meeting. San Diego, 2000.

44. Sjaastad O, Batnes J, Haugen S. The Vaga Study. An outline of the design. Cephalalgia 1999; 19: 24–30.

45. Kumar KL, Bordiuk JD. Hemicrania continua: a therapeutic dilemma. Headache 1991; 31: 345.

46. Sjaastad O, Antonaci F. Chronic paroxysmal hemicrania (CPH) and hemicrania continua: transition from one stage to another. Headache 1993; 33: 551–4.

47. Peres MFP, Zukerman E. Hemicrania continua responsive to rofecoxib. Cephalalgia 2000; 20: 130–1.

48. Antonaci F, Pareja JA, Caminero AB, Sjaastad O. Chronic paroxysmal hemicrania continua: lack of efficacy of sumatriptan. Headache 1998; 38: 197–200.

49. Espada F, Morales-Asín F, Escalza I et al. Hemicrania continua: nine new cases. Cephalalgia 1999; 19: 442 (Abstract).

50. Newman LC, Goadsby PJ. Unusual primary headache disorders. In: Silberstein SD, Lipton RB, Dalessio DJ, eds. Wolff's headache and other head pain. 7th edn. New York: Oxford University Press, 2001, 310–24.

51. Katsarava Z, Fritsche G, Diener HC, Limmroth V. Drug-induced headache (DIH): following the use of different triptans. Cephalalgia 2000, 20: 293 (Abstract).

52. Mathew NT. Drug induced headache. Neurol Clin 1990; 8: 903–12.

53. Diamond S, Dalessio DJ. Drug abuse in headache. In: Diamond S, Dalessio DJ, eds. The Practicing Physician's Approach to Headache. 3rd edn. Baltimore: Williams & Wilkins, 1982,

54. Saper JR. Ergotamine dependence. Headache 1987; 27: 435–8.

55. Saper JR. Chronic headache syndromes. Neurol Clin 1989; 7: 387–412.

56. Saper JR, Jones JM. Ergotamine tartrate dependency: features and possible mechanisms. Clin Neuropharmacol 1986; 9: 244–56.

57. Andersson PG. Ergotism: the clinical picture. In: Diener HC, Wilkinson MS, eds. Drug-Induced Headache. Berlin: Springer, 1988, 16–19.

58. Rapoport AM, Weeks RE, Sheftell FD et al. The 'analgesic washout period': a critical variable evaluation in the evaluation of headache treatment efficacy. Neurology 1986; 36: 100–1.

59. Baumgartner C, Wessly P, Bingol C et al. Long-term prognosis of analgesic withdrawal in patients with drug-induced headaches. Headache 1989; 29: 510–14.

60. Dichgans J, Diener HD, Gerber WD et al. Analgetika-induzierter dauerkopfschmerz. Dtsch Med Wochenschr 1984; 109: 369–73.

61. Rapoport AM. Analgesic rebound headache. Headache 1988; 28: 662–5.

62. Kudrow L. Paradoxical effects of frequent analgesic use. Adv Neurol 1982; 33: 335–41.

63. Diener HC, Dichgans J, Scholz E et al. Analgesic-induced chronic headache: long-term results of withdrawal therapy. J Neurol 1989; 236: 9–14.

64. Rasmussen BK, Jensen R, Olesen J. Impact of headache on sickness absence and utilization of medical services. J Epidemiol Community Health 1992; 46: 443–6.

65. Isler H. Headache drugs provoking chronic headache: historical aspects and common misunderstandings. In: Diener HC, Wilkinson M, eds. Drug-Induced Headache. Berlin: Springer-Verlag, 1988, 87–94.

66. Micieli G, Manzoni GC, Granella F et al. Clinical and epidemiological observations on drug abuse in headache patients. In: Diener HC, Wilkinson M, eds. Drug-Induced Headache. Berlin: Springer-Verlag, 1988, 20–8.

67. Silverman K, Evans SM, Strain EC, Griffiths RR. Withdrawal syndrome after the double-blind cessation of caffeine consumption. N Eng J Med 1992; 327: 1109–14.

68. Potter DL, Hart DE, Calder CS, Storey JR. A double-blind, randomized, placebo-controlled, parallel study to determine the efficacy of topiramate in the prophylactic treatment of migraine. Neurology 2000; 54: A15 (Abstract).

69. Wilkinson M. Introduction. In: Diener

HC, Wilkinson M, eds. Drug-Induced Headache. Berlin: Springer-Verlag, 1988, 1–2.

70. Silberstein SD. Chronic daily headache and tension-type headache. Neurology 1993; 43: 1644–9.

71. Catarci T, Fiacco F, Argentino C. Ergotamine-induced headache can be sustained by sumatriptan daily intake. Cephalalgia 1994; 14: 374–5.

72. Silberstein SD. Drug-induced headache. Neurol Clin N Amer 1998; 16: 107–23.

73. Merikangas KR, Angst J, Isler H. Migraine and psychopathology: results of the Zurich cohort study of young adults. Arch Gen Psychiatry 1990; 47: 849–53.

74. Breslau N, Davis GC. Migraine, physical health and psychiatric disorders: a prospective epidemiologic study of young adults. J Psychiatric Res 1993; 27: 211–21.

75. Lake AE, Saper JR, Madden SF, Kreeger C. Comprehensive inpatient treatment for intractable migraine: a prospective long-term outcome study. Headache 1993; 33: 55–62.

76. Mitsikostas DD, Thomas AM. Comorbidity of headache and depressive disorders. Cephalalgia 1999; 19: 211–17.

77. Verri AP, Cecchini P, Galli C et al. Psychiatric comorbidity in chronic daily headache. Cephalalgia 1998; 18: 45–9.

78. Curioso EP, Young WB, Shechter AL, Kaiser RS. Psychiatric comorbidity predicts outcome in chronic daily headache patients. Neurology 1999; 52: A471 (Abstract).

79. Tekle Haimanot R, Seraw B, Forsgren L et al. Migraine, chronic tension-type headache, and cluster headache in an Ethiopian rural community. Cephalalgia 1995; 15: 482–8.

80. Rasmussen BK. Epidemiology of headache. Cephalalgia 1995; 15: 45–68.

81. Wang SJ, Fuh JL, Lu SR et al. Chronic daily headache in Chinese elderly: prevalence, risk factors and biannual follow-up. Neurology 2000; 54: 314–19.

82. Post RM, Silberstein SD. Shared mechanisms in affective illness, epilepsy, and migraine. Neurology 1994; 44: S37–47.

83. Isler H. Migraine treatment as a cause of chronic migraine. In: Rose FC, ed. Advances in Migraine Research and Therapy. New York: Raven Press, 1982, 159–64.

84. Silberstein SD, Saper JR, Freitag F. Migraine: Diagnosis and treatment. In: Silberstein SD, Lipton RB, Dalessio DJ, eds. Wolff's headache and other head pain. 7th edn. New York: Oxford

University Press, 2001, 121–237.

85. Raskin NH. Repetitive intravenous dihydroergotamine as therapy for intractable migraine. Neurology 1986; 36: 995–7.

86. Diener HC, Pfaffenrath V, Soyka D, Gerber WD. Therapie des medikamenten-induzierten dauerkopfschmerzes. Münch Med Wschr 1992; 134: 159–62.

87. Tavola T, Gala C, Conte G, Invernizzi G. Traditional Chinese acupuncture in tension-type headache: a controlled study. Pain 1992; 48: 325–9.

88. Silberstein SD. Treatment of headache in primary care practice. Am J Med 1984; 77: 65–72.

89. Silberstein SD, Lipton RB. Overview of diagnosis and treatment of migraine. Neurology 1994; 44: 6–16.

90. Bussone G, Sandrini G, Patruno G et al. Effectiveness of fluoxetine on pain and depression in chronic headache disorders. In: Nappi G, Bono G, Sandrini G, Martignoni E, Micieli G, eds. Headache and Depression: Serotonin Pathways as a Common Clue. New York: Raven Press, 1991, 265–72.

91. Couch JR, Ziegler DK, Hassainein R. Amitriptyline in the prophylaxis of migraine. Arch Neurol 1976; 26: 121–7.

92. Diamond S, Baltes B. Chronic tension headache treated with amitriptyline: a double blind study. Headache 1971; 11: 110–16.

93. Holland J, Holland C, Kudrow L. Low dose amitriptyline prophylaxis in chronic scalp muscle contraction headache. Proceedings of the First International Headache Congress. Munich, September, 1983.

94. Lance JW, Curran DA. Treatment of chronic tension headache. Lancet 1964; 1: 1236–9.

95. Pluvinage R. Le traitement des migraines et des céphalées psychogènes par l'amitriptyline. Sem Hop 1978; 54: 713–16.

96. Pfaffenrath V, Kellhammer U, Pollmann W. Combination headache: practical experience with a combination of beta-blocker and an antidepressive. Cephalalgia 1986; 6: 25–32.

97. Pfaffenrath V, Diener HC, Isler H et al. Efficacy and tolerability of amitriptylinoxide in the treatment of chronic tension-type headache: a multicentre controlled study. Cephalalgia 1994; 14: 149–55.

98. Holroyd KA, Nash JM, Pingel JD. A comparison of pharmacologic (amitriptyline HCl) and nonpharmacologic (cognitive–behavioral) therapies for chronic tension headaches. J Consulting Clin Psychology 1991; 59: 387–93.

99. Gobel H, Hamouz V, Hansen C et al. Chronic tension-type headache: amitriptyline reduces clinical headache-duration and experimental pain sensitivity but does not alter pericranial muscle activity readings. Pain 1994; 59: 241–9.

100. Saper JR, Silberstein SD, Lake AE, Winters ME. Double-blind trial of fluoxetine: chronic daily headache and migraine. Headache 1994; 34: 497–502.

101. Manna V, Bolino F, DiCicco L. Chronic tension-type headache, mood depression and serotonin. Headache 1994; 34: 44–9.

102. Palmer KJ, Benfield P. Fluvoxamine: an overview of its pharmacologic properties and a review of its use in nondepressive disorders. CNS Drugs 1994; 1: 57–87.

103. Langemark M, Olesen J. Sulpiride and paroxetine in the treatment of chronic tension-type headache. Headache 1994; 34: 20–4.

104. Mathew NT. Prophylaxis of migraine and mixed headache. A randomized controlled study. Headache 1981; 21: 105–9.

105. Bright RA, Everitt DE. Beta-blockers and depression. Evidence against association. JAMA 1992; 267: 1783–7.

106. Jensen R, Brinck T, Olesen J. Sodium valproate has a prophylactic effect in migraine without aura. Neurology 1994; 44: 647–51.

107. Mathew NT, Saper JR, Silberstein SD et al. Migraine prophylaxis with divalproex. Arch Neurol 1995; 52: 281–6.

108. Hering R, Kuritzky A. Sodium valproate in the prophylactic treatment of migraine: a double-blind study versus placebo. Cephalalgia 1992; 12: 81–4.

109. Klapper J. Divalproex sodium in the prophylactic treatment of migraine. Headache 1995; 35: 290 (Abstract).

110. Mathew NT, Ali S. Valproate in the treatment of persistent chronic daily headache. An open label study. Headache 1991; 31: 71–4.

111. Shuaib A, Ahmed F, Muratoglu M, Kochanski P. Topiramate in migraine prophylaxis: a pilot study. Cephalalgia 1999; 19: 379 (Abstract).

112. Miller DS, Talbot CA, Simpson W, Korey A. A comparison of naproxen sodium, acetaminophen and placebo in the treatment of muscle contraction headache. Headache 1987; 27: 392–6.

113. Johnson ES, Tfelt-Hansen P. Nonsteroidal antiinflammatory drugs. In: Olesen J, Tfelt-Hansen P, Welch KMA, eds. The Headaches. New York: Raven Press, 1993, 391–5.

114. Mylecharane EJ, Tfelt-Hansen P. Miscellaneous drugs. In: Olesen J, Tfelt-Hansen P, Welch KMA, eds. The Headaches. New York: Raven Press, 1993: 397–402.

115. Kangasniemi PJ, Nyrke T, Lang AH, Petersen E. Femoxetine–a new 5HT uptake inhibitor–and propranolol in the prophylactic treatment of migraine. Acta Neurol Scand 1983; 68: 262–7.

116. Scholz E, Gerber WD, Diener HC, Langohr HD. Dihydroergotamine vs flunarizine vs nifedipine vs metoprolol vs propranolol in migraine prophylaxis: a comparative study based on time series analysis. In: Scholz E, Gerber WD, Diener HC, Langohr HD, eds. Advances in Headache Research. In Rose CF ed. London: John Libbey & Co., 1987, 139–45.

117. Smuts JA, Baker MK, Smuts HM et al. Botulinum toxin type A as prophylactic treatment in chronic tension-type headache. Cephalalgia 1999; 19: 454 (Abstract).

118. Gobel H, Lindner V, Krack P et al. Treatment of chronic tension-type headache with botulinum toxin. Cephalalgia 1999; 19: 455 (Abstract).

119. Silberstein SD, Silberstein JR. Chronic daily headache: prognosis following inpatient treatment with repetitive IV DHE. Headache 1992; 32: 439–45.

chapter 9

Trigeminal autonomic cephalgias I – cluster headache: diagnosis and treatment

Trigeminal autonomic cephalalgias (TACs) consist of a group of headache syndromes usually marked by cyclical episodes of severe head pain with cranial autonomic activation.[1] Cluster headache is the most common of the TACs; while rare relative to other primary headaches, its prevalence is similar in northern climates to multiple sclerosis.[2] Cluster headache is clearly a problem that can best be managed by neurologists and headache specialists. It is a distinct clinical and epidemiological entity, named by Friedman and Mikropoulos in 1958.[3] Its importance as a primary headache derives from its extraordinary morbidity. The pain is devastating and the syndrome is both unique and rewarding to manage; as a consequence, physicians with an interest in head pain should be acquainted with the condition. The other TACs that may be confused with cluster headache (Table 9.1) have distinct treatment responses and will be dealt with in Chapter 10. These disorders are less common, and probably less well recognized.

Cluster headache is a relatively well-characterized syndrome clinically,[4] whose description dates back hundreds of years.[5] Isler provides a very interesting description by Gerhard van Swieten in 1745.[6]

> A healthy, robust man of middle age (was suffering from) trouble-some pain which came on every day at the same hour at the same spot above the orbit of the left eye, where the nerve emerges from the opening of the frontal bone; after a short time the left eye began to redden, and to overflow with tears; then he felt as if his eye was slowly forced out of its orbit with so much pain, that he nearly went mad. After a few hours all these evils ceased, and nothing in the eye appeared at all changed.

The historical aspects of cluster headache have been dealt with,[7] and there are excellent texts on the subject.[8,9] Very clear English-language descriptions of this syndrome can be dated to the mid-20th century, with landmark descriptions of its periodicity by Ekbom[10] and temporal clustering by Kunkle.[11] Many creative terms have been used for the disorder, which is a reflection of the curiosity it has fostered amongst medical practitioners[12] The names have very often revealed accurate views

about some of the condition's pathophysiology (Table 9.2).

Clinical features

The image of the tortured cluster headache sufferer rocking or pacing in the dark, with tears streaming from one eye and a face contorted in exquisite pain, is distinctive and compelling in medicine. The individual attack, which lasts on average 60–90 minutes, is called a cluster headache or cluster attack. Attacks occur in series that last for weeks or months (called cluster periods or bouts), with the attack frequency ranging from one every other day to eight a day. The cluster periods are separated by remissions that usually last months or years.[2] On average, a cluster period lasts 6–12 weeks while a remission lasts 12 months.[8,13] Considerable variations, both between patients and in individuals, are characteristic. About 10% of patients have chronic symptoms with no significant remission periods. The International Headache Society (IHS) criteria[4] for cluster require at least five attacks of severe, unilateral, orbital, suborbital, and/or temporal pain that last 15–180 minutes if untreated and are associated with at least one of the following: conjunctival injection, lacrimation, nasal congestion, rhinorrhea, forehead and facial sweating, miosis, ptosis, or eyelid edema.

Cluster headache attacks are stereotypical. They are generally shorter than migraine. The pain is almost invariably unilateral and very severe; it is usually located in or around the eye or in the temporal region. It is often described in such graphic terms as boring, tearing, or burning, or with descriptive metaphors liking it to 'a hot poker in the eye' or to the feeling 'the eye is being pushed out'. Patients who have both cluster headache and migraine state that their cluster headache attacks are more severe than their migraines. Cluster headache patients who have had other painful experiences, such as kidney stones or childbirth, readily report that the pain of cluster headache is worse. The attack frequency is from one a day or every second day to two or more a day. It is usually said that eight per day is a maximum; certainly the headache frequency makes the other TACs, such as

● **Table 9.1** Cluster headache, other TACs, and short-lasting head pains

Trigeminal autonomic cephalalgias (TACs)	Other short-lasting head pains
• Cluster headache • Paroxysmal hemicrania • SUNCT* syndrome • Hemicrania Continua	• Primary stabbing headache† • Benign cough headache • Hypnic headache • Trigeminal neuralgia

*Shortlasting unilateral neuralgiform headache attacks with conjunctival injection and tearing
†Currently known as Idiopathic Stabbing Headache but due for change in the second edition of the International Headache Society classification

● **Table 9.2** Older Terms for Cluster headache

- Erythroprosopalgia of Bing[146]
- Ciliary neuralgia[147]
- Migrainous neuralgia (Harris)[148]
- Erythromelalgia of the head[146]
- Horton's headache[10]
- Histaminic cephalalgia[87]
- Petrosal neuralgia (Gardner) or sphenopalatine neuralgia[149]
- Vidian neuralgia[150]
- Sluder's neuralgia[149]
- Hemicrania angioparalytica[151]

paroxysmal hemicrania, become more likely (see Chapter 10). Once a cluster period begins, many patients find that individual headache attacks can be triggered or precipitated by ingestion of alcohol and by other vasodilators, notably nitroglycerin[14] and histamine. Alcohol rarely precipitates an attack during a remission period; most sufferers will avoid alcohol as soon as a drink triggers an attack and will remain abstinent until the cluster period is over. It is noteworthy that typical migraine aura may be seen in cluster headache[15] in as many as 15% of patients.[16] It usually comes with the pain and should not necessarily put clinicians off the diagnosis of cluster headache; even attacks with hemiplegia have now been reported.[16]

Gastrointestinal symptoms were not felt to be typical of cluster headache attacks: while vomiting is rare, nausea occurs in as many as 40% of patients. In some patients, nausea may be secondary to drug ingestion. The reported frequency of photophobia in patients with cluster headache varies from 5% to 72%, while phonophobia was reported only occasionally, in 12–39% of cluster headache cases.[13,17] However, recent quantitative data suggest that cluster headache patients have as much sensitivity to light and sound as migraine patients (who are markedly more sensitive than controls).[18]

In contrast to migraineurs, cluster headache patients are restless and occasionally even violent during an attack. Most are unwilling to lie down but prefer to pace about or sit and rock back and forth. Some will exert pressure on the painful area with a hand or place either an icepack or a hotpack over the affected eye and temple. Many will isolate themselves from family members or leave the house to get into cold or fresh air for the duration of the attack. Violent, destructive behavior that may even result in self-inflicted injuries may occur, but this is rare. Some contemplate suicide during an attack, while others have been known to beg a family member to end their suffering.

The IHS further subdivided episodic cluster headache based on whether or not the periodicity was determined. Episodic cluster headache has clear inter-bout intervals of at least 2 weeks, while chronic cluster headache does not. The revised IHS classification that is due out in 2002 or 2003 is likely to require a 1-month inter-bout interval. The IHS subdivided chronic cluster headache depending on whether or not the current chronic bout had been preceded by episodic cluster headache. Such distinctions may be helpful with prognostication.[19,20] Chronic cluster headache can be a dreadful problem that drives otherwise normal people to extraordinary acts. Fortunately the disease is giving up its pathophysiological secrets and new, previously unconsidered therapeutic options, are being studied (see below).

A signature feature of cluster headache, apart from cycling, and indeed for the entire array of the TACs, is the association with autonomic symptoms. These features include lacrimation and nasal congestion, suggestive of cranial parasympathetic activation, and miosis and ptosis, suggestive of a Horner's syndrome (Table 9.3). The IHS

• **Table 9.3** *Diagnostic features of cluster headache modified from the International Headache Society [4] with the proposed change**

Cluster headache has two key forms-
1. **Episodic:** Occurs in periods lasting 7 days to 1 year separated by pain-free periods lasting 1 month
2. **Chronic:** Attacks occur for more than 1 year without remission or with remissions lasting less than 1 month.

Headaches must have each of:
- Severe unilateral orbital, supraorbital, temporal pain lasting 15 minutes to 3 hours;
- Frequency: one every second day to eight per day;
- Associated with one of:
  - lacrimation
  - nasal congestion
  - rhinorrhea
  - forehead/facial sweating
  - miosis
  - ptosis
  - eyelid edema
  - conjunctival injection
  - sense of restlessness or agitation during headache*

• **Table 9.4** *Secondary headache in the differential diagnosis of cluster headache*

Vascular
Vertebral artery dissection[152] or aneurysm[153]
Pseudoaneursym of intracavernous carotid a.[29]
Aneurysm of anterior communicating artery[154]
Carotid aneurysm[154]
Occipital lobe AVM[155]
AVM middle cerebral territory[156]
Giant cell arteritis

Caudal medulla or cervical spinal cord
High cervical meningioma[157]
Unilateral cervical cord infarction[158]
Lateral medullary infarction[159]

Intracranial lesions
Pituitary adenoma[160] (prolactinoma[154])
Meningioma of the lesser wing of sphenoid[161]

Facial lesions
Facial trauma[162]
Orbitosphenoidal aspergillosis[163]

Orbital or sinus
Tolosa-Hunt syndrome
Maxillary sinusitis

Other
Head or neck injury[164]
Raeder's paratrigeminal neuralgia
SUNCT syndrome

AVM, arteriovenous malformation; SUNCT, short lasting unilateral neuralgiform headache attacks with conjunctival injection and tearing

system requires, and good clinical practice dictates, that the syndrome is diagnosed when there are no other inter-current illnesses that could be responsible.

Physical characteristics

The typical heavy facial features of many of those subject to cluster headache were noted by Graham.[21] Deep nasolabial furrows, 'peau d'orange' skin, and telangiectasia led to the description of 'leonine facies'. Women with cluster headache often have a masculine appearance, according to Kudrow.[22] Many of the characteristic facial features believed typical of those subject to cluster headache are most likely owing to heavy tobacco use, which are also characteristic of this population. Kudrow [23] reported that two-thirds of the patients in his large series had hazel-colored eyes. He also noted that many of those who are subject to cluster headache are tall – about 3 inches above average.

Differential diagnosis

Before a final diagnosis of cluster can be made, other primary disorders that might be confused with cluster headache, and secondary headache disorders that mimic cluster headache, need to be considered (Table 9.4).

Much of the confusion with regard to cluster headache surrounds the symptoms of cranial autonomic activation, such as lacrimation or conjunctival injection. It is a physiological fact that significant trigeminal nociceptive input will activate the cranial parasympathetic outflow by a reflex mechanism in the brainstem.[24,25] Recognition of this fact makes it is easier to diagnose underlying conditions. Migraine may present with recurrent unilateral headache with ipsilateral autonomic symptoms, particularly during severe attacks. However, the frequency and duration of cluster headache attacks differ from migraine. Cluster headache attacks are short-lived (90–120 minutes) compared to migraine, which can last from 4–72 hours. Cluster attacks are almost always unilateral, frequently nocturnal, can occur several times a day, and are associated with less nausea, vomiting, and aura than migraine. Alcohol typically triggers an attack of cluster headache in 20–30 minutes while headache is often delayed in migraineurs.

Cluster headache must be differentiated from the other TACs (see Chapter 10; Table 9.1), particularly paroxysmal hemicrania, if the attacks are relatively short and the frequency above a few a day. In clinical practice, we recommend a trial of indomethacin (indometacin) for patients who have episodic cluster headache and do not respond readily to the treatments described below, and for all patients with chronic cluster headache. Furthermore, for reasons yet to be elucidated, obstructive sleep apnea is rather common in cluster headache,[26,27] and probing for the condition is often clinically rewarding; we recommend it strongly. Hemicrania continua can be mistaken for cluster headache if the history focuses on short-lived unilateral exacerbations of pain and misses the chronic low level of pain between exacerbations.

There are a number of secondary mimics of cluster headache. Giant cell arteritis (GCA) pain is usually continuous but may wax and wane, and is often associated with systemic symptoms, such as fever, polymyalgia, and weight loss. Ptosis in GCA may be confused with the autonomic feature of cluster headache. Trigeminal neuralgia is characterized by paroxysmal electric shock-like jabs of unilateral pain, most commonly limited to the distribution of the second or third divisions of the trigeminal nerve. The pain can be triggered by stimulation of limited areas of facial skin or oral mucosa. In an acute attack, the cluster headache sufferer is typically agitated and moves about, in contrast to the migraineur, who is typically quiescent. Sinusitis, glaucoma, intracranial aneurysms, tumors, arteriovenous malformations, dissection of the cervicocephalic cerebral blood vessels (carotid or vertebral), and even cervical cord lesions (meningioma) or infarctions can mimic cluster headache. In many of these instances, however, the history and examination disclose features that suggest a secondary cause of headache, and the history lacks the typical stereotyped periodicity of attack and remission phases.[2]

In most patients with typical cluster headache, there is no organic cause, but a few patients have had lesions responsible for their headaches. One series followed 11 patients with facial trauma with soft-tissue injury. In all but one patient, the injury involved the trigeminal territory. Although the attacks had the clinical appearance of cluster headache, with ipsilateral autonomic features, they were refractory to treatment and did not show the usual periodicity or remissions. In our experience, the trauma is usually in the ophthalmic division of the trigeminal nerve, most particularly involving the supraorbital nerve. Cluster-like headaches have also been reported to occur in patients who have lesions involving the posterior and anterior circulation (Table 9.4). It has been suggested that these lesions might irritate the C_{1-2} fibers that innervate the dura mater.[29] Certainly lesions involving structures that are innervated by branches of C_2 will trigger cranial autonomic activation in humans[28] and experimental animals;[30] indeed C_2 activation can sensitize trigeminal neurons that receive input from intracranial vessels.[31] The various sites of the lesions do not support the view that the cavernous sinus is the key locus of pathology in cluster headaches,[32,33] while recent functional data demonstrate that cavernous sinus involvement is a general feature of ophthalmic division pain and not specific for cluster headache.[34]

Epidemiology

Ekbom et al[35] studied 18-year-old Swedish army recruits and found the prevalence of cluster headache to be 0.09%. Kudrow extrapolated these results to distribution of age at onset obtained from headache clinic data to yield a rate of approximately 0.4%.[36] In Minnesota, the age-adjusted incidence of cluster headache was 15.6 per 100 000 person-years for men and 4.0 per 100 000 person-years for women. Cluster headache affects men more frequently than women, with a ratio of about 4 : 1,[16,37] it is substantially similar in females.[38] The mean age of onset is 27–31 years,[39] approximately 10 years later than that of migraine. Kudrow[8] found cluster headache, in his clinic, to be disproportionately more prevalent among black than white patients, and particularly so among black women, where the male : female ratio was 3 : 1.

Kudraw[8] studied 495 patients with cluster headache. Of the males (405) 27.4% were found to have at least one affected first-degree relative, and for the females (90) 37%. Of the patients' parents (990), 1.8% had cluster headache, which is considerably more than the population prevalence. Recent studies report between 14-fold[40] and 39-fold[41] increases in the risk of cluster headache among first-degree relatives. It seems likely that there is some inherited basis for cluster headache,[42] and certainly twins with cluster headache have been identified.[43–45]

Pathophysiology

The pathophysiology of cluster headache is better understood now than when the first edition of this book was written. Some of the features of cluster headache overlap with those of other primary vascular headaches, such as migraine, and have a similar neurobiology, which is covered in Chapter 5. Pain is usually centered about the eye and is reported as retro-orbital or temporal. This implies involvement of the ophthalmic (first) division of the trigeminal nerve. The pain may be referred to the first division by an intracranial process. It has been suggested, on anatomical grounds,[32] that this may be an inflammatory or vasculitic process in or around the cavernous sinus.[33] The cavernous sinus is a point of intersection of the first division of the trigeminal nerve and the cranial sympathetic and cranial parasympathetic nerves (Figure 9.1). Given the pain (trigeminal nerve), the signs of sympathetic dysfunction (the Horner's syndrome of miosis and ptosis), and the parasympathetic overactivity (lacrimation, nasal congestion, and injection of the eye), the cavernous sinus site is an attractive possibility. Until recently, few patients have been imaged during acute cluster headache. A case of Ekbom's reported in 1970[46] showed carotid narrowing on angiography, while a later case captured supraorbital changes.[47] Availability of magnetic resonance angiography (MRA) and positron emission tomography (PET) have shed new light on this problem, and we feel it is most likely that cluster headache is primarily a brain disorder with sec-

ondary changes in the cranial circulation resulting from trigeminal–autonomic activation.

Functional imaging and cluster headache

Until the mid-1980s, most studies of cluster headache were done with single photon emission computed tomography (SPECT). The results of this semi-quantitative method have been quite heterogeneous, some reporting an increase,[48,49] some a decrease,[50] and some no differences in cortical blood flow.[51,52] The variations were probably due to methodological differences. Spontaneous and glyceryl trinitrate- (nitroglycerin) provoked attacks are reported to be accompanied by a bilateral decrease in middle cerebral artery blood flow velocities implying vasodilation.[53,54] A PET study by Di Piero and co-workers[55] considered cluster headache patients out of the active period and normal volunteers using the cold-water pressor test. They demonstrated changes in pain transmission systems out of the active period of the disease, suggesting a possible involvement of central tonic pain mechanisms in the pathogenesis of cluster headache. To some extent this has been corroborated by a recent electrophysiological study.[55a]

In 1996, the first PET study in acute cluster headache was reported.[56] The authors investigated four patients, and their findings supported their earlier work,[57] which suggested a preference for the non-dominant hemisphere, especially for the anterior cingulate cortex, in affective processing of chronic ongoing pain syndromes. In a subsequent study of nine patients with cluster headache, the acute attack was compared to the headache-free state.[58] The observed areas of activation fell into three broad groups:

- areas known to be involved in pain processing or responses to pain, such as cingulate and insula cortex and contralateral thalamus;
- areas activated specifically in cluster headache but not in other causes of head pain, notably the posterior hypothalamic gray matter;
- a region outside the brain consistent with the internal carotid artery.

The latter area was confirmed to be the internal carotid artery using MRA,[59] and can be seen in both nitroglycerin-triggered and spontaneous attacks of cluster headache.[59,60]

These data demonstrate that cluster headache and migraine share some processing pathways, as might be expected, but may be distinguished on a functional neuroanatomical basis by areas of activation specific to the clinical syndrome. Remarkably, when a patient with both migraine and cluster headache was scanned during a migraine, the pattern of activation was that of migraine

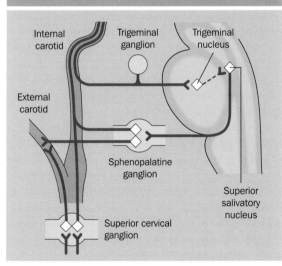

NEURAL INNERVATION OF THE CRANIAL CIRCULATION

Internal carotid
Trigeminal ganglion
Trigeminal nucleus
External carotid
Sphenopalatine ganglion
Superior salivatory nucleus
Superior cervical ganglion

● **Figure 9.1** *Neural innervation of the carotid arteries relevant to cluster headache. Sympathetic fibres arise in the superior cervical ganglion and follow the external and internal carotid arteries. The parasympathetic fibres arise in the superior salivatory nucleus in the pons and project to the sphenopalatine (pterygopalatine in humans) ganglion, as well as the otic and some carotid miniganglia. There is a reflex loop between the trigeminal innervation, that arises in the trigeminal ganglion, which activates the parasympathetic fibres.*

(brainstem) not cluster (posterior hypothalamic gray matter) headache.[61] The posterior hypothalamic gray matter is not activated with nitroglycerin triggering when the patient is out of the cluster bout.[60] Moreover, experimental pain in the first division of the trigeminal nerve induced by injection of capsaicin into the forehead produces carotid dilation and activation of brain areas concerned with pain, but not posterior hypothalamic activation.[62] Furthermore, MRA demonstrates that the carotid dilation with capsaicin injection in normal volunteers is seen only when pain is induced in the forehead, not when capsaicin is injected into the skin over the jaw or on the leg.[25] Pain in the trigeminal distribution produces carotid dilation through a normal trigeminal–autonomic reflex pathway;[34] it is the over-expression of this reflex pathway in TACs that is abnormal.

Linking the biology of cluster headache to clinical practice – posterior hypothalamic gray matter

The key pathophysiological processes of cluster headache take place within the central nervous system. The most curious feature of the disorder is its episodic nature, from which the very apt name, cluster headache, is derived. During the cluster periods, patients note that their headaches turn on and off like clockwork, respecting some daily (circadian) rhythm that has the stamp of the biological clock; patients will often awaken with headache at the same time every night. Moreover, the occurrence of cluster periods often follow half-yearly, yearly, or even biennial cycles of recurrent bouts, one of the most fascinating cycling processes of human biology. These processes implicate involvement of the suprachiasmatic region, and unraveling the neurobiology will tell us much about human biological clocks.

Cluster periods are more likely with the summer and winter solstices and less likely around the equinoxes. In many Western countries, clocks are shifted for daylight saving time, which may contribute to this phenomenon. Perhaps some central permissive process entrains or releases the trigeminovascular pain system. The PET imaging studies described above demonstrate unilateral activation in the hypothalamic gray matter ipsilateral to the headache side during the cluster pain,[58] but not during other forms of severe trigeminal pain. This dissociation implies a central locus for the basic pathophysiology of the disorder. While migraine and cluster headache share much in the expression of the pain, their underlying generation distinguishes them. It is the central nervous system's triggering or driving process that ultimately characterizes the primary headache syndromes. The finding of increased gray matter in the region of the posterior hypothalamic gray matter in patients with cluster headache,[63] and a report suggesting that stimulation of the region is an effective treatment of chronic cluster headache,[64] ushers in an entirely new era in terms of the pathophysiology, but perhaps more importantly in terms of completely revised thinking about management.

Treatment

Pharmacological treatment for cluster headache can be abortive (acute; Table 9.5), prophylactic (preventive; Table 9.6), or a combination of both methods. Acute treatment is directed at managing the individual attack. Preventive treatment is directed at controlling the frequency of attacks and is thus employed in both the episodic and chronic forms of the disorder. Patients should be instructed to avoid afternoon naps and alcoholic beverages, including wine and beer, since alcohol induces acute attacks during active cluster periods. They should be cautioned about prolonged exposure to volatile substances, such as solvents, gasoline, or oil-based paints, during cluster periods. Dietary influences, with the exception of alcohol, appear to have little importance in cluster headache. High altitude hypoxemia (levels above 5000 feet) may induce attacks during cluster periods. Cluster attacks due to high altitude may be prevented by oral administration of acetazolamide, 250 mg twice a day for 4 days, starting 2 days before the high altitude is reached.

Management of acute attacks (Table 9.5)

An overriding problem in acute cluster headache therapy is that the attacks begin rapidly, peak very quickly, and subside over less than 2 or 3 hours. To be of any value, a therapy must therefore be rapid in onset. Oral preparations that are used for migraine may not be effective; indeed, treating cluster headache as a *form* of migraine is a very considerable therapeutic mistake. Acute cluster headache is perhaps the worst pain known to humans; it follows that its relief is a responsibility that transcends financial considerations. In our view, withholding expensive but effective treatments in cluster headache is simply unethical. The options for acute treatment are oxygen, triptans, ergot derivatives and intranasal lidocaine.

Oxygen

Oxygen inhalation, a standard acute treatment for cluster headache, was first used by Horton.[65] Given via a non-

● **Table 9.5** *Abortive treatment*

	Efficacy	Tolerability	Clinical Use
100% oxygen (7–12 L/min) for 15–20 minutes	Aborts headache in 70% in <15 minutes	Very well-tolerated	First line choice; inconvenient
Sumatriptan 20 mg I.N.	Effective	Triptan AEs; contraindicated in cardiovascular disease	First line choice
Sumatriptan 6 mg S.C.	Highly effective		First line choice
Dihydroergotamine 1.0 mg I.M. or I.V.	Effective	Contraindicated in cardiovascular disease	First line choice
Lidocaine I.N. (4–6%)	Questionable	Fair to good	Limited

I.N., intranasally; S.C., subcutaneously; AEs, adverse effects; I.M., intramuscularly; I.V., intravenously

● **Table 9.6** *Prophylactic treatment*

Short-term prevention Episodic cluster headache	**Long-term prevention** *Episodic cluster headache – prolonged bouts* *chronic cluster headache*
• Corticosteroids (i.e. prednisolone, prednisone) • Methysergide • Daily (nocturnal) ergotamine • Verapamil • Greater occipital nerve injection • Pizotifen*	• Verapamil • Lithium • Methysergide • Divalproex sodium* • Pizotifen* • ?Topiramate • ?Gabapentin • ?Melatonin

? = unproven but promising
* = questionable efficacy

rebreathing mask at a flow rate of 7–12 L/minute for 15–20 minutes, it is effective in approximately 70% of patients, and may work within 5 minutes.[66,67] In clinical practice, it may take as long as 15–20 minutes to be effective, and our experience is that studies have somewhat overestimated its response rate, although a subspecialty practice base may select it for treatment-refractory patients. Oxygen is an extremely safe, cost-effective treatment. In some patients, oxygen may delay rather than abort the attack, and pain may return. Oxygen's effectiveness may depend on the timing of its administration: it may be most effective when given at the maximum intensity of the pain,[68] although some patients report it is more effective when used early. High flow rate, high oxygen percentage, and allowing a reasonable time period of inhalation are all key elements in the success of the treatment.

In most countries, small portable cylinders are available. These can be taken in the car, to work, or kept at the bedside for nighttime attacks. Some patients find it inconvenient to keep oxygen available during cluster periods.

In a placebo-controlled study, hyperbaric oxygen (2 atm) given for 30 minutes aborted an acute attack of cluster within 5–13 minutes in six of seven patients, while none of the placebo group had relief. In the long-term, three patients reported complete interruption and three patients partial interruption of their cluster cycle.[69] Other authors have reported similar benefits of hyperbaric oxygen.[70,71] In clinical practice, we see no clear benefit for hyperbaric treatment over standard high flow/high concentration oxygen. If hyperbaric oxygen disrupts the cluster cycle that would be valuable.

PATHOGENESIS OF CLUSTER HEADACHE

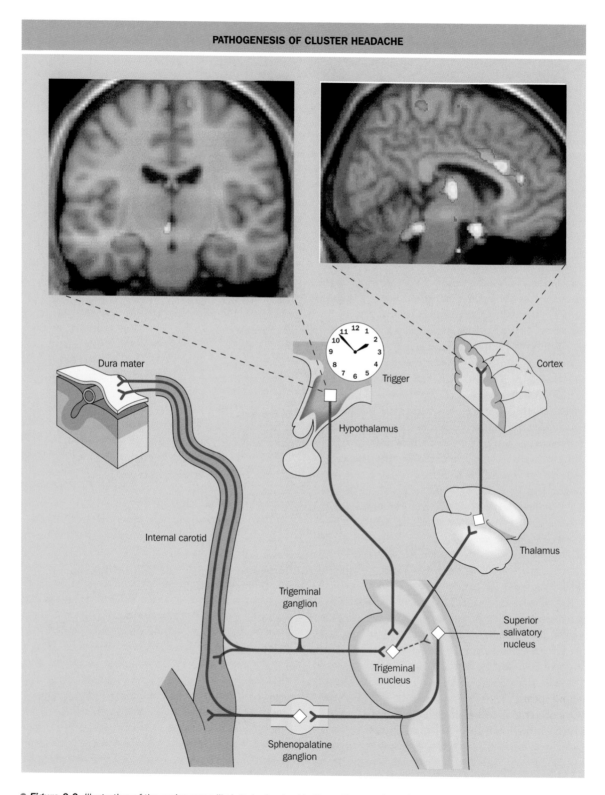

● **Figure 9.2** *Illustration of the major areas likely to be involved in the pathogenesis and expression of cluster headache. The hypothalamic gray is likely from PET[58] studies to be the basic site of dysfunction which interacts with the trigemino-parasympathetic pathways to produce the pain and autonomic symptomatology.*

Triptans (serotonin, 5-HT$_{1B/1D}$ agonists)
Sumatriptan

Sumatriptan is available in various countries as a 6-mg subcutaneous injection, a 20-mg nasal spray, a 25-mg suppository, and 25-mg, 50-mg and 100-mg oral tablets. In a double-blind, placebo-controlled study, sumatriptan (6 mg subcutaneously) was more effective than placebo in acute cluster headache. A response was noted by 10 minutes, and 74% of treated patients were pain-free by 15 minutes.[72] Sumatriptan usually continues to be effective with repeated use for several months.[73] While generally well tolerated, sumatriptan is contraindicated in patients with ischemic heart disease or uncontrolled hypertension.[74] A 6-mg subcutaneous sumatriptan injection is a remarkably effective treatment. It works rapidly and efficiently, often producing a benefit in 5–7 minutes after administration.[75] The current auto-injector device is easy to use and needleless devices are promised. Patients do not seem to develop tachyphylaxis even over long bouts of cluster headache.[76] Rebound headache is not a problem in cluster headache with the exception of patients who also have a personal history of migraine. The mechanism of action of sumatriptan in cluster headache is likely to be similar to that described in migraine (see Chapter 5), although a case of cluster headache responsive to sumatriptan even after complete trigeminal root section is now documented.[77] The peripheral and central sites of action of the class are illustrated in Figure 9.3.

Sumatriptan nasal spray has been studied in an open label fashion and had modest effects.[78,79] A double-blind, placebo-controlled, cross-over study of sumatriptan 20 mg intranasally has also shown efficacy greater than placebo.[80]

Preemptive treatment with sumatriptan in a regimen of 100 mg three times daily does not alter either the timing or the frequency of headaches.[81] These data are in accordance with published data for migraine with aura that has shown pretreating patients with the injectable form of sumatriptan prior to headache does not prevent headache,[82] and results in lower overall efficacy for the oral form.[83]

Zolmitriptan

It has been shown that zolmitriptan 5 mg and 10 mg orally were effective treatments of acute cluster headache versus placebo, but only in patients with the episodic form.[84] For most patients oral zolmitriptan is not practical, but the results suggest that the intranasal formulation,[85] which has much better pharmacokinetics,[86] might offer a useful therapeutic option to cluster headache patients.

POTENTIAL SITES OF ACTION OF THE TRIPTANS

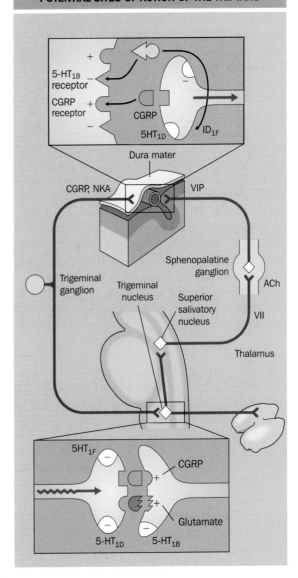

● **Figure 9.3** *Illustration of the possible sites of action of the triptans both peripherally and within the central nervous system.*

Ergot derivatives
Dihydroergotamine

Dihydroergotamine (DHE), available in injectable and intranasal forms, is effective in relieving acute attacks of cluster headache. Parenteral DHE (1 mg intramuscularly)[87] and intranasal DHE[88] are effective for some, but not all, patients. Intravenous injection gives more rapid relief than intramuscular injection, with benefit in less than 10 minutes. Andersson and Jespersen[88] conducted a double-blind comparative trial of DHE nasal spray (1 mg). DHE did not change the duration or frequency of the attacks, but it did decrease pain intensity. Since DHE as a nasal spray has a 40% bioavailability, administration of a higher dose may be more effective for the treatment of cluster headache.

Ergotamine

Ergotamine tartrate (available as a tablet, suppository, or, in some countries, as an inhalant) may only partially ameliorate an acute cluster attack because of the pharmacokinetics of the preparation. Some patients may respond to rectal ergotamine. We feel that ergotamine is no longer a first-line treatment for acute cluster headache.

Topical local anesthetics

Local intranasal anesthetic agents, such as cocaine[89,90] or lidocaine,[91,92] have been reported to be effective. Cocaine has no advantage, and is not preferentially utilized. Lidocaine 4–6% nasal drops (1 ml) may be used and repeated once after 15 minutes.[92] We find it a useful adjunct but rarely use it as the primary therapy for acute attacks.

Other agents
Analgesics and narcotics

Non-parenteral analgesics and narcotics have little role in the treatment of cluster headache, although they may be useful for some patients who are unresponsive to oxygen and have ischemic heart disease. The opiate butorphanol can be administered by a nasal spray and is sometimes a useful strategy although controlled studies are not available. Caution to avoid overuse syndromes is required. This compound is a sedative as well as an analgesic; this can be a useful combination for patients who have attacks of cluster headache that awaken them from sleep, and, in that setting, could be a very useful option. It has no cardiovascular risks and is thus a medically safe option in patients for whom vasoconstrictor compounds are contraindicated or oxygen has failed to be useful.

Promising approaches

Local steroid and anesthetic injection of the ipsilateral greater occipital nerve[93] has been reported to be effective in cluster headache. It has some utility in the acute setting, but we have also found it to have short-term preventive effects. Octreotide, a synthetic somatostatin analogue, has also been reported to be useful in cluster headache.[94,95] It would provide an interesting approach since it has no vascular effects, and may illustrate a new principle. It is clear that somatostatin can inhibit neurons in the trigeminal nucleus caudalis in rat,[96] and other forms of headache respond to somatostatin.[97,98] We predict that somatostatin agonists may be effective in both cluster headache and migraine; controlled studies are required.

Prophylactic pharmacotherapy of cluster headache

Preventive treatment in cluster headache is aimed at both shortening bouts[99] and controlling attack frequency. All the treatments are largely empirical, although many are very effective.[2] Most cluster patients require prophylactic therapy at some point since:

1) attacks are frequent, severe, of rapid onset, and often too short-lived for acute medication to take effect;
2) acute treatment may only postpone the attack;
3) treating frequent attacks with abortives may result in medication overuse;
4) failing to stop the cluster period early may prolong the suffering for months.[100]

Medications generally accepted as effective in the prophylactic treatment of cluster headache include ergotamine, methysergide, corticosteroids, verapamil, and lithium carbonate. Chlorpromazine, although it has been reported to be effective,[101] β-blockers, antidepressants, and histamine desensitization are probably ineffective as prophylaxis. It has been suggested that divalproex (valproate),[102] gabapentin[103,104] and topiramate[105] are effective in cluster headache, although clear evidence is lacking and clinical experience is mixed. Corticosteroids are not appropriate for the treatment of chronic cluster headache in the long-term. Reports of indometacin-sensitive cluster headache[106,107] may have documented cases of paroxysmal hemicrania (See Chapter 10). The goal of prophylactic therapy is to produce a rapid remission of headaches and to maintain that remission with minimal side-effects until the cluster period is over.

The principles of prophylactic pharmacotherapy are as follows:

1) start medications early in the cluster period;
2) continue the drugs until the patient is headache-free for at least 2 weeks;
3) taper the drugs rather than abruptly withdrawing them;
4) restart the drugs at the beginning of the next cluster period.[100]

Because preventive treatments become effective over days to weeks and are rarely completely effective, abortive agents, such as oxygen, sumatriptan, DHE, or intranasal lidocaine should almost always be used to treat break-through attacks.

The medication choice will depend on:

1) previous drug response;
2) prior adverse drug reactions;
3) contraindications to drug use;
4) type of cluster (episodic or chronic) and length of bout;
5) frequency and timing of attacks (nocturnal versus diurnal);
6) the patient's age and lifestyle.

Preventive therapies in cluster headache can be classified as being either short-term or long-term. The distinction high-lights the fact that some drugs work quickly, but may have undesirable long-term side-effects; these are used for short-term prophylaxis. Other medicines are slower in onset but more easy to use in the medium to long term. The distinction is important for patients with episodic cluster headache of long bout duration who are treated with similar drugs to patients with chronic cluster headache. As a principle, single optimized drugs are preferred, but combining two or more drugs may be necessary.

Short-term preventatives

Corticosteroids

Treating cluster headache with a short burst of oral corti-costeroids has been recommended for some years[108] and is certainly effective. The effect is usually rapid in onset, but headache often reappears as the dose is dropped. Corticosteroids are an excellent short-term solution but are not appropriate in the long term. Adverse effects include insomnia, restlessness, personality changes, hypona-tremia, edema, hyperglycemia, osteoporosis, myopathy, and gastric ulcers. Patients must be warned about the problem of osteonecrosis (ON) of the femoral head, and at other common sites (femoral condyles, head of humerus, scaphoid, lunate and talus).[109] The shortest course of prednisolone reported to be associated with ON of the femoral head was a 30-day course of 16 mg/day.[110] Fur-thermore, courses of adrenocorticotropic hormone[111] have produced ON after 16 days and dexamethasone at 16 mg per day after 7 days.[112] Mirzai et al[109] have taken the view that dexamethasone was, therefore, more problematic, and that an inter-use interval of less than 12 months was also a problem. Taken together, 21–28-day courses of oral prednisolone or prednisone (60–100 mg/day for 7–10 days with a 5–10 mg/day taper) seem entirely reasonable and largely safe, when restricted to once a year.

Ergotamine

Ergotamine tartrate is an agonist at 5-HT$_{1B/1D}$ receptors, as is sumatriptan. It shares many of sumatriptan's pre-clinical actions.[113] Ergotamine tartrate, up to 4 mg (in divided doses), is effective and probably poses only a small risk of rebound headache, which may occur in patients with a family history of migraine. Ergotamine is particularly useful in controlling nocturnal attacks when taken at bedtime.[11,87,114]

Methysergide

Methysergide maleate is a congener of methylergonovine and lysergic acid diethylamide. It is widely distributed throughout the body, crosses the blood–brain barrier, and binds to serotonin receptors in the brain. It has affinity for 5-HT$_1$ and 5-HT$_2$ receptors. Methysergide is effective in 65–69% of patients who have episodic cluster headache.[8,115] Response rates are lower in chronic cluster. This drug is indicated in younger patients, who are without the potential risk of artherosclerotic heart disease. Side-effects include muscle cramps, nausea, diarrhea, and abdominal discomfort; these often occur initially, but usually subside over several days.[116,117] Prolonged treat-ment has been associated with fibrotic reactions (retroperitoneal, pleural, pulmonary, and cardiac valvular), although this is rare.[118] The rapid onset of effect, and the fibrotic complications, with the necessity to take breaks from therapy every 6 months for 1 month, makes methy-sergide more suitable in patients with relatively short bouts of cluster headache. If methysergide use is prolonged and a drug holiday is omitted, periodic renal profiling, chest X-ray, echocardiogram, and magnetic resonance imaging of the abdomen must be performed.

Long-term preventive agents

Calcium-channel blockers

The calcium antagonists are a group of chemically hetero-geneous drugs that were developed as cardiovascular agents. They interact with the L-type voltage-gated calcium channel,[119] although flunarizine may interact with the P/Q channel[120] that has been implicated in familial hemiplegic migraine.[121] The clear evidence is for the use of verapamil. We do not use nimodipine, although there is some open-label evidence for its use.[122,123]

Verapamil

Verapamil has been studied in the treatment of cluster headache, and many, including the authors, believe it is the prophylactic drug of choice when cluster headache bouts are prolonged.[123-125] Doses range from 240–960 mg daily. The maximum approved dose is 480 mg per day but many patients with cluster headache require higher doses. We recommend careful monitoring as the dose is escalated, particularly beyond 480 mg per day. Constipation is the most common side-effect. Other symptoms include ankle edema, dizziness, nausea, hypotension, gum hypertrophy and fatigue. Gum hypertrophy may result in tooth loss and should prompt careful withdrawal of verapamil and dental review. Verapamil can cause heart block by slowing conduction in the atrioventricular node[126] as demonstrated by prolongation of the A–H interval.[127] Given that the PR interval on the ECG is made up of atrial conduction, A–H and His bundle conduction, it may be difficult to monitor subtle early effects as the verapamil dose is increased. This question needs study in this group of patients, but it seems appropriate to do a baseline ECG and then repeat the ECG 10 days after a dose change, usually made in 80 mg increments, when doses exceed 240 mg daily. Verapamil can be combined with ergotamine or lithium. When verapamil and lithium are used together, there may be increased sensitivity to lithium.[128] In one double-blind trial, verapamil was found to be as effective as lithium.[125]

Lithium carbonate

Lithium's mode of action in cluster headache (and in manic-depressive illness) is unknown. It alters circadian rhythms and reduces random eye movement sleep. It has been suggested that the lithium-induced depletion of inositol results in decreased production of the second messenger inositol triphosphate, reducing neuronal activity. Lithium is rapidly and almost completely absorbed. Lithium carbonate is more effective in chronic than in episodic cluster headache,[129,130] although this may simply be a reflection of the time necessary for it to have a useful effect rather than any biological difference. Seventy-eight percent of patients with chronic headache and 63% of patients with episodic cluster headache respond. The usual initial dose of lithium is 300 mg b.i.d., but higher doses may be required. Lithium has a long half-life (24 hours) and takes about 1 week to reach steady-state levels, at which time (and periodically thereafter) a lithium level should be obtained. Lithium is often effective at a blood level of 0.4–0.8 mol/l (less than the usual therapeutic dose for mania). A therapeutic response is often seen within 1 week. Some patients may require an additional preventive agent, such as ergotamine or verapamil, along with lithium, and some patients eventually become resistant to lithium. Side-effects of lithium include slight weakness, mild nausea, thirst (which usually subsides), tremor, lethargy, slurred speech, and blurred vision. Toxicity is manifested by nausea, vomiting, anorexia, diarrhea, and neurologic signs or symptoms: confusion, nystagmus, ataxia, extrapyramidal signs, and seizures. Concomitant use of sodium-depleting diuretics should be avoided, as sodium depletion will result in high lithium levels and neurotoxicity; given the conditions in outlined Chapter 10, it should be noted that concurrent use of indometacin can increase the lithium level. Hypothyroidism and polyuria (nephrogenic diabetes insipidus) can occur with long-term use. Polymorphonuclear leukocytosis may occur and be mistaken for occult infection.

Possibly effective and promising treatments

Divalproex sodium

Divalproex sodium (250–3000 mg/day) has been reported to be effective in cluster headache.[102] Treatment was well tolerated with only nausea reported. A controlled study is needed and preliminary indications are that it was no better than placebo. Lethargy, tremor, weight gain, and hair loss are some of the common side-effects. Pancreatitis and liver function abnormalities are rare severe adverse events. Blood counts and liver function should be obtained prior to treatment. Follow-up monitoring is not necessary unless the patient is symptomatic.

Topiramate

Topiramate (50–200 mg/day) was associated with rapid improvement in 10 cluster headache patients in an open-label study.[105] Starting at a low dosage and making small increments can minimize both the total daily dosage and the potential for side-effects. Somnolence, dizziness, ataxia, and cognitive symptoms are the most commonly-reported side-effects. Topiramate is a weak carbonic anhydrase inhibitor, and renal calculi and paresthesias have been reported. In a second open trial 21 patients were treated with topiramate up to 200 mg/day. Eleven had complete remission in 1–27 days and another five patients had more than a 50% reduction in attack frequency.[131] A controlled study is indicated.

Pizotifen

Pizotifen has been reported to be of benefit in cluster headache.[132–134] Widely used in the United Kingdom and Canada for migraine prevention, it is not available in the United States. Modern controlled trials are not available and it is generally not held to be very useful in cluster headache.

Capsaicin

Capsaicin desensitizes sensory neurons by depleting substance P. In a double-blind, placebo-controlled study using capsaicin (0.025% cream b.i.d.) applied intranasally via a cotton-tipped applicator on the side of headache for 7 days, patients who received the active drug had significantly less frequent and less severe attacks.[135]

Indometacin

Indometacin is the treatment of choice for paroxysmal hemicrania (see Chapter 10). Some patients with cluster headache have been suggested to respond to it.[106,107] Objective evidence for this is lacking, and a placebo-controlled trial is warranted.

Melatonin

Based on the circadian periodicity of cluster headache and changes that were reported in plasma levels,[136] a placebo-controlled, parallel-group study of 10 mg of melatonin daily was conducted.[137] The authors found melatonin superior to placebo in this small study. This question should be reconsidered given the current biological understanding of cluster headache.

Some treatment protocols

Treatment and dosage must be individualized. Many clinicians start treatment of both episodic and chronic cluster headache with the long-term preventive verapamil at 120–480 mg/day. When there is a clear history of shorter bouts (less than 8 weeks) one can start with ergotamine tartrate 1–4 mg/day, particularly for patients with nocturnal attacks, who should take a dose at bedtime. However, this precludes the use of sumatriptan for acute attacks and is thus becoming less attractive as a strategy. Similarly, corticosteroids give a quick response to patients and can bring short but welcome relief when daily attacks are frequent. For patients with short bouts it can be used alone. For patients with longer bouts it can be started with verapamil to prevent attacks as verapamil's benefits evolve. Corticosteroids can then be tapered after 2–4 weeks. Ergotamine can be used alone or in combination with verapamil. Methysergide 1–3 mg three to four times a day is an effective alternative, especially in younger patients. Methysergide should not be combined with ergotamine. Lithium or valproate can be used next, alone or in combination with verapamil. Pizotifen is preferred by some, when it is available, before verapamil, but this would not be our approach. For longer-term treatment, particularly in chronic cluster headache, verapamil or lithium, alone or in combination, would be our drug of choice. In resistant cases, triple therapy using ergotamine, verapamil, and lithium or methysergide, verapamil, and lithium may be considered.

Acetazolamide may be a useful pretreatment for patients whose attacks are triggered by altitude, such as a ski trip. Kudrow suggests 250 mg twice daily for four days commencing 2 days prior to reaching high altitudes.

The treatment-resistant patient and options for surgical procedures

Cluster headache patients may become refractory to both acute and preventive therapies, or have an intercurrent illness (particularly ischemic heart disease) that makes medical therapy difficult or impossible. Such patients are candidates for an ablative neurosurgical procedure. Management of these refractory cases can be very difficult, requiring time, patience, and experience with what is a relatively rare situation. It is our view that ablative procedures in cluster headache should be done exclusively in headache centers where medical therapy can be truly optimized and surgeons have sufficient experience to provide patients with reliable results.

Dihydroergotamine given repetitively intravenously every 8-hours in an inpatient setting is an effective treatment for intractable cluster headache, rendering most patients headache-free during treatment. This approach will provide weeks or months in which to consider the options without the pressure of a patient in daily agony. Most such patients will have received multiple medications, including ergotamine (oral and suppository), steroids, and even intramuscular DHE, but remain refractory until intravenous DHE therapy is initiated.[138] Histamine desensitization has been used to treat patients with intractable cluster headache with mixed results.[139] Local steroid and anesthetic injection of the ipsilateral occipital nerve has been advocated, with headache relief for 5–73 days.[93] Many patients required more than one injection. In our experience, and that of others, local steroid injections can be effective and buy valuable time while devising a further plan of management.

In our experience, approximately 10% of patients with chronic cluster headache do not respond to prophylactic pharmacotherapy or have significant contraindications to effective preventive or acute agents. These patients are candidates for surgical consideration.

Indications for surgical treatment include:

1) strictly unilateral headache;
2) total resistance to medical therapy or significant contraindications to effective medical therapy;
3) a stable personality profile with no addictive potential.

Sphenopalatine ganglionectomy

When sphenopalatine ganglionectomy[140] was attempted in 13 patients with severe intractable cluster headaches, only two patients had complete relief at 1-year follow-up, and seven patients had little relief. This is in keeping with our impression of this procedure. However, it has virtually zero morbidity and is thus the first choice of the ablative procedures.

Trigeminal surgery

It is not at all clear what the best way forward is after a failed sphenopalatine ganglionectomy. It has been our practice to offer radiofrequency thermocoagulation of the trigeminal ganglion. The overall results have been encouraging, with almost 75% of patients becoming free of cluster headache attacks.[141,142] However, complications include anesthesia dolorosa, transient corneal infection, transient diplopia, and recurrent sty. Recurrence of pain is possible after a number of years, and repeat surgery may be necessary. Glycerol injection has been proposed for the treatment of intractable cluster headache. This procedure affords significant pain relief and corneal safety.[143,144] The main problem with this approach is control of the lesion size and inadvertent spread of the glycerol intracranially. For these reasons, we do not advocate this approach.

Gamma knife radiosurgery

Gamma knife radiosurgery was reported to be effective in six medically recalcitrant cluster headache patients.[145] The time-to-effective-relief was either immediate or within 1 week. Four patients were pain-free at follow-up after more than 8 months. This study has not yet been duplicated, and the overall efficacy, safety, and durability of the procedure is as yet unknown. However, it is a noninvasive procedure with fewer side-effects than ablative surgery and may represent a viable alternative in some patients prior to a destructive procedure.

The future

The demonstration of activations in the posterior hypothalamic gray matter during acute attacks of cluster headache with PET,[58] and the subsequent demonstration of structural changes in that region,[63] have suggested that this brain region may be fundamental in the generation of acute cluster headache. A patient with chronic cluster headache had a stimulator placed into this region, rendering the patient headache free.[64] This observation needs repetition and examination, since a reversible, essentially very low-morbidity treatment aimed at the responsible brain region would completely revolutionize the management of intractable cluster headache. This finding provides a sense of optimism to patients whose life is otherwise very clearly hell on earth.

References

1. Goadsby PJ, Lipton RB. A review of paroxysmal hemicranias, SUNCT syndrome and other short-lasting headaches with autonomic features, including new cases. Brain 1997; 120: 193–209.
2. Dodick DW, Rozen TD, Goadsby PJ, Silberstein SD. Cluster headache. Cephalalgia 2000; 20: 787–803.
3. Friedman AP, Mikropoulos HE. Cluster headache. Neurology 1958; 8: 653.
4. Headache Classification Committee of the International Headache Society. Classification and diagnostic criteria for headache disorders, cranial neuralgia, and facial pain. Cephalalgia 1988; 8: 1–96.
5. Koehler PJ. Prevalence of headache in Tulp's observationes medicae (1641) with a description of cluster headache. Cephalalgia 1993; 13: 318–20.
6. Isler H. Episodic cluster headache from a textbook of 1745: Van Swieten's classic description. Cephalalgia 1993; 13: 172–4.
7. Sjaastad O. Cluster Headache Syndrome. London: Saunders, 1992.
8. Kudrow L. Cluster Headache: Mechanisms and Management. New York: Oxford University Press, 1980.
9. Olesen J, Goadsby PJ. Cluster Headache and Related Conditions. Oxford: Oxford University Press, 1999.
10. Ekbom K. Ergotamine tartrate orally in Horton's histaminic cephalalgia (also called Harris's ciliary neuralgia). Acta Psychiatr Scand 1947; 46: 106.
11. Kunkle EC, Pfeiffer JB, Wilhoit WM, Hamrick LW. Recurrent brief headache in 'cluster' pattern. In: Merritt HH, ed. Transactions of the American Neurological Association. 77th Annual Meeting, Atlantic City, N.J.: American Neurological Association 1952, 240–3.
12. Horton BT, MacLean AR, Craig WM. A new syndrome of vascular headache: results of treatment with histamine: preliminary report. Mayo Clin Proc 1939; 14: 257–60.
13. Ekbom K. A clinical comparison of cluster headache and migraine. Acta Neurol Scand 1970; 46: 1.
14. Ekbom K. Nitroglycerin as a provocative agent in cluster headache. Arch Neurol 1968; 19: 487–93.
15. Silberstein SD, Niknam R, Rozen TD, Young WB. Cluster headache with aura. Neurology 2000; 54: 219–20.
16. Bahra A, May A, Goadsby PJ. Cluster headache: a prospective clinical study in 230 patients with diagnostic implications. Neurology 2002;58: 354–61.
16a. Siow HC, Young WB, Peres MF, Rozen TD, Silberstein SD. Hemiplegic cluster. Headache 2002; 42: 136–9.
17. Nappi G, Micieli G, Cavallini A et al. Accompanying symptoms of cluster attacks: their relevance to the diagnostic criteria. Cephalalgia 1992; 3: 165–8.
18. Vingen JV, Pareja JA, Stovner LJ. Increased sensitivity to light and sound during cluster headache bout. In: Olesen J, Goadsby PJ, eds. Cluster Headache and Related Conditions. Oxford: Oxford University Press, 1998, 207–11.
19. Manzoni GC, Micieli G, Granella F et al. Cluster headache – course over ten years in 189 patients. Cephalalgia 1991; 11: 169–74.
20. Sjostrand C, Waldenlind E, Ekbom K. A follow-up study of 60 patients after an assumed first period of cluster headache. Cephalalgia 2000; 20: 653–7.
21. Graham JR. Cluster headache.

Presentation at the International Symposium on Headache, Chicago. 1969.

22. Kudrow L. Cluster headache: diagnosis, management, and treatment. In: Dalessio DJ, Silberstein SD, eds. Wolff's Headache and Other Head Pain. 6th edn. Oxford: Oxford University Press, 1993, 171–97.

23. Kudrow L. Cluster headache: diagnosis and management. Headache 1979; 19: 142–50.

24. Goadsby PJ, Duckworth JW. Effect of stimulation of trigeminal ganglion on regional cerebral blood flow in cats. Am J Physiol 1987; 253: R270–4.

25. May A, Buchel C, Turner R, Goadsby PJ. MR angiography in facial and other pain: neurovascular mechanisms of trigeminal sensation. J Cereb Blood Flow Metabol 2001; 21: 1171–6.

26. Kudrow L, McGinty DJ, Phillips ER, Stevenson M. Sleep apnea in cluster headache. Cephalalgia 1984; 4: 33–8.

27. Chervin RD, Zellek N, Lin X et al. Sleep disordered breathing in patients with cluster headache. Neurology 2000; 54: 2302–6.

28. Giffin N, Goadsby PJ. Basilar artery aneurysm with autonomic features: an interesting pathophysiological problem. J Neurol Neurosurg Psychiatry 2001; 71: 805–8.

29. Koenigsberg AD, Solomon GD, Kosmorsky DO. Pseudoaneurysm within the cavernous sinus presenting as cluster headache. Headache 1994; 34: 111–13.

30. Vincent MB, Ekman R, Edvinsson L et al. Reduction of calcitonin gene-related peptide in the jugular blood following electrical stimulation of rat greater occipital nerve. Cephalalgia 1992; 12: 275–9.

31. Bartsch T, Goadsby PJ. Stimulation of the greater occipital nerve (GON) enhances responses of dural responsive convergent neurons in the trigeminocervical complex in the rat. Cephalalgia 2001; 21: 401–2.

32. Moskowitz MA. Cluster headache: evidence for a pathophysiologic focus in the superior pericarotid cavernous sinus plexus. Headache 1988; 28: 584–6.

33. Hardebo JE. How cluster headache is explained as an intracavernous inflammatory process lesioning sympathetic fibres. Headache 1994; 34: 125–31.

34. May A, Goadsby PJ. The trigeminovascular system in humans: pathophysiological implications for primary headache syndromes of the neural influences on the cerebral circulation. J Cereb Blood Flow Metabol 1999; 19: 115–27.

35. Ekbom K, Ahlborg B, Schele R. Prevalence of migraine and cluster headache in Swedish men of 18. Headache 1978; 18: 9–19.

36. Kudrow L. Cluster headache. In: Blau JN, ed. Headache: Clinical, Therapeutic, Conceptual, and Research Aspects. London: Chapman & Hall, 1987, 113–19.

37. Manzoni GC. Gender ratio of cluster headache over the years: a possible role of changes in lifestyle. Cephalalgia 1998; 18: 138–42.

38. Rozen TD, Niknam R, Shechter AL et al. Cluster headache in women: clinical characteristics and comparison to cluster headache in men. J Neurol Neurosurg Psychiatry 2001; 70: 613–17.

39. Manzoni EC, Terzano MG, Bono G et al. Cluster headache – clinical findings in 180 patients. Cephalalgia 1983; 3: 21–30.

40. Russell MB, Andersson PG, Thomsen LL, Iselius L. Cluster headache is an autosomal dominantly inherited disorder in some families: a complex segregation analysis. J Med Genet 1995; 32: 954–6.

41. Leone M, Russell MB, Rigamonti A et al. Increased familial risk of cluster headache. Neurology 2001; 56: 1233–6.

42. Russell MB, Andersson PG, Iselius L. Cluster headache is an inherited disorder in some families. Headache 1996; 36: 608–12.

43. Roberge C, Bouchard JP, Simard D, Gagne R. Cluster headache in twins. Neurology 1992; 42: 1255–6.

44. Sjaastad O, Shen JM, Stovner LJ, Elsas T. Cluster headache in identical twins. Headache 1993; 33: 214–17.

45. Couturier EG, Hering R, Steiner TJ. The first report of cluster headache in identical twins. Neurology 1991; 41: 761.

46. Ekbom K, Greitz T. Carotid angiography in cluster headache. Acta Radiologica 1970; 10: 177–86.

47. Waldenlind E, Ekbom K, Torhall J. MR-angiography during spontaneous attacks of cluster headache: a case report. Headache 1993; 33: 291–5.

48. Norris JW, Hachinski VC, Cooper PW. Cerebral blood flow changes in cluster headache. Acta Neurol Scand 1976; 54: 371–4.

49. Sakai F, Meyer JS. Regional cerebral hemodynamics during migraine and cluster headaches measured by the 133-Xe inhalation method. Headache 1978; 18: 122–32.

50. Nelson RF, du Boulay GH, Marshall J et al. Cerebral blood flow studies in patients with cluster headache. Headache 1980; 20: 184–9.

51. Henry PY, Vernhiet J, Orgogozo JM, Caille JM. Cerebral blood flow in migraine and cluster headache.

Compartmental analysis and reactivity to anesthetic depression. Res Clin Stud Headache 1978; 6: 81–8.

52. Krabbe AA, Henriksen L, Olesen J. Tomographic determination of cerebral blood flow during attacks of cluster headache. Cephalalgia 1984; 4: 17–23.

53. Dahl A, Russell D, Nyberg-Hansen R, Rootwelt K. Cluster headache: transcranial doppler ultrasound and RCBF studies. Cephalalgia 1990; 10: 87–94.

54. Tegeler CH, Davidai G, Gengo FM et al. Middle cerebral artery velocity correlates with nitroglycerin-induced headache onset. J Neuroimag 1996; 6: 81–6.

55. Di Piero V, Fiacco F, Tombari D, Pantano P. Tonic pain: a SPET study in normal subjects and cluster headache patients. Pain 1997; 70: 185–91.

55a. Nappi G, Sandrini G, Alfonsi E, Proietti Cecchini A, Michieli G, Moglia A. Impaired circadian rhythmicity of nociceptive reflex thresholds in cluster headache. Headache 2002; 42: 125–31.

56. Hsieh JC, Hannerz J, Ingvar M. Right lateralized central processing for pain of nitroglycerin induced cluster headache. Pain 1996; 67: 59–68.

57. Hsieh JC, Belfrage M, Elander SS et al. Central representation of chronic ongoing neuropathic pain studied by positron emission tomography. Pain 1995; 63: 225–36.

58. May A, Bahra A, Buchel C et al. Hypothalamic activation in cluster headache attacks. Lancet 1998; 352: 275–8.

59. May A, Buchel C, Bahra A et al. Intracranial vessels in trigeminal transmitted pain: a PET study. Neuroimage 1999; 9: 453–60.

60. May A, Bahra A, Buchel C et al. PET and MRA findings in cluster headache and MRA in experimental pain. Neurology 2000; 55: 1328–35.

61. Bahra A, Matharu MS, Buchel C et al. Brainstem activation specific to migraine headache. Lancet 2001; 357: 1016–17.

62. May A, Kaube H, Buchel C et al. Experimental cranial pain elicited by capsaicin: A PET study. Pain 1998; 74: 61–6.

63. May A, Ashburner J, Buchel C et al. Correlation between structural and functional changes in brain in an idiopathic headache syndrome. Nature Med 1999; 5: 836–8.

64. Leone M, Franzini A. Stereotactic stimulation of the posterior hypothalamic gray matter in a patient with intractable cluster headache. N Eng J Med 2001; 345: 1428–9.

65. Horton BT. Histaminic cephalalgia:

differential diagnosis and treatment. Mayo Clin Proc 1956; 31: 325–33.

66. Kudrow L. Response of cluster headache attacks to oxygen inhalation. Headache 1981; 21: 1–4.

67. Fogan L. Treatment of cluster headache. A double-blind comparison of oxygen air inhalation. Arch Neurol 1985; 42: 362–3.

68. Igarashi H, Sakai F, Tazaki Y. The mechanism by which oxygen interrupts cluster headache. Cephalalgia 1991; 11: 238–9.

69. Di Sabato F, Fusco BM, Pelaia P, Giacovazzo M. Hyperbaric oxygen therapy in cluster headache. Pain 1993; 52: 243–5.

70. Weiss LD. Treatment of cluster headache patient in a hyperbaric chamber. Headache 1989; 29: 109–10.

71. Porta M, Granella F, Coppola A. Treatment of cluster headache attacks with hyperbaric oxygen. Cephalalgia 1991; 11: 236–7.

72. Ekbom K. Treatment of acute cluster headache with sumatriptan. N Eng J Med 1991; 325: 322–6.

73. Ekbom K, Cole JA. Subcutaneous sumatriptan in the acute treatment of cluster headache attacks. Can J Neurol Sci 1993; 20: 30.

74. Goadsby PJ. Cluster headache and the clinical profile of sumatriptan. Eur Neurol 1994; 34: S35–9.

75. Ekbom K, Monstad I, Prusinski A et al. Subcutaneous sumatriptan in the acute treatment of cluster headache: a dose comparison study. The Sumatriptan Cluster Headache Study Group. Acta Neurol Scand 1993; 88: 63–9.

76. Ekbom K, Waldenlind E, Cole JA et al. Sumatriptan in chronic cluster headache: results of continuous treatment for eleven months. Cephalalgia 1992; 12: 254–6.

77. Matharu MS, Goadsby PJ. Persistence of attacks of cluster headache after trigeminal nerve root section. Brain 2002: in press.

78. Hardebo JE, Dahlof C. Sumatriptan nasal spray (20 mg/dose) in the acute treatment of cluster headache. Cephalalgia 1998; 18: 487–9.

79. Hofer SS, Kinze S, Einhaupl KM, Arnold G. Treatment of acute cluster headache with 20 mg sumatriptan nasal spray: an open pilot study. Cephalalgia 2000; 20: 330.

80. van Vliet JA, Bahra A, Martin V et al. Intranasal sumatriptan is effective in the treatment of acute cluster headache: a double-blind, placebo-controlled, crossover study. Cephalalgia 2001; 21: 270–1.

81. Monstad I, Krabbe A, Micieli G. Preemptive oral treatment with sumatriptan during a cluster period.

Headache 1995; 35: 607–13.

82. Bates D, Ashford E, Dawson R et al. Subcutaneous sumatriptan during the migraine aura. Neurology 1994; 44: 1587–92.

83. Goadsby PJ. The effect of migraine aura during an attack on treatment outcome: results from the sumatriptan naratriptan aggregated patient (SNAP). SNAP Database Study Group. Cephalalgia 2001; 21: 416.

84. Bahra A, Gawel MJ, Hardebo JE et al. Oral zolmitriptan is effective in the acute treatment of cluster headache. Neurology 2000; 54: 1832–9.

85. Dowson AJ, Hansen SB, Farkkila AM. Zolmitriptan nasal spray is fast acting and highly effective in the acute treatment of migraine. Neurology 2000; 7: 82.

86. Sorensen J, Bergstrom M, Antoni A et al. Distribution of 11C-zolmitriptan nasal spray assessed by positron emission tomography (PET). Eur J Neurology 2000; 7: 82

87. Horton BT. Histaminic cephalalgia. Lancet 1952; 2: 92–8.

88. Andersson PG, Jespersen LT. Dihydroergotamine nasal spray in the treatment of attacks of cluster headache. Cephalalgia 1986; 6: 51–4.

89. Barre F. Cocaine as an abortive agent in cluster headache. Headache 1982; 22: 69–73.

90. Costa A, Pucci E, Antonaci F et al. The effect of intranasal cocaine and lidocaine on nitroglycerin induced attacks in cluster headache. Cephalalgia 2000; 20: 85–91.

91. Robbins L. Intranasal lidocaine for cluster headache. Headache 1995; 35: 83–4.

92. Kitrelle JP, Grouse DS, Seybold ME. Cluster headache: local anesthetic abortive agents. Arch Neurol 1985; 42: 496–8.

93. Anthony M. The role of the occipital nerve in unilateral headache. In: Rose FC, ed. Current Problems in Neurology: Four Advances in Headache Research. London: John Libbey, 1987, 257–62.

94. Otsuka F, Kageyama J, Ogura T, Makino H. Cluster headache dependent upon octreotide injection. Headache 2001; 41: 629.

95. Sicuteri F, Geppetti P, Marabini S, Lembeck F. Pain relief by somatostatin in attacks of cluster headache. Pain 1984; 18: 359–65.

96. Bereiter DA. Morphine and somatostatin analogue reduce c-Fos expression in trigeminal subnucleus caudalis produced by corneal stimulation in the rat. Neurosci 1997; 77: 863–74.

97. Misolni N, Mario R, Bronstein M. Headache in acromegaly; dramatic improvement with somatostatin

analogue SMS 209–995. Clin J Pain 1990; 6: 243–5.

98. Williams G, Ball J, Bloom S, Joplin GF. Improvement in headache associated with prolactinoma during treatment with somatostatin analogue: an 'N of 1' study. N Eng J Med 1986; 315: 1166–7.

99. de Carolis P, De Capoa D, Agati R et al. Episodic cluster headache: short and long-term results of prophylactic treatment. Headache 1988; 28: 475–6.

100. Mathew NT. Cluster headache. Neurology 1992; 42: 32–6.

101. Caviness VS, O'Brien P. Cluster headache: response to chlorpromazine. Headache 1980; 20: 128–31.

102. Hering R, Kuritzky A. Sodium valproate in the treatment of cluster headache: an open clinical trail. Cephalalgia 1989; 9: 195–8.

103. Leandri M, Luzzani M, Cruccu G, Gottlieb A. Drug-resistant cluster headache responding to gabapentin: a pilot study. Cephalalgia 2001; 21: 744–6.

104. Ahmed F. Chronic cluster headache responding to gabapentin: a case report. Cephalalgia 2000; 20: 252–3.

105. Wheeler S, Carrazana EJ. Topiramate-treated cluster headache. Neurology 1999; 53: 234–6.

106. Diamond S, Mogabgab ER, Diamond M. Cluster headache variant: spectrum of a new headache syndrome responsive to indomethacin. In: Rose FC, ed. Advances in Migraine Research and Therapy. New York: Raven Press, 1982, 57–65.

107. Gearney DP. Indomethacin-responsive episodic cluster headache. J Neurol Neurosurg Psychiatry 1983; 46: 860–1.

108. Jammes JL. The treatment of cluster headaches with prednisone. Dis Nerv Sys 1975; 36: 375–6.

109. Mirzai R, Chang C, Greenspan A, Gershwin ME. The pathogenesis of osteonecrosis and the relationships to corticosteroids. J Asthma 1999; 36: 77–95.

110. Fischer DE, Bickel WH. Corticosteroid-induced avascular necrosis. J Bone Joint Surg 1971; 53A: 859–64.

111. Good AE. Bilateral aseptic necrosis of the femur following a sixteen day course of corticotropin. J Am Med Assoc 1974; 228: 497–9.

112. Anderton JM, Helm R. Multiple joint osteonecrosis following short-term steroid therapy. J Bone Joint Surg 1982; 64A: 139–42.

113. Tfelt-Hansen P, Saxena PR, Dahlof C et al. Ergotamine in the acute treatment of migraine: a review and European consensus. Brain 2000; 123: 9–18.

114. Symonds C. Migrainous variants. Trans Med Soc London 1952; 67: 237–50.

115. Curran DA, Hinterberger H, Lance JW. Methysergide: research clinical studies. Headache 1967; 1: 74–122.

116. Graham JR. Methysergide for the prevention of headache. N Eng J Med 1964; 270: 132–9.

117. Lance JW, Fine RD, Curran DA. An evaluation of methysergide in the prevention of migraine and other vascular headaches. Med J Aust 1963; 1: 814–18.

118. Graham JR, Suby HI, LeCompte PR, Sadowsky NL. Fibrotic disorders associated with methysergide therapy for headache. N Engl J Med 1966; 274: 360–8.

119. Stea A, Soong TW, Snutch TP. Voltage gated calcium channels. In: North RA, ed. Handbook of Receptors and Channels. Ligand and voltage gated ion channels. Boca Ratan, FL: CRC Press, 1995: 113–53.

120. Geer JJ, Dooley DJ, Adams ME. K(+)-stimulated 45Ca2+ flux into rat neocortical minislices is blocked by omega-Aga-IVa and the dual Na+/Ca2+ channel blockers lidoflazine and flunarizine. Neurosci Let 1993; 158: 97–100.

121. Ophoff RA, Terwindt GM, Vergouwe MN. Familial hemiplegic migraine and episodic ataxia type-2 are caused by mutations in the Ca2+ channel gene CACNLA4. Cell 1996; 87: 543–52.

122. de Carolis P, Baldrati A, Agati R. Nimodipine in episodic cluster headache: results and methodological considerations. Headache 1987; 27: 397–9.

123. Meyer JS, Hardenberg J. Clinical effectiveness of calcium entry blockers in prophylactic treatment of migraine and cluster headaches. Headache 1983; 23: 266–77.

124. Gabai IJ, Spierings ELH. Prophylactic treatment of cluster headache with verapamil. Headache 1989; 29: 167–8.

125. Bussone G, Leone M, Peccarisi C. Double blind comparison of lithium and verapamil in cluster headache prophylaxis. Headache 1990; 30: 411–17.

126. Singh BN, Nademanee K. Use of calcium antagonists for cardiac arrhythmias. Am J Cardiol 1987; 59: 153B-162B.

127. Naylor WG. Calcium Antagonists. London: Academic Press, 1988.

128. Solomon SD, Lipton RB, Newman LC. Prophylactic therapy of cluster headaches. Clin Neuropharmacol 1991; 14: 116–30.

129. Mathew NT. Clinical subtypes of cluster headache and response to lithium therapy. Headache 1978; 18: 26–30.

130. Ekbom K. Lithium for cluster headache: review of literature and preliminary results of long term treatment. Headache 1981; 21: 132–9.

131. Lainez MJ, Pascual J, Santonta JM et al. Topiramate in the prophylactic treatment of cluster headache. Cephalalgia 2001; 21: 500 (Abstract).

132. Sicuteri F, Franchi G, Del Bianco PL. An antaminic drug, BC 105, in the prophylaxis of migraine. Int Arch Allergy 1967; 31: 78–93.

133. Speight TM, Avery GS. Pizotifen (BC-105): a review of its pharmacological properties and its therapeutic efficacy in vascular headaches. Am J Med Sci 1972; 240: 327–31.

134. Ekbom K. Prophylactic treatment of cluster headache with a new serotonin agonist, BC 105. Acta Neurol Scand 1969; 45: 601–10.

135. Marks DR, Rapoport A, Padla D. A double-blind placebo-controlled trial of intranasal capsaicin for cluster headache. Cephalalgia 1993; 13: 114–16.

136. Leone M, Bussone G. Melatonin in cluster headache: rationale for use and possible therapeutic potential. CNS Drugs 1998; 9: 7–16.

137. Leone M, D'Amico D, Moschiano F et al. Melatonin versus placebo in the prophylaxis of cluster headache: a double-blind pilot study with parallel groups. Cephalalgia 1996; 16: 494–6.

138. Mather P, Silberstein SD, Schulman E. The treatment of cluster headache with repetitive intravenous dihydroergotamine. Headache 1991; 31: 525–32.

139. Diamond S, Freitag FG, Prager J. Treatment of intractable cluster. Headache 1986; 42–6.

140. Meyer JS, Binns PM, Ericsson AD. Sphenopalatine ganglionectomy for cluster headache. Arch Otolaryngol 1970; 92: 475–84.

141. Mathew NT, Hurt W. Percutaneous radiofrequency trigeminal gangliorhizolysis in intractable cluster headache. Headache 1988; 28: 328–31.

142. Onofrio BM. Radiofrequency percutaneous Gasserian ganglion lesions. Results in 140 patients with trigeminal pain. J Neurosurg 1975; 42: 132–9.

143. Pieper DR, Dickerson J, Hassenbusch SJ. Percutaneous retrogasserian glycerol rhizolysis for treatment of chronic intractable cluster headaches: long-term results. Neurosurg 2000; 46: 363–8.

144. Hassenbush SJ, Kunkel RS, Kosmorsky GS. Trigeminal cisternal injection of glycerol for treatment of chronic intractable cluster headaches. Neurosurgery 1991; 29: 504–8.

145. Ford RG, Ford KT, Swaid S et al. Gamma knife treatment of refractory cluster headache. Headache 1998; 38: 1–9.

146. Bing R. Uber traumatische erythromelalgie und erthroprosopalgie. Nervenarzt 1930; 3: 506–12.

147. Romberg MH. Lehrbuch der nervenkrankheiten des menschen. Berlin: Dunker, 1840.

148. Harris W. Ciliary (migrainous) neuralgia and its treatment. Br Med J 1936; 1: 457–60.

149. Sluder G. The syndrome of sphenopalatine ganglion neurosis. Am J Med 1910; 140: 868–78.

150. Vail HH. Vidian neuralgia. Ann Otol Rhinol Laryngol 1932; 41: 837–56.

151. Eulenburg A. Lehrbuch der nervenkrankheiten. Berlin: Hirschwald, 1878.

152. Cremer P, Halmagyi GM, Goadsby PJ. Secondary cluster headache responsive to sumatriptan. J Neurol Neurosurg Psychiatry 1995; 59: 633–4.

153. West P, Todman D. Chronic cluster headache associated with vertebral artery aneurysm. Headache 1991; 31: 210–12.

154. Greve E, Mai J. Cluster headache like headaches: a symptomatic feature? Cephalalgia 1988; 8: 79–82.

155. Mani S, Deeter J. Arteriovenous malformation of the brain presenting as a cluster headache – a case report. Headache 1982; 22: 184–5.

156. Muoz C, Tejedor ED, Frank A, Barreiro P. Cluster headache syndrome associated with middle cerebral artery arteriovenous malformation. Cephalalgia 1996; 16: 202–5.

157. Kuritzky A. Cluster headache-like pain caused by an upper cervical meningioma. Cephalalgia 1984; 4: 185–6.

158. de la Sayette V, Schaeffer S, Coskun O et al. Cluster headache-like attack as an opening symptom of a unilateral infarction of the cervical cord: persistent anaesthesia and dysaesthesia to cold stimuli. J Neurol Neurosurg Psychiatry 1999; 66: 397–400.

159. Cid C, Berciano J, Pascual J. Retroocular headache with autonomic features resembling 'continuous' cluster headache in a lateral medullary infarction. J Neurol Neurosurg Psychiatry 2000; 69: 134–41.

160. Tfelt-Hansen P, Paulson OB, Krabbe AE. Invasive adenoma of the pituitary gland and chronic migrainous neuralgia. A rare coincidence or a causal relationship? Cephalalgia 1982; 2: 25–8.

161. Hannerz J. A case of parasellar meningioma mimicking cluster headache. Cephalalgia 1989; 9: 265–9.

162. Lance JW. Mechanism and Management of Headache. London: Butterworth Scientific, 1993.

163. Heidegger S, Mattfeldt T, Rieber A et al. Orbitosphenoidal aspergillus infection mimicking cluster headache: a case report. Cephalalgia 1997; 17: 676–9.

164. Hunter CR, Mayfield FH. Role of the upper cervical roots in the production of pain in the head. Am J Surg 1949; 78: 743–9.

chapter 10

Trigeminal autonomic cephalgias II-(paroxysmal hemicrania and SUNCT) and other short-lasting headache (hypnic headache)

Trigeminal autonomic cephalgias (TACs) consist of a group of headache syndromes marked by head pain in the distribution of the trigeminal nerve with cranial autonomic activation.[1] The most common TAC, cluster headache, is covered in Chapter 9. The present chapter concerns two other TACs: paroxysmal hemicrania and short-lasting unilateral neuralgiform headache attacks with conjunctival injection and tearing (SUNCT). Hemicrania continua, which may be classified with the TACs in the revision of the International Headache Society (IHS) Classification, is dealt with under the primary chronic daily headaches (see Chapter 8). For simplicity, this chapter will also cover hypnic headache, although autonomic activation is not a feature of this disorder, the brevity of attacks makes it part of the differential diagnosis (Table 10.1). Structural disease may give rise to short-lived headaches that are sometimes triggered by a Valsalva maneuver or a postural change. Mass lesions, including those that interfere with cerebrospinal fluid egress, and pathology in the posterior fossa or base of the skull are particularly associated with short-lived Valsalva or cough-related headache.[2] Even subarachnoid hemorrhage can give rise to brief headache. The secondary headaches are dealt with in Part III, and we have therefore placed the other primary headaches (cough, exertional and sexual headache) in that section to compare and contrast them with their important secondary differential diagnoses.

Paroxysmal hemicrania

Sjaastad et al[3] first reported eight cases (seven of whom were female) of a frequent, unilateral, severe but short-lasting headache without remission, for which he coined the term chronic paroxysmal hemicrania (CPH). The mean daily frequency of attacks varied from seven to 22, with the pain persisting from 5 to 45 minutes on each occasion. The site and associated autonomic phenomena were similar to cluster headache, but the attacks of CPH were suppressed completely by indomethacin. A subsequent review of 84 cases showed a history of remission in 35 cases, whereas 49 were chronic.[4] For symmetry with the cluster headache nomenclature, we support the use of the terms episodic paroxysmal hemicrania, as coined by Kudrow et al,[5] for the remitting form, and chronic paroxysmal hemicrania for the unremitting form. We refer to the group as paroxysmal hemicrania (PH).

PH usually begins in adulthood,[6] with a mean age of 34 years and a range of 6–81 years.[4] Females tend more usually to be affected than males in a ratio of 3 : 1. The disorder has no apparent racial boundaries.[7] The pain is usually in the distribution of the ophthalmic division of the trigeminal nerve, but it has also been reported in the occipital region. The syndrome is almost invariably unilateral, but one patient who responded to indomethacin had bilateral pain.[8] The pain is excruciating and may be throbbing as it builds up, although it is usually stabbing or boring. In contrast to patients with cluster headache, patients with CPH usually sit quietly and hold their heads or take to bed, behavior that is rare in cluster headache.[9] Patients may have soreness or tenderness in the interval between attacks, especially if the attacks are frequent. This is not a special feature of PH, but a generic feature of severe, frequent headache, and may be expected with the significant nociceptive load being placed on the trigeminal pain system. This feature can make the differential diagnosis with hemicrania continua rather difficult (Chapter 8). To make a diagnosis when the situation is unclear, we ask patients to keep a detailed pain diary and balance the prominence of the exacerbations and their associated features. The 2–45 minute duration[10] is shorter than the typical 30–180 minute duration for cluster headache,[11] and the overlap can create diagnostic problems. The associated autonomic symptoms are almost completely accounted for by cranial parasympathetic activation (as in cluster headache),[12] except for the ptosis, which is likely to be a partial Horner's syndrome due to a functional sympathetic deficit.[13] Parasympathetic activation may cause edema of the wall of the internal carotid artery and subsequent compression of the cervical sympathetic nerves as they pass through the base of the skull. Attacks may be precipitated by mechanical stimulation, particularly head movement, in some patients.[14–16] Rarely, PH may be

● **Table 10.1** *Primary Headache- cluster headache, other TACs and short-lasting headaches*

Trigeminal autonomic cephalgias (TACs)	Other short-lasting headaches
• Cluster headache • Paroxysmal hemicrania • SUNCT† syndrome • Hemicrania continua*	• Primary stabbing headache‡ • Trigeminal neuralgia • Benign cough headache • Benign exertional headache • Benign sex headache • Hypnic headache

†Shortlasting unilateral neuralgiform headache attacks with conjunctival injection and tearing
‡Currently known as idiopathic stabbing headache but due for change in the second edition of the International Headache Society Classification
*Discussed with chronic daily headache in this text

accompanied by a typical migrainous aura,[17] as has been noted for cluster headache.[9,18]

Children with PH have been reported,[19–21] although at least one case has been considered to be cluster headache.[22] We have seen a 4-year-old girl with an otherwise typical indomethacin-sensitive headache whom we have followed for 3 years, and a 6-year-old boy, again with a typical history and treatment response. Indomethacin continued to be effective in both, and with time the dose has been lowered.

The essential features of PH (Table 10.2) are:

• female preponderance;
• unilateral, usually fronto–temporal, very severe pain;
• short-lasting attacks (2–45 minutes);
• very frequent attacks (usually more than five a day);
• marked cranial autonomic features ipsilateral to the pain;
• robust, quick (less than 72 hours), excellent response to indomethacin.

Pareja[23] has reported patients with unilateral paroxysmal hemicrania which swap sides from attack to attack. Attacks of autonomic features without pain are also reported.[23,24] This has been observed in cluster headache after trigeminal nerve section,[25] and is excellent evidence that these are primarily central nervous system (CNS) disorders. Some recent cases have broadened our understanding of PH. Boes et al[26] reported otalgia and an interesting sensation of fullness of the external auditory meatus responding to indomethacin, and there has been some interesting speculation from Dodick about extra-trigeminal pain in episodic PH.[27] A typical case responding to acetazolamide has been reported.[28] We doubt that the full clinical dimensions of PH have been defined.

Pathophysiology and investigations

The pathophysiology of PH is unknown. The comparative rarity of the syndrome and the short-lasting nature of the individual attacks make PH a difficult disorder to study. The available observations suggest many similarities to cluster headache.

Blood and neuropeptide changes

Alterations in cylic release of catecholamines and β-endorphin occur in CPH[29] and are similar to those reported in

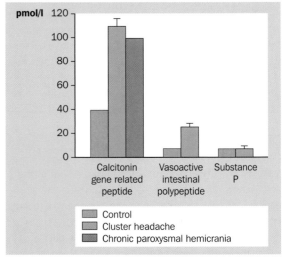

● **Figure 10.1** *This figure demonstrates the changes in calcitonin gene-related peptide (CGRP), vasoactive intestinal polypeptide (VIP) and substance P cluster headache and chronic paroxysmal hemicrania (CPH). The level of elevation of CGRP and VIP in the CPH patient is comparable with that seen in cluster headache patients.[30]*

● **Table 10.2** *Proposed Revised International Headache Society Diagnostic Criteria for paroxysmal hemicrania*

3.1 Diagnostic criteria:
    A. At least 20 attacks fulfilling B–E.
    B. Attacks of severe, unilateral, orbital, supraorbital, or temporal pain lasting 2–30 minutes.
    C. Attack frequency above five a day for more than half of the time, although periods with lower frequency may occur.
    D. Pain is associated with at least one of the following signs/symptoms on the pain side:
        1. Conjunctival injection
        2. Lacrimation
        3. Nasal congestion
        4. Rhinorrhea
        5. Ptosis
        6. Eyelid edema
    E. Headache is stopped completely by indomethacin.
    F. Not attributable to another disorder.
3.2.1 *Episodic paroxysmal hemicrania*
    Description: Occurs in periods lasting 7 days to 1 year separated by pain-free periods lasting 1 month or more.
    Diagnostic criteria:
    A. All alphabetical headings of 3.1.
    B. At least two periods of headaches lasting (untreated patients) from 7 days to 1 year and separated by remissions of at least 1 month.
3.2.2 *Chronic paroxysmal hemicrania*
    Description: Attacks occur for more than 1 year without remission or with remissions lasting less than 1 month.
    Diagnostic criteria:
    A. All alphabetical headings of 3.1.
    B. Absence of remission phases for 1 year or more or with remissions lasting less than 1 month.

cluster headache. An increased level of calcitonin gene-related peptide (CGRP) and vasoactive intestinal polypeptide (VIP) in the cranial venous blood of a patient with CPH has been reported (Figure 10.1). The levels returned to normal after successful treatment with indomethacin.[30] These data are discussed below. Other observations in CPH include relative thrombocythemia[31] and increased phosphatidylserine labelling in neutrophils.[32] The relevance of these changes is not clear. Blood dyscrasias would not be a widespread experience of physicians treating primary headache syndromes, and the neutrophil studies seem of doubtful significance.

Electrophysiologic and autonomic studies

Patients with CPH are reported to have reduced pain thresholds, reduced corneal reflex thresholds, and normal blink reflexes.[33] Autonomic function studies, including salivation and nasal secretion, are normal.[34] Facial sweating is normal in CPH[35] in contrast to cluster headache.[36] The pupil ipsilateral to the pain (measured by pupillometry) is consistently smaller than its unaffected counterpart,[37] most likely reflecting a partial Horner's syndrome. Similar findings were observed in studies of patients with cluster headache.[38] Bradycardia has been observed in CPH, and one of five patients studied developed a bundle branch block and atrial

fibrillation during attacks.[39] Whether the bradycardia is a response to the severe pain or is part of an underlying autonomic problem requires further study. Event-related potentials, which have been reported to be abnormal in migraine,[40] are normal in PH,[41] as is cognitive processing.[42]

Blood flow studies

Facial thermographic studies have shown cold spots over either the supraorbital margin or the inner canthus interictally,[43] or increased temperature over the affected area during the headache.[13] Mongini et al's thermographic results[43] were identical for patients with CPH and cluster headache. Cerebral blood flow studies of carbon dioxide reactivity, as measured by transcranial Doppler, were abnormal in three patients,[44] while a single patient had increased ocular blood flow during attacks.[45] The limited numbers of patients makes a judgment about their significance difficult. The modest changes that are seen are in line with what is reported in regional or transcranial Doppler studies in cluster headache, wherein the numbers of patients studied have been more convincing.[46] The ocular blood flow changes observed in patients with CPH are similar to those in cluster headache patients although, in comparison with normals, cluster headache patients had relatively reduced flow between attacks.[45]

Imaging

Magnetic resonance imaging (MRI) studies of patients with CPH have been normal,[47] but segmental narrowing of ophthalmic veins on orbital phlebography has been reported.[47] These changes are similar to those seen in patients with cluster headache[48,49] and Tolosa–Hunt syndrome (see Chapter 6).[50–53] The findings on orbital phlebography are neither specific nor likely to be pathophysiologically relevant. The test has no practical place in patient management.

There are, therefore, no specific diagnostic investigations in PH. The only clear conclusion from the pathophysiological and imaging studies is that attacks are associated with parasympathetic activation most likely mediated through the greater superficial petrosal outflow with an associated mild partial Horner's syndrome. There is little to suggest a fundamental neurobiological separation between PH and cluster headache with regard to the final common pathways activated. The shorter attack duration, greater attack frequency, and different effect of indomethacin perhaps point to differences in the generation and thus to CNS mechanisms for these disorders.

Differential diagnosis

The differential diagnosis of PH includes the other primary short-lasting headaches (Table 10.1) and the secondary causes of PH (Table 10.3).[54–69] Because secondary PH, as a proportion of all PH, has been relatively frequently reported, probably as a form of publication bias, the clinician is committed to investigate to identify or exclude treatable underlying causes. In addition, the list of associations is likely to be spuriously long with coincidences being reported. Resolving this issue will require a better understanding of the disease pathophysiology. A reasonably complete screen of a patient with PH, considering the associated clinical problems reported, would include a blood count, looking for thrombocythemia,[55] an erythrocyte sedimentation rate (ESR), vasculitic investigations,[55] and a brain imaging procedure, looking for an intracranial tumor such as a lesion in the region of the sella turcica[54,70] or elsewhere.[55] Other structural mimics of PH include an arteriovenous malformation,[56] cavernous sinus meningioma[57] or parotid epidermoid.[58] Secondary PH is more likely if the patient requires high doses (>200 mg/day) of indomethacin,[57] although we have seen patients requiring high doses initially to induce a remission, and then being maintained on lower doses. Should the pain become bilateral, a lumbar puncture should be carried out to look for intracranial hypertension, even though there has been a response to indomethacin.[59] The latter may occur because indomethacin, among its actions, will lower intracranial pressure.[71,72] If bundle branch block or atrial fibrillation is suspected, an electrocardiogram and Holter monitor should be performed.[39] A chest X-ray should be considered to look for a Pancoast tumor.[73]

It is worth noting in the differential diagnosis of PH that it may coexist with trigeminal neuralgia and that PH-tic syndrome has been reported.[60–64] Both episodic PH and CPH can coexist with trigeminal neuralgia,[65] and we favor the term PH-tic syndrome to cover both.[74] The clinical utility of being aware of this syndrome, whether there is an important biological association or not, is that both components require individual treatment, such as with the combination of indomethacin and carbamazepine. Another unexplored clinical coexistence is a report of PH with cough headache;[75] fortunately indomethacin is a treatment strategy for both problems.

Treatment

The standard initial treatment of PH is indomethacin 25 mg three times daily. We recommend increasing to 50 mg three times daily if the patient has no response after 1 week, and to wait a further 2 weeks before pushing to 75 mg three times daily for 3 weeks. Patients with no response to 225 mg of indomethacin daily are unlikely to respond. Occasionally patients with a partial response require higher doses or modification of timing to improve relief. Slow-release indomethacin preparations at night help prevent nocturnal breakthrough headaches. One way of foreshortening the oral indomethacin trial is to conduct an indomethacin test by injection, either open-label[76] or placebo-controlled (Matharu and Goadsby, unpublished data). In the medium- to long-term, some patients with gastrointestinal side-effects require treatment with gastroprotective agents, such as H_2-blockers or proton pump

---

● **Table 10.3** Secondary paroxysmal hemicrania and the clinical associations

- Gangliocytoma of the sella turcica[54]
- Collagen vascular disease[55]
- Frontal lobe tumor[55]
- Cerebrovascular disease[56]
- Cavernous sinus meningioma[57]
- Parotid epidermoid[58]
- Raised intracranial pressure[59]
- Coexistent primary headache
  - PH-tic syndrome[60–65]
  - Cluster headache[66–68]
  - Migraine[68,69]

inhibitors. There seems to be no tachyphylaxis to the effects of indomethacin.[77] The IHS criteria require a response to indomethacin to make the diagnosis.[11] Although this is unattractive in many ways, in the absence of a biological marker it is at least pragmatic. PH responds to other drugs, although less effectively. These include other nonsteroidal antiinflammatory drugs (NSAIDs), such as naproxen[78] and calcium-channel blockers, especially verapamil[79-81] (perhaps analogous to their use in cluster headache). One patient with an otherwise convincing clinical picture of PH failed to respond to indomethacin 300 mg, but did respond to acetazolamide 250 mg three times daily.[28] Sumatriptan has been reported to benefit a patient with bilateral CPH[60] and a unilateral case,[82] although it was ineffective in other cases[83,84] In our experience, in contrast to its striking effects in cluster headache,[85] sumatriptan is not reliably effective for PH. The lack of a response may be owing to the very short duration of the headache, or indeed, when it is effective the short attack may be reported as a positive response. Both the sumatriptan response and a controlled or at least systematic use of oxygen would be welcome in PH to determine the real effects in comparison to those seen with the treatment of cluster headache. Similarly, the issue of whether verapamil is helpful in PH requires a careful study. There is a report of the COX-II inhibitor celecoxib being useful in PH,[86] we have found this a somewhat variable effect.

Case study

A 35-year-old woman presented with an 8-year history of bouts of headache. She described stabbing, severe, left frontal and retro-orbital pains that would last 1–2 minutes and occur three to five times a day. The attacks were associated with marked watering of the left eye and left-sided ptosis. She had no nasal stuffiness or migrainous features. She would typically move rather than be still during an attack. The attacks came in bouts of 6 months with intervening breaks of 10–12 months. She had used numerous medications, including corticosteroids, methysergide, lithium, propranolol, pizotifen, amitriptyline, and ergotamine, with no benefit. When first seen she was 2 months into a bout. She was started on indomethacin 25 mg three times daily, and her headaches ceased completely after 3 days. The drug was stopped 2 weeks later, and the attacks recurred within 2 days. Indomethacin was restarted and the attacks again settled rapidly.

Short-lasting unilateral neuralgiform headache attacks with conjunctival injection and tearing (SUNCT)

This form of short-lasting headache is also among the rarest of headache syndromes and again has remarkable autonomic associations.[87] Several clinical features differentiate SUNCT from other short-lasting headaches (Table 10.4). A case seen by one of the authors will illustrate the clinical picture.

Case study

A 56-year-old woman presented with a 5-year history of daily, episodic, short-lasting headaches. Attacks occurred up to five times a day and lasted 15–20 seconds each. The attacks, which were left-sided, moderately severe, and retro-orbital, were associated with marked tearing and redness of the ipsilateral eye and mild rhinorrhea. The patient had no nausea, photophobia, or phonophobia. There was no history of migraine or family history of headache. She had no physical signs on examination of the nervous system and she was normotensive. MRI of the brain was normal.

She had used amitriptyline, propranolol, pizotifen, methysergide, lithium, and verapamil without success. The latter lengthened the attacks and made the pain more severe. The patient had had a trial of steroids and used ergots and sumatriptan without success. She also had an unsuccessful trial of indomethacin, valproate, and carbamazepine. She was refractory to treatment when lost to follow-up.

Clinical features

Patients who suffer from SUNCT are usually men,[88] with a male : female ratio of 17:2.[89] The pain occurs in paroxysms that last 5–250 seconds,[90] although longer, duller interictal pains have been reported, and two patients have had attacks that lasted up to 2 hours.[91] Although patients may have as many as 30 episodes an hour, five to six attacks an hour is more usual. The frequency may also vary in bouts. One man, who suffered from as many as 20 attacks a day, reduced to a frequency of once or twice in 1–4 weeks,[92] while another patient had almost continuous attacks for up to 3 hours.[93] Attacks over days in an almost status-like pattern are reported.[94] Intravenous lidocaine is an extremely useful therapeutic option in managing these devastating attacks in clinical practice. A systematic study of attack frequency demonstrated a mean of 28 attacks a

● **Table 10.4** *Proposed International Headache Society (IHS) diagnostic criteria for SUNCT**

Diagnostic criteria

A. At least 20 attacks fulfilling B–E
B. Attacks of unilateral moderately severe orbital, or temporal stabbing, or throbbing pain lasting from 10–120 secs
C. Attack frequency from 3 to 200 per day
D. Pain is associated with conjunctival injection and lacrimation
E. Not attributable to another disorder
Comment: At least one of the following signs or symptoms may be seen on the affected side.
  1. Nasal congestion
  2. Rhinorrhea
  3. Eyelid edema

* Clinical note: The literature clearly suggests that secondary SUNCT is most likely be due to a posterior fossa lesion.

day, with a range of six to 77.[91] The conjunctival injection seen with SUNCT is often the most prominent autonomic feature, although tearing may also be very obvious. Other less prominent autonomic stigmata include rhinorrhea or forehead sweating. The attacks may become bilateral, but the most severe pain remains unilateral. Most cases have some associated precipitating factors, which may be mechanical movements of the neck,[95,96] a feature that is seen often in TACs, including cluster headache (Table 10.1).

Secondary SUNCT and associations

The literature reports a number of patients with secondary SUNCT syndromes, which are invariably lesions involving the posterior fossa. Two reported patients had homolateral cerebellopontine angle arteriovenous malformations diagnosed on MRI,[97,98] while another had a cavernous hemangioma of the brainstem seen only on MRI.[99] We[100] and others[101] have noted structural deformity involving the posterior fossa to present as a SUNCT-like syndrome. A posterior fossa lesion causing otherwise typical SUNCT has also been noted in human immunodeficiency virus/acquired immunodeficiency syndrome (Graff-Radford, personal communication). These cases highlight the need for cranial MRI in the work-up of a suspected case of SUNCT.

SUNCT and trigeminal neuralgia

The connections between posterior structures and the trigeminal system proper are well documented in the laboratory (see Chapter 5) and are readily seen in clinical practice. Just as PH-tic or cluster-tic syndromes have been reported (see above), there has been a discussion in the literature concerning the relationship between SUNCT and trigeminal neuralgia. However, because SUNCT and trigeminal neuralgia are both short-lasting triggerable headaches, reports of the coexistence or transformation

between the two syndromes[102] begs a more interesting question. Based on evolution of the clinical phenotype from trigeminal neuralgia to SUNCT, it has been argued that these conditions can transform one to another, trigeminal neuralgia to SUNCT. Benoliel and Sharav[103] reported six cases of what was classified as trigeminal neuralgia with lacrimation together with 16 without lacrimation. Descriptions of trigeminal neuralgia with lacrimation can be found in the writings of Gowers,[104] Collier[105] and Kinnier-Wilson.[106] Bouhassira et al[107] argued that SUNCT may be a form of *transformed* trigeminal neuralgia based on the shared phenomenology. The carbamazepine response in trigeminal neuralgia is generally very rewarding, and SUNCT patients comment that carbamazepine is helpful, as did case 6 of Benoliel and Sharav.[103] Sjaastad et al[108] have made comments on the distinction between SUNCT and trigeminal neuralgia by reporting the characteristics of first division trigeminal neuralgia and accepting some degree of autonomic activation. Both conditions are relatively short-lasting, having attacks in seconds, and may have few or many attacks a day. However, SUNCT typically has prominent cranial autonomic symptoms,[88] such as tearing and conjunctival injection, which has been proposed to be activation of the trigeminal-autonomic reflex.[46] We have seen lacrimation with experimental head pain from capsaicin injection,[109] and it is recognized with other forms of secondary trigeminal neuropathic pain.[110] There is a considerable experimental animal literature to document that stimulation of trigeminal afferents can result in cranial autonomic outflow (see Chapter 5), the trigeminal autonomic reflex.[46] It thus could be concluded that some degree of cranial parasympathetic activation is a normal physiological response to nociceptive input in the first division of the trigeminal nerve.

If we accept that first division nociceptive input results in cranial parasympathetic activation of some degree, perhaps subclinical, because of the unique physiologic connections with the first division of the trigeminal nerve,[111] then we would expect to see such symptoms in trigeminal neuralgia, or indeed experimental pain, and we do. Indeed these symptoms are sometimes seen in migraine, and can result in appropriate neuropeptide marker release.[112] It could then be suggested that the key feature of trigeminal autonomic syndromes, such as SUNCT, is the degree of cranial autonomic activation, which may relate to central disinhibition of this reflex. Certainly, there are direct hypothalamic–trigeminal connections,[113] and the unifying finding for SUNCT[114] and cluster headache[115] seems to be hypothalamic activation (Figure 10.2). Operationally, this leads to the clinical markers of the degree of cranial parasympathetic activation being excessive for SUNCT in addition to a lack of refractory period after stimulation, and the response to classical treatment with carbamazepine and the finding of an aberrant vascular loop in trigeminal neuralgia. This is not ideal and more data are required to better differentiate these conditions.

Pathophysiology and investigations

Orbital phlebography is reported to be abnormal in patients with SUNCT, with a narrowed superior ophthalmic vein homolateral to the pain.[116] This finding led to the suggestion that SUNCT may be a form of orbital venous vasculitis,[117] although there are similar reports in cluster headache, Tolosa–Hunt syndrome, and PH (see above).

Forehead sweating, which is normal in CPH, is usually increased during bouts of SUNCT.[118] Pupillometry and pharmacological approaches have revealed no abnormalities.[119] Since conjunctival injection occurs during SUNCT, it is not surprising that intraocular pressure and corneal temperatures are elevated during attacks.[120] This most likely reflects marked parasympathetic activation with local vasodilation. Bradycardia in association with attacks of SUNCT[121] may similarly indicate increased parasympathetic outflow. Systolic blood pressure is sometimes elevated,[122] although ventilatory function is normal.[123] The parasympathetic manifestations favor a central pathogenesis for SUNCT as a manifestation of the trigeminovascular reflex,[124] rather than a peripheral vasculitic cause. Transcranial Doppler and single-photon emission computed tomography (SPECT) studies have not demonstrated convincing changes in the vasomotor activity[125] or cerebral blood flow[126] during attacks of pain. One patient who experienced multiple attacks that could be averaged to identify significant areas of brain activation was studied using functional MRI (fMRI). The pattern seen was increased posterior hypothalamic blood flow[114] in a region very similar to that identified in patients with acute cluster headache (Figure 10.2).[115]

Treatment

SUNCT is remarkably refractory to treatment (Table 10.5). Most drugs used in the treatment of other short-lasting

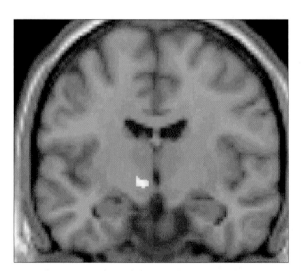
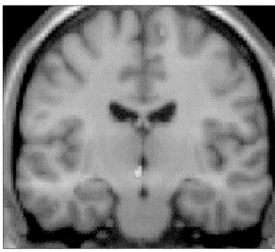

● **Figure 10.2** *Comparison of spontaneous pain attacks and rest – (no pain) conditions in a patient with SUNCT (BOLD-f MRI; left side)[114] and cluster headache (PET; right side).[115] The activations during the attack are shown as statistical parametric maps which show the areas of significant rCBF increases (p < 0.001) in colour superimposed on an anatomical reference derived from a T1-weighted MR image. The left side of the picture is the left side of the brain. Significant activation was detected next to the third ventricle slightly lateralized to the left and rostral to the aqueduct. The activation is ipsilateral to the pain side and lies in the diencephalcn in the posterior hypothalamic gray matter.*

headaches are not useful in SUNCT. Drugs and procedures reported to be either useful or without effect in SUNCT, based on the authors' personal experience and the literature,[127] are recorded in Table 10.5. Two patients with a provisional diagnosis of SUNCT that responded to sumatriptan most likely represent a spontaneous remission and are only described in a limited way.[128] Indomethacin is not useful for SUNCT.

Hypnic headache

Hypnic headache was first described by Raskin.[129] The patients were between 67 and 84 years of age and had headaches of a moderately severe nature that typically came on a few hours after going to sleep. These headaches last from 15 to 30 minutes (Table 10.6). They are typically generalized, although they may be unilateral,[130–134] and can

be throbbing.[135] Patients may report falling back to sleep only to be awakened by a further attack a few hours later, with up to three repetitions of this pattern over the night. In a large and very carefully presented series of Dodick et al's[136] 19 patients, 16 (84%) were female and the mean age at onset was 61 ± 9 years. Headaches were bilateral in two-thirds and unilateral in one-third, while 80% of cases had mild or moderate pain. Three patients reported similar headaches when falling asleep during the day. None had photophobia or phonophobia.[136]

Management

Patients with this form of headache generally respond to a bedtime dose of lithium carbonate (200–600 mg)[129,135] and for those that do not tolerate this, verapamil or methysergide at bedtime may be alternative strategies. Two patients who responded to flunarizine 5 mg at night have been reported.[131] Dodick et al[136] reported that one to two

● **Table 10.5** Treatments of SUNCT

Treatment	Dose (maximum/day)	Response	Number of reported patients
Pharmacological			
Aspirin	1800 mg	–	6
Paracetamol	4 g	–	6
Indomethacin (indometacin)	200 mg	–	3
Naproxen	1 g	–	3
Ibuprofen	1200 mg	–	7
Ergotamine (oral)	3 mg	–	1
Dihydroergotamine (ivi)	3 mg	–	5
Sumatriptan (oral)	300 mg	–*	1
Sumatriptan (sc)	6 mg	–	7
Prednisolone (oral)	100 mg	–	4
Methysergide	8 mg	–	5
Verapamil	480 mg	**	5
Valproate	1500 mg	–*	3
Lithium	900 mg	–	3
Propranolol	160 mg	–	2
Amitriptyline	100 mg	–	10
Carbamazepine	1200 mg	+	5
Lamotrigine	200 mg	+	3
Topiramate	200 mg	+	5
Procedures or infusions			
Lidocaine (4 mg/min ivi)		+	4
Greater occipital nerve block		–	4

* One patient with slight improvement
** Treatment worsened condition
– treatment had no effect
+ open label treatment helpful

cups of coffee or 60 mg of caffeine orally at bedtime was helpful. We find about one-third of patients respond to nighttime caffeine. We successfully controlled a patient who was poorly tolerant of lithium using verapamil at night (160 mg), and others have reported a case controlled by indomethacin.[137] This is an important observation in the context of TAC.[1] Other strategies are important since lithium may have significant side-effects in the age group affected by hypnic headache.

Differential diagnosis of short-lasting headaches

The differential diagnosis of the short-lasting headaches can be clinically challenging (Table 10.7); however, these can be devastating conditions with very considerable clinical rewards from correct diagnosis and treatment. The TACs (cluster headache, PH, and SUNCT syndrome) present a distinct group to be differentiated from short-

---

● **Table 10.6** *Proposed Diagnostic Criteria for Hypnic Headache*

Description: Attacks of pain that may be unilateral or bilateral and always occur after falling asleep.
Diagnostic criteria:

A. Head pain is preferentially bilateral and awakens patient from sleep.
B. Head pain lasts from 15 up to 180 minutes.
C. Head pain occurs at least 15 times per month at least from 15 up to 180 minutes.
D. None or only one of the following:
   1. Nausea
   2. Photophobia
   3. Phonophobia
E. Not attributable to another disorder.

Comment. The syndrome is usually seen in patients above the age of 60 years. The pain is usually mild to moderate. Duration of the attack longer than 180 minutes was reported in some cases. Intracranial disorders, trigeminal-autonomic cephalgias have to be excluded.

● **Table 10.7** *Differential Diagnosis of Short-Lasting Headaches*

Feature	Cluster headache	Paroxysmal hemicrania	SUNCT†	Idiopathic stabbing headache††	Trigeminal neuralgia	Hypnic headache
Gender (M:F)	4:1	1:3	8:1	F > M	F > M	5:3
Pain						
-type	Boring	Boring	Stabbing	Stabbing	Stabbing	Throbbing
-severity	Very	Very	Severe	Severe	Very	Moderate
-location	Orbital	Orbital	Orbital	Any	V2/V3>V1	Generalized
Duration	15–180 min	2–45 min	15–120 s	<30 s	<1 s	15–30 min
Frequency	1–8/day	1–40/day	1/day–30/hr	any	any	1–3/night
Autonomic	+	+	+	−	-††	−
Trigger	Alcohol nitrates	Alcohol nitrates	Cutaneous	None	Cutaneous	Sleep
Indomethacin	?	+	−	+	−	†

†Short-lasting unilateral neuralgiform headache attacks with conjunctival injection and tearing.
††Cranial autonomic activation may be seen in first division trigeminal neuralgia
‡Currently known as idiopathic stabbing headache but due for change in the second edition of the International Headache Society Classification to primary stabbing headache.

lasting headaches that do not have prominent cranial autonomic syndromes, notably trigeminal neuralgia, idiopathic (primary) stabbing headache, and hypnic headache. By determining the cycling pattern, the length and frequency of attacks, and the timing of the bouts, most patients can be classified. The importance of clinical classification of this group is threefold. First, the clinical phenotype determines the likely secondary causes to consider and the appropriate investigations to order. Secondly, the appropriate classification gives clarity to the patient, with a clear diagnosis, and allows the physician to draw on available literature to comment on natural history. Thirdly, the correct diagnosis determines the therapy. Therapy can be excellent if the diagnosis is correct but useless if it is not. These headaches are an example of headache at its best in clinical practice.

References

1. Goadsby PJ, Lipton RB. A review of paroxysmal hemicranias, SUNCT syndrome and other short-lasting headaches with autonomic features, including new cases. Brain 1997; 120(Part 1): 193–209.
2. Pascual J, Igessias F, Oterino A, Vazquez-Barquero A. Cough, exertional, and sexual headaches: an analysis of 72 benign and symptomatic cases. Neurology 1996; 46: 1520–4.
3. Sjaastad O, Apfelbaum R, Caskey W et al. Chronic paroxysmal hemicrania (CPH). The clinical manifestations. A review. Ups J Med Sci Suppl 1980; 31: 27–33.
4. Antonaci F, Sjaastad O. Chronic paroxysmal hemicrania (CPH): a review of the clinical manifestations. Headache 1989; 29: 648–56.
5. Kudrow L, Esperanca P, Vijayan N. Episodic paroxysmal hemicrania. Cephalalgia 1987; 42: 964–6.
6. Sjaastad O. Chronic paroxysmal hemicrania. In: Vinken PJ, Bruyn GW, Klawans HL, Rose FC, eds. Handbook of Clinical Neurology. Amsterdam: Elsevier Science, 1986: 257–66.
7. Joubert J, Powell D, Djikowski J. Chronic paroxysmal hemicrania in South African Black. A case report. Cephalalgia 1987; 7: 193–6.
8. Pollmann W, Pfaffenrath V. Chronic paroxysmal hemicrania: the first possible bilateral case. Cephalalgia 1986; 6: 55–7.
9. Bahra A, May A, Goadsby PJ. Cluster headache: a prospective clinical study in 230 patients with diagnostic implications. Neurology. 2002; 58; 354–61.
10. Russell D. Chronic paroxysmal hemicrania: severity, duration and time of occurrence of attacks. Cephalalgia 1984; 4: 53–6.
11. Headache Classification Committee of the International Headache Society. Classification and diagnostic criteria for headache disorders, cranial neuralgia, and facial pain. Cephalalgia 1988; 8(Suppl 7): 1–96.
12. Goadsby PJ, Edvinsson L. Human in vivo evidence for trigeminovascular activation in cluster headache. Brain 1994; 117: 427–34.
13. Drummond PD. Tomographic and pupillary asymmetry in chronic paroxysmal hemicrania. A case study. Cephalalgia 1985; 5: 133–6.
14. Sjaastad O, Egge K, Horven I. Chronic paroxysmal hemicrania. V. Mechanical precipitation of attacks. Headache 1979; 19: 31–6.
15. Sjaastad O, Russell D, Saunte C, Horven I. Chronic paroxysmal hemicrania. VI. Precipitation of attacks. Further studies on the precipitation mechanism. Cephalalgia 1982; 2: 211–14.
16. Sjaastad O, Saunte C, Graham JR. Chronic paroxysmal hemicrania. VII. Mechanical precipitation of attacks: new cases and localization of trigger points. Cephalalgia 1984; 4: 113–18.
17. Matharu MJ, Goadsby PJ. Post-traumatic chronic paroxysmal hemicrania (CPH) with aura. Neurology 2001; 56: 273–5.
18. Silberstein SD, Niknam R, Rozen TD, Young WB. Cluster headache with aura. Neurology 2000; 54: 219–20.
19. Kudrow DB, Kudrow L. Successful aspirin prophylaxis in a child with chronic paroxysmal hemicrania. Headache 1989; 29: 280–1.
20. Broeske D, Lenn NJ, Cantos E. Chronic paroxysmal hemicrania in a young child: possible relation to ipsilateral occipital infarction. J Child Neurol 1993; 8: 235–6.
21. Gladstein J, Holden EW, Peralta L. Chronic paroxysmal hemicrania in a child. Headache 1994; 34: 519–20.
22. Solomon S, Newman LC. Chronic paroxysmal hemicrania in a child? Headache 1995; 35: 234.
23. Pareja JA. Chronic paroxysmal hemicrania: dissociation of the pain and autonomic features. Headache 1995; 35: 111–13.
24. Bogucki A, Szymanska R, Braciak W. Chronic paroxysmal hemicrania: lack of pre-chronic stage. Cephalalgia 1984; 4: 187–9.
25. Matharu MS, Goadsby PJ. Persistence of attacks of cluster headache after trigeminal nerve root section. Brain. 2002; 125: 976–84.
26. Boes CJ, Swanson JW, Dodick DW. Chronic paroxysmal hemicrania presenting as otalgia with a sensation of external acoustic meatus obstruction: two cases and a pathophysiologic hypothesis. Headache 1998; 38: 787–91.
27. Dodick DW. Extratrigeminal episodic paroxysmal hemicrania. Further clinical evidence of functionally relevant brain stem connections. Headache 1998; 38: 794–8.
28. Warner JS, Wamil AW, McLean MJ. Acetazolamide for the treatment of chronic paroxysmal hemicrania. Headache 1994; 34: 597–9.
29. Micieli G, Cavallini A, Facchinetti F et al. Chronic paroxysmal hemicrania: a chronobiological study (case report). Cephalalgia 1989; 9: 281–6.
30. Goadsby PJ, Edvinsson L. Neuropeptide changes in a case of chronic paroxysmal hemicrania – evidence for trigeminoparasympathetic activation. Cephalalgia 1996; 16: 448–50.
31. MacMillan JC, Nukada H. Chronic paroxysmal hemicrania. N Z Med J 1989; 102: 251–2.
32. Fragoso YD, Seim S, Stovner LJ et al. Arachidonic acid metabolism in polymorphonuclear cells in headaches. A methodological study. Cephalalgia 1988; 8: 149–55.
33. Antonaci F, Sandrini G, Danilov A, Sand T. Neurophysiological studies in chronic paroxysmal hemicrania and hemicrania continua. Headache 1994; 34: 479–83.
34. Saunte C. Chronic paroxysmal hemicrania: salivation, tearing and nasal secretion. Cephalalgia 1984; 4: 25–32.
35. Antonaci F. The sweating pattern in hemicrania continua. A comparison with chronic paroxysmal hemicrania. Funct Neurology 1991; 6: 371–5.

36. Drummond PD, Lance JW. Pathological sweating and flushing accompanying the trigeminal lacrimation reflex in patients with cluster headache and in patients with a confirmed site of cervical sympathetic deficit. Evidence for parasympathetic cross-innervation. Brain 1992; 115: 1429–45.

37. Soyka D, Taneri Z, Oestreich W, Schmidt R. Flunarizine IV in the acute treatment of common or classical migraine attacks – a placebo-controlled double-blind trial. Headache 1989; 29: 21–7.

38. Drummond PD. Autonomic disturbances in cluster headache. Brain 1988; 111: 1199–209.

39. Russell D, Storstein L. Chronic paroxysmal hemicrania: heart rate changes and ECG rhythm disturbances. A computerized analysis of 24 ambulatory ECG recordings. Cephalalgia 1984; 4: 135–44.

40. Wang W, Schoenen J. Interictal potentiation of passive 'oddball' auditory event-related potentials in migraine. Cephalalgia 1998; 18: 261–5.

41. Evers S, Bauer B, Suhr B et al. Cognitive processing in primary headache: a study of event-related potentials. Neurology 1997; 48: 108–13.

42. Evers S, Bauer B, Suhr B et al. Cognitive processing is involved in cluster headache but not in chronic paroxysmal hemicrania. Neurology 1999; 53: 357–63.

43. Mongini F, Caselli C, Macri V, Tetti C. Thermographic findings in craniofacial pain. Headache 1990; 30: 497–504.

44. Shen JM. Transcranial doppler sonography in chronic paroxysmal hemicrania. Headache 1993; 33: 493–6.

45. Horven I, Russell D, Sjaastad O. Ocular blood flow changes in cluster headache and chronic paroxysmal hemicrania. Headache 1989; 29: 373–6.

46. May A, Goadsby PJ. The trigeminovascular system in humans: pathophysiological implications for primary headache syndromes of the neural influences on the cerebral circulation. J Cereb Blood Flow Metabol 1999; 19: 115–27.

47. Antonaci F. Chronic paroxysmal hemicrania and hemicrania continua: orbital phlebography and MRI studies. Headache 1994; 34: 32–4.

48. Hannerz J, Ericson R, Bergstroud G. Orbital phlebography in patients with cluster headache. Cephalalgia 1987; 7: 207–11.

49. Hannerz J. Orbital phlebography and signs of inflammation in episodic and chronic cluster headache. Headache

50. Hannerz J. Pathoanatomic studies in a case of Tolosa–Hunt syndrome. Cephalalgia 1988; 8: 25–30.

51. Hoes MJAM, Bruyn GW, Vievoye GJ. The Tolosa–Hunt syndrome – literature review: seven new cases and hypothesis. Cephalalgia 1981; 1: 181–94.

52. Tolosa E. Periarteritic lesions of the carotid siphon with the clinical features of a carotid infraclinoidal aneurysm. J Neurol Neurosurg Psychiatry 1954; 17: 300–2.

53. Hunt WE, Meagher JN, LeFever HE, Zeman W. Painful ophthalmoplegia. Its relation to indolent inflammation of the cavernous sinus. Neurology 1961; 11: 56–62.

54. Vijayan N. Symptomatic chronic paroxysmal hemicrania. Cephalalgia 1992; 12: 111–13.

55. Medina JL. Organic headaches mimicking chronic paroxysmal hemicrania. Headache 1992; 32: 73–4.

56. Newman LC, Herskoviz S, Lipton R, Solomon S. Chronic paroxysmal headache: two cases with cerebrovascular disease. Headache 1992; 32: 75–6.

57. Sjaastad O, Stovner LJ, Stolt-Nielsen A et al. CPH and hemicrania continua: requirements of high dose indomethacin dosages – an ominous sign? Headache 1995; 35: 363–7.

58. Mariano HS, Bigal ME, Bordini CA, Speciali JG. Chronic paroxysmal hemicrania (CPH)-like syndrome as a first manifestation of cerebral metastasis of parotid epidermoid carcinoma: a case report. Cephalalgia 1999; 19: 442–2.

59. Hannerz J, Jogestrand T. Intracranial hypertension and sumatriptan efficacy in case of chronic paroxysmal hemicrania with became bilateral. (The mechanism of indomethacin in CPH). Headache 1993; 33: 320–3.

60. Hannerz J. Trigeminal neuralgia with chronic paroxysmal hemicrania: the CPH-tic syndrome. Cephalalgia 1993; 13: 361–4.

61. Caminero AB, Pareja JA, Dobato JL. Chronic paroxysmal hemicrania-tic syndrome. Cephalalgia 1998; 18: 159–61.

62. Hannerz J. The second case of chronic paroxysmal hemicrania-tic syndrome. Cephalalgia 1998; 18: 124.

63. Martinez-Salio A, Porta-Etessam J, Perez-Martinez D et al. Case reports: chronic paroxysmal hemicrania-tic syndrome. Headache 2000; 40: 682–5.

64. Zukerman E, Peres MF, Kaup AO et al. Chronic paroxysmal hemicrania-tic

syndrome. Neurology 2000; 54: 1524–6.

65. Boes CJ, Matharu MS, Goadsby PJ. The paroxysmal hemicrania-tic syndrome. Cephalalgia. 2002; (In Press)

66. Tehindrazanarivelo AD, Visy JM, Bousser MG. Ipsilateral cluster headache and chronic paroxysmal hemicrania: two case reports. Cephalalgia 1992; 12: 318–20.

67. Centonze V, Bassi A, Causarano V et al. Simultaneous occurrence of ipsilateral cluster headache and chronic paroxysmal hemicrania: a case report. Headache 2000; 40: 54–6.

68. Pearce SH, Cox JG, Pearce JM. Chronic paroxysmal hemicrania, episodic cluster headache and classic migraine in one patient. J Neurol Neurosurg Psychiatry 1987; 50: 1699–700.

69. Pareja J. Chronic paroxysmal hemicrania coexisting with migraine. Differential response to pharmacological treatment. Headache 1992; 32: 77–8.

70. Gawel MJ, Rothbart P. Chronic paroxysmal hemicrania which appears to arise from either third ventricle pathology or internal carotid artery pathology. Cephalalgia 1992; 12: 327.

71. Harrigan MR, Tuteja S, Neudeck BL. Indomethacin in the management of elevated intracranial pressure: a review. J Neurotrauma 1997; 14: 637–50.

72. Forderreuther S, Straube A. Indomethacin reduces CSF pressure in intracranial hypertension. Neurology 2000; 55: 1043–5.

73. Delreux V, Kevers L, Callewaert A. Hemicranie paroxystique inaugurant un syndrome de pancoast. Rev Neurol 1989; 145: 151–2.

74. Goadsby PJ, Lipton RB. Paroxysmal hemicrania-tic syndrome. Headache 2001; 41: 608–9.

75. Mateo I, Pascual J. Coexistence of chronic paroxysmal hemicrania and benign cough headache. Headache 1999; 39: 437–8.

76. Antonaci F, Pareja JA, Caminero AB, Sjaastad O. Chronic paroxysmal hemicrania and hemicrania continua. Parenteral indomethacin: the 'indotest'. Headache 1998; 38: 122–8.

77. Sjaastad O, Antonaci F. Chronic paroxysmal hemicrania: a case report. Long lasting remission in the chronic stage. Cephalalgia 1987; 7: 203–5.

78. Hannerz J, Ericson K, Bergstrand G. Chronic paroxysmal hemicrania: orbital phlebography and steroid treatment. A case report. Cephalalgia 1987; 7: 189–92.

79. Schlake HP, Bottger IG, Grotemeyer KH et al. Single photon emission tomography (SPECT) with 99 mTc-HMPAO (hexamethyl propyleneamino oxime) in chronic paroxysmal

hemicrania – a case report. Cephalalgia 1990; 10: 311–15.

80. Shabbir N. Adolescent chronic paroxysmal hemicrania responsive to verapamil monotherapy. Headache 1994; 34: 209–10.

81. Evers S, Husstedt IW. Alternatives in drug treatment of chronic paroxysmal hemicrania. Headache 1996; 36: 429–32.

82. Pascual J, Quijano J. A case of chronic paroxysmal hemicrania responding to subcutaneous sumatriptan. J Neurol Neurosurg Psychiatry 1998; 65: 407.

83. Dahlof C. Subcutaneous sumatriptan does not abort attacks of chronic paroxysmal hemicrania (CPH). Headache 1993; 33: 201–2.

84. Antonaci F, Pareja JA, Caminero AB, Sjaastad O. Chronic paroxysmal hemicrania continua: lack of efficacy of sumatriptan. Headache 1998; 38: 197–200.

85. Goadsby PJ. Cluster headache and the clinical profile of sumatriptan. Eur Neurol 1994; 34: S35–S39.

86. Mathew NT, Kailasam J, Fischer A. Responsiveness to celecoxib in chronic paroxysmal hemicrania. Neurology 2000; 55: 316.

87. Sjaastad O, Saunte C, Salvesen R. Short-lasting unilateral neuralgiform headache attacks with conjunctival injection, tearing, sweating, and rhinorrhea. Cephalalgia 1989; 9: 147–56.

88. Pareja JA, Sjaastad O. SUNCT syndrome. A clinical review. Headache 1997; 47: 195–202.

89. Pareja JA, Sjaastad O. SUNCT syndrome in the female. Headache 1994; 34: 217–20.

90. Pareja JA, Ming JM, Kruszewski P et al. SUNCT syndrome: duration, frequency and temporal distribution of attacks. Headache 1996; 36: 161–5.

91. Pareja JA, Joubert J, Sjaastad O. SUNCT syndrome. Atypical temporal patterns. Headache 1996; 36: 108–10.

92. Sjaastad O, Zhao JM, Kruszewski P, Stovner LJ. Short-lasting unilateral neuralgiform headache attacks with conjunctival injection, tearing, etc. (SUNCT): III. Another Norwegian case. Headache 1991; 31: 175–7.

93. Pareja JA, Pareja J, Palomo T et al. SUNCT syndrome: repetitive and overlapping attacks. Headache 1994; 34: 114–16.

94. Pareja JA, Caballero V, Sjaastad O. SUNCT syndrome. Status-like pattern. Headache 1996; 36: 622–4.

95. Becser N, Berky M. SUNCT syndrome: a Hungarian case. Headache 1995; 35: 158–60.

96. Calvo JF, Tinetti N, Leston J. SUNCT. The first Argentinian case. J Neurol Sci 1997; 150(suppl): S34.

97. Bussone G, Leone M, Volta GD et al. Short-lasting unilateral neuralgiform headache attacks with tearing and conjunctival injection: the first symptomatic case. Cephalalgia 1991; 11: 123–7.

98. De Benedittis G. SUNCT syndrome associated with cavernous angioma of the brain stem. Cephalalgia 1996; 16: 503–6.

99. Morales F, Mostacero E, Marta J, Sanchez S. Vascular malformation of the cerebellopontine angle associated with SUNCT syndrome. Cephalalgia 1994; 14: 301–2.

100. ter Berg JW, Goadsby PJ. Significance of atypical presentation of symptomatic SUNCT: a case report. J Neurol Neurosurg Psychiatry 2001; 70: 244–6.

101. Moris G, Ribacoba R, Solar DN, Vidal JA. SUNCT syndrome and seborrheic dermatitis associated with craneosynostosis. Cephalalgia 2001; 21: 157–9.

102. Sesso RM. SUNCT syndrome or trigeminal neuralgia with lacrimation and conjunctival injection? Cephalalgia 2001; 21: 151–3.

103. Benoliel R, Sharav Y. Paroxysmal hemicrania. Case studies and review of the literature. Oral Surg Oral Med Oral Pathol Oral Radiol Endod 1998; 85: 285–92.

104. Gowers WR. A manual of diseases of the nervous system. Philadelphia: P. Blakiston, Son & Co, 1888.

105. Collier J. Diseases of the nervous system. In: Price FW, ed. A textbook of the Practice of Medicine. London: Hodder and Stoughton, 1922.

106. Kinnier-Wilson SA. Neuritis. In: Bruce AN, ed. London: Edward Arnold, 1940, 380–91.

107. Bouhassira D, Attal N, Esteve M, Chauvin M. SUNCT syndrome. A case of transformation from trigeminal neuralgia. Cephalalgia 1994; 14: 168–70.

108. Sjaastad O, Pareja JA, Zukerman E et al. Trigeminal neuralgia. Clinical manifestations of first division involvement. Headache 1997; 37: 346–57.

109. May A, Buchel C, Turner R et al. Neurovascular dilatation of intracranial vessels in experimental headache. Cephalalgia 1999; 19: 464–5.

110. Raeder JG. 'Paratrigeminal' paralysis of the oculopupillary sympathetic. Brain 1924; 47: 149–58.

111. May A, Buchel C, Turner R, Goadsby PJ. MR angiography in facial and other pain: neurovascular mechanisms of trigeminal sensation. J Cereb Blood Flow Metabol 2001; 21: 1171–6.

112. Goadsby PJ, Edvinsson L, Ekman R. Vasoactive peptide release in the extracerebral circulation of humans during migraine headache. Ann Neurol 1990; 28: 183–7.

113. Malick A, Burstein R. Cells of origin of the trigeminohypothalamic tract in the rat. J Comparative Neurol 1998; 400: 125–44.

114. May A, Bahra A, Buchel C et al. Functional magnetic resonance imaging in spontaneous attacks of SUNCT: short-lasting neuralgiform headache with conjunctival injection and tearing. Ann Neurol 1999; 46: 791–4.

115. May A, Bahra A, Buchel C et al. Hypothalamic activation in cluster headache attacks. Lancet 1998; 352: 275–8.

116. Kruszewski P. Short-lasting, unilateral, neuralgiform headache attacks with conjunctival injection and tearing (SUNCT syndrome): V. Orbital phlebography. Cephalalgia 1992; 12: 387–9.

117. Hannerz J, Greitz D, Hansson P, Ericson K. SUNCT may be another manifestation of orbital venous vasculitis. Headache 1992; 32: 384–9.

118. Kruszewski P, Zhao JM, Shen JM, Sjaastad O. SUNCT syndrome: forehead sweating pattern. Cephalalgia 1993; 13: 108–13.

119. Zhao JM, Sjaastad O. SUNCT syndrome: VIII. Pupillary reaction and corneal sensitivity. Funct Neurol 1993; 8: 409–14.

120. Sjaastad O, Kruszewski P, Fostad K et al. SUNCT syndrome: VII. Ocular and related variables. Headache 1992; 32: 489–95.

121. Kruszewski P, Sand T, Shen JM, Sjaastad O. Short-lasting, unilateral, neuralgiform headache attacks with conjunctival injection and tearing (SUNCT syndrome): IV. Respiratory sinus arrhythmia during and outside paroxysms. Headache 1992; 32: 377–83.

122. Kruszewski P, Fasano ML, Brubakk AO et al. Short-lasting, unilateral, neuralgiform headache attacks with conjunctival injection, tearing, and subclinical forehead sweating (SUNCT syndrome): II. Changes in heart rate and arterial blood pressure during pain paroxysms. Headache 1991; 31: 399–405.

123. Kruszewski P, White LR, Shen JM. Respiratory studies in SUNCT syndrome. Headache 1995; 35: 344–8.

124. Goadsby PJ, Zagami AS, Lambert GA. Neural processing of craniovascular pain: synthesis of the central structures involved in migraine. Headache 1991; 31: 365–71.

125. Shen JM, Johnsen HJ. SUNCT syndrome: estimation of cerebral blood flow velocity with transcranial doppler ultrasonography. Headache 1994; 34:

25–31.

126. Poughias L, Aasly J. SUNCT syndrome: cerebral SPECT images during attacks. Headache 1995; 35: 143–5.

127. Pareja JA, Kruszewski P, Sjaastad O. SUNCT syndrome: trials of drugs and anesthetic blockades. Headache 1995; 35: 138–42.

128. Ghose RR. SUNCT syndrome. Med J Aust 1995; 162: 667–8.

129. Raskin NH. The hypnic headache syndrome. Headache 1988; 28: 534–6.

130. Gould JD, Silberstein SD. Unilateral hypnic headache: a case study.

Neurology 1997; 49: 1749–51.

131. Morales-Asin F, Mauri JA, Iniquez C et al. The hypnic headache syndrome: report of three new cases. Cephalalgia 1998; 18: 157–8.

132. Vieira-Dias M, Esperanca P. Hypnic headache: report of two cases. Headache 2001; 41: 726–7.

133. Trucco M, Maggioni F, Badino R, Zanchin G. Hypnic headache syndrome; report of a new Italian case. Cephalalgia 2000; 20: 312.

134. Centonze V, D'Amico D, Usai S et al. First Italian case of hypnic headache, with literature review and discussion of

nosology. Cephalalgia 2001; 21: 71–4.

135. Newman LC, Lipton RB, Solomon S. The hypnic headache syndrome: a benign headache disorder of the elderly. Neurology 1990; 40: 1904–5.

136. Dodick DW, Mosek AC, Campbell JK. The hypnic ('alarm clock') headache syndrome. Cephalalgia 1998; 18: 152–65.

137. Ivanez V, Soler R, Barreiro P. Hypnic headache syndrome: a case with good response to indomethacin. Cephalalgia 1998; 18: 225–6.

Secondary headache disorders

chapter 11

Post-traumatic headache

Introduction

Post-traumatic headache, a new secondary headache that arises after head injury, is often a part of the post-traumatic syndrome. It can follow a mild-to-moderate closed head injury even when the patient has experienced no loss of consciousness. In addition to headache, symptoms of the post-concussion syndrome include depression, irritability, memory impairment, loss of libido, dizziness or vertigo, alcohol intolerance, and attention and concentration difficulties.[1]

Definitions

Minor head injury and minor traumatic brain injury are difficult to define, compared with moderate or severe injury in which structural damage is evident. Recent definitions have used the Glasgow Coma Scale[2] score (Table 11.1) to determine the severity of a traumatic brain injury. Minor head injury has been variously defined.[3-5] The American Congress of Rehabilitation Medicine defined minor traumatic brain injury as 'a traumatically induced physiological disruption of brain function' with at least one of the following:

(1) any period of loss of consciousness;
(2) any memory loss for events just before or after the accident;
(3) any alteration in mental state at the time of the accident; and
(4) focal neurological deficits that may or may not be transient.

The injury should not result in a loss of consciousness of greater than 30 minutes, an initial Glasgow coma scale score of less than 13 (after 30 minutes), or posttraumatic amnesia exceeding 24 hours.[4]

Concussion has also been variously defined. The American Academy of Neurology modified the Cantu criteria for their practice parameter:[6,7]

(1) Grade 1: confusion with no amnesia and no loss of consciousness;
(2) Grade 2: confusion with amnesia and no loss of consciousness;
(3) Grade 3: loss of consciousness.[8] Concussion is defined as a 'trauma-induced alteration in mental status that may or may not involve loss of consciousness'.

These definitions allow a range of severity and treatment protocols to be considered when evaluating patients and athletes with concussion.[5]

Most physicians agree that some patients have headache as a sequela to cranial trauma, but this relationship is hotly debated. The frequency, characteristics and risk factors of post-traumatic headache are disputed. The arguments are complicated by the medico-legal issues which sometimes mix science with the self-interest of various stakeholders. Cranial trauma of many kinds can induce headache that persists long after the trauma; this has been reported with motor vehicle accidents, blunt trauma, such as falling from a horse, or even iatrogenic trauma, such as from a craniotomy. Moreover, the discussion becomes more complex as one attempts to classify the various clinical presentations that may be seen after cranial trauma. We believe that patients present with headache syndromes following head injury and that these patients require clinical management.

Epidemiology

Motor vehicle accidents account for 45% of head injury, falls for 30%, and occupational and recreational accidents for 20%.[9] Patients with mild head injury, defined as a Glasgow coma scale of 13–15 (Table 11.1), are hospitalized at a rate of approximately 200/100 000 per year.[10] Post-traumatic headache develops in many of these patients.[11–17] Whiplash refers to the sequence of extension, flexion, and lateral motions of the neck that follows impact, with or without direct trauma to the head. Its symptoms, which are similar to post-traumatic syndrome and post-traumatic headache, include neck pain,

● **Table 11.1** Glasgow coma scale

Eye opening (E)		Best motor response (M)	
Spontaneous	4	Obeys	6
To sound	3	Localizes	5
To pain	2	Withdraws	4
None	1	Abnormal flexion	3
Verbal response (V)		Extends	2
		None	1
Oriented	5		
Confused	4		
Inappropriate	3		
Incomprehensible	2	Score equals sum (of)	
None	1	E+M+V and ranges between 3–15	

headaches, dizziness, and paraesthaesias. Cognitive and psychological sequelae are extremely common. It is important to distinguish a post-traumatic headache, initiated by head injury, from exacerbation of a pre-existing headache disorder following head injury. Head injury may initiate de novo headache in an individual without a predisposition or may be a precipitating factor of a primary headache disorder in an individual with a biological predisposition; these logically distinguishable circumstances may be difficult to distinguish clinically.

Clinical features

Symptoms of post-traumatic syndrome may develop immediately or they may be delayed (or not initially recognized) following trauma. Head, neck, and shoulder pain usually begins within 24–48 hours of the injury, while local tenderness at the site of trauma often occurs immediately. Pain can develop in the frontal or occipital region months after the injury. The International Headache Society (IHS) criteria for post-traumatic headache[18] (Table 11.2) are not primarily concerned with the headache's clinical features, but with the temporal relationship of the headache to the trauma. The IHS criteria for post-traumatic headache require the onset of headache within two weeks of either the head injury itself or within 2 weeks of regaining consciousness following the head injury. However, in clinical practice it is often difficult to determine when the headache actually started, since head pain may be obscured by other aspects of clinical presentation.

A variety of pain patterns that resemble the primary headache disorders may develop after head injury. The most frequently seen pattern resembles tension-type headache (TTH) and occurs in 85% of patients. It is characterized by generalized, persistent, bilateral, mild-to-moderate pain.[19] The headaches may be exacerbated by very mild physical or mental activity.[20] In one study,[21] headaches were mild in 30% of patients, moderate in 52%, and severe in 18%, and the pain was occipital in 51% of patients, frontal in 44%, and generalized in 11% of patients. The studies do not report the frequency of the headaches, their temporal profile or the associated symptoms (such as nausea and photophobia) which accompany the pain. Haas[22] used the IHS criteria for primary headache disorders to categorize 30 post-traumatic headache patients. Eight patients' headaches were classified as migraine, 12 as chronic TTH, two as analgesic abuse headache, seven as 'probable analgesic abuse headache,' and one was unclassifiable. Couch et al[23] compared 106 patients with post-traumatic chronic daily

● **Table 11.2** IHS criteria for post-traumatic headache[18]

5.1   Acute post-traumatic headache

5.1.1 With significant head trauma and/or confirmatory signs

Diagnostic criteria:

A Significance of head trauma documented by at least one of the following:

   1 Loss of consciousness

   2 Post-traumatic amnesia lasting more than 10 minutes

   3 At least two of the following exhibit relevant abnormality: clinical neurological examination, X-ray of skull, neuroimaging, evoked potentials, spinal fluid examination, vestibular function test, neuropsychological testing

B Headache occurs less than 14 days after regaining consciousness (or after the trauma, if there has been no loss of consciousness)

C Headache disappears within 8 weeks after regaining consciousness (or after trauma, if there has been no loss of consciousness)

5.1.2 With minor head trauma and no confirmatory signs

Diagnostic criteria:

A Head trauma that does not satisfy 5.1.1 A

B Headache occurs less than 14 days after injury

C Headache disappears within 8 weeks after injury

5.2   Chronic post-traumatic headache

A Significance of head trauma documented by at least one of the following:

   1 Loss of consciousness

   2 Post-traumatic amnesia lasting more than 10 minutes

   3 At least two of the following exhibit relevant abnormality: clinical neurological examination, X-ray of skull, neuroimaging, evoked potentials, spinal fluid examination, vestibular function test, neuropsychological testing

B Headache occurs less than 14 days after regaining consciousness (or after the trauma, if there has been no loss of consciousness)

C Headache continues for more than 8 weeks after regaining consciousness (or after trauma, if there has been no loss of consciousness)

5.2.2 With minor head trauma and no confirmatory signs

Diagnostic criteria

A Head trauma that does not satisfy 5.1.1 A

B Headache occurs less than 14 days after injury

C Headache continues for more than 8 weeks after injury

headache to a similar number of idiopathic chronic daily headache patients and found no significant differences among 19 headache characteristics.

Migraine with or without aura may be triggered by impact.[24] Alternatively, a pattern of recurring migraine-like headaches may begin at some time after a head injury.[11,19,25–27] In one study,[25] 35 patients had newly-acquired migraine with or without aura, beginning within a few days of mild head injury or whiplash injury. Most

● **Table 11.3** *Sequelae of mild head injury*

Headaches	Psychological and somatic complaints
Tension-type	Irritability
Migraine	Anxiety
Cluster	Depression
Low cerebrospinal pressure	Personality change
Occipital neuralgia	Fatigue
Idiopathic intracranial	Sleep disturbance
hypotension	Decreased libido
Supraorbital and infraorbital	Decreased appetite
neuralgia	**Rare sequelae**
Cervicogenic	
Temporomandibular joint	Subdural and epidural
syndrome or dysfunction	haematomas
Local neuroma	Seizures
Mixed	Transient global amnesia
Cranial nerve symptoms and signs	Tremor
	Dystonia
Dizziness	
Vertigo	
Tinnitus	
Hearing loss	
Blurred vision	
Diplopia	
Convergence insufficiency	
Light and noise sensitivity	
Diminished taste and smell	

patients experienced two or three attacks per week. Amitriptyline and propranolol are dramatically effective in 71% of patients. Some patients have post-traumatic headache with features of chronic (transformed) migraine.[28]

Since trauma can trigger typical primary headaches, such as migraine, TTH, or cluster headache, the IHS advised a fourth digit code to account for such a situation. Diagnosing a clinically typical post-traumatic headache is difficult. The essence of the diagnosis is that the cranial trauma triggered the headache from which the patient suffers. The headache is often mixed with symptoms of the post-traumatic syndrome, a symptom complex that also includes vertigo, blurred vision, and cognitive complaints. Post-traumatic syndrome symptoms (Table 11.3) may be delayed or develop immediately following trauma. Local occipital tenderness occurs immediately, while head, neck, and shoulder pain usually begins within 24–48 hours of the injury. Pain in the frontal or occipitocervical region may occur and may be associated with the other headache types.

Orthostatic headache can occur secondary to intracranial hypotension, with features similar to those of a post-lumbar puncture headache. Intracranial hypotension could result from a cerebrospinal fluid (CSF) leak through a dural root sleeve tear or a cribriform plate fracture. Idiopathic intracranial hypertension (pseudotumour) with and without papilloedema has also been reported as a consequence of head injury.[29]

Dysautonomic cephalalgia can follow injury to the carotid sheath. This rare, severe, unilateral headache is localized to the frontotemporal area and is associated with ipsilateral increased facial sweating and pupillary dilation.[1,30]

Temporomandibular joint injury may occur. Symptoms include incomplete jaw opening, clicking on lateral movements, jaw pain with mastication or prolonged talking, and pain on palpation of the jaw joint or the muscles of mastication. Temporomandibular joint dysfunction may be a headache trigger.

Non-headache symptoms of the post-traumatic syndrome

Impaired memory and difficulty concentrating are common in the post-traumatic syndrome.[17] Some patients have neurocognitive deficits and a documented inability to process information.[31] Many have difficulty processing different stimuli simultaneously and appear absent-minded because they must devote their full concentration to the task at hand. Other frequently reported symptoms include anger, depression, irritability and personality changes.

Non-specific dizziness and episodic and positional vertigo are commonly associated with post-traumatic headache.[32] Sleep disturbances, including insomnia and daytime drowsiness, are frequent. Non-specific staring episodes, non-vestibular dizziness and periodic loss of consciousness are rare.

Risk factors

Age, gender, and certain mechanical factors are risks for a poor outcome after head injury or whiplash injury. Women have a 1.9-fold increased risk of post-traumatic headache compared with men.[33] Increased age is associated with a less rapid and less complete recovery.[34–36] Post-traumatic headache is more likely if the head is inclined or rotated prior to impact, if a rear-end collision occurred, or the occupant was unprepared.[37] The relationship between the severity of the injury and the severity or incidence of the post-traumatic headache is uncertain. The persistence of the headache does not correlate with the duration of unconsciousness, post-traumatic amnesia, skull fracture, electroencephalogram (EEG) abnormalities, or bloody CSF.[21,32]

Pathophysiology

Post-traumatic headache is a group of trauma-induced disorders with overlapping symptoms. Multiple mechanisms may contribute to the development of headache. Peripheral nerve injury may result in neuropathic pain; soft tissue or skeletal injuries may initiate or trigger chronic daily headache; and injury to the neck, jaw and tissues of the scalp cause pain that is referred into the head.

Head injury causes shear forces to the brain that can produce diffuse axonal injury. Direct impact is not necessary.[38] Diffuse axonal injury is most common in the corpus callosum, internal capsule, fornices, dorsolateral midbrain, and pons.[39] Head injury usually involves a combination of translational and rotational forces. Restricted rotation makes it more difficult to produce a concussion in animals.[40] Unsynchronized rotations often develop between the cerebral hemispheres and the cerebellum,[40] making axons in the upper brainstem particularly vulnerable to diffuse axonal injury. Midbrain haemorrhage can result. Ischaemic brain injury, abnormal cerebrovascular autoregulation, and vasospasm may follow severe headache (Figure 11.1).

Testing

Neuroimaging

Most hospitalized patients with mild or moderate head injury have magnetic resonance imaging (MRI) abnormalities. These abnormalities ameliorate, with many resolving within 1 month.[41] Because of the risk of subsequent deterioration, all patients with mild behavioural abnormalities, equivocal findings on examination, or a Glasgow coma scale of <15 should undergo neuroimaging. With subacute or chronic post-traumatic syndrome, however, guidelines are less clear. If neuroimaging was not done, brain computed tomography (CT) or MRI should be performed to exclude chronic subdural haematoma, hydrocephalus, or a structural lesion unrelated to the trauma. If neck pain is prominent and persistent, a cervical MRI may be indicated, but if the neurological examination is normal or severe radicular symptoms are absent, an abnormal MRI usually does not change therapy. Of concern is a possible fracture or dislocation of the cervical spine, and the patient should have cervical spine films to rule out this problem.

Single photon emission computed tomography (SPECT)

Single photon emission computed tomography (SPECT) observes the physiological behaviour of the brain. In the acute phase of head injury, technetium-99m hexamethyl-propyleneamineoxime (Tc-HMPAO) SPECT is more sensitive than CT and is helpful in predicting outcome.[42–44] In 20 patients with head injury, Tc-HMPAO SPECT showed abnormalities in 60%, whereas only 25% had abnormalities on CT.[45] In 12 patients with mild-to-moderate head injury 1–9 years after injury, Tc-HMPAO SPECT was abnormal in 10 patients, while CT was abnormal in six patients.[46]

Electroencephalography (EEG)

The EEG is usually of little value in evaluating post-traumatic headache. While often abnormal immediately after injury, it normalizes within minutes to weeks. Persistent findings that were once considered abnormal are now considered normal variants with the same incidence found in the general population.[47]

Evoked potentials

Short latency somatosensory evoked potentials have not been shown to be of value in head injury.[48] On the other hand, brainstem auditory evoked potentials have been found to be abnormal in 10–20% of patients with head injury and post-concussion syndrome. While the brainstem auditory evoked potential separates groups of patients with post-traumatic headache from groups of controls, it does not differentiate an individual with post-traumatic headache from one without post-traumatic headache.

Blood testing: S-100 and ApOE

The S-100 is a marker of brain injury in head trauma and

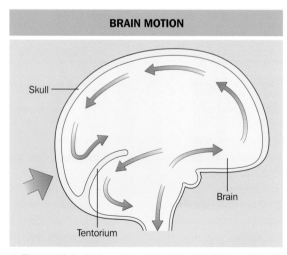

BRAIN MOTION

Skull

Brain

Tentorium

● **Figure 11.1** *Brain motion. (From Ward C. Status of head injury modeling. Head and Neck Injury Criteria, Washington D.C., USA, Department of Transportation, 1981.)*

correlates with the Glasgow coma scale on admission.[49] In hospitalized mild head injury patients, S-100 was detectable in 28% of patients, 36% of whom had contusions on MRI. In patients with detectable S-100 levels, there was a trend toward impaired neuropsychological functioning on measures of attention, memory, and information processing speed. Carriers of the ApoE4 genotype experience more severe neuropsychological sequela following head injury[50] though the relationship to headache is not clear.

Neuropsychological testing

Neuropsychological testing in patients with head injury is often markedly abnormal early on and improves or resolves with time. Abnormalities are found in information processing, auditory vigilance, reaction time, sustained divided and distributed attention, visual and verbal memory, design fluency imagination, and analytic capacity.

Neuropsychological tests were performed on 30 patients with post-traumatic syndrome after whiplash injury. Deficits in attention and concentration resolved within 6 weeks. Visual memory, imagination, and analytic capacity were recovered within the next 6 weeks. Verbal memory abstraction, cognitive selectivity, and information processing speed took more than 12 weeks to recover.[51] This suggests that a hierarchy of functional recovery follows mild head injury.

The paced auditory serial addition test is a widely used test of information processing that is often abnormal shortly after head injury. Patients are presented with a random series of digits at intervals of either 1–2 to 2–4 seconds (same interval for entire test), and are asked to add the most recently presented number to the one before. The score is expressed as the percentage correct at each rate or as the mean correct response per second. It has been given serially over 8 weeks postinjury and demonstrates cognitive recovery to normal. Paced auditory serial addition test recovery, however, was delayed in head injury patients with post-traumatic syndrome compared with a nonpost-traumatic syndrome control group.[31]

Relationship between cranial trauma and headache

Migraine,[25] cluster headache, or chronic daily headache syndromes can occur after even trivial head injury.[24] Post-traumatic headache is more common in patients with a history of headache.[33,52] Post-traumatic headache usually lasts for 3–5 years and then abates[53] independent of financial compensation.[21,54,55] Since 10% of most populations studied have migraine, and many more suffer from other headache types (see Chapter 3), the association

between trauma and headache could at times be one of chance. We think not, but the question is difficult to resolve. It has been suggested that post-traumatic headache may be seen up to 24 months after the injury, and that as many as 12% of patients acquire their headaches more than 6 months after the trauma.[36] The problem with such assertions is that we do not know how many people would acquire a headache in a suitable control group. The IHS thus set a somewhat arbitrary limit that the headache should come on within 2 weeks of the head injury. While this criterion is *ad hoc*, it is useful in practice and provides a legal guideline. If cranial trauma induces a headache process, it seems likely that it would have a relatively short latency from a physiological point of view; certainly the concept that a headache starting years after cranial trauma has a causative relationship to the trauma seems difficult to accept. Considering evidence from known triggers, such as nitroglycerine,[56] which takes typically 4–8 hours to trigger migraine, or premonitory symptoms in migraine that have been documented to occur three days before the attack, limits greater than 2 weeks have no biological precedent in headache. One might suggest reducing the triggering time to one week, but this should only be done with new, properly controlled studies.

Diagnosis

The diagnosis of post-traumatic headache and post-traumatic syndrome, therefore, is established by symptoms that are consistent with the syndrome and onset that is related to trauma. The differential diagnoses include subdural or epidural haematoma, CSF hypotension, cerebral vein thrombosis, cavernous sinus thrombosis, cervical or carotid artery dissection, cerebral haemorrhage, epilepsy, and hydrocephalus.

Management

Management of post-traumatic headache is dictated by the clinical syndrome. Structural problems, such as low CSF pressure syndromes, must be excluded by neuroimaging and a careful history and physical examination. Patients with post-traumatic headache are often misunderstood. They may be distressed and require support and an objective, comprehensive approach to treatment. An explanation of the existence and recognition of the syndrome can be very therapeutic.

A recognizable primary headache syndrome (e.g.

migraine or cluster headache) that has been triggered by cranial trauma is managed in the usual manner. Cervical and soft tissue injuries should be identified and treated, as should anxiety, depression, and cognitive dysfunction. Post-traumatic chronic daily headache is very difficult to treat, but again the management principles are as outlined in Chapter 8.

Few studies have evaluated specific drug treatments for post-traumatic headache. Most have involved the use of the antidepressant, amitriptyline. We have found tricyclics, such as amitriptyline and imipramine, as well as valproate, to be extremely useful in these patients. Like many patients with chronic daily headache syndromes, medication overuse can be a complicating variable that must be addressed if treatment is to be successful. Perhaps the most effective tool is a careful and straightforward explanation of the syndrome. Explaining to patients that, when disturbed, the pain-producing structures of the brain can effectively 'wind themselves up' to produce the pain that was triggered by, but persists independent of, the original trauma can help them cope with what must seem a bizarre situation.

Sumatriptan and zolmitriptan are effective for the migrainous exacerbation of post-traumatic headache, but not for the baseline headache.[57] Repetitive intravenous dihydroergotamine is effective for post-traumatic headache that meets the criteria of chronic daily headache[58,59] and appeared to improve cognitive function in one study.[59] Intravenous chlorpromazine has been effective in acute post-traumatic headache. One must be on the lookout for analgesic and ergotamine overuse[60] in patients with daily or near-daily headache; preventive medications should be used preferentially and abortive medications limited.

Physical modalities, such as physical therapy, exercise, chiropractic treatment, and massage, have been beneficial for some patients, particularly when the headache is related to, or occurs in association with, cervical trauma. Cervical orthoses, electrotherapy, and heat and cold have been used successfully, particularly in the acute stage, to improve function. These methods have not been rigorously tested, but such data would be of great value in planning treatment regimens. In one open study, manual therapy was more successful than cold packs in relieving chronic post-traumatic headache.[61] After the initial, acute phase, exercise programmes are important to prevent deconditioning and a decrease in the overall level of functioning.

Outcome

Since prognostic studies have used different study designs, varying subject characteristics, and various definitions of head injury, accurately ascertaining the prognosis of post-traumatic headache is difficult. One month after mild head injury, 31%[62] to 90%[63] of patients had headache. Two to three months post-injury, 32%[64] to 78%[10] of patients had headache. One year after injury, the range was 8%[65] to 35%.[66] Two to four years after injury, three studies show that 20–24% of patients had persistent headache.

Approximately one-third of patients are unable to return to work after head injury.[67] In one study, 34% of previously employed patients admitted to a hospital had not returned to work 3 months after injury. Older patients with higher levels of education and employment, greater income, and higher socioeconomic status are, however, likely to return to work.[17]

In the post-traumatic headache patient, two processes may occur simultaneously. The first process is diffuse axonal injury, which is due to acceleration/deceleration forces. When diffuse axonal injury is more severe, it is associated with abnormalities on MRI, positron emission tomography, SPECT, and certain neuropsychological tests. Clinical improvement may occur over several months, with these tests normalizing or improving. A second process, separate from diffuse axonal injury, may be responsible for the persistent headache, psychopathology, and neurocognitive deficits that occur after head injury. This process is often heralded by more severe early headache. A pre-existing factor or vulnerability may be a necessary precondition for this process to present itself fully in a given individual.

References

1. Young WB, Packard RC, Ramadan N. Headaches associated with head trauma. In: Silberstein SD, Lipton RB, Dalessio DJ, eds. Wolff's Headache and Other Head Pain. 7th edn. New York: Oxford University Press, 2001, 325–48.
2. Teasdale G, Jennett B. Assessment of coma and impaired consciousness: a practical scale. Lancet 1984; 2: 81–4.
3. Rimel RW. Disability caused by minor head injury. J Head Trauma Rehabil 1981; 6: 86–7.
4. Anonymous. Definition of mild traumatic brain injury. J Head Trauma Rehabil 1993; 6: 87.
5. Packard RC. Epidemiology and pathogenesis of posttraumatic headache. J Head Trauma Rehabil 1999; 14: 9–21.
6. Cantu RC. Return to play guidelines after a head injury. Clinics Sports Med 1998; 17: 45–60.
7. Cantu BC. Head and spine injuries in the young athlete. Clin Sports Med 1988; 7: 459–72.
8. Kelly JP, Rosenberg JH. Diagnosis and management of concussion in sports. Neurology 1997; 48: 575–80.
9. Jennett B, Frankowski RF. The epidemiology of head injury. In: Braakman R, ed. Handbook of Clinical Neurology. New York: Elsevier, 1990, 1–7.
10. Kraus JF, McArthur DL, Silberman TA. Epidemiology of mild brain injury. Sem Neurol 1994; 14: 1–7.
11. Evans RW. The postconcussion syndrome and the sequelae of mild head injury. Neurol Clin 1992; 10: 815–47.
12. Raskin NH. Posttraumatic headache: the postconcussion syndrome. In: Raskin NH, ed. Headache. New York: Churchill Livingstone, 1988.
13. Brenner C, Friedman AP. Posttraumatic headache. J Neurosurg 1944; 1: 379–91.
14. Elkind AH. Posttraumatic headache. In: Diamond S, Dalessio DJ, eds. The practicing physician's approach to headache. 5th edn. Baltimore: Williams and Wilkins, 1992, 146–61.
15. Speed WG. Psychiatric aspects of posttraumatic headaches. In: Adler C, Adler S, Packard R, eds. Psychiatric aspects of headache. Baltimore: Williams and Wilkins, 1987, 210–17.
16. Gfeller JD, Chibnall JT, Duckro PN. Postconcussion symptoms and cognitive functioning in posttraumatic headache patients. Headache 1994; 34: 503–7.
17. Rimel RW, Giordani B, Barth JT et al. Disability caused by minor head injury. Neurosurgery 1981; 9: 221–8.
18. Headache Classification Committee of the International Headache Society. Classification and diagnostic criteria for headache disorders, cranial neuralgia, and facial pain. Cephalalgia 1988; 8: 1–96.
19. Mandel S. Minor head injury may not be 'minor'. Postgrad Med J 1989; 85: 213–15.
20. Kelly R. Headache after cranial trauma. In: Hopkins A, ed. Headache: problems in diagnosis and management. London: Saunders, 1988: 219.
21. De Benedittis G, De Santis A. Chronic posttraumatic headache: clinical, psychopathological features and outcome determinants. J Neurosurg Sci 1983; 27: 177–86.
22. Haas DC. Classification of chronic posttraumatic headache. Cephalalgia 1995; 15: 162.
23. Couch JR, Samuel S, Leviston T, Teagram H. Can head injury by itself produce the syndrome of chronic daily headache. American Headache Society 42nd Annual Scientific Meeting, June 23–25, 2000.
24. Haas DC, Lourie T. Trauma-triggered migraine: an explanation for common neurologic attacks after mild head injury. Neurosurg 1988; 68: 181–8.
25. Weiss HD, Stern BJ, Goldbert J. Posttraumatic migraine: chronic migraine precipitated by minor head or neck trauma. Headache 1991; 31: 451–6.
26. Binder LM. Persisting symptoms after mild head injury: a review of the postconcussive syndrome. J Clin Exp Neuropsychol 1986; 8: 323–46.
27. Winston KR. Whiplash and its relationship to migraine. Headache 1987; 27: 452–7.
28. Saper JR. Headache disorders: current concepts in treatment strategies. Littleton: Wright-PSG, 1983.
29. Silberstein SD, Marcelis J. Pseudotumor cerebri without papilledema. Headache 1990; 30: 304.
30. Vijayan N. A new posttraumatic headache syndrome. Headache 1977; 17: 19–22.
31. Gronwall D, Wrightson P. Delayed recovery of intellectual function after minor head injury. Lancet 1974; 2: 605–9.
32. Lidvall HF, Linderoth B, Norlin B. Causes of the postconcussional syndrome. Acta Neurol Scand 1974; 40: 1–143.
33. Jensen OK, Nielsen FF. The influence of sex and pretraumatic headache on the incidence and severity of headache after head injury. Cephalalgia 1990; 10: 285–93.
34. Bohnen N, Twinjnstra A, Jolles J. Posttraumatic and emotional symptoms in different subgroups of patients with mild head injury. Brain Injury 1992; 6: 481–7.
35. McClelland RJ, Fenton GW, Rutherford W. The postconcussional syndrome revisited. J Royal Soc Med 1994; 87: 508–10.
36. Cartlidge N, Shaw D, eds. Head Injury. Philadelphia: WB Saunders, 1981, 95–154.
37. Mendelson G. Not 'cured by a verdict'. Med J Aust 1982; 2: 132–4.
38. Gennarelli TA. Mechanisms of brain injury. J Emerg Med 1993; 1: 5–11.
39. Blumbergs PC, Jones NR, North JB. Diffuse axonal injury in head trauma. J Neurol Neurosurg Psychiatry 1989; 52: 838–41.
40. Elson LM, Ward CC. Mechanisms and pathophysiology of mild head injury. Sem Neurol 1994; 14: 8–18.
41. Levin HS, Amparo E, Eisenberg HM. Magnetic resonance imaging and computerized tomography in relation to the neurobehavioral sequelae of mild and moderate head injuries. J Neurosurg 1987; 66: 706–13.
42. Abdel-Dayem HM, Sadek SA, Kouris K. Changes in cerebral perfusion after acute head injury: comparison of CT with Tc-99m-PAO SPECT. Radiology 1987; 165: 221–6.
43. Reid RH, Gulenchyn K, Ballinger JR. Cerebral perfusion imaging with Tc-HM-PAO following cerebral trauma. Clin Nucl Med 1990; 15: 383–8.
44. Abdel-Dayem HM, Masdeu J, O'Connell R. Brain perfusion abnormalities following minor/moderate closed head injury: comparison between early and late imaging in two groups of patients. Eur J Nucl Med 1994; 21: 750.
45. Gray BG, Ichise M, Chung D. Technetium-99m-HMPAO SPECT in the evaluation of patients with remote history of traumatic brain injury: a comparison with X-ray computed tomography. J Nucl Med 1992; 33: 52–8.
46. Krelina M, Reid R, Ballinger J. Regional cerebral blood flow in patients with remote close-head injuries. Can J Neurol Sci 1989; 2: 279 (Abstract).
47. Schoenhuber R, Gentilini M. Neurophysiologic assessment of mild head injury. In: Levin HS, Eisenberg HM, Benton AL, eds. Mild head injury. New York: Oxford University Press, 1989, 142–50.
48. Bricolo AP, Turella GS. Electrophysiology of head injury. In: Braakman R, ed. Handbook of Clinical Neurology. New York: Elsevier, 1990, 181–206.
49. Herrmann M, Curio N, Jost S, Wunderlich MT et al. Protein S-100B and neuron specific enolase as early neurobiochemical markers of the severity of traumatic brain injury. Restorative

Neurol Neurosci 1999; 14: 109–14.

50. Lichtman SW, Seliger G, Tycko B, Marder K. Apolipoprotein E and functional recovery from brain injury following postacute rehabilitation. Neurology 2000; 55: 1536–9.

51. Keidel M, Yaguez L, Wilhelm H, Diener HC. Prospective follow-up of neuropsychologic deficiency after cervicocephalic acceleration trauma. (German). Nervenarzt 1992; 63: 731–40.

52. Russell MB, Olesen J. Migraine associated with head trauma and its relation to migraine. Eur J Neurol 1996; 3: 424–8.

53. Medina JL. Efficacy of an individualized outpatient program in the treatment of chronic posttraumatic headache. Headache 1992; 32: 180–3.

54. Packard RC, Ham LP. Posttraumatic headache: determining chronicity. Headache 1993; 33: 133–4.

55. Packard RC. Posttraumatic headache: permanency and relationship to legal settlement. Headache 1992; 32:

496–500.

56. Thomsen LL, Kruuse C, Iversen HK, Olesen J. A nitric oxide donor (nitroglycerine) triggers genuine migraine attacks. Neurology 1994; 1: 73–80.

57. Gawel MJ, Rothbart P, Jacobs H. Subcutaneous sumatriptan in the treatment of acute episodes of posttraumatic headache. Headache 1993; 33: 96–7.

58. McBeath JG, Nanda A. Use of dihydroergotamine in patients with postconcussion syndrome. Headache 1994; 34: 148–51.

59. Young WB, Hopkins MM, Janyszek B, Primavera JP. Repetitive intravenous DHE in the treatment of refractory posttraumatic headache. Headache 1994; 34: 297 (Abstract).

60. Herd A, Ludwig L. Relief of posttraumatic headache by intravenous chlorpromazine. J Emerg Med 1994; 12: 849–51.

61. Jensen OK, Nielsen FF, Vosmar L. An open study comparing manual therapy

with the use of cold packs in the treatment of posttraumatic headache. Cephalalgia 1990; 10: 241–50.

62. Munderhoud JM, Boclens ME, Huizenga J. Treatment of minor head injuries. Clin Neurol Neurosurg 1980; 82: 127–40.

63. Denker PG. The postconcussion syndrome: prognosis and evaluation of the organic factors. NY State J Med 1944; 44: 379–84.

64. Denny-Brown D. Disability arising from closed head injury. JAMA 1945; 127: 429–36.

65. Rutherford WH, Merrett JD, McDonald JR. Symptoms of one year following concussion from minor head injuries. Injury 1978; 10: 225–30.

66. Dencker SJ, Lofving BA. A psychometric study of identical twins discordant for closed head injury. Acta Psychiatr Neurol Scand 1958; 33.

67. Rutherford WH, Merrett JD, McDonald JR. Sequelae of concussion caused by minor head injuries. Lancet 1977; 1: 1–4.

chapter 12

Headache associated with nonvascular intracranial disorders

Introduction

Headache is a very common clinical manifestation of both reduced and increased intracranial pressure. Any disruption of cerebrospinal fluid (CSF) production, flow, or absorption may lead to alterations in intracranial pressure and headache. Clinical syndromes in altered intracranial pressure include postlumbar puncture headache, spontaneous intracranial hypotension, brain tumor, idiopathic intracranial hypertension, hydrocephalus, intracranial hemorrhage, and subdural hematoma. Mass lesions can influence pain-sensitive intracranial structures by invasion, inflammation, irritation or traction; in addition they may impede CSF flow, or directly increase pressure by mass effect, all of which can produce headache. Some disorders produce unique symptoms that aid in their diagnosis; for example, the orthostatic headache that is characteristic of intracranial hypotension or the cough headache associated with hindbrain abnormalities.

The International Headache Society (IHS)[1] classifies most of these conditions in a group referred to as 'headache associated with nonvascular intracranial disorder [7.0]' (Table 12.1). Intracranial disorders may also produce exacerbation of a preexisting headache; this circumstance is outside the scope of discussion for this chapter.

In this chapter, we will first review the production and flow of CSF. We will then consider the causes of intracranial hypotension and the headache disorders associated with reduced intracranial pressure. We will discuss the headaches of increased intracranial pressure associated with space-occupying structural lesions. Next we will consider the headaches of intracranial hypertension in the absence of space-occupying lesions. We will discuss the secondary forms and exertional and cough headache as

well as the primary disorders that are in their differential diagnosis.

Cerebrospinal fluid dynamics

History

Galen first described the ventricular cavities in the 2nd century, but it was left to Contugno, in 1764, to describe the CSF. Earlier anatomists did not encounter CSF because decapitation, performed before dissection, allowed it to escape. In 1825, Magendie tapped the cisterna magna in animals, named the CSF, and discovered the foramen between the IVth ventricle and the subarachnoid space that now bears his name.[2]

Dandy's work supported the view that the CSF originated from the choroid plexus and the perivascular spaces of the brain. Key and Retzius demonstrated that the CSF passes from the subarachnoid space through the Pacchionian bodies into the cerebral venous sinuses (Figure 12.1).[2]

Lumbar puncture was introduced by Quinke in 1891. Using a percutaneous needle with a stylet, Quinke measured the components of CSF and its pressure in normal and disease states. Bier first described postlumbar puncture headache in 1898. Following injection of cocaine into

● **Table 12.1** *Headache associated with nonvascular intracranial disorder*

Diagnostic criteria
1. Symptoms and/or signs of intracranial disorder.
2. Confirmation by appropriate investigation.
3. Headache as a new symptom or of a new type occurs temporally related to intracranial disorder.

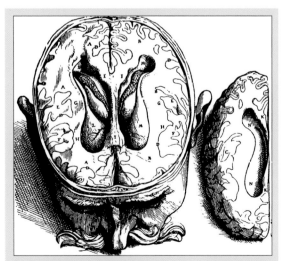

● **Figure 12.1** *A view of the brain from Andreas Vesalius' Fabrica, showing the ventricles.*

his own subarachnoid space, he developed a violent postural headache.[3] Schaltenbrand,[4] a German neurologist, first described spontaneous intracranial hypotension, which he termed spontaneous aliquorrhea, in 1938. Woltman, at the Mayo Clinic, was the first to describe the syndrome in the United States.[5]

Production, flow, absorption, and pressure

The major source of CSF is the choroid plexus; however, some CSF is formed in extrachoroidal sites. The choroid plexus of the lateral ventricle is continuous with that of the IIIrd ventricle, but separate from that of the IVth ventricle. Both active transport and serum dialysis are involved in CSF production (Figure 12.2).[6]

Based on autopsy and other old data, CSF volume was estimated to be 150 ml. However, recent magnetic resonance imaging (MRI) volumetric studies have demonstrated significant variations, particularly with age.[7] Mean ± standard deviation (SD) cranial CSF volume has been calculated as 157 ± 59 ml for both sexes and for all persons aged 24–80 years (more for men, less for women, and much lower for younger than older persons, who have more generous ventricular volumes and larger CSF cisterns.[8]

The estimated rate of CSF formation in humans is 0.37 ± 0.1 ml/min or 500 ml/day. This rate is unaffected by intracranial pressures over a broad range (of −10 to 240 mm H_2O).[6] The total CSF volume is renewed every 6–8 hours.

The zero reference level of lumbar CSF pressure is the right atrial pressure level. In normal subjects, CSF pressure varies with respiration over a range of 2–5 mm H_2O and with the cardiac cycle over a 1–2 mm H_2O range. In humans, in the lateral recumbent position, the average CSF pressure is 150 mm H_2O, with a range of 70–200 mm H_2O.[2,6] Corbett and Mehta[9] recorded CSF pressures between 200 and 250 mm H_2O in normal non-obese controls, suggesting that the upper limit of normal may be 250 mm H_2O. When CSF pressure falls below 50–90 mm H_2O, symptoms of intracranial hypotension occur. At times, the CSF pressure is not measurable and CSF can only be obtained by aspiration.[2,6,10,11] If simultaneous pressures are taken from the cerebral ventricles, the cisterna magna, and the lumbar sac during a change from the recumbent to the erect posture, there is a significant change in pressure throughout the system. The pressure rises to 375–565 mm H_2O in the lumbar sac, becomes 0 mm H_2O at the level of the cisterna magna, and can fall to −85 mm H_2O in the ventricles (Figure 12.3).[6,12–15]

The factors that determine CSF pressure are listed in Table 12.2. Of these, transmitted venous pressure is the most important determinant.[6] Intracranial pressure can be elevated by any of the mechanisms in Table 12.3. A mass lesion can produce elevated intracranial pressure when it:

CSF PATHWAYS

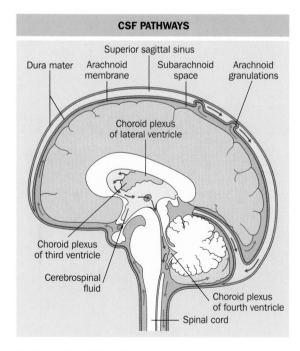

● **Figure 12.2** CSF pathways.

CSF PRESSURES IN THE FOUR GROUPS

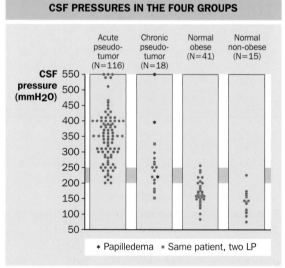

● **Figure 12.3** CSF pressures in the four groups. Three patients in the chronic group still had papilledema (asterisks). One patient in the chronic group had two lumbar punctures (squares). One lumbar puncture was normal and the other showed elevated pressure.

Table 12.2 *Factors determining CSF pressure*

1. CSF secretion pressure.
2. CSF absorption rate.
3. Intracranial arterial pressure.
4. Intracranial venous pressure.
5. Brain bulk.
6. Hydrostatic pressure.
7. Presence of intact surrounding/coverings.

Table 12.3 *Mechanisms for elevated intracranial pressure*

1. Increased CSF production or secretion pressure.
2. Decreased CSF absorption.
3. Increased venous pressure.
4. Obstruction of normal CSF flow.
5. Increase in brain bulk: mass lesion/cerebral edema.
6. Increased bulk or pressure in dura.
7. Combination of above.

- reaches a critical size;
- obstructs the intracranial venous system producing increased venous pressure; or
- obstructs the CSF pathways.

According to the Monro–Kellie doctrine, increased intracranial volume leads to increased intracranial pressure. Since an adult's skull has rigid walls, it forms a closed chamber, and a small exit, the foramen magnum, provides the only outlet for CSF into the vertebral canal.

When monitored continuously with isovolumetric pressure transducers, patients with intracranial hypertension show frequent, rapid pressure fluctuations. In addition to the fluctuations with respiration and cardiac cycles described above, plateau waves, which are acute elevations of pressure that last 5–20 minutes and can reach levels as high as 600–1300 mm H_2O, may occur (Figure 12.4).

When intracranial hypotension is present, intracranial CSF pressure falls as individuals move from the recumbent to the upright position. This produces increased traction on the supporting structures of the brain (the blood vessels and dural sinuses), which may cause headache in the upright position. Secondary compensatory venous dilation may contribute to the headache as well.[11,16] Intracranial CSF volume loss, as measured by MRI, occurs mainly in the cortical sulci and has been correlated with postlumbar puncture low CSF pressure headache. Venous dilation par-

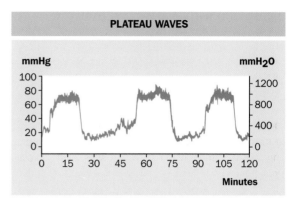

PLATEAU WAVES

● **Figure 12.4** *Plateau waves as visualized with an intracranial pressure transducer in a patient with a malignant brain tumor. During the waves a rapid increase in signs of cerebral dysfunction was noted.*

tially compensates for the volume loss.[17] Jugular compression, which causes more venous dilation but increases intracranial pressure, aggravates low pressure headache. A downward displacement of the brain with incisural or cerebellar tonsillar herniation that could be mistaken for a Chiari malformation (Figure 12.5) has been described in some studies.[17–19] In addition, descent of the brainstem, flattening of the basis pontis, and bowing of the optic chiasm over the pituitary gland may occur. The downward displacement is limited by the recumbent position required for neuroimaging; these findings might be even greater in the upright position. These MRI abnormalities often resolve with headache improvement.[20–23] Thus, headache may result from painful venous dilation, displacement of and traction on pain-sensitive intracranial structures, or both.

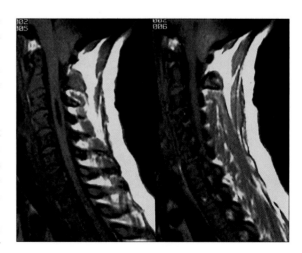

● **Figure 12.5** *Chiari malformation.*

Intracranial hypotension and low pressure headache

Headache is the most common clinical symptom of intracranial hypotension (Table 12.4). Unlike intracranial hypertension, where headache occurs in 30–80% of symptomatic patients, headache is present in most patients with symptomatic intracranial hypotension.[10] Symptomatic intracranial hypotension without headache typically occurs in elderly individuals with CSF shunting (usually for a communicating hydrocephalus) and excessive drainage. (Evidence of sinking of the brain is typically absent, perhaps because the effects of brain atrophy and reduced CSF volume balance out.[24]) The headache, when present, is typically bilateral.[11] It is accentuated by the erect position and relieved with recumbency (orthostatic headache). The pain is moderate or severe, dull or throbbing in nature, and usually not relieved with analgesics. Head-shaking, coughing, straining, sneezing, and jugular compression aggravate the pain. The more severe the headache, the more likely the patient is to have dizziness, nausea, vomiting, and tinnitus. The longer the patient has been upright, the longer it takes the headache to subside with recumbency.[25] Physical examination is usually normal; however, there may be mild neck stiffness and a slow pulse rate ('vagus pulse') may be present. CSF pressure usually ranges from 0–65 mm H_2O. The CSF composition is usually normal, but protein may be slightly elevated and a few red blood cells may be present.[10]

Many patients who have low CSF pressure have a non-postural headache in addition to their postural headache.[26] Some patients do not have definite orthostatic headaches but instead have constant, lingering headaches that are worse when they are upright and less intense when they are recumbent. Less frequently the opposite is noted: an initially lingering headache that transfers into a typical orthostatic headache days or weeks later. When CSF leak is intermittent, the headache may also be intermittent and have variable features.[11]

Intracranial hypotension can be divided into two categories (Table 12.5):

- spontaneous, with no obvious evidence of CSF leak or systemic illness; and
- symptomatic, which may be associated with a CSF leak.[27]

The IHS[1] classifies low CSF pressure headache as one that 'occurs or worsens less than 15 minutes after assuming the upright position and disappears or improves less than 30 minutes after resuming the recumbent position'.

Table 12.4 *Features of low CSF pressure headache*

Pain: Aggravated by upright position; relieved with recumbency. Aggravated by head shaking and jugular compression.

Associated symptoms: Anorexia, blurry vision, change in hearing, horizontal diplopia, neck or interscapular pain, facial numbness, galactorrhea, arm radiculopathy, nausea, vomiting, dizziness, tinnitus, photophobia, anorexia, and generalized malaise.

Physical examination: Within normal limits (rare neck stiffness, slow pulse rate ('vagus pulse'))

Lumbar puncture: CSF opening pressure from 0 to 70 mm H_2O in the lateral decubitus position

Table 12.5 *Causes of low CSF pressure headache syndrome*

1. Spontaneous intracranial hypotension.
2. Symptomatic
   - A. Lumbar puncture: diagnostic, myelographic and spinal anesthesia
   - B. Traumatic: head or back trauma
     - 1) With CSF leak (dural tear, traumatic nerve root avulsion)
     - 2) Without CSF leak
   - C. Postoperative: craniotomy, spinal surgery, postpneumonectomy (thoracoarachnoid fistula)
     - 1) With CSF leak
     - 2) Without CSF leak
   - D. Spontaneous CSF leak: CSF rhinorrhea, occult pituitary tumor, dural tear.
   - E. Systemic illnesses: dehydration, diabetic coma, hyperpnea, meningoencephalitis, uremia, severe systemic infection.

The most common cause of intracranial hypotension is lumbar puncture. Head or back trauma, craniotomy, and spinal surgery can produce CSF hypotension as a result of a dural tear or traumatic avulsion of a nerve root that results in a CSF leak.[28–30] In addition, craniotomy and trauma can produce intracranial hypotension that is unassociated with a CSF leak. This may be a result of decreased CSF formation, decreased cerebral blood flow, or both.[31] Low pressure syndromes can occur secondary to CSF rhinorrhoea, which may be spontaneous, posttraumatic, or due to a pituitary tumor. Spontaneous dural tears must be ruled out in all cases of spontaneous intracranial hypotension. A systemic medical illness, including severe dehydration, hyperpnoea, meningoencephalitis, uremia, a severe systemic infection, or infusion of hypertonic solution, can cause CSF hypotension. Postural headache can also occur in patients who have had CSF shunts. This is one of the complications of treating idiopathic intracranial hypertension.[32,33] Other causes of spontaneous positional headache, such as a colloid cyst of the IIIrd ventricle, need to be ruled out.[34]

Postlumbar puncture headache is believed to be caused by low CSF volume (and pressure) secondary to CSF leakage. In fact, dural holes and subdural collections of CSF have been observed at laminectomy or autopsy performed postlumbar puncture.[2,35] Kunkle induced postlumbar puncture headache in normal subjects by draining CSF.[36] Headache appeared when pressure was reduced by removing 20 ml of CSF. The estimated intracranial pressure fell to between -220 and -290 mm H_2O from a normal -100 mm H_2O in the sitting position. Performing spinal drainage on a patient who had a prior section of the Vth and IXth cranial nerves and upper cervical nerves on the left side did not produce left-sided headache.[2] No direct correlation exists between the level of pressure on a subsequent lumbar puncture and the presence of either low- or high-pressure headache, but a correlation exists between CSF volume loss and headache.[17] Jugular compression increases headache severity despite increasing intracranial pressure, suggesting that the headache is caused by intracranial hypovolemia, not hypotension.[37] As the low-volume (pressure) headache improves, the associated tinnitus and feeling of ear blockage disappear. An anatomical connection between the subarachnoid space and the cochlea would allow development of labyrinthine hypotension and cochlear symptoms.[2]

The headache of CSF volume depletion is a consequence of descent of the brain. CSF reduces the weight of the floating brain within the cranial cavity to less than 50 g. Even at this reduced weight, the brain must be supported within the cranium. Some of the weight is shared by suspension from above, mostly by the cerebral veins that end in the sagittal sinus and, to a lesser extent, by the cerebellar veins that end in the transverse and straight sinuses. The cerebellar tentorium, the large vessels of the base, and the skull base provide support from below. Various anchoring structures of the brain are pain-sensitive, and pain can be provoked when these structures are subjected to traction or distortion.[38] Sinking of the brain leads to traction or distortion of these structures and, therefore, the appearance of orthostatic or primarily orthostatic headaches.

The same mechanism may be responsible for the cranial nerve palsies, the visual blurring or visual field defects, or even the dizziness or altered hearing that are fairly common in affected patients. Another possible mechanism for the dizziness or disturbed hearing, however, may be altered pressure in the perilymphatic fluid. Stupor, encephalopathy, cerebellar size, and Parkinsonism may result from compression of diencephalon, posterior fossae, and midline structures. Various clinical manifestations and their proposed mechanisms are listed in Table 12.4. Pain at different levels of the spine (cervical, thoracic, and lumbar) is not uncommon but does usually indicate the level of the leak.

Headache follows lumbar puncture in 15–30% of patients. Onset varies from 15 minutes to 4 days following lumbar puncture, but it can take as long as 12 days to manifest. Untreated, the headache typically resolves in 2–14 days (most commonly 4–8 days) but may last for months or even years.[35]

The volume of CSF leakage after lumbar puncture, measured by MRI, does not correlate with the occurrence of postlumbar puncture headache.[39] Postlumbar puncture headache is more common in younger patients and in women, who are affected twice as often as men.[25,35,37,40–42] This sex difference is most marked in younger women in most, but not all, studies.[25] A lower incidence of postlumbar puncture headache in patients with higher opening pressures has been reported but not confirmed.[41,42] Patients who had headaches before lumbar puncture were more likely to report postlumbar puncture headache.[42] Race, quantity of CSF removed, a bloody tap, multiple perforations of the dura, or the qualifications of the operator do not influence the incidence of postlumbar puncture headache (Table 12.6).[35,42] The incidence is dependent upon the type of procedure: surgical lumbar puncture, 13%; obstetrical procedure, 18%; and diagnostic procedure, 32%.[43] Torrey observed that postlumbar puncture headache was rare among schizophrenic patients, perhaps due to their insensitivity to pain.[44] This

● Table 12.6 *Post-LP headache*

Contributing factors
- Prior headache
- Female gender
- Type of procedure
- Size and type of needle

Noncontributing factors
- Race
- Quantity of CSF removed
- Bloody tap
- Multiple perforations of the dura
- Qualifications of the operator

finding was not confirmed in another study.[45] A low frequency of postlumbar puncture headache has been reported in demented patients.[46]

Vilming et al[41] reported a 7% incidence of short duration, nonpostural, postlumbar puncture headache. This type of headache has not been included in past series of postlumbar puncture headache, and it is uncertain whether it is a low-grade postlumbar puncture headache or is totally unrelated. Rare neurologic sequelae include IIIrd, IVth, VIth, and VIIIth nerve palsies causing diplopia, tinnitus, and bilateral deafness.[47] Most patients with postlumbar puncture headache improve spontaneously.

There is no evidence that postlumbar puncture headache is prevented by keeping the patient supine after the lumbar puncture, keeping the patient prone after the lumbar puncture, removing the needle with the patient prone and head down, or maintaining adequate hydration.[2,25,35] In fact, prolonged recumbency may increase the risk of postlumbar puncture headache.[42] Evidence suggests that using a small gauge (smaller than 22) needle may decrease the incidence of postlumbar puncture headache in most[37,48–50] but not all[51] studies. However, using this size of needle for a diagnostic lumbar puncture is difficult. A nontraumatic lumbar puncture needle that reportedly is associated with a low incidence of postlumbar puncture headache has been developed.[52,53]

A distinction must be made between a patient with an orthostatic headache that is relieved by recumbency and a patient with a headache that is aggravated by movement or assuming the upright posture. If the headache is orthostatic and the patient does not have orthostatic hypotension, then the diagnosis is intracranial hypotension, the causes of which are listed in Table 12.5.

The clinical syndrome of spontaneous intracranial hypotension is similar to that of postlumbar puncture headache. Schaltenbrand described three possible mechanisms to explain the pathophysiology of spontaneous intracranial hypotension:

- decreased CSF production;
- increased CSF absorption; and
- CSF leakage from cryptic small dural tears.[4]

By definition, there is intracranial hypotension but no evidence of central nervous system (CNS) trauma or prior lumbar puncture. Cases of spontaneous intracranial hypotension have been reported in which the radionuclide cisternogram showed rapid uptake in the bladder and kidneys and rapid transport of isotope with no evidence of CSF leak.[27,54–56] Rando and Fishman reported rapid uptake in the bladder and kidney in two cases of spontaneous intracranial hypotension secondary to CSF spinal leaks.[57] They believe that hyperabsorption is due to an occult CSF leak and that increased CSF absorption only occurs with elevated intracranial pressure.

Slowing of isotope flow, which is evidence for decreased CSF production, has also been reported.[58–61] This could lead to brain sagging with compression of the pituitary–hypothalamic axis and further reduction in CSF production.[60] Slit-like ventricles and tight basilar cisterns have been reported on computed tomography (CT) scan in patients with spontaneous intracranial hypotension, leading to speculation that this contributed to decreased CSF production.[33] However, small ventricles owing to a compensatory increase in brain volume is most likely a result, rather than a cause, of decreased CSF production.

Occult CSF leakage is probably the major cause of idiopathic intracranial hypotension.[62] A history of minor trauma is often elicited.[63] In 39 Mayo Clinic cases, 52% of patients had a history of minor trauma or an inciting event.[23] These included falling onto the buttocks,[58,64] a sudden twist or stretch,[62,65] sexual intercourse or orgasm,[66] a sudden sneeze or paroxysmal coughing,[67] vigorous exercise,[68] or strenuous effort during racket sports.[69] Traumatic rupture of spinal epidural cysts (formed during development), perineural cysts, or a nerve sheath tear[19,57,62–64,69,70] could then produce a cryptic CSF leak. CSF can also leak into the petrous or ethmoidal regions[71] or through the cribriform, and the patient may swallow the fluid and be unaware of the leak.

The Mayo Clinic[23] series had an equal representation of men and women. The true incidence of spontaneous low CSF pressure headache is unknown. This syndrome is often under-recognized since the neurologic examination is normal and headache is such a common complaint.

The diagnosis of low CSF pressure (Table 12.7) is easily

> ● **Table 12.7** *Findings in intracranial hypotension*
>
> - Reduced CSF opening pressure (opening pressure from 0 to 65 mm H_2O in the lateral decubitus position)
> - CSF pleocytosis and increased protein concentrations
> - Diffuse pachymeningeal gadolinium enhancement
> - Subdural fluid collections
> - Slit ventricles with tight basilar cisterns
> - Enlarged pituitary
> - Engorged cerebral venous sinuses
> - Imaging evidence of descent of the brain
>   - Flattening of optic chiasm
>   - Obliteration of prepontine or perichiasmatic cisterns
>   - Descent of the cerebellar tonsils (may mimic Type I Chiari)
>   - Crowding of posterior fossa

made when orthostatic headache is present, particularly if there is an obvious aetiology, such as head or back trauma, a recent lumbar puncture, a recent craniotomy, or an associated medical illness (Table 12.5).

If no obvious cause is apparent or the diagnosis is uncertain, lumbar puncture at the time of radioisotope cisternography or ionic myelography is indicated, following an MRI with and without gadolinium. Lumbar punctures can be difficult in these patients, with either traumatic or 'dry' taps. Some patients require cisternal taps for fluid collection. When the CSF pressure is below atmospheric pressure, a 'sucking noise' may be heard when the stylet is removed from the lumbar puncture needle, and air may be visible within the lateral ventricles on X-ray.[23] The opening pressure usually ranges from 0–70 mm H_2O. However, in the Mayo Clinic series in spontaneous intracranial hypotension, the opening pressure was at times in the normal range, especially if the measurement was made after a period of recumbency.[23]

CSF analysis is benign in low-pressure headache. Reported abnormalities include a moderate pleocytosis, the presence of red blood cells, and elevated protein. The elevated protein may be due to disruption of normal hydrostatic and oncotic pressure across the venous sinus and arachnoid villi, resulting in serum protein passing into the CSF.[16,57,72]

Radioisotope cisternography or ionic myelography is done to identify CSF leaks that may have resulted from a dural tear.[73] Occult CSF rhinorrhoea should be searched for by examining the collection of radioisotope in the nose using numbered cotton pledgets. A radioactive tracer is instilled into the lumbar subarachnoid space. Its pattern of distribution is followed by scanning the entire neuraxis with a gamma camera at 4, 8, and 24 hours. CSF normally

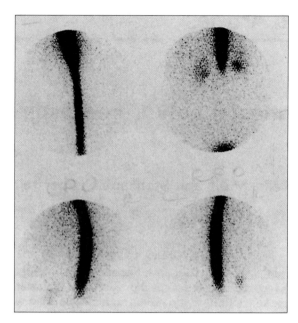

● **Figure 12.6.** *Scintigraph at 45 minutes showing early bladder and kidney uptake. No evidence of CSF leak. (Reproduced from ref. 23, with permission.)*

flows upward to the cerebral convexities and the sylvian fissures.[27] Early isotope accumulation in the bladder and kidneys or leakage outside the subarachnoid space is abnormal and should be looked for (Figure 12.6).

CSF hyperabsorption is one explanation for intracranial hypotension.[54,56,74] However, the early appearance of tracer in the bladder is usually secondary to an occult CSF leak and not due to hyperabsorption.[57] Water-soluble myelography and CT myelography have been used to help localize the site(s) of CSF leakage, and some leaks may still be missed. Although CT myelography has a somewhat higher yield, the yield of both studies may be suboptimal.[71] Nonionic (pantopaque) myelography, which is no longer available, revealed dural tears even when cisternography and ionic myelography were normal. If no secondary cause is present and no dural leak can be demonstrated, spontaneous intracranial hypotension should be considered.[4,27,61,62,75] However, the inability to detect a leak despite early filling of the bladder does not necessarily mean the mechanism is hyperabsorption.

Neuroimaging in intracranial hypotension (MRI, myelography, CT myelography)

Diffuse meningeal enhancement (DME) on enhanced gadolinium MRI is the most common MRI abnormality in CSF leaks and CSF volume depletion (Figure 12.7, Tables 12.7 and 12.8).[21] Meningeal enhancement occurs with

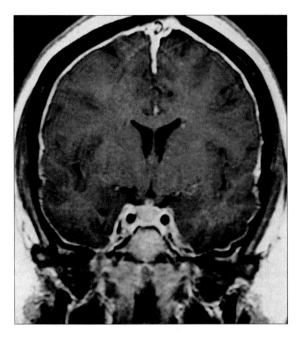

● **Figure 12.7** *Diffuse meningeal enhancement. (Reproduced from ref. 163, with permission.)*

● **Table 12.8** *Diffuse meningeal enhancement*

- Both supra- and infratentorial
- Pachymeningeal
- No enhancement of depths or cortical sulci
- No brainstem enhancement

severe posttraumatic,[76] positional,[19,20,77,78] spontaneous, and postlumbar puncture headache. One spontaneous case had a negative meningeal biopsy.[20] After the patient recovered, the meningeal enhancement disappeared. Before DME was a recognized feature of spontaneous intracranial hypotension, patients often had extensive testing to rule out other causes of meningeal enhancement, such as meningeal carcinomatosis, meningitis, subarachnoid hemorrhage, neuroborreliosis, and neurosarcoidosis.[77,79]

Diffuse pachymeningeal enhancement is limited to the pachymeninges, without any evidence of leptomeningeal involvement. The enhancement is both supratentorial and infratentorial. It is nonnodular, linear, and typically uninterrupted.[21,80] It is of variable thickness, often being thick and obvious, but sometimes very thin. DME may improve or resolve with headache resolution.[19,21,77,79,81] Mokri's group

has reviewed many of the radiologic features of low CSF volume headache.[79,80,82,83]

Descent of the brain or 'sagging' or 'sinking' of the brain is also a common MRI finding and is manifested by descent of the cerebellar tonsils (which may sometimes mimic type 1 Chiari malformation),[84] decrease in the size of the prepontine cistern, inferior displacement of the optic chiasm, effacement of perichiasmatic cisterns, and crowding of the posterior fossa (Figure 12.5).

Subdural fluid collections are usually but not always bilateral. These are thin (2–7 mm in maximal thickness) without compression or effacement of the underlying sulci.

Decrease in the size of the ventricles, or 'ventricular collapse', is not always obvious and is best noted when a head MRI obtained after recovery is compared with a previous MRI taken during the symptomatic phase.

MRI abnormalities result from CSF volume depletion. Loss of CSF volume leads to sinking of the brain and descent of the cerebellar tonsils, collapse and decrease in the size of the ventricles, decrease in the size of the subarachnoid cisterns, flattening of the optic chiasm, and crowding of the posterior fossa. The CSF volume loss is compensated for by an increase in intracranial blood volume as well as subdural fluid collected. Intracranial blood volume mainly involves the venous system and is manifested by meningeal venous hyperemia. Because leptomeninges have blood–brain barriers and pachymeninges do not, it is the pachymeninges that enhance with gadolinium.[7,19,85] Other manifestations of compensatory venous hypervolemia include engorgement of the venous sinuses and pituitary gland and prominence and engorgement of the spinal epidural venous plexus.

Myelography with water-soluble contrast material, especially when followed by CT scanning (CT myelography), is the most accurate test for demonstrating the site of CSF leaks.[82] It can demonstrate extra-arachnoid or extradural contrast, as well as penetration of contrast (and therefore the leaked CSF) in the paraspinal soft tissues. This sometimes presents as elongated collections in the epidural space within the spinal canal and on axial CT cuts may appear as 'dog ear-shaped' collections located ventral or dorsal to the thecal sac. CT and CT myelography also show meningeal diverticula of various sizes. Myelography also provides an opportunity to measure the CSF opening pressure and obtain fluid for analysis.

Biopsy

The justification for subjecting patients to meningeal biopsy no longer exists. The information on biopsy dates back to the initial observations of meningeal enhancement on MRI, when clinicians were not confident about the association of pachymeningeal enhancement and CSF leaks or intracranial hypotension.[18,20,21,76,77] Then, understandably, patients were vigorously investigated for various types of meningeal disease, particularly meningeal inflammation, infection, and meningeal carcinomatosis.

Meningeal biopsy has shown normal appearance of the dura on gross examination. The leptomeninges also appear normal, except in some of the long-standing cases, wherein the arachnoid may appear thickened or opaque. Microscopically, the dura appears entirely normal on its epidural aspect. However, a fairly thin zone of fibroblasts and thin-walled blood vessels in an amorphous matrix resembling an organized hygroma is typically noted in the subdural aspect of the dura. Arachnoidal cell hyperplasia may be seen in chronic cases. No particular cellular infiltration or inflammatory change is noted. Dural meningeal abnormalities probably represent secondary reactive phenomena most likely related to the changes in CSF volume or pressure.[80]

Chen et al[86] used color Doppler flow imaging to measure superior ophthalmic vein blood flow in patients with suspected intracranial hypotension (orthostatic headache and clinical features of intracranial hypotension). The mean diameter of the superior ophthalmic vein was substantially larger in the patients with intracranial hypotension (3.9 (SD 0.2) mm) than in the healthy controls (2.6 (SD 0.4) mm) and the headache controls (2.7 (SD 0.2) mm) ($p < 0.0001$). The mean maximum flow velocity was significantly higher in the intracranial hypotension group (17.0 (SD 3.4) cm/s) than in the healthy controls (7.9 (SD 1.1) cm/s) and the other patients (7.3 (SD 1.7) cm/s) ($p < 0.0001$). Seven patients with intracranial hypotension were reassessed after being treated with an epidural blood patch. The clinical symptoms were relieved and there was a striking reversal of the superior ophthalmic vein flow. Superior ophthalmic vein blood flow measured by color doppler flow imaging may provide a practical, simple, and non-invasive diagnostic method for suspected intracranial hypotension.

The clinical-imaging spectrum of CSF volume depletion

Mokri and Bahram[7] have described four clinical syndromes in CSF volume depletion (Table 12.9).

I. Classic form: headaches (typically orthostatic), low CSF pressure, and typical MRI abnormalities are noted.
II. Normal-pressure: typical clinical manifestations and imaging abnormalities are present, but despite documented CSF leak, CSF opening pressures are consistently within limits of normal.[83]
III. Normal meninges: despite typical clinical manifestations and documented CSF leak and low CSF pressures, meninges appear normal on MR imaging.[7]
IV. No headache: typical MRI abnormalities are present and CSF pressure is low, but headaches are curiously absent despite documented CSF volume depletion as the result of CSF leak or CSF shunt overdrainage.[77]

'CSF volume depletion' may reflect this clinical-imaging spectrum more accurately than 'intracranial hypotension'.

Treatment

Many treatment modalities exist for intracranial hypotension, including bed rest, peripheral intravascular volume expansion, steroids, caffeine, blood patch, abdominal binder, and continuous intrathecal saline infusion (Table 12.10).[33,55,67,87–90] The treatment should be based on the cause (Table 12.5). Any associated illness should be

---

● **Table 12.9** *Low CSF volume syndromes*

	Headache	DPME	SB	Subdural	Low Pressure
Type I (Classic)	+	+	+/−	+/−	+
Type II (Normal pressure)	+	+	+/−	+/−	−
Type III (No DPME)	+	−	+/−	+/−	+/−
Type IV (No headache)	-	+	+/−	+/−	+/−

Reproduced with permission from Mokri and Bahram.[7]
DPME, diffuse pachymeningeal enhancement
SB, sagging brain

Table 12.10 *Treatment of low-CSF pressure headache*

Nonpharmacologic
    Bed rest
    Abdominal binder
Intravenous and oral pharmacologic
    Caffeine, theophylline
    Corticosteroids, ACTH
Epidural interventions
    Blood patch
    Sodium chloride
    Dextran patch
    Injection of fibrin glue
    Morphine sulphate
Surgical repair of the leak

treated and if a CSF leak exists, it should be treated appropriately and repaired if it is accessible and can be identified. The treatment of postlumbar puncture headache and spontaneous intracranial hypotension are similar. Postcraniotomy hypotension will not be discussed. Treatment of low CSF pressure headache begins with non-invasive therapeutic modalities (Table 12.10) of bed rest and an abdominal binder. If these modalities are pro-longed, however, they are not cost-effective; therefore, if there is no improvement, intravenous or oral caffeine can be used and may produce significant relief.

Caffeine produces intracerebral arterial constriction, probably by blockading brain adenosine receptors.[25] Caffeine sodium benzoate 500 mg intravenously was dramatically effective in 75% of patients with low CSF pressure who had undergone previous lumbar puncture.[87] A second dose 2 hours later raised the success rate to 85%. In an open study, 2 litres of intravenous Ringer's lactate solution containing 500 mg of caffeine sodium benzoate was given at a rate of 1 litre for the first hour and then 1 litre over 2 hours. Both could be repeated after 4 hours. The total response rate in 18 patients was 75%.[91]

In a placebo-controlled, double-blind study,[33] postpartum patients were given oral caffeine (300 mg): 120% the dose of caffeine in caffeine sodium benzoate (250 mg caffeine, 250 mg sodium benzoate). Beneficial effects were rapid, with 70% of patients experiencing relief within 4 hours and no symptom recurrence.[92]

A brief trial of steroids and caffeine, bed rest, or an abdominal binder may be beneficial. If relief is not obtained within 24 hours, a quick steroid taper is recommended because of potential side-effects. If the patient continues to be symptomatic after a noninvasive medical approach, a blood patch is indicated.

With a 96.8% success rate, the blood patch, originally described by Gormley in 1960,[93] is the most successful treatment for low CSF pressure headache.[94–96] It is performed by infusing 10–20 ml of autologous blood in the epidural space under sterile conditions. A prospective study conducted to evaluate the efficacy of different volumes of blood found no difference between 10 ml and 10–15 ml of blood (determined by patient height). The blood patch was initially successful in 91% of patients 2 hours after the procedure. Long-term, 87% were satisfied, but only 61% had both immediate and permanent relief. Results did not differ according to the volume injected.[97] Many investigators have performed blood patches for spontaneous intracranial hypotension and have described similar results. The presumed mechanism of action of the blood patch is an immediate gelatinous tamponade of the dural leak followed by fibrin deposition and fibroblastic activity. The blood patch can tolerate a pressure as high as 40 mm Hg soon after coagulation.[97] Collagen deposition and scar formation are complete within 3 weeks. However, this mechanism has recently been challenged by several investigators who have noted a recurrence of orthostatic headache 4–6 months after a successful blood patch.[25] They propose that compression of the dural sac with an increment in CSF pressure may serve as a signal that deactivates the low CSF pressure headache, possibly by antagonizing adenosine receptors.[25]

MRI at 30 minutes and 3 hours has shown the extradural blood patch to have a mass effect, compressing the dural sac and displacing the conus medullaris and cauda equina. The main bulk of the clot occupied four or five vertebral levels, with a thinner spread cephalad and caudad. Initially some blood entered the CSF and changed the MRI signal, but this concentrated to a focal dural clot by 3 hours. After 7 hours, the mass effect had disappeared (Figure 12.8).[98]

If the headache of intracranial hypotension recurs, a repeat blood patch should be performed or a continuous intrathecal saline infusion attempted.[90,94] In the latter procedure, an epidural catheter is placed at the L2–3 level and a saline infusion begun at a rate of 20 ml/hour and continued for as long as 72 hours.

A retrospective study of 196 patients treated with the epidural blood patch revealed no major complications. Thirty-seven percent had pain at the injection site, 12% had leg pain, 10% had sensory disturbances in the lower extremities, 8% had gait disturbances, and 8% had leg weakness. These symptoms were mild and transient.[99]

Increased intracranial pressure

Many disorders are associated with the syndrome of increased intracranial pressure (Table 12.11). Intracranial

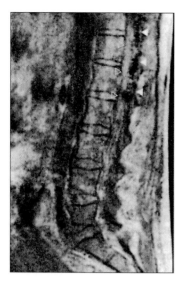

Figure 12.8
Midline T1
weighted sagittal
section (GE
500/14/90)
showing normal
appearances
before blood patch.
(Reproduced from
ref. 164, with
permission.)

Table 12.12 Mechanisms for headache with increased intracranial pressure

1. Traction on pain-sensitive intracerebral vessels (venous sinuses and arteries at the base of the brain).
2. Transient herniation of hippocampal gyri.
3. Traction on cranial or cervical nerves, or elevation of intracranial pressure.

Postulated mechanisms for headache are listed in Table 12.12. A convexity meningioma may distort the adjacent middle meningeal artery and cause pain, which may be referred to the ipsilateral frontotemporal region (Figure 12.9). A posterior fossa tumor may impinge upon the VIIth cranial nerve, producing a headache that is referred to the ipsilateral ear.

Although increased CSF pressure is not necessary for headache development, it clearly plays a role in some patients with CNS neoplasms, acute obstructive hydrocephalus, and idiopathic intracranial hypertension. The rate of the change in pressure may be critical. Sudden increases in intracranial pressure caused by tumors obstructing the foramen of Monro or the cerebral aqueduct may cause abrupt, severe headache associated with gait disturbance, syncope, incontinence, or visual obscurations.

hypertension may be idiopathic (no clear identifiable cause) or symptomatic. It is often difficult to correlate the clinical features with the underlying pathological process, since increased intracranial pressure is not always associated with either headache or papilledema, and no direct correlation exists between the degree of pressure elevation and the presence of headache. Headache does not usually occur with mild-to-moderate elevations of intracranial pressure when there is no associated traction or distortion of pain-sensitive structures; however, this is not the case in at least two conditions (acute hydrocephalus and essential intracranial hypertension).

Intracranial neoplasms

Headache occurs at presentation in up to 20% of patients with brain tumors and develops in the course of the disease in 60%. Headache is a rare initial symptom in

Table 12.11 Syndromes of increased intracranial pressure

1. Primary
   A. Idiopathic intracranial hypertension with papilledema
   B. Idiopathic intracranial hypertension without papilledema
2. Secondary
   A. Hydrocephalus
   B. Mass lesion
      Neoplasm
      Stroke – hematoma
   C. Meningitis/encephalitis
   D. Trauma
   E. Major intracranial and extracranial venous obstruction
   F. Drugs: vitamin A, nalidixic acid, anabolic steroids, steroid withdrawal
   G. Systemic disease: renal disease, hypoparathyroidism, systemic lupus erythematosus

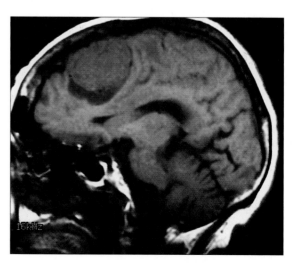

Figure 12.9 Meningioma.

patients with pituitary tumors, craniopharyngiomas, or cerebellopontine angle tumors.[100,101] Headache is a very common initial symptom with infratentorial tumors (other than cerebellopontine angle tumors), occurring in 80–85% of patients.[102,103] Elevation of intracranial pressure is not necessary to produce headache. In one older, pre-CT series of 72 brain-tumor patients, headache occurred in those patients without elevated intracranial pressure as often as it did in those with elevated intracranial pressure.[101] The headache is usually bilateral, but it can occur only on the side of the tumor.[100,101] Supratentorial tumors that impinge on structures innervated by the ophthalmic division of the Vth cranial nerve may produce frontotemporal headache, while posterior fossa tumors may compress the IXth and Xth cranial nerves and produce occipitonuchal pain. Metastatic brain tumors may invade the meninges (meningeal carcinomatosis) and produce generalized headache and other signs of meningeal irritation. Occasionally, brain tumors produce a migraine-like headache, even with a visual aura. The severe headaches can be aggravated by Valsalva, position change, or exertion and probably result from sudden increases in intracranial pressure or traction on pain-sensitive structures, such as the dura, cranial nerves, or large venous sinuses.[104]

One pre-CT/MRI series looked at the characteristic headache features of 221 patients who had brain tumors, only 60% of whom had headache. Tumor location had no significant bearing on the presence or absence of headache. Pain intensity was mild to moderate in 63% of patients and severe in 37%. The headaches were intermittent in 85% of patients, throbbing in 15%, aggravated by changing position in 20% and by coughing or exertion in 25%, and on the side of the tumor in 30%. Five patients had exertional headaches. Half the patients had nausea or vomiting. Twenty-five percent had headache during sleep, on arising, or both. Increased intracranial pressure was observed in 42% of patients with headache and in 6% of patients without headache.[105]

In a survey of 778 patients with cerebral tumor, headache was the earliest or principal symptom in 54%. No difference in headache frequency was noted between rapidly-growing and slow-growing tumors. The headache can occur intermittently and mimic migraine.[106]

In a recent series of 111 consecutive patients with primary (34%) or metastatic (66%) brain tumor, diagnosis was based on neuroimaging.[107] Increased intracranial pressure was defined by the presence of papilledema, obstructive hydrocephalus, communicating hydrocephalus from leptomeningeal metastasis, or a lumbar puncture opening pressure >250 mm H_2O of CSF. Headache was present in 48% of both primary and metastatic tumors.

The pain was similar to tension-type headache (TTH) in 77% of patients, to migraine in 9%, and to other headache types in 14%. Unlike true TTH, brain-tumor headaches were worsened by bending in 32% of patients and nausea or vomiting was present in 40%.[107]

Eighty-six percent of patients with increased intracranial pressure usually had headaches that were typically frontal and pressure-like or aching. Only 1% of patients had a unilateral headache. The headache was constant in 61% of patients. The pain was severe, associated with nausea and vomiting, and resistant to common analgesics. Ataxia was present in 61% of patients. In contrast, only 36% of patients who had a supratentorial tumor without increased intracranial pressure had headaches. These headaches were milder and more likely to be intermittent (however, they were constant in 20% of patients). Nausea, vomiting, and ataxia were much less common.[107]

Patients with a history of prior headaches were more likely to have headaches with their brain tumor. In many cases, this headache was similar in character to the prior headache, but it was more severe, more frequent, or associated with neurologic signs or symptoms. In a prospective study of patients with brain tumor, only 8% had headache as their first and isolated clinical manifestation at the time of diagnosis. Thirty-one percent had headache, but only one of the original patients continued to have headache as an isolated symptom.[108] The prevalence of headache as an initial symptom of brain tumor has decreased in many series due to earlier detection by neuroimaging (Figure 12.10).

Other space-occupying lesions

In other space-occupying lesions, such as subdural hematomas and brain abscesses, headache is an earlier and more frequent symptom. Eighty-one percent of McKissock's[109] 216 patients with chronic subdural hematoma had headache; only 11% of acute and 53% of subacute subdural hematoma patients had headache. The difference in headache prevalence between patients with tumor and patients with subdural hematoma is believed to be due to the more rapid evolution and greater extent of the hematomas. The lesser occurrence of headache in patients with acute and subacute subdural hematomas compared with patients with chronic subdural hematomas may be due to the underlying traumatic cerebral changes in the former, which obtund consciousness early and make it difficult to elicit a history of headache (Figure 12.11). In brain abscesses, a progressively severe, intractable headache is common. It was present in 70–90% of patients in one published clinical series (Figure 12.12).[110] The higher headache prevalence in patients with abscesses, compared with those with tumors, may be due

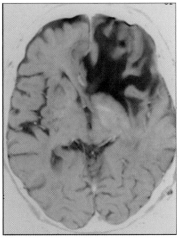

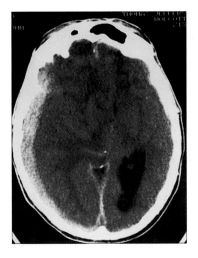

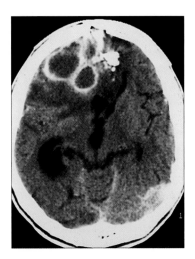

● *Figure 12.10* Glioma.   ● *Figure 12.11* Subdural.   ● *Figure 12.12* Brain abscess.

to the faster evolution, the associated meningeal reaction, and the occasional low-grade fever that may accompany abscesses (see Chapter 14).

Uncommon headaches

Paroxysmal headaches are a unique feature experienced by some patients who have a colloid cyst of the third ventricle or other pedunculated tumor that may obstruct CSF flow. These headaches are often sudden in onset, reach peak intensity in seconds, and are brief. They may also resolve quickly and may be precipitated (and relieved) by changes in position. They may be a cause of brief losses of consciousness or 'drop attacks'. Patients may walk unsteadily between headaches.

Cough or exertional headache is a transient, severe headache precipitated by Valsalva maneuver or running. These headaches are usually brief and poorly localized. Brain tumors have been identified in 2–11% of patients who have these types of headaches.[111,112]

Headaches may be caused by metastasis to the skull base. Five syndromes based on location have been defined.[113] These include:

(1) orbital syndrome, which consists of a dull supraorbital ache that may be followed by diplopia, proptosis, and later visual loss;
(2) parasellar syndrome (metastasis to the sella turcica, cavernous sinus), which consists of unilateral frontal headache, periorbital edema, ocular paresis, and ophthalmic trigeminal sensory loss;
(3) gasserian ganglion syndrome, which is characterized as a dull ache in the cheek, jaw, or forehead, occasional trigeminal neuralgia-like

pain, and loss of sensation in the V_2 and V_3 sensory distribution;
(4) jugular foramen syndrome, which consists of unilateral, dull, aching, retroauricular pain, hoarseness, and dysphagia; and
(5) occipital condyle syndrome, which consists of severe, unilateral, occipital headaches that are aggravated by neck flexion. Patients may also complain of dysarthria and dysphagia. Ipsilateral tongue atrophy is common.[10]

Headaches occur as a symptom of brain tumor more commonly in children (over 90%) than in adults (≈60%), perhaps owing to the greater prevalence of posterior fossa tumors in children.[114] The following characteristics occur frequently in children with brain tumors: headache awakening the child from sleep or present on awakening, severe or prolonged headache, increased severity or frequency of headache, and increased frequency of vomiting. Most of the children (94%) who had headaches had neurologic signs. In 96%, diagnostic clues appeared within 4 months of the onset of headache.[115]

Rossi and Vassella[116] compared 600 children with migraine with 67 children with brain tumors. Characteristic features in the brain-tumor group were nocturnal headache or headache present on arising, both associated with vomiting and increased headache frequency. These symptoms were present in 32% of the brain-tumor group and 10% of the childhood-migraine group. Nocturnal headache or headache present on arising associated with vomiting or progressive neurologic symptoms or signs occurred in 65 of the 67 children with brain tumor within 2 months of headache onset. Zammarano et al[117] found five of 2416 tumor patients who presented with migraine-like headache had no other signs of tumor. Changes in cognition may be the first sign of brain tumor. Children with headache must be followed to establish that they have normal growth and intellectual and motor development.

In Kennedy and Nathwani's[118] brain-tumor series, headache was the presenting symptom in 53% of children, but most had other symptoms and signs as well, and 46% had papilledema. The median duration of headache before tumor diagnosis in these children was 5 months.[119] In this series, brain-tumor headaches could mimic migraine or TTH, sometimes for years.

In 1991, the Childhood Brain Tumor Consortium published their retrospective record review on the incidence of headache in children with CNS tumors. The overall incidence of headache was 62%, ranging from 70% in patients who had infratentorial lesions, to 58% in patients who had supratentorial tumors, to 35% in patients with spinal canal tumors, approximately the incidence of benign headache in elementary school children. Headache was typically associated with other signs or symptoms and was an isolated symptom in less than 1%. Symptoms of intracranial tumor included abnormal academic performance, difficulty walking, back or abdominal pain, bladder symptoms, increasing head circumference, and failure to thrive. Regardless of tumor location, headache frequency increases in the (individual) child through age 7 years, then levels off. The low percentage of headache in the very young may be due to the expansile nature of the infant skull or may be an artefact of the inability of young children to communicate the source of their discomfort.[120]

Fourteen to 32 months following successful combined whole brain radiotherapy and chemotherapy of their posterior fossa or pineal tumors, four children developed episodic, severe hemicranial headaches associated with nausea and transient visual loss, hemisensory deficit, dysphasia, or hemiparesis.[121] These children had no prior history of similar headaches, no family history of migraine, and no evidence of tumor recurrence. The cause of these migrainous manifestations is unclear. Headache in treated brain-tumor patients does not necessarily mean tumor recurrence.

Intracranial hypertension in the absence of a space-occupying lesion

Intracranial hypertension may be either idiopathic, with no clear identifiable cause, or symptomatic, a result of venous sinus occlusion, radical neck dissection, hypoparathyroidism, vitamin A intoxication, systemic lupus erythematosus, renal disease, or drug side-effects (nalidixic acid, danocrine, or steroid withdrawal) (Table 12.11).[122]

The syndrome of idiopathic intracranial hypertension, also known as 'pseudotumor cerebri' or 'benign intracranial hypertension', is a condition of increased intracranial pressure of unknown cause that occurs predominantly in obese women of childbearing age (Table 12.11). A definitive diagnosis cannot be made without excluding brain tumors and other intracranial mass lesions, infections, hypertensive encephalopathy, pulmonary encephalopathy (related to chronic carbon dioxide toxicity), and obstruction of the cerebral ventricles. The adjective 'benign' is no longer employed because, although spontaneous recovery usually occurs, this is not invariable and permanent visual loss may occur. In fact, visual loss occurs in 80% of patients, and blindness occurs in 10%.[123,124] The symptoms of idiopathic intracranial hypertension are those of generalized increased intracranial pressure, with headache occurring in most, but not all, patients. Idiopathic intracranial hypertension can cause unilateral, bilateral, frontal, or occipital headache, although bifrontotemporal headache is the most common.[125] Unilateral headache with increased CSF pressure due to idiopathic intracranial hypertension may be an exacerbation of a migraine diathesis or a new local phenomenon. Transient visual obscuration (TVO),[126] an episode of visual clouding in one or both eyes, usually lasting seconds, occurs with all forms of increased intracranial pressure with papilledema but is not a specific symptom. TVO can occur in patients without increased intracranial pressure who have elevated optic discs from other causes, such as disc edema, nerve sheath tumor, drusen, or coloboma. Other common symptoms include pulsatile tinnitus, diplopia, and visual loss. Some patients report shoulder and arm pain (perhaps secondary to nerve root dilation) and retroorbital pain.[123] Signs include papilledema and VIth nerve palsy.

Idiopathic intracranial hypertension occurs with a frequency of about one case per 100 000 per year in the general population and 19.3 cases per 100 000 per year in obese women aged 20–44 years.[127] The patient with idiopathic intracranial hypertension is commonly a young, obese woman with chronic daily headaches, normal laboratory studies, a normal neurologic examination (except for papilledema), and an empty sella (Table 12.13, Figures 12.13 and 12.14).

No evidence links idiopathic intracranial hypertension with pregnancy, hypertension, diabetes, thyroid disease, iron-deficiency anemia, or tetracycline or oral contraceptive use. Arterial hypertension may be overreported in obese patients with idiopathic intracranial hypertension if a large blood pressure cuff is not used.[123] Symptomatic intracranial hypertension can be secondary to changes in cranial venous outflow, which may influence intracranial pressure by:

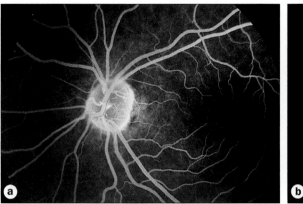
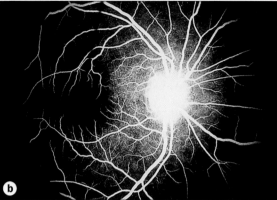

● *Figure 12.13* *Papilledema fundi. (a) Normal. (b) Papilledema.*

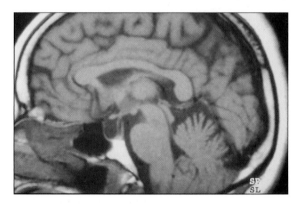

● *Figure 12.14* *Empty sella.*

- increasing cerebral blood volume;
- producing brain edema; and
- impairing CSF absorption.

Intracranial venous outflow obstruction can be caused by chronic otitis, head trauma, tumors, hypercoagulable states, and cerebral edema.[128] Extracranial venous outflow obstruction occurs with surgical ligation and further compression of venous outflow. Cranial venous outflow hypertension can also occur without obstruction in patients with arteriovenous malformations, cardiac failure, and pulmonary failure. The pathophysiology of idiopathic intracranial hypertension is unknown. Postulated mechanisms are listed in Table 12.14. Some studies suggest that interstitial brain edema and a decreased rate of absorption at the arachnoid villi are the major contributors.[129–137] The disturbances of CSF hydrodynamics in idiopathic intracranial hypertension persist for years.[138]

Malm et al[138] believe that increased CSF pressure in idiopathic intracranial hypertension is a result of either a

● **Table 12.13** *Features of idiopathic intracranial hypertension*

1. Headache: chronic tension-type headache with migrainous features, may be present upon awakening. Can be intermittent or absent.
2. Associated features: pulsatile tinnitus, transient visual obscurations, diplopia, visual loss, shoulder and arm pain.
3. Patients: predominantly obese women aged 20–50 years.
4. Physical and neurologic examinations: within normal limits, except for papilledema, visual loss, obesity, and a VIth nerve palsy.
5. Neuroradiology: CT or MRI show no evidence of intracranial mass, hydrocephalus, or venous sinus thrombosis. (Empty sella may be present.)
6. Lumbar puncture: demonstrates increased CSF pressure with a normal composition. (May show decreased protein.)
7. No other causes of increased CSF pressure present.

● **Table 12.14** *Pathophysiology of idiopathic intracranial hypertension*

1. Increased rate of CSF formation
2. Increased intracranial venous pressure
3. Decreased rate of CSF absorption
4. Increase in brain interstitial fluid (edema).

rise in venous sagittal sinus pressure secondary to extracellular edema causing venous obstruction or a low conductance for CSF reabsorption that produces a compensatory increase in CSF pressure. King et al[139] evaluated nine idiopathic intracranial hypertension patients using cerebral venography and manometry. Elevated

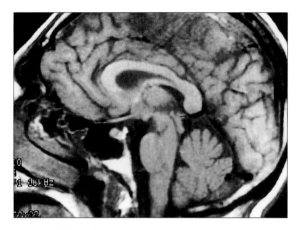

● *Figure 12.15* Venous obstruction.

venous pressure was found in the superior sagittal and proximal transverse sinuses, which dropped at the level of the lateral third of the transverse sinus. The abnormality, not as well demonstrated on venography, resembled mural thrombosis. Two patients with intracranial hypertension due to minocycline did not have venous hypertension. The authors suggested that most patients with idiopathic intracranial hypertension have partial venous outflow obstructions,[139] blurring the distinction between idiopathic and symptomatic causes (Figure 12.15).

Using angiography and manometry, Karahalios et al[140] studied ten patients with idiopathic intracranial hypertension. Five patients had dural venous outflow obstruction on venography while five had normal anatomy. Pressure was elevated in the superior sagittal sinus in all patients. A high-pressure gradient was observed across the stenosis in those patients with obstruction. In those without obstruction, the right atrial pressure was elevated. Angioplasty or infusion of thrombolytic agents improved outlet obstruction but not the clinical picture. The authors suggested that elevated intracranial venous pressure may be the universal mechanism of idiopathic intracranial hypertension, and that all cases are symptomatic. Our major concern with this observation is the absence of any sign of right heart failure in the patients with elevated right atrial pressure.

Headache owing to idiopathic intracranial hypertension occurs in about 75% of cases. It is more common in patients who present to neurologists (in Weisberg's series 100% had headache) than in those who present to ophthalmologists with visual loss or to otolaryngologists with tinnitus.[141] Although their headaches may be very severe, patients with idiopathic intracranial hypertension are, on the whole, not particularly ill. Somnolence, fever, or other systemic symptoms should suggest venous sinus occlusion

or some other cause of increased pressure. If the patient has been headache-prone in the past, the headaches of idiopathic intracranial hypertension may be qualitatively similar but more constant and severe. Patients who have idiopathic intracranial hypertension usually have daily, continuous headaches that qualify as chronic daily headaches.

Wall[125] recently described the headache of idiopathic intracranial hypertension. Most of the patients had severe daily headaches that they described as more severe and different from previous headaches. The headaches commonly awakened the patient from sleep, were pulsating in character, and had associated symptoms of nausea, vomiting, and pulsatile tinnitus and the common feature of retroocular pain with eye movement.

Most of the patients in Wall's study were women (93%) and obese (93%). The mean age was 31 years. Headache was reported by 92% of patients: of those, 73% had chronic daily headache, 93% said it was the most severe ever, and 83% said it was pulsatile. Nausea occurred in 57% of patients, vomiting in 38%, and orbital pain in 43%. TVO was present in 71%, diplopia in 38%, and visual loss in 31%.[125]

Pain on eye movement, while not a common feature of migraine, occurs in up to 20% of patients with idiopathic intracranial hypertension.[123,125] The typical ocular pain is retrobulbar and bilateral, in contrast to the unilateral pain on eye movement that is associated with the visual loss that occurs with optic neuritis.

Another feature of idiopathic intracranial hypertension is a cranial bruit that may be audible to observers. The bruit, caused by turbulence in the major venous sinuses, may be soft- or high-pitched and is best auscultated with the bell over the mastoid or the temporalis while the mouth is held open.[142]

Occasionally, patients with idiopathic intracranial hypertension are found to have papilledema while being examined for another purpose. Five to 10% of patients are essentially asymptomatic.[142] Loss of visual field and visual acuity are the only significant complications of idiopathic intracranial hypertension with papilledema. Ophthalmologic examination should include intraocular pressure, visual fields (Goldmann or Humphrey), optic disc photos, visual acuity, and a search for a relative afferent pupil.[142]

Papilledema is the hallmark sign of idiopathic intracranial hypertension, but rarely patients with increased intracranial pressure do not have papilledema.[143–145] Examination of the dilated ocular fundus using indirect ophthalmoscopy is necessary to be certain there is no optic disc edema.

Recognizing early papilledema can be difficult. The

earliest sign is optic disc elevation, which, however, may also occur as a normal variant. The earliest objective signs of papilledema are (1) edema in the peripapillary region that obscures the details of the adjacent nerve fiber layer; (2) coarsening and irregularity of this nerve fiber layer; (3) loss of spontaneous venous pulsations after previous documentation of their presence; and (4) associated choroidal folds. When papilledema is difficult to determine, repeated examinations or serial optic disc stereo photographs are useful.

Papilledema is the cause of most of the visual loss that occurs with idiopathic intracranial hypertension. Although there is a significant correlation between high grade papilledema and atrophic papilledema and visual loss[146,147] in the individual patient, the severity of visual loss cannot be predicted from the severity of the papilledema. A partial explanation for this is that the amount of papilledema decreases with axonal death from optic nerve compression. Horizontal diplopia occurs in about one of three patients with idiopathic intracranial hypertension, and VIth nerve palsies are present in 10–20% of patients in large series. A relative afferent pupillary defect, which occurs in about 25% of patients, is a sensitive sign of a unilateral optic neuropathy. It is usually absent in idiopathic intracranial hypertension, since its existence depends on asymmetry of visual loss and the optic neuropathy of idiopathic intracranial hypertension is usually fairly symmetric. Visual acuity is usually unaffected in patients with papilledema except when the condition is long-standing. A better measure of central visual loss is contrast sensitivity testing. As opposed to Snellen acuity, it reveals deficits in 50–75% of eyes tested.

Most patients with papilledema (50–94%) have visual loss,[124] which is asymptomatic in 25–50% of patients. However, it is important to measure since it serves as a marker for therapeutic intervention. Perimetry is the main measure used to determine the course of therapy. The visual field defects found in idiopathic intracranial hypertension are the same types as those that are reported to occur in papilledema due to other causes. These 'disc-related defects' are the same type as those found in glaucoma, although they occur with different frequencies. The most common defects are enlargement of the physiologic blind spot, loss of inferonasal portions of the visual field, and constriction of isopters. Other defects are central, paracentral and cecocentral scotomas, arcuate scotomas, altitudinal patterns of loss, and other nerve fiber bundle defects. The loss of visual field may be progressive and severe and lead to blindness. The onset of visual loss is usually gradual; however, acute, severe visual loss can occur.

Idiopathic intracranial hypertension without papilledema

Intracranial hypertension can occur without papilledema.[122,144,148,149] The clinical, historical, radiographic, and demographic characteristics are identical to patients with papilledema except for:

- possible association with prior head trauma or meningitis;
- extended delay in diagnosis, which requires lumbar puncture in the absence of papilledema; and
- no evidence of the visual loss seen in patients with idiopathic intracranial hypertension with papilledema.

Patients, particularly obese women, who have chronic daily headache and symptoms of increased intracranial pressure (i.e. pulsatile tinnitus, a history of head trauma or meningitis, an empty sella on neuroimaging studies, or a headache that is unrelieved by standard therapy) should have a diagnostic lumbar puncture.

Why papilledema is absent in these cases of intracranial hypertension is not known. Congenital or acquired optic nerve sheath defects, 'chronic idiopathic intracranial hypertension' with resolution of papilledema, or early idiopathic intracranial hypertension are alternative explanations.

In a spinal fluid examination study of 85 patients with refractory transformed migraine, 12 patients had elevated CSF pressures, which ranged from 230 to 450 mm H_2O.[145] Ten of the twelve were women and half were obese. This observation supports our position that a subset of patients with chronic daily headache, who fit the stereotype of the obese female of childbearing age, may have idiopathic intracranial hypertension without papilledema. These patients may respond to chronic daily headache treatment, but often, although not always, respond better if the elevated CSF pressure is treated. These patients would not have been identified if a lumbar puncture had not been performed.[150]

Treatment

The treatment of elevated intracranial pressure depends on the underlying cause. In many cases, the history, clinical examination, and neuroradiographic studies define the syndrome, and distinctive therapy can be initiated. Thus, arterio-venous malformation, abscess, cerebral neoplasm, cerebral infarct, acute meningitis, subarachnoid hemorrhage, subdural hematoma, and acute obstructive hydrocephalus may be treated with appropriate surgical (drainage, shunt) or medical (antibiotics, hyperventilation, steroids, hypertonic osmotic diuretics) intervention.

In patients with idiopathic intracranial hypertension (with or without papilledema), chronic meningitis, and some cases of subarachnoid hemorrhage, diagnosis is based on lumbar puncture following neuroimaging (paying attention to empty sella and sinus thrombosis). If lumbar puncture is unremarkable and intracranial pressure is elevated to greater than 200 mm H_2O (in nonobese subjects), then idiopathic intracranial hypertension is the likely diagnosis. Routine blood chemistries (PT, PTT, ANA, VDRL, FIA-Abs, SMA 12/6, thyroxine, and thyroid-stimulating hormone) are helpful.

Once the diagnosis of idiopathic intracranial hypertension is made, secondary causes should be sought and eliminated. Over fifty diseases, conditions, toxins, or pharmaceuticals have been associated with idiopathic intracranial hypertension. Obese patients should be encouraged to lose weight. If the patient is asymptomatic and has no visual loss, then no treatment is indicated, but careful ophthalmologic follow-up is needed. If the only complaint is headache and there is either no papilledema or papilledema with no visual loss, then the idiopathic intracranial hypertension should be treated aggressively.

Weight loss is a cornerstone in the management of idiopathic intracranial hypertension. Newborg treated nine patients with a strict low-calorie rice diet (fluid and salt restriction and a total caloric intake of 400–1000 calories per day). All patients had reversal of their papilledema. The benefits to visual fields and visual acuity were not ascertained.[151] Resolution of idiopathic intracranial hypertension can also occur following surgically-induced weight loss (gastric exclusion procedure)[152,153] in morbidly obese women.

There is a subset of idiopathic intracranial hypertension patients with orthostatic edema,[154] for whom a low salt diet and fluid restriction may be beneficial. This is especially true for patients who lose only a small percentage of their total body mass yet have resolution of their optic disc edema.

Headache associated with idiopathic intracranial hypertension and papilledema frequently responds to standard headache treatment (Table 12.15). Surgical treatment of idiopathic intracranial hypertension has been directed toward preventing visual loss. Many patients experience headache improvement following optic nerve sheath fenestration (ONSF).

If rigorous headache therapy is unsuccessful, or if there is visual loss, then a 4- to 6-week trial of furosemide (frusemide) or a potent carbonic anhydrase inhibitor (acetazolamide) should be given. The starting dose is 500 mg twice daily, which can be increased up to 2 g daily. Side-effects include nausea, depression, acral and

Table 12.15 Treatment of idiopathic intracranial hypertension

1. Eliminate symptomatic causes.
2. Weight loss (if patient is obese).
3. Standard headache treatment.
4. Carbonic anhydrase inhibitors and loop diuretics.
5. Short course of high dose corticosteroids.
6. Serial lumbar punctures.
7. Lumboperitoneal or ventriculoperitoneal shunt.
8. Optic nerve sheath fenestration.

perioral numbness and tingling, and renal stones. Rare cases of hepatic failure have been reported with the use of carbonic anhydrase inhibitors. Patients thus treated develop a compensated metabolic acidosis, which serves as a marker of compliance. Furosemide (40–160 mg/day) with potassium supplementation may also reduce the headache.[155] These drugs decrease elevated intracranial pressure. The use of high dose steroids (prednisone or dexamethasone) is controversial but may be effective in idiopathic intracranial hypertension. Rebound headache is common when steroids are withdrawn.

Lumbar puncture typically relieves headache in idiopathic intracranial hypertension; however, a postlumbar puncture headache occasionally occurs. Lack of headache improvement following the first or subsequent lumbar puncture may be because the headache is generated by a mechanism other than CSF pressure or a venous sinus occlusion. In some of our intractable headache patients, the relationship between the CSF pressure and the headache becomes uncertain. At times, lumbar puncture reduces the pressure and relieves the headache, and at other times the headache does not improve. Since CSF is rapidly replaced, prolonged symptomatic relief may reflect a persistent CSF leak. Alternatively, transient reduction of CSF pressure may allow decompression of the arachnoid villi, allowing for prolonged enhanced CSF absorption. Patients with idiopathic intracranial hypertension who have visual loss or a severe incapacitating headache that does not respond to medical therapy or repeated lumbar punctures may need surgical management.

Some suggest treating idiopathic intracranial hypertension with a lumboperitoneal shunt, but this has a high re-operation rate and the potential for a hindbrain herniation and a new headache to develop. Others believe ventriculoperitoneal shunt is the preferred shunting procedure. Eggenberger et al[156] retrospectively reviewed the efficacy of lumboperitoneal shunt in 27 patients with idiopathic intracranial hypertension. A functioning shunt always alleviated symptoms. None of the patients had low pressure headache or abdominal pain for the first 2 months. However, 56% of patients required shunt revision. Other than shunt failure, there were no major complications. In the series, 67% of the patients were shunted for intractable headache; all had headache improvement or relief postoperatively. Shunt revision was performed for obstruction (in 65% of patients) or secondary intracranial hypotension (in 15.1%). Two patients had asymptomatic tonsillar herniation, neither of whom were re-operated.

ONSF entails surgical incision of the dura covering the intraorbital optic nerve. The proposed mechanism is improved optic nerve axoplasmic flow and continuous intraorbital CSF drainage. Sixty-five to 76% of patients get relief from medically-uncontrolled headache with ONSF. Although ONSF has been performed on patients with unilateral papilledema, to our knowledge it is untried in patients with idiopathic intracranial hypertension without papilledema. Without threatened vision loss, the small risk of visual loss due to the surgery probably outweighs the potential benefits.

Exertional and cough headaches

Although coughing and exertion rarely provoke headache, they can aggravate any type of headache. However, transient, severe head pain upon coughing, sneezing, weight-lifting, bending, straining at stool or stooping defines cough headache. Originally described by Tinel[157] in 1932 as 'la céphalée à l'effort' and later by Symonds,[111] cough headache mainly affects middle-aged men. It runs its course over a few years and is uncommon in the clinic. For example, at the Mayo Clinic, Rooke diagnosed cough headache only 93 times over a 14-year period.[112] He proposed the broader term 'benign exertional headache' for any headache that is precipitated by exertion, has an acute onset, and is unassociated with structural CNS disease, thus combining cough and exertional headache. In a population-based study,[158] benign cough headache and benign exertional headache each had a prevalence of about 1%.

The most recent classification of these disorders was done by the IHS[1] (Tables 12.16 and 12.17). The IHS separates 'benign cough headache' and 'benign exertional headache', since these entities have different clinical features, diagnostic evaluations, and treatment responses.[159,160]

Headache associated with sexual activity describes bilateral headaches precipitated by masturbation or coitus, also in the absence of any intracranial disorder. Benign

● **Table 12.16** Benign cough headache

- Benign cough headache is a bilateral headache of sudden onset, lasting less than one minute, precipitated by coughing.
- It may be prevented by avoiding coughing.
- It may be diagnosed only after structural lesions such as posterior fossa tumor have been excluded by neuroimaging.

● **Table 12.17** Benign exertional headache

- Benign exertional headache is specifically brought on by physical exercise.
- It is bilateral, throbbing in nature at onset, and may develop migrainous features in patients susceptible to migraine.
- It lasts from 5 minutes to 24 hours.
- It is prevented by avoiding excessive exertion, particularly in hot weather or at high altitude.
- It is not associated with any systemic or intracranial disorder.

● **Table 12.18** Headache associated with sexual activity

Headache is:
- precipitated by sexual excitement
- bilateral at onset
- prevented or eased by ceasing sexual activity before orgasm
- not associated with any intracranial disorder such as aneurysm.
Dull type
A dull ache in the head and neck that intensifies as sexual excitement increases.
Explosive type
A sudden severe ('explosive') headache occurring at orgasm.
Postural type
Postural headache resembling that of low CSF pressure developing after coitus.

sexual headache is now a well-defined entity with three types recognized in the IHS classification (Table 12.18).[1] They are described according to the presumed clinical pathophysiological mechanism. The most frequent, type 2, begins suddenly at the time of orgasm and is thought to be related to hemodynamic changes. It is often associated with exertional headache. Cough, exertional, or sexual headache may be a manifestation of subarachnoid hemorrhage; when this diagnosis is suspected, work-up includes an emergency non-contrast CT and a lumbar puncture if the CT is negative or equivocal (see Chapter 13). Angina may also present as exertional headache without chest pain, a condition termed cardiac cephalgia.[161]

Benign and symptomatic cough headache

Benign cough headache is uncommon. The mean age of onset is 55 years, with a range of 19–73 years. Patients over 40 years of age are twice as likely to have this headache, and it occurs four times more often in men than in women.[112] The pain begins immediately[111,162] or within seconds after coughing, sneezing, or a Valsalva maneuvre (lifting, straining at stool, blowing, crying, or singing).[157,163,164] The pain is severe in intensity, with a bursting, explosive, or splitting quality that lasts a few seconds or minutes. The headache is usually bilateral, with maximal pain at the vertex or in the occipital, frontal, or temporal region. Bending the head or lying down may be impossible.[165] The headache is not generally associated with nausea or vomiting, and the neurologic examination is usually normal. Vomiting suggests an organic basis for the headache.[160] As many as 25% of cases have an antecedent respiratory infection.[111,112,166] Most patients are pain-free between attacks of head pain, but in some cases the paroxysms are followed by dull, aching pain that may persist for hours; five of the 21 patients reported by Symonds had such additional headaches.[111] As these patients often express their complaint as a continuous headache, they should be asked directly about the role of exertion as a trigger factor.

Age at onset is significantly lower for symptomatic cough headache than for benign cough headache (Table 12.19) Pascual et al[159] found that symptomatic cough headache could be precipitated by laughing, weight-lifting, or acute body or head postural changes in addition to coughing. Symptomatic cough headache can be caused by a hindbrain abnormality, such as an Arnold–Chiari malformation, posterior fossa meningioma, midbrain cyst, basilar impression, acoustic neurinoma, and brain tumor.[105,167,168] In the Pascual et al series, headache was the only symptom, at first, of Arnold-Chiari type I malformation in three patients; however, all patients had or eventually developed posterior fossa signs or syringomyelia. Besides beginning earlier in life than benign cough headache, symptomatic cough headache does not respond to indomethacin (indometacin). If a patient does not respond to indomethacin, has posterior fossa signs, or is younger than 50 years of age, MRI must be done. Cough headache can be confused with other disorders, such as exertional headache, effort migraine, and coital headache.[166,169] In fact, 40% of patients with coital headache of the vascular type had exertional headache, suggesting a relationship between these entities.[170]

Benign and symptomatic exertional headache

Benign exertional headache begins almost 40 years earlier than benign cough headache. The pain is typically throbbing, lasts from 5 minutes to 24 hours, and is provoked by physical exercise. The pain usually begins during exertion, is non-explosive, and can be either bilateral or unilateral.

Symptomatic exertional headache is usually severe, bilateral, and explosive in onset. Twelve of the patients in the study performed by Pascual et al[159] presented because of acute headache that coincided with physical exercise. Etiologies included subarachnoid hemorrhage, sinusitis, and brain mass.

● **Table 12.19** Symptomatic cough headache

Parameter	Cough headache		Exertional headache		Sexual headache	
	Benign	Symptomatic	Benign	Symptomatic	Benign	Symptomatic
Patients (n)	13	17	16	12	13	1
Age, range (years)	67 ± 11, 44–81	39 ± 14, 15–63	24 ± 11, 10–48	42 ± 14, 18–61	41 ± 9, 24–57	60
Sex (% men)	77	59	88	43	85	100
Duration	Secs to 30 min	Seconds to days	Min to 2 days	1 day to 1 month	1 min to 3 hours	10 days
Bilateral localization	92%	94%	56%	100%	77%	Yes
Quality	Sharp, stabbing	Bursting, stabbing	Pulsating	Explosive, pulsating	Explosive + pulsating	Explosive + pulsating
Other manifestations	No	Posterior fossa signs	Nausea, photophobia	Nausea, vomiting, double vision, neck rigidity	None	Vomiting, neck rigidity
Diagnosis	Idiopathic	Chiari Type I malformation	Idiopathic	SAH, sinusitis, brain metastases	Idiopathic	SAH

Modified from Pascual et al.[159]

Benign and symptomatic sexual headache

Benign sexual headache (explosive type 2) begins later than benign exertional headache and earlier than benign cough headache. The headache is usually bilateral, but it can be unilateral. The pain is usually severe and explosive with occasional throbbing and stabbing. Its duration varies, lasting from less than 1 minute to 3 hours (average 30 minutes). The frequency of the episodes is directly related to the frequency of sexual intercourse or masturbation. Up to one-third of patients have similar episodes with physical exertion.

Explosive headache that occurs during coitus can be due to a subarachnoid hemorrhage or the conditions discussed in the differential diagnosis of cough and exertional headaches.

Differentiated symptomatic and benign exertional, cough and sexual headaches

Rooke[112] followed 103 patients who had exertional headache but no detectable intracranial disease on initial examination. After three or more years of follow-up, 10 patients subsequently developed organic intracranial lesions; 30 of the remaining 93 had complete headache relief within 5 years. The remainder improved or were headache-free after 10 years. This pre-CT era study emphasizes the importance of careful evaluation for organic disease.

Apart from Rooke's series,[112] the largest series of headaches of sudden onset provoked by cough, physical exercise, or sexual excitement was performed by Pascual et al.[159] Benign and symptomatic cases differed in several clinical aspects. Symptomatic cough headache began earlier in life, tended to last longer, and was more frequent than benign cough headache. Chiari type I malformation was the only cause. Subacute hemorrhage, sinusitis, and brain metastases were the causes of symptomatic exertional headache. Of the 219 cases of exertional and cough headache reviewed by Sands et al,[160] 48 had an identifiable organic etiology. Table 12.20 summarizes cases of cough and exertional headache, grouping together etiologically-related cases from several selected series. The group with posterior fossa space-occupying lesions includes cases with Arnold–Chiari deformity and hindbrain herniation. Posttraumatic and postcraniotomy cases were also grouped together. From Sands's review, one cannot accurately estimate how many patients with exertional headache have structural disease.[111,112,157,162,164,165,167,169,171–173]

Symptomatic exertional and sexual headaches began later in life and lasted longer than benign exertional and sexual headaches. Male predominance was not present in the symptomatic exertional headache group. Furthermore,

● **Table 12.20** Aetiologies for cough and exertional headache in literature.[141]

Condition	Patients, n (%)
Structural (organic)	48
Posterior fossa space-occupying lesions	18 (37.5)
After trauma or after craniotomy	13 (27.0)
Supratentorial space-occupying lesions	9 (18.7)
Basilar impression/platybasia	6 (12.5)
Syrinx	2 (4.2)
Benign exertional headache	171
Total	**219**

all patients with symptomatic headaches had manifestations of meningeal irritation or intracranial hypertension. Patients with subarachnoid bleeding had only had one headache episode. Neuroradiologic studies could be avoided in patients who fit the following profile: men around the third decade of life with clinically typical benign sexual or exertional headaches, a normal neurologic examination, and short-duration, multiple episodes of pulsating pain of short duration that responded to specific acute and preventive migraine treatment. However, all other patients must have a brain CT (and a CSF examination if the CT scan is normal). Benign cough headache and benign exertional headache are separate conditions. Besides the different precipitants (sudden Valsalva maneuvres and sustained physical exercise, respectively), benign cough headache begins later than benign exertional headache. Cough headache starts 43 years later, on average, than exertional headache, and, while the youngest patient with benign cough headache in Pascual's series was 44 years old, the oldest patient with benign exertional headache was 48 years of age. Benign cough headache tended to be shorter than benign exertional headache and the pain quality and response to treatment were different. Benign cough headache was described as sharp or stabbing and responsive to indomethacin, whereas benign exertional headache was pulsating, tended to last longer, and improved with ergotamine or propranolol. It is not uncommon for patients to experience both benign sexual headache and benign exertional headache; this occurred in 31% of patients in the Pascual et al series.

Other types of headache may be exacerbated by exertion. Severe migraine, postlumbar puncture headache, and, rarely, pseudotumor cerebri may be aggravated by coughing.[10] Paroxysmal headache may also occur in patients with IIIrd ventricular colloid cysts that produce intermittent obstruction of CSF flow through the foramen of Monroe resulting in abrupt increases of intracranial pressure. Patients who have lateral ventricular tumors, craniopharyngiomas, pinealomas, and tumors of the cerebellum and cerebrum also experience similar headache. Phaeochromocytomas[10,174,175] may also cause paroxysmal headache, especially during exercise. In Rooke's series of 303 patients with intracranial lesions, however, none of the 27 patients with an unruptured cerebral aneurysm or vascular anomaly complained of exertional headache.

Van den Bergh[176] reported two patients with Arnold–Chiari malformation (defined as descent of the hindbrain into the cervical canal, with meningomyelocele absent and hydrocephalus rare) who had headache paroxysms brought on by coughing, sneezing, and laughing. In Arnold–Chiari malformation, a ball-valve mechanism may be responsible for CSF passing more easily from the spine to the cranium than vice versa. Lumbar CSF pressure waves following a cough occur sooner and rise higher than cisternal pressure waves; the lumbar pressure waves also fall sooner and lower. Therefore, there is one phase during which the lumbar pressure exceeds the cisternal pressure, followed by a phase in which the cisternal pressure is greater than the lumbar pressure; this is aggravated by the ball-valve effect and can produce cough headache.[176 177]

Stevens et al[178] retrospectively studied 141 patients who had adult Arnold–Chiari malformation. Headache was present in 41 patients and was considered a symptom only if it was exacerbated by head movement, exercise, or coughing.

Outcomes of preoperative cough- and posture-related headache showed no relationship to tonsillar descent or any other imaging parameter, including the size of the cisterna magna, yet the latter feature was significantly improved in 62.6% of cases. Cough- and posture-related headache, like drop attacks, are thought to result from intermittent tonsillar impaction in the foramen magnum. Therefore, the lack of association of such features with small or obliterated cisterna magna or low-lying tonsils both pre- and postoperatively suggests that the origin of these symptoms is more complex.[178]

The long-term outlook for these patients is favorable. If the headaches are frequent or severe, prophylactic therapy is required, as the short duration of the headaches renders acute therapy impractical. Some patients respond dramatically to indomethacin in doses of 25–150 mg daily.[165] If the patient has gastrointestinal intolerance to indomethacin, concomitant treatment with misoprostol, sucralfate, or antacids may be helpful. When indomethacin fails, naproxen, ergonovine, and phenelzine may be useful, but propranolol is not.[166]

Acetazolamide 1125–2000 mg per day[179] and methysergide[180,181] have been reported to be effective in open-label trials. Several authors have written of the occasional efficacy of lumbar puncture.[111,112,182] Raskin noted the effectiveness of 40 ml lumbar puncture in six of 14 patients.[182] Three had immediate relief after the procedure and the other three obtained relief over 2 days. One of the responders redeveloped cough headache 6 weeks after the initial lumbar puncture but responded completely to a repeat spinal tap. Six of the eight who failed lumbar puncture responded to indomethacin.

References

1. Headache Classification Committee of the International Headache Society. Classification and diagnostic criteria for headache disorders, cranial neuralgia, and facial pain. Cephalalgia 1988; 8: 1–96.
2. Fishman RA. Cerebrospinal fluid in diseases of the nervous system. 2nd edn, Philadelphia: WB Saunders Company, 1992.
3. Morewood GH. A rational approach to the cause, prevention and treatment of postdural puncture headache. Can Med Assoc J 1993; 148: 1087–93.
4. Schaltenbrand G. Neure Anschauen zor Pathophysiologie der Liquorzirkulation. Zentralb Nforchir 1938; 3: 290–300.
5. Woltman HW. Headache: a consideration of some of the more common types. Med Clin N Amer 1940; 24: 1159–70.
6. Milhorat TH. Hydrocephalus and the cerebrospinal fluid. Baltimore: Williams and Wilkins, 1972.
7. Mokri B, Bahram MD. Spontaneous cerebrospinal fluid leaks: from intracranial hypotension to cerebrospinal fluid hypovolemia – evolution of a concept. Mayo Clin Proc 1999; 74: 1113–23.
8. Matsumae M, Kikinis R, Morocz IA et al. Age-related changes in intracranial compartment volumes in normal adults assessed by magnetic resonance imaging. J Neurosurg 1996; 84: 982–91.
9. Corbett JJ, Mehta MP. Cerebrospinal fluid pressure in normal obese subjects and patients with pseudotumor cerebri. Neurology 1983; 33: 1386–8.
10. Wall M, Silberstein SD, Aiken RD. Headache associated with abnormalities in intracranial structure or function: high cerebrospinal fluid pressure headache and brain tumor. In: Silberstein SD, Lipton RB, Dalessio DJ, eds. Wolff's Headache and Other Head Pain. 7th edn. New York: Oxford University Press, 2001,393–416.
11. Mokri B. Headache associated with abnormalities in intracranial structure or function: low cerebrospinal fluid pressure headache. In: Silberstein SD, Lipton RB, Dalessio DJ, eds. Wolff's Headache and Other Head Pain. 7th edn. New York: Oxford University Press, 2001,417–33.
12. Von Storch T, Carmichael A, Banks T. Factors producing lumbar cerebrospinal fluid pressure in many in the erect position. Arch Neurol Psychiatry 1937; 38: 1158.
13. Loman J. Components of cerebrospinal fluid pressure as affected by changes in posture. Arch Neurol Psychiatry 1934; 31: 679–81.

14. Loman J, Myerson A, Goldman D. Effects of alteration of posture on cerebrospinal fluid pressure. Arch Neurol Psychiatry 1935; 33: 1279–84.

15. Freemont-Smith F, Kubie L. Relation of vascular hydrostatic pressure and osmotic pressure to cerebrospinal fluid pressure. Assoc Res Nerv Dis Proc 1929; 8: 154.

16. Cass W, Edelist G. Post spinal headache. JAMA 1974; 227: 786–7.

17. Grant R, Condon B, Hart I, Teasdale GM. Changes in intracranial CSF volume after lumbar puncture and their relationship to post-LP headache. J Neurol Neurosurg Psychiatry 1991; 54: 440–2.

18. Good DC, Ghobrial M. Pathologic changes associated with intracranial hypotension and meningeal enhancement on MRI. Neurology 1993; 43: 2698–700.

19. Fishman RA, Dillon WP. Dural enhancement and cerebral displacement secondary to intracranial hypotension. Neurology 1993; 43: 609–11.

20. Pannullo S, Reich J, Posner J. Meningeal enhancement associated with low intracranial pressure. Neurology 1992; 42: 430.

21. Pannullo SC, Reich JB, Krol G et al. MRI changes in intracranial hypotension. Neurology 1993; 43: 919–26.

22. Kasner SE, Rosenfield J, Farber RE. Spontaneous intracranial hypotension: headache with a reversible Arnold–Chiari malformation. Headache 1995; 35: 557–9.

23. Lay CL, Campbell JK, Mokri B. Low cerebrospinal fluid pressure headache. In: Goadsby PJ, Silberstein SD, eds. Headache. Boston: Butterworth-Heinemann, 1997, 355–68.

24. Mokri B, Atkinson JL. False pituitary tumor in CSF leaks. Neurology 2000; 55: 573–75.

25. Raskin NH. Headaches caused by alterations of structure or homeostasis. In: Raskin NH, ed. Headache. New York: Churchill Livingstone, 1988, 283–316.

26. Vilming ST, Kloster R. Postlumbar puncture headache: clinical features and suggestions for diagnostic criteria. Cephalalgia 1997; 17: 778–84.

27. Marcelis J, Silberstein SD. Spontaneous low cerebrospinal fluid pressure headache. Headache 1990; 30: 192–6.

28. Sharrock NE. Postural headache following thoracic somatic paravertebral nerve block. Anesthesiology 1980; 52: 360–2.

29. Kieffer SA, Wolff JM, Prentice WB, Loken MK. Scinticisternography in individuals without known neurological

disease. Am J Roentgenol Radium Ther Nucl Med 1971; 112: 225–36.

30. Front D, Penning L. Subcutaneous extravasation of CSF demonstration by scinticisternography. Nuclear Med 1973; 15: 200–1.

31. Bell WB, Joynt RJ, Sahs AL. Low spinal fluid pressure syndromes. Neurology 1960; 10: 512–21.

32. Major O, Fedorcsak I, Sipos L et al. Slit-ventricle syndrome in shunt operated children. Acta Neurochirurgica 1994; 127: 69–72.

33. Murros K, Fogelholm R. Spontaneous intracranial hypotension with slit ventricles. J Neurol Neurosurg Psychiatry 1983; 46: 1149–51.

34. Young WB, Silberstein SD. Paroxysmal headache caused by colloid cyst of the third ventricle: case report and review of the literature. Headache 1997; 37: 15–20.

35. Tourtellote WW, Haerer A, Heller GL et al. Postlumbar puncture headaches. Springfield: Charles C Thomas, 1964.

36. Kunkle EL, Ray BS, Wolff HG. Experimental studies on headache: analysis of the headache associated with changes in intracranial pressure. Arch Neurol Psychiatry 1943; 49: 323–59.

37. Raskin NH. Lumbar puncture headache: a review. Headache 1990; 30: 197–200.

38. Fay T. Mechanism of headache. Arch Neurol Psychiatry 1937; 37: 471–4.

39. Iqbal J, Davis LE, Orrison WW. An MRI study of lumbar puncture headaches. Headache 1995; 35: 420–2.

40. Dripps RD, Vandam LD. Long term follow-up of patients who received 10 098 spinal anesthetics. JAMA 1954; 156: 1486–91.

41. Vilming ST, Schrader H, Monstad I. The significance of age, sex, and cerebrospinal fluid pressure in post lumbar puncture headache. Cephalalgia 1989; 9: 99–106.

42. Kuntz KM, Kokmen E, Stevens JC et al. Postlumbar puncture headaches: experience in 501 consecutive procedures. Neurology 1992; 42: 1884–7.

43. DiGiovanni AJ, Dunbar BS. Epidural injections of autologous blood for postlumbar-puncture headache. Anesth Analg 1970; 49: 268–71.

44. Torrey EF. Headaches after lumbar puncture and insensitivity to pain in psychiatric patients. N Engl J Med 1979; 301: 110.

45. Daniels AM, Sallie R. Headache, lumbar puncture, and expectation. Lancet 1981; I: 1003.

46. Blennow K, Wallin A, Häger O. Low frequency of postlumbar puncture headache in demented patients. Acta Neurol Scand 1993; 88: 221–3.

47. Reid JA, Thorburn J. Headache after spinal anaesthesia. Br J Anaesth 1991; 67: 674–7.

48. Lynch J, Krings-Ernst I, Strick K et al. Use of a 25-gauge Whitacre needle to reduce the incidence of postdural puncture headache. Br J Anaesth 1991; 67: 690–3.

49. Rasmussen BS, Blom L, Hansen P, Mikkelsen SJ. Postspinal headache in young and elderly patients. Two randomised, double-blind studies that compare 20- and 25-gauge needles. Anaesthesia 1989; 44: 571–3.

50. Geurts JW, Haanschoten MC, Van Wijk RM et al. Post-dural headache in young patients. A comparative study between the use of 0.52 mm (25-gauge) and 0.33 mm (29-gauge) spinal needles. Acta Anaesthesiol Scand 1990; 34: 350–3.

51. McGann GM, Gleeson FV, Kelly I et al. The influence of needle size on postmyelography headache: a controlled trial. Br J Radiol 1992; 65: 1102–4.

52. Engelhardt A, Oheim S, Neundorrfer B. Post lumbar puncture headache: experiences with an 'atraumatic' needle. Cephalalgia 1991; 11: 356–7.

53. Braune HJ, Huffman G. A prospective double-blind clinical trial, comparing the sharp Quincke needle (22G) with an 'atraumatic' needle (22G) in the induction of postlumbar puncture headache. Acta Neurol Scand 1992; 86: 50–4.

54. Labadie EL, Antwerp JV, Bamford CR. Abnormal lumbar isotope cisternography in an unusual case of spontaneous hypoliquorrheic headache. Neurology 1976; 26: 135–9.

55. Kraemer G, Hanns HC, Eissner D. CSF hyperabsorption: a cause of spontaneous low CSF pressure headache (abstract). Neurology 1987, 238.

56. Molins A, Alvarez J, Somalla J et al. Cisternographic pattern of spontaneous liquoral hypotension. Cephalalgia 1990; 10: 59–65.

57. Rando TA, Fishman RA. Spontaneous intracranial hypotension: report of two cases and review of the literature. Neurology 1992; 42: 481–7.

58. Bell WE, Joynt RJ, Sahs AL. Low spinal fluid pressure syndromes. Neurology 1958; 8: 157–63.

59. Teng P, Papatheodorou C. Primary cerebrospinal fluid hypotension. Los Angeles Neurol Soc 1968; 33: 121–8.

60. Yamamoto M, Suehiro T, Nakata H et al. Primary low cerebrospinal fluid pressure syndrome associated with galactorrhea. Intern Med 1993; 32: 228–31.

61. Huber M. Spontaneous hypoliquorrhea:

seven observations. Schweiz Arch Neurol Neurochir Psychiatry 1970; 106: 9–23.

62. Lasater GM. Primary intracranial hypotension. Headache 1970; 10: 63–6.

63. Lake AP, Minckler J, Scanlan RL. Spinal epidural cyst: theories of pathogenesis. J Neurosurg 1974; 40: 774–8.

64. Nosik WA. Intracranial hypotension secondary to lumbar nerve sleeve tear. JAMA 1955; 157: 1110–11.

65. Horton JC, Fishman RA. Neurovisual findings in the syndrome of spontaneous intracranial hypotension from aural cerebrospinal fluid leak. Ophthalmology 1994; 101: 244–51.

66. Paulson GW, Klawans HL. Benign orgasmic cephalalgia. Headache 1974; 13: 181–7.

67. Baker CC. Headache due to spontaneous low spinal fluid pressure. Minn Med 1983; 66: 325–8.

68. Capobianco DJ, Kuczler FJ. Case report: primary intracranial hypotension. Mil Med 1990; 155: 64–6.

69. Garcia-Albea E, Cabrera F, Tejeiro J et al. Delayed postexertional headache, intracranial hypotension and racket sports (letter). J Neurol Neurosurg Psychiatry 1992; 55: 975.

70. Farraraccio BE. Positional headache due to spontaneous intracranial hypotension. S Med J 1992; 85: 57.

71. Fernandez E. Headaches associated with low spinal fluid pressure. Headache 1990; 30: 122–8.

72. Sipe JC, Zyroff J, Waltz TA. Primary intracranial hypotension and bilateral isodense subdural hematomas. Neurology 1981; 31: 334–7.

73. Vilming ST, Campbell JK. Low cerebrospinal fluid pressure. In: Olesen J, Tfelt-Hansen P, Welch KM, eds. The Headaches. 2nd edn. Philadelphia: Lippincott Williams & Wilkins, 2000; 831–40.

74. Weber WE, Heidendal GA, De Krom MC. Primary intracranial hypotension and abnormal radionuclide cisternography. Report of a case and review of the literature. Clin Neurol Neurosurg 1991; 93: 55–60.

75. Lindquist T, Moberg E. Spontaneous hypoliquorrhea. Acta Med Scand 1949; 132: 556–61.

76. Sable SG, Ramadan NM. Meningeal enhancement and low CSF pressure headache. An MRI study. Cephalalgia 1991; 11: 275–6.

77. Hochman MS, Naidich TP, Kobetz SA, Fernandez-Maitin A. Spontaneous intracranial hypotension with pachymeningeal enhancement on MRI. Neurology 1992; 42: 1628–30.

78. Bourekas EC, Jonathan SL, Lanzieri CF. Postcontrast meningeal MR enhancement secondary to intracranial hypotension caused by lumbar puncture. J Comput Assist Tomogr 1995; 19: 299–301.

79. Mokri B, Krueger BR, Miller GM, Piepgras DG. Meningeal gadolinium enhancement in low-pressure headaches. J Neuroimag 1993; 3: 11–15.

80. Mokri B, Parisi JE, Scheithauer BW et al. Meningeal biopsy in intracranial hypotension: meningeal enhancement on MRI. Neurology 1995; 45: 1801–7.

81. Berlit P, Berg-Dammer E, Kuehne B. Abducens nerve palsy in spontaneous intracranial hypotension (scientific note). Neurology 1994; 44: 1552.

82. Mokri B, Piepgras DG, Miller GM. Syndrome of orthostatic headaches and diffuse pachymeningeal gadolinium enhancement. Mayo Clin Proc 1997; 72: 400–13.

83. Mokri B, Hunter SF, Atkinson JL, Piepgras DG. Orthostatic headaches caused by CSF leak but with normal CSF pressures. Neurology 1998; 51: 786–90.

84. Atkinson JL, Weinshenker BG, Miller GM et al. Acquired Chiari I malformation secondary to spontaneous cerebrospinal fluid leakage and chronic intracranial hypotension syndrome in seven cases. J Neurosurg 1998; 88: 237–42.

85. Haines DE, Harkey HL, al-Mefty O. The 'subdural' space: a new look at an outdated concept. Neurosurg 1993; 32: 111–20.

86. Chen CC, Luo CL, Wang SJ, et al. Colour doppler imaging for diagnosis of intracranial hypotension. Lancet 1999; 354: 826–9.

87. Sechzer PH, Abel L. Post-spinal anesthesia headache treated with caffeine. Curr Ther Res 1978; 24: 307–12.

88. Gaukroger PB, Brownridge P. Epidural blood patch in treatment of spontaneous low CSF pressure headache. Pain 1987; 29: 119–22.

89. Parris WCV. Use of epidural blood patch in treating chronic headache. Can J Anaesth 1987; 34: 403–6.

90. Peterson RC, Freeman DP, Knox CA, Gibson BE. Successful treatment of spontaneous low cerebrospinal fluid pressure headache (abstract). Ann Neurol 1987; 22: 148.

91. Jarvis AP, Greenawalt JW, Fagraeus L. Intravenous caffeine for postdural puncture headache. Anesth Analg 1986; 65: 316–17.

92. Camann WR, Murray RS, Mushlin PS, Lambert DH. Effects of oral caffeine on postdural puncture headache. Anesth Analg 1990; 70: 181–4.

93. Gormley JB. Treatment of post-spinal headache. Anesthesiology 1960; 21: 565–6.

94. Bart AJ, Wheeler AS. Comparison of epidural saline infusion and epidural blood placement in the treatment of post lumbar puncture headache. Anesthesiology 1978; 48: 221–3.

95. Milette PC, Paqacz A, Charest C. Epidural blood patch for the treatment of chronic headache after myelography. J Can Assoc Radiol 1982; 33: 236–8.

96. Ostheimer GW, Palahniuk RJ, Shnider SM. Epidural blood patch for postlumbar-puncture headache. Anesthesiology 1974; 41: 307–8.

97. Taivainen T, Pitkanen M, Tuominen M, Rosenberg PH. Efficacy of epidural blood patch for postdural puncture headache. Acta Anaesthesiol Scand 1993; 37: 702–5.

98. Beards SC, Jackson A, Griffiths AG, Horsman EL. Magnetic resonance imaging of extradural blood patches: appearances from 30 min to 18 h. Br J Anaesth 1993; 71: 182–8.

99. Tarkkila PJ, Miralles JA, Palomaki EA. The subjective complications and efficiency of the epidural blood patch in the treatment of postdural puncture headache. Reg Anaesth 1989; 14: 247–50.

100. Jaeckle KA. Clinical presentations and therapy of nervous system tumors. In: Bradley WG, Daroff RB, Fenichel GM, Marsden CD, eds. Neurology in Clinical Practice. Boston: Butterworth-Heinemann, 1991, 1008–30.

101. Lavyne MH, Patterson RH. Headache and brain tumor. In: Dalessio DJ, ed. Wolff's Headache and Other Head Pain. 5th edn. New York: Oxford University Press, 1987, 343–9.

102. Kunkle EC, Pfeiffer JB, Wilholt WM, Hamrick LD Jr. Recurrent brief headache in 'cluster' pattern. Trans Am Neurol Assoc 1942; 77: 240–3.

103. Northfield DWC. Some observations on headache. Brain 1938; 77: 240–3.

104. Ray BS, Wolff HG. Experimental studies on headache. Pain sensitive structures of the head and their significance in headache. Arch Surg 1940; 41: 813–56.

105. Rushton JG, Rooke ED. Brain tumor headache. Headache 1962; 2: 147–52.

106. Heyck H. Examinations and differential diagnosis of headache. In: Vinken BT, Bruyn GW, eds. Handbook of Clinical Neurology. New York: John Wiley & Sons 1968: 25–36.

107. Forsyth PA, Posner JB. Headaches in patients with brain tumors. A study of 111 patients. Neurology 1993; 43: 1678–83.

108. Vazquez-Barquero A, Ibanez FJ, Herrera S. Isolated headache as the presenting

clinical manifestation of intracranial tumor: a perspective study. Cephalalgia 1994; 14: 270–2.

109. McKissock W. Subdural hematoma. A review of 389 cases. Lancet 1960; 1: 1365–70.

110. Britt RH. Brain abscess. In: Wilkins RH, Rengachary SS, eds. Neurosurgery. New York: McGraw Hill, 1985; 1928–56.

111. Symonds C. Cough headache. Brain 1956; 79: 557–68.

112. Rooke ED. Benign exertional headache. Med Clin N Amer 1968; 52: 801–8.

113. Greenberg HS, Deck MD, Vikram B et al. Metastasis to the base of the skull: clinical findings in 43 patients. Neurology 1981; 31: 530–7.

114. Zulch KJ, Mennel HD, Zimmerman V. Intracranial hypertension. In: Vinken BJ, Bruyn GW eds. Handbook of Clinical Neurology. New York: Elsevier. 1974: 89–149.

115. Honig PJ, Charney EB. Children with brain tumor headaches. Am J Dis Child 1982; 136: 121–4.

116. Rossi LN, Vassella F. Headache in children with brain tumor. Childs Nerv Syst 1998; 5: 307–9.

117. Zammarano CB, D'Ancona ML, Miceli MC. Headache and cerebral neoplasm in childhood. In: Lanzi G, Balottin U, Cernibori A, eds. Headache in Children and Adolescents. Amsterdam: Elsevier, 1989; 177–8.

118. Kennedy CR, Nathwani A. Headache as a presenting feature of brain tumors in children. Cephalalgia 1995; 15: 15.

119. Galicich JH, Sundaresan N. Metastatic brain tumors. In: Wilkins RH, Rengachary SS, eds. Neurosurgery. New York: McGraw-Hill, 1985; 600.

120. Childhood Brain Tumor Consortium. The epidemiology of headache among children with brain tumor: headache in children with brain tumors. J Neurooncol 1991; 10: 31–46.

121. Shuper A, Packer RJ, Vezina LG. Complicated migraine-like episodes in children following cranial irradiation and chemotherapy. Neurology 1995; 45: 1837–40.

122. Marcelis J, Silberstein SD. Idiopathic intracranial hypertension without papilledema. Arch Neurol 1991; 48: 392–9.

123. Giuseffi V, Wall M, Siegal PZ, Rojas PB. Symptoms and disease associations in idiopathic intracranial hypertension (pseudotumor cerebri): a case control study. Neurology 1991; 41: 239–44.

124. Wall M, George D. Idiopathic intracranial hypertension: a prospective study of 50 patients. Brain 1991; 114: 155–80.

125. Wall M. The headache profile of idiopathic intracranial hypertension.

Cephalalgia 1990; 10: 331–5.

126. Sadun AA, Currie JN, Lessell S. Transient visual obscurations with elevated optic discs. Ann Neurol 1984; 16: 489–94.

127. Durcan FJ, Corbett JJ, Wall M. The incidence of pseudotumor cerebri: population studies in Iowa and Louisiana. Arch Neurol 1988; 45: 875–7.

128. Johnston I, Hawke S, Kalmagyi M, Antyeo C. The pseudotumor syndrome. Arch Neurol 1991; 48: 740–7.

129. Borgesen SE, Gjerris F. Relationships between intracranial pressure, ventricular size, and resistance to CSF outflow. Neurosurg 1987; 67: 534–9.

130. van Alphen HAM. Migraine, a result of increased CSF pressure: a new pathophysiologic concept (preliminary report). Neurosurg Rev 1986; 9: 121–4.

131. Gjerris F, Sorenson S, Vorstrup S, Paulson OB. Intracranial pressure, conductance to cerebrospinal fluid outflow, and cerebral blood flow in patients with benign intracranial hypertension (pseudotumor cerebri). Ann Neurol 1985; 17: 158–62.

132. Fishman RA. The pathophysiology of pseudotumor cerebri. An unsolved puzzle. Neurology 1984; 41: 257–8.

133. Bjerre P, Lindholm J, Gyldensted C. Pseudotumor cerebri: a theory on etiology and pathogenesis. Acta Neurol Scand 1982; 66: 472–81.

134. Donaldson JO, Binstock ML. Pseudotumor cerebri in an obese woman with Turner syndrome. Neurology 1981; 31: 758–60.

135. Janny P, Chazal J, Colnet G et al. Benign intracranial hypertension and disorders of CSF absorption. Surg Neurol 1981; 15: 168–74.

136. Fishman RA. Pathophysiology of pseudotumor. Ann Neurol 1979; 15: 168–74.

137. Johnston I. Reduced CSF absorption syndrome. Reappraisal of benign intracranial hypertension and related conditions. Lancet 1973; 8: 2418–21.

138. Malm J, Kristensen B, Markgren P, Ekstedt J. CSF hydrodynamics in idiopathic intracranial hypertension: a long-term study. Neurology 1992; 42: 851–8.

139. King JO, Mitchell PJ, Thomson KR, Tress BM. Cerebral venography and manometry in idiopathic intracranial hypertension. Neurology 1995; 45: 2224–8.

140. Karahalios DG, Rekate HL, Khayata MH, Apostolides PJ. Elevated intracranial venous pressure as a universal mechanism in pseudotumor cerebri of varying etiologies. Neurology 1996; 46: 198–202.

141. Weisberg LA. Benign intracranial

hypertension. Medicine 1975; 54: 197–207.

142. Corbett JJ. Headache due to idiopathic intracranial hypertension. In: Goadsby P, Silberstein SD, eds. Blue Books of Practical Neurology: Headache. Boston: Butterworth Heinemann, 1997, 279–83.

143. Wang SJ, Silberstein SD, Patterson S, Young WB. Idiopathic intracranial hypertension without papilledema: a case–control study in a headache center. Neurology 1998; 51: 245–9.

144. Spence JD, Amacher AL, Willis NR. Benign intracranial hypertension without papilledema: role of 24 hour cerebrospinal fluid pressure monitoring in diagnosis and management. Neurosurgery 1980; 7: 326–36.

145. Mathew NT, Ravinshankar K, Sanin LC. Coexistence of migraine and idiopathic intracranial hypertension without papilledema. Neurology 1996; 46: 1226–30.

146. Wall M, White WN. Asymmetric papilledema in idiopathic intracranial hypertension: prospective interocular comparison of sensory visual function. Invest Ophthalmol Vis Sci 1998; 39: 134–42.

147. Orcutt JC, Page NG, Sanders MD. Factors affecting visual loss in benign intracranial hypertension. Ophthalmol 1984; 91: 1303–12.

148. Scanarini M, Mingrino S, d'Avella D, Della Corte V. Benign intracranial hypertension without papilledema: a case report. Neurosurgery 1979; 5: 376–7.

149. Lipton HL, Michelson PE. Pseudotumor cerebri syndrome without papilledema. JAMA 1972; 220: 1591–2.

150. Silberstein SD, Corbett JJ. The forgotten lumbar puncture. Cephalalgia 1993; 13: 212–13.

151. Newborg B. Pseudotumor cerebri treated by rice reduction diet. Arch Inter Med 1974; 133: 802–7.

152. Amaral JF, Tsiaris W, Morgan T, Thompson WR. Reversal of benign intracranial hypertension by surgically induced weight loss. Arch Surg 1987; 122: 946–9.

153. Sugerman HJ, Felton WL, Sismanis A et al. Gastric surgery for pseudotumor cerebri associated with severe obesity. Ann Surg 1999; 229: 634–40.

154. Friedman DI, Streeten DH. Idiopathic intracranial hypertension and orthostatic edema may share a common pathogenesis. Neurology 1998; 50: 1099–104.

155. Corbett JJ, Thompson HS. The rational management of idiopathic intracranial hypertension. Arch Neurol 1991; 46: 1049–51.

156. Eggenberger ER, Miller NR, Vitale S. Lumboperitoneal shunt for the

treatment of pseudotumor cerebri. Neurology 1996; 46: 1524–30.

157. Tinel J. Un syndrome d'algie veineuse intracrânienne. La céphalée à l'effort. Prat Med Fr 1932; 13: 113–19.

158. Rasmussen BK, Jensen R, Schroll M, Olesen J. Epidemiology of headache in a general population – a prevalence study. J Clin Epidemiol 1991; 44: 1147–57.

159. Pascual J, Igessias F, Oterino A, Vazquez-Barquero A. Cough, exertional, and sexual headaches: an analysis of 72 benign and symptomatic cases. Neurology 1996; 46: 1520–4.

160. Sands GH, Newman L, Lipton R. Cough, exertional, and other miscellaneous headaches. Med Clin N Amer 1991; 75: 733–46.

161. Lipton RB, Lowenkopf T, Bajwa ZH et al. Cardiac cephalalgia: a malignant form of exertional headache. Neurology 1997; 49: 813–16.

162. Nick J. La céphalée d'effort. A propos d'une série de 43 cases. Sem Hop Paris 1980; 56: 621–8.

163. Tinel J. La céphalée à l'effort. Syndrome de distension douloureuse des veines intracrâniennes. Médicine (Paris) 1932; 13: 113–18.

164. Nightingale S, Williams B. Hindbrain hernia headache. Lancet 1987; 1: 731–4.

165. Mathew NT. Indomethacin responsive headache syndromes. Headache 1981; 21: 147–50.

166. Raskin NH. The indomethacin-responsive syndromes. In: Raskin NH, ed. Headache. New York: Churchill Livingstone, 1988; 255–68.

167. Williams B. Cough headache due to craniospinal pressure dissociation. Arch Neurol 1980; 37: 226–30.

168. Raskin N. Headaches associated with organic diseases of the nervous system. Med Clin N Amer 1978; 62: 459–66.

169. Ekbom K. Cough headache. In: Vinkin PJ, Bruyn GW, Klawans HL, eds. Headache (Handbook of Clinical Neurology). New York: Elsevier Science Publishing, 1986, 67–371.

170. Silbert PL, Edis RH, Stewart-Wynne EG, Gubbay SS. Benign vascular sexual headache and exertional headache: interrelationships and long term prognosis. J Neurol Neurosurg Psychiatry 1991; 54: 417–21.

171. Ibbotson S. Weight-lifter's headache. Br J Sports Med 1987; 21: 138.

172. Paulson GW. Weightlifter's headache. Headache 1983; 23: 193–4.

173. Powell B. Weight lifter's cephalalgia. Ann Emerg Med 1982; 11: 449–51.

174. Lance JW, Hinterberger H. Symptoms of pheochromocytoma with particular reference to headache correlated with catecholamine production. Arch Neurol 1976; 33: 281–8.

175. Paulson GW, Zipf RE, Beekman JF. Pheochromocytoma causing exercise-related headache and pulmonary edema. Ann Neurol 1979; 5: 96–9.

176. Van den Bergh V, Amery WK, Waelkens J. Trigger factors in migraine: a study conducted by the Belgian migraine society. Headache 1987; 27: 191–6.

177. Williams B. Cerebrospinal fluid pressure changes in response to coughing. Brain 1976; 99: 331–46.

178. Stevens JM, Serva WAD, Kendall BE et al. Chiari malformation in adults: relation of morphological aspects to clinical features and operative outcome. J Neurol Neurosurg Psychiatry 1993; 56: 1072–7.

179. Wang SJ, Fuh JL, Lu SR. Benign cough headache is responsive to acetazolamide. Neurology 2000; 55: 149–50.

180. Bahra A, Goadsby PJ. Cough headache responsive to methysergide. Cephalalgia 1998; 18: 495–6.

181. Calandre L, Hernandez-Lain AH, Lopez-Valdes EL. Benign Valsalva's maneuver-related headache: an MRI study of six cases. Headache 1996; 36: 251–3.

182. Raskin NH. The cough headache syndrome: treatment. Neurology 1995; 45: 1784.

chapter 13

Headache associated with vascular disease: migraine and stroke

Introduction

Headache and cerebrovascular disease may be associated in a number of ways. Because primary headache disorders and cerebrovascular disease each produce head pain, focal neurologic deficits and alterations in cerebral blood flow, these disorders sometimes present diagnostic challenges. In addition, one headache disorder (migraine) is a risk factor for stroke in some populations. Here we will first consider the relationship of migraine and stroke. We will then discuss the headaches associated with a number of stroke types including transient ischemic attacks, ischemic stroke (thrombotic, embolic, lacunar), intracerebral hemorrhage and subarachnoid hemorrhage.[1–3] Then we will discuss headache in other vascular disorders including cortical vein thrombosis, carotid dissection and primary vasculitis of the nervous system. We will summarize the headaches associated with endarterectomy and close with comments on the clinical and pathophysiologic implications of the links between migraine and stroke.

Association of migraine and stroke

Migraine and stroke have a long-studied and complex set of inter-relationships. Charcot[4,5] noted that migraine aura persisted on occasion and suggested that migraine and stroke may be associated. Since then, the relationships between these disorders have challenged clinicians and scientists. The migraine aura can mimic transient ischemic attacks (TIAs). Conversely, in stroke, headache may occur as a preictal, ictal, or postictal feature.[1–3] In addition to the problem of differential diagnosis, there are causal relationships between migraine and stroke on several levels. Here we categorize the various relationships between stroke and migraine using a revision of the method of Welch and Levine. (Table 13.1).[6] We consider true migrainous infarction, migraine as a risk factor for stroke, stroke with clinical features of migraine, and difficult-to-classify scenarios.

Migraine may cause stroke directly in a condition referred to as true migrainous infarction. In this condition, a patient with migraine with aura develops a persistent neurologic deficit or a radiographic stroke in a pattern consistent with the neurologic deficit of the aura. Hospital series suggest that 1–17% of strokes in patients who are under 50 years of age are attributed to migraine.[7,8] In general, the relationship between migraine and stroke is stronger for migraine with aura[9,10] than for migraine without aura. Strokes related to migraine are more likely in the distribution of the posterior cerebral artery.[11,12] The evidence suggests that migraine-associated stroke is unlikely to arise from atherosclerotic disease. Bougousslavsky et al[13] reported that 9% of patients who had a stroke during an attack of migraine with aura had arterial lesions; in contrast, arterial lesions were found in 91% of migraine with aura patients who experienced a stroke remote from a migrainous event and in 82% of patients who had a stroke and had no history of migraine. The low prevalence of arterial lesions suggests that mechanisms other than focal arterial pathology may underlie migrainous infarction.

To identify factors associated with migrainous infarction, Rothrock et al[10] compared the clinical features of 310 migraineurs and 30 patients with acute migrainous stroke. They found no significant differences in gender, mean age of migraine onset, mitral valve prolapse, hypertension, active smoking, or active estrogen use. Migraine with aura was substantially overrepresented in patients with migrainous stroke (80%) compared with migraine patients without stroke. In this study, migrainous infarction carried a poor prognosis. Six recurrent ischemic infarcts (all migraine-associated) were diagnosed in 28 patients, who were followed for a mean of 25.3 months. No strokes occurred in 173 of the control migraine patients who were followed for at least 1 year. As the two groups were similar in this vascular risk profile, migraine with aura may be an independent risk factor for stroke.

Table 13.1 *Classification of migraine-related stroke.*[6]

Category	Feature
I	Coexisting stroke and migraine
II	Stroke with clinical features of migraine
	A Symptomatic migraine
	B Migraine mimic
III	Migraine-induced stroke
	A Without risk factors
	B With risk factors
IV	Uncertain

Migraine as a risk factor for stroke (migraine coexistent with stroke)

In this condition, 'a clearly defined clinical stroke syndrome must occur remotely in time from a typical attack of migraine'.[6] In this category, migraine may contribute to the risk of stroke through an unspecified mechanism. Mitral valve prolapse is comorbid with both migraine and stroke, which may help account for the association between migraine and stroke.

The case–control design has been used to examine migraine as a risk factor for stroke. The Collaborative Group for the Study of Stroke in Young Women compared hospitalized stroke patients with both community- and hospital-based controls.[14] There was a twofold increase in the risk of stroke for women with migraine when compared with community controls but not relative to hospital controls; thus the study was inconclusive. A hospital-based, case–control study of 89 patients found an association between migraine and stroke; after adjusting for vascular risk factors, however, this was no longer statistically significant.[15] Tzourio et al[16,17] reported that migraine was associated with a fourfold increased risk of stroke in women under the age of 45 years. A strong association between stroke and migraine occurs in women under 45 years of age for migraine without aura (odds ratio, OR = 3.0) and migraine with aura (OR = 6.2). The risk is significantly increased in women with migraine who smoke more than one pack a day (OR = 10.2) or use oral contraceptives (OR = 13.9).

Carolei et al[18] conducted a case–control study of 308 patients aged 15–44 years with either TIA or stroke, and 591 prospectively-recruited age- and sex-matched controls to evaluate the relationship of migraine and stroke. For each case, a hospital control and population control were randomly selected. A history of migraine was more frequent in patients than in controls (14.9% vs. 9.1%; adjusted OR = 1.9, 95% confidence interval (CI) = 1.1–3.1). In the prospectively-designed subgroup analyses, a history of migraine reached the highest odds ratio (3.7, 95% CI = 1.5–9) and was the only significant risk factor for TIA or stroke in women under the age of 35 years ($p = 0.003$). A history of migraine was not associated with stroke risk in men or in patients over 35 years of age; however, recognized atherosclerotic risk factors were statistically significant in these groups, suggesting different risk profiles for cerebral ischemic events in younger women and older men.[18] Previous migraine with aura was more frequent in stroke patients compared with controls (OR = 8.6, 95% CI = 1–75). These epidemiologic studies do not provide information on the temporal relationship of the stroke to a migraine attack, nor do they fully assess other confounding stroke mechanisms. This makes inferences about causality and mechanisms difficult.

Migraine-related stroke was evaluated as part of the prospective Physicians' Health Study, a randomized, double-blind, placebo-controlled trial of aspirin and beta-carotene. The study enrolled 22 071 male physicians.[19] In this study, 6.7% of the participants reported that they had migraine, but no distinction was made between migraine with or without aura. After adjusting for age, aspirin use, and other vascular risk factors, the relative risk (RR) of total stroke was 1.84 (95% CI = 1.06–3.20), comparing those who reported migraine with those who did not. For ischemic stroke, the RR was 2.00 (95% CI = 1.10–3.64). The accuracy of self-diagnosed migraine is not certain, and this may influence study results. Neither the occurrence of stroke during migraine nor the relationship of stroke to type of migraine was assessed in this study.

The most recent case–control studies, summarized in Table 13.2, suggest that migraine is a risk factor for ischemic stroke in young women, with a RR around 3.[16,18,20–22] The risk is higher in migraine with aura, with RR ranging from 4[22] to 6[20] to 9.[18] It is markedly increased by smoking (RR 10) and by the use of oral contraceptives (RR 16).[20,22] These risk factors are synergistic (have a more than additive effect), since the OR for ischemic stroke in young female migraineurs who take oral contraceptives and smoke reaches 34.4 (3.27–3.61).[22]

The absolute risk of stroke, which is normally very low in young women, is substantially increased by the presence of migraine. Therefore, young women with migraine should be considered a target group for stroke prevention. Other vascular risk factors, and potential protective factors, need to be considered. In contrast to young women, there is no good evidence that migraine is a risk factor in older age groups.[23]

Stroke with clinical features of migraine

In this category, a secondary headache that resembles migraine arises in the context of cerebrovascular disease. Welch and Levine[6] distinguish two subtypes: symptomatic migraine and migraine mimic. In the symptomatic group, a structural central nervous system (CNS) lesion, such as arteriovenous malformation, produces typical episodes of migraine with aura. The symptoms of migraine with aura may result from triggering of the aura process by the structural abnormality.

Migraine mimic includes cases of acute stroke accompanied by both headache and focal neurologic symptoms that are difficult to distinguish from migraine with aura. The differential diagnosis is difficult in patients who continue to have migraine with aura late in life, when the inci-

Table 13.2 *The association between migraine and stroke in young women: recent case–control studies.*

Authors	Patients	Diagnosis of migraine	Risk of stroke in migraine patients
Tzourio et al[16]	212 patients aged 15–80 years with ischemic stroke 212 hospitalized controls matched for sex, age, and history of hypertension	Direct interview by neurologists, IHS criteria	OR = 4.3 (1.2, 16.3) in women < 45 years
Tzourio et al[21]	72 females aged 15–44 years hospitalized for an ischemic stroke 173 hospitalized controls matched for age	Direct interview by neurologists, IHS criteria	MWA: OR = 3.0 (1.5, 5.8) MA: OR = 6.2 (2.11,18.0)
Lidegaard[22]	692 females aged 15–44 years in a national registry of ischemic stroke 1584 population-based controls matched for age	Questionnaire	OR = 2.8 ($p < 0.001$)
Carolei et al[18]	308 patients aged 15–44 years hospitalized for transient ischemic attack or stroke 591 hospitalized controls	Direct interview by neurologists, IHS criteria	OR = 3.7 (1.5, 9) in women < 35 years MA: OR 8.6 (1, 75)
Chang et al[23]	291 females aged 20–44 years with stroke 736 age and hospital matched controls	Questionnaire Modified IHS criteria	OR = 3.5 (1.3, 9.6) MWA: OR = 2.9 (0.6, 13.5) MA: OR = 3.8 (1.2, 11.5)

IHS = International Headache Society, OR = Odds ratio,
MWA = Migraine without aura, MA = Migraine with aura

Table from Bousser et al[26]

dence of cerebrovascular disease increases. Carotid dissection, which occurs more commonly in migraineurs, can also produce symptoms that mimic a migraine attack but results in an ischemic stroke.

The International Headache Society (IHS) criteria include a disorder termed 'migrainous cerebral infarction' (IHS 1.6.2).[24] We recommend a revision of that definition as outlined below:

- Patients previously fulfill criteria for migraine with aura
- The present attack is typical of previous attacks
- A neuroimaging procedure demonstrates an ischemic infarction in the relevant area
- Alternative causes of stroke are ruled out by appropriate investigations, including imaging procedures for the relevant arteries, echocardiography (preferably transesophageal), and antiphospholipid antibody (APL) syndromes.

These criteria are similar to those prepared by the IHS and to the criteria developed by Welch and Levine for 'migraine induced stroke'.[6] The diagnosis of migrainous cerebral infarction should be supported by appropriate investigations to rule out other causes of cerebral infarction. Iglesias and Bousser[26] performed an extensive review of over 200 cases of migrainous infarcts reported before 1988. When they applied IHS criteria, requiring minimum 'appro-

priate investigations' (transthoracic echocardiography (TTE) and cerebral angiogaphy (any variety)), the number of migrainous infarcts dramatically shrank to 40. This would further decrease if blood tests such as APL were required as 'appropriate investigations'. The absence of another cause does not imply, by default, that migraine is the cause.[25] Neither does the presence of another cause exclude a role for migraine in the etiology of the stroke.

Migrainous infarcts exist but they are rare and vastly overdiagnosed.[6,26–32] Until we have specific diagnostic tools for migraine, it is good clinical practice to use restrictive criteria so as not to overlook other potentially treatable causes.

Uncertain classification

In some patients migraine and stroke appear together, but the nature of the causal relationship, if any, is difficult to firmly establish. For example, a patient may have a typical migraine with aura, take a vasoactive drug such as ergotamine, and then develop a cerebral infarction. In this sequence, it is not clear if the stroke was a consequence of the migraine itself (migrainous cerebral infarction), a result of the treatment with vasoconstrictive medication, or an interaction between the two. As a second example, consider a patient with migraine and frequent or prolonged aura who has a stroke during cerebral angiography. Migraine-like headaches and stroke may also be associated with the APL syndrome, systemic vasculitides, oral contraceptive use, or mitochondrial encephalopathy with lactic acidosis and stroke-like episodes (MELAS). A causal relationship between migraine and stroke is difficult to prove in patients with these or other confounding variables.

Mechanisms of the comorbidity of migraine and stroke

Migraine can produce stroke in several ways:

- Stroke may arise as a consequence of the migraine attack itself, due, for example, to reduced regional cerebral blood flow (rCBF)[33-35] or platelet dysfunction.[36-38]
- Stroke may result from a condition comorbid with migraine, such as carotid dissection,[39] mitral valve prolapse,[40,41] or APL syndrome,[41,43] which are themselves risk factors for stroke.
- Both migraine and stroke may result from an underlying disorder such as MELAS[44,45] or cerebral autosomal dominant arteriopathy with subcortical infarcts and leukoencephalopathy (CADASIL).[46]

Migraine with aura is characterized by impaired cerebrovascular reactivity and decreased rCBF.[33,47-49] These hemodynamic changes are believed to be a consequence of primary neuronal events.[50] The process is thought to be analogous to the spreading cortical depression of Leão,[51] in which a wave of neuronal depression is associated with a reduction in rCBF (see Chapter 5). Olesen and colleagues[47,49] have described similar cerebral blood flow (CBF) changes, known as spreading oligemia, during the aura of migraine in humans. Between attacks, CBF studies suggest that there may be cortical flow asymmetries and differences in cerebrovascular reactivity in migraine with aura patients versus control subjects.[52,53] It is uncertain whether this is part of the physiology or the result of repeated attacks of migraine with aura.

The decrease in rCBF secondary to arteriolar vasoconstriction may be accompanied by sluggish blood flow in dilated intracerebral conductance vessels. Migraine is not associated with an increase in the major conventional risk factors for ischemic stroke,[54] but may be associated with newly-suggested risk factors, such as mitral valve prolapse,[30] patent foramen ovale,[55] hereditary thrombophilia[56] (particularly factor V Leiden mutation),[57-59] or increased platelet aggregation.[60] Caplan[5] reviewed patients with migraine and vertebrobasilar ischemia and concluded that posterior circulation ischemia is common in migraineurs and is not always benign.

Angiography in migraine sufferers revealed severe narrowing in both the vertebral and basilar arteries and occlusion of the basilar or posterior cerebral arteries. This was interpreted as spasm but is very similar to the characteristic 'string sign' of carotid dissection.[61,62] In fact, migraine is a risk factor for dissection.[63] Another possibility is that migraine produces 'pseudo-occlusion' due to vasoconstriction ('spasm') severe enough to prevent anterograde flow. Alternatively, prolonged vasoconstriction could also lead to hemostasis and in situ thrombosis. Moskowitz,[64] in his model of neurogenic inflammation, showed that platelet aggregation occurs in the lumen of blood vessels. Thus, pathologic activation of the trigeminovascular system could result in structural changes of the cerebral vessels, linking the mechanism for headache pain and the potential for cerebral ischemia.

During migraine attacks, migraineurs may undergo severe vasoconstriction in the vertebral and basilar arteries.[5,65,66] Transcranial Doppler ultrasonography demonstrates persistent increased flow velocities, presumed secondary to focal arterial narrowing, in migraineurs.[67,68] Migraine-induced vasoconstriction could lead to chronic structural changes in blood vessels. Levine and Ramadan[69] have suggested that repeated episodes of migraine-induced vasoconstriction and vasodilation may weaken the internal elastic lamina of cerebral vessels and predispose to arterial dissection. Dissection is more common in migraineurs; therefore, migraine may be a risk factor for stroke because of morphologic changes in cerebral blood vessels. It is also possible for stroke to produce migraine-like headache. Olesen et al[70] analysed CBF changes in ischemia-induced (symptomatic) migraine (which is similar to migraine mimic) and migraine-induced ischemic infarction. They studied 15 consecutive patients and concluded that symptomatic migraine may be more frequent than true migrainous infarction, although the distinction could not be made in all cases. Areas with decreased CBF may be more susceptible to spreading cortical depression giving rise to migraine aura. Although migraine is a risk factor for ischemic stroke, more often cerebral ischemia appears to trigger migraine-like headache. Recurrent migraine with aura may be a residual symptom of stroke due to a decreased migraine threshold. A genetic predisposition to migraine,[71] the location and extent of a stroke, and the persistence of small, marginally perfused cortical areas are possible factors to determine the development of migraine with aura after stroke.[70]

Both migraine and stroke produce cerebral metabolic derangements with elements in common. Both disorders produce elevated CBF levels of gamma-aminobutyric acid and cyclic adenosine monophosphate.[72] Migraine-like headaches and stroke-like episodes are both components of MELAS, a mitochondrial disorder due to a mutation in mitochondrial tRNA that results in abnormal oxidative metabolism.[44,45] It is possible that some cases of status migraine without other neurologic manifestation may be a forme fruste of the mitochondrial disorders, although there are no reported cases published that establish this. More severe involvement may produce migrainous stroke due to endothelial dysfunction-induced cerebral angiopathy resulting from impaired energy metabolism.

CADASIL, an inherited arterial disease of the brain,[73] and familial hemiplegic migraine both map to chromosome 19.[74] Familial hemiplegic migraine is distinguished from CADASIL by its early onset, relatively benign prognosis, and normal magnetic resonance imaging (MRI) findings. The main clinical presentation of CADASIL is recurrent subcortical ischemic events, either transient or (more often) permanent.[75] The vascular presentation is not constant and other symptoms, such as dementia, depression, or migraine with aura, can occur. Although these symptoms are usually associated with a history of recurrent strokes, they may be the prominent, or only, manifestation of the disease. Vascular dementia is found in one-third of affected family members and as many as 90% of subjects before death. Attacks of migraine with aura occur in 22% of cases, while its prevalence in the general population is about 6% (see Chapter 6).

White matter abnormalities, possibly ischemic in nature, have been reported in patients with migraine, particularly migraine with aura. Migraine with aura and white matter abnormalities could be a consequence of the same underlying pathophysiologic mechanism that occurs in the mitochondrial diseases (see Chapter 6).

Migrainous infarcts should be differentiated from very long-lasting deficits that can occur after a migrainous attack without computed tomography (CT) or MRI evidence of infarcts and with complete recovery. This has been documented in migraine with aura,[76] and particularly in familial hemiplegic migraine, an autosomal dominant variety of migraine with aura in which hemiplegia, often associated with aphasia, hemianopia, drowsiness, and sometimes coma, can last up to several weeks and then resolve without sequelae.[77–82]

Headaches in stroke syndromes

Ischemic stroke

The headache of ischemic stroke, like that of intracerebral hemorrhage, is accompanied by focal neurologic signs, or alterations in consciousness, or both, that allow it to be differentiated from a primary headache. Headache accompanies ischemic stroke in from 17%[1] to 34%[83] of cases. It may be more frequent in vertebrobasilar than carotid territory strokes and is infrequent in subcortical infarcts and lacunes due to single perforator disease.[83,84] The cause of headache in ischemic stroke is not well understood. The probability of acute-onset headache is directly related to vertebrobasilar stroke and a past history of migraine and inversely related to lacunar stroke.[83] The location of the stroke and a prior history of headache are the best predictions of a headache with an ischemic stroke, but stroke location does not predict headache location. The headache of ischemic stroke is usually unilateral and less likely to be severe or associated with vomiting than the headache of subarachnoid or intracerebral hemorrhage.[1]

Intracerebral hemorrhage

In intracerebral (intraparenchymal) hemorrhage, the headache is usually associated with the rapid development of focal neurologic signs and/or alterations in consciousness, which allows this headache to be differentiated from a primary headache. Headache is present in intracerebral hemorrhage in 60–80% of patients able to speak and is more common in cerebellar and lobar hemorrhages than in thalamic, caudate, capsuloputaminal, or brainstem hemorrhages.[85] Meningeal signs, hematoma location, and female gender were more predictive of headache than hematoma volume. This suggests that headache is more often related to subarachnoid blood and to local anatomic effects than to intracranial hypertension.[85]

The headache of intracerebral hemorrhage is often unilateral and increases gradually in intensity.[84] Nausea, vomiting, and severe hypertension are often associated features. Headache laterality predicts the side of the hemorrhage with an 80% predictive value[85] but otherwise has limited value for predicting hemorrhage location.[1,85]

The headache of cerebellar hemorrhage is often acute and can be severe and maximal at onset, mimicking the headache of subarachnoid hemorrhage (SAH).[86,87] Occipital location and associated neck stiffness are common.[85,88] Orthostatic headache with aggravation by the upright position and alleviation by lying down can occur.[86]

Subarachnoid hemorrhage and thunderclap headache

The headache of SAH is often sudden in onset, reaching maximum intensity within 1 minute. The headache is usually but not inevitably severe. An acute neurologic event must be considered when patients present with severe, acute-onset headache, although migraine can present in this manner (Figure 13.1).[89]

SAH from a ruptured aneurysm occurs in 28 000 people a year in North America.[90] The classical presentation of an aneurysmal SAH is an acute-onset, severe headache associated with a stiff neck, photophobia, nausea, vomiting, and perhaps obtundation or coma; it is easily differentiated from migraine. This catastrophic presentation is often preceded by a minor hemorrhage that can signal the increased likelihood of a major rupture, often within hours to weeks; these 'warning leaks' may be difficult to diagnose.[90–95] In most series of patients with 'minor leaks' related to SAH, headache, nausea, or vomiting are commonly identified retrospectively; loss of consciousness is less common, and seizures or cranial nerve findings are rare. In one study, non-exertional activities preceding the SAH were more frequent than exertional activities.[92] Harling et al[96] could not clinically differentiate between SAH and other benign headaches in patients presenting with the sudden onset of their worst headache ever. Both the SAH and non-SAH groups had neck stiffness and photophobia, but the SAH group had significantly more vomiting.

An extensive neurologic evaluation, including CT and lumbar puncture, is indicated in patients presenting with their first or worst headache, particularly if it is associated with focal neurologic signs, stiff neck, or changes in cognition. CT, which would be performed by most physicians under these clinical circumstances, can miss subarachnoid blood. CT is very accurate if done in close proximity to the hemorrhage. As the subarachnoid blood clears, the CT scan becomes increasingly insensitive.[97] A lumbar puncture can confidently diagnose SAH, and its omission can be detrimental to the patient.[98] Day and Raskin[99] reported a case of thunderclap headache in which angiography showed an aneurysm and arterial spasm, but the CT scan was normal and the cerebrospinal fluid (CSF) bloodless. Several prospective studies had suggested that thunderclap headache in the setting of a normal CT and lumber puncture, in close proximity to the event, is usually benign and angiography probably not necessary.[96,100]

Wijdicks et al[100] prospectively followed 71 patients with severe, sudden-onset thunderclap headaches who had normal CT and CSF findings. All but two patients were admitted to the hospital within 2 days of the headache; only seven patients (10%) reported a previous similar headache. Neurologic examination was normal except for questionable meningismus in 10 patients (14%). Four patients underwent angiography, which was normal. The patients were followed for a mean 3.3 years; none developed evidence of subsequent SAH. Recurrent headaches developed in 12 patients, beginning as early as 1 day and as long as 4 years after the initial one. Four patients were readmitted and still had normal CT and CSF studies; of these, two patients had normal angiography. A total of 31 patients (44%) developed tension-type headaches or migraine without aura during the follow-up period.

Harling et al[96] prospectively followed 14 patients who presented to a regional neurosurgical unit with a sudden headache that was suggestive of SAH but with normal CSF and CT scan. It was not possible, on clinical grounds alone, to distinguish these patients from those who had bled. These patients were followed for a minimum of 18 months. One patient had no further headache, four had musculoskeletal pain, five had psychogenic pain, and four had migraine-type headaches. None developed an unequivocal SAH, and the investigators concluded that angiography cannot be justified in patients with thunderclap headache.

Markus[101] compared the clinical features of thunderclap headache to SAH in a prospective series of 55

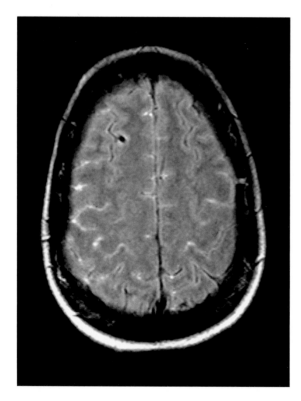

● **Figure 13.1** CT scan showing acute hemorrhage.

patients who presented to a district general hospital with a provisional diagnosis of SAH. Criteria for thunderclap headache included a headache starting within seconds and reaching maximum intensity within 1 minute and a normal CSF examination within 48 hours of headache onset. The clinical features were compared to those of patients who presented to a regional neurosurgical unit with SAH without focal neurologic symptoms or impairment of consciousness. The thunderclap headache was described as the worst headache the patients had ever experienced. The most common locations were occipital (50%) and frontal (38%). Three patients had previously experienced a similar thunderclap headache. No patient in the thunderclap group (n = 18) had developed a SAH at 24 months' follow-up. This was the evidence for the absence of an unruptured aneurysm.

Hughes[102] reported two cases of thunderclap headache due to unruptured aneurysms. Case 1 was a healthy, 32-year-old man who presented with a severe, abrupt-onset, left-sided headache. When evaluated 12 days after the ictus, the headache was gone, CT was negative and lumbar puncture showed nine red blood cells. A left middle cerebral artery trifurcation aneurysm was found; no evidence of recent hemorrhage was found at surgery. Case 2 was a 48-year-old woman who presented with a severe, abrupt-onset headache that was different from her usual migraine. She had a large left posterior cerebral artery aneurysm that showed no evidence of rupture at surgery.

Ng and Pulst[103] reported a 53-year-old woman who presented with the acute onset of the worst headache of her life. Examination, CT, and lumbar puncture were normal. The patient was discharged after 36 hours of observation, but she was re-admitted 2 days later with recurring, persistent headaches. The next day she was found unresponsive. An angiogram showed a distal right internal carotid artery aneurysm. She died shortly thereafter.

Raps et al[104] looked at the clinical spectrum of unruptured intracranial aneurysms, performing a retrospective study of 111 patients (with 132 unruptured aneurysms) who presented to a tertiary referral center. Aneurysms were defined as unruptured by the absence of visible hemorrhage on CT scan, lack of xanthochromia or red blood cells on CSF examination and by visual inspection at the time of surgery. The study included 85 women and 26 men with a mean age of 51.2 years. Fifty-four symptomatic patients were identified; 19 had acute symptoms: ischemia (n = 7), headache (n = 7), seizures (n = 3), and cranial neuropathy (n = 23) and 35 had chronic symptoms attributed to mass effect, including headache (n = 18) and visual loss (n = 10).

Acute severe thunderclap headache, comparable to SAH but without nuchal rigidity, was seen in 6.3% (7/111) of the patients with unruptured aneurysms, most of which were located in the anterior circle of Willis.[104] Thus cataclysmic headache may serve as the symptom of both a ruptured and an unruptured aneurysm. The mechanism for acute headache is likely to involve the vessel wall and may include acute expansion, intraluminal bleeding, or occult hemorrhage. While this study shows conclusively that an unruptured aneurysm can cause thunderclap headache, it does not allow an estimate of the prevalence of this phenomenon in the population due to selection bias.

Intracranial berry aneurysm occurs in 1–2% of the adult population.[104] If < 7% of these in a selected series present with thunderclap headache, the prevalence of this headache type in the general population is no more than 0.1%. The age range is 10–70 years and frequency of recurrence is uncertain. Migraine is an episodic disorder with a 1-year prevalence of about 12%. If 5% of migraineurs had an attack of acute-onset headache, prevalence would be about 0.6%, which is approximately an order of magnitude higher than that of thunderclap headache from unruptured aneurysm. This could, in part, account for the failure of clinical prospective series of thunderclap headache to detect large numbers of unruptured aneurysms. In addition, the criterion for detection is rupture, not angiography. Thus, patients followed for 3 years still could have an unruptured aneurysm (the risk for rupture is only 1% annually.)

In summary, unruptured aneurysm can cause thunderclap headache. The true frequency of unruptured aneurysms among patients with thunderclap headache is unknown. All patients with a possible unruptured aneurysm should have magnetic resonance angiography (MRA). The routine use of cerebral angiography is not recommended because of the risk of permanent (0.1%) and transient (1.2%) deficits in this low-yield population, but angiography is justified in high risk patients.[105]

Headaches associated with vascular procedures

Postcarotid endarterectomy headache

Postcarotid endarterectomy headache is defined by the IHS as an ipsilateral headache that begins within 2 days of carotid endarterectomy, in the absence of carotid occlusion or dissection.[106] The most frequent type of headache that occurs after carotid endarterectomy is a mild, diffuse, nonspecific headache that is not associated with focal deficits, seizures, or increased systemic blood pressure.[107]

This self-limited syndrome occurs in as many as 60% of cases, usually in the 5 days following surgery, particularly during the first two postoperative days. The headache is usually bilateral and frontal, although unilateral headaches occur. This pressure pain is usually mild or moderate and requires no treatment. Its temporal profile is highly variable and may be continuous or intermittent, with a mean duration of 3 days.[25,107]

The second type of postcarotid endarterectomy headache is an episodic, short-lasting pain with trigeminal-autonomic features (see Chapters 9 & 10).[107–109] It is an ipsilateral headache that occurs 12–120 hours after carotid surgery (mean 49.5 hours). The attacks occur once or twice daily and last 2–3 hours. There are no prodromata. The pain is pulsating, moderate or severe, and located mainly in the retroocular and temporoparietal regions. Associated autonomic features are present in various combinations and may include ipsilateral conjunctival injection, lacrimation, rhinorrhea, nasal stuffiness, and Horner's syndrome. In most cases, the pain resolves spontaneously in 2–25 days (mean 14 days). This headache has been related to decreased sympathetic activity.[110]

The third type of headache is part of the 'cerebral hyperperfusion syndrome' that mainly occurs after correction of a very high-grade stenosis in patients with chronic cerebral ischemia.[108,111–115] It is a severe, unilateral, throbbing pain that begins after a mean latent interval of 3 days after surgery. It often precedes the onset of seizures, contralateral focal deficits, and an increase in systemic blood pressure on around the seventh postoperative day.[25]

Headache during intracranial endovascular procedures

Headache has been reported after balloon inflation or embolization of arteriovenous malformations or aneurysms.[116,117] It is a severe, unilateral pain of abrupt onset that occurs shortly after the procedure and is ipsilateral to the occluded artery. It is localized to specific areas according to the artery involved: the temple for the proximal middle cerebral artery, the retroorbital area for the middle of the middle cerebral artery stem, the lateral part of the neck for the upper vertebral artery, and the vertex and occiput for the inferior portion of the basilar artery. This pain is nonthrobbing and not associated with other symptoms. It is most likely due to distention of the arterial wall and provides a good model of pure vascular headache. By contrast, pain is not mentioned in the largest series (23 patients) so far published of angioplasty for atherosclerotic intracranial stenosis.[118]

Headaches associated with other forms of vascular disorders

Cerebral venous thrombosis

Cerebral venous thrombosis (CVT) has a wide spectrum of clinical presentations and an unpredictable but usually favorable outcome.[25] Headache is the most frequent symptom of CVT; it is present in 80–90% of cases and is often the initial and sometimes the only symptom.[119–122] The headache has no specific characteristics. It is often diffuse, but it can be unilateral, localized to any region of the head, or even limited to the neck. It varies in severity, ranging from a mild sensation of heaviness to excruciating pain.[25] The mode of onset is usually subacute (> 2 but ≤ 30 days), but can be sudden. The headache is usually constant, but it can be intermittent, particularly initially, and can even occur in attacks. The headache may be a consequence of intracranial hypertension due to impaired CSF absorption or a consequence of venous occlusion. There are four main patterns and some unusual presentations.[123]

The first pattern, headache with isolated intracranial hypertension, has a characteristic presentation. The headache is progressive over days or weeks. It is almost always associated with papilledema and, less frequently, with sixth-nerve palsy, tinnitus, and transient visual obscurations. It mimics idiopathic intracranial hypertension (pseudotumor cerebri) and accounted for 40% of Bousser et al's 160 patients.[25]

The second pattern is headache with focal signs, usually due to venous infarction. Acute cases mimic arterial strokes, with the rapid onset of neurologic deficits. There is also a chronic presentation, with progressive neurologic deficits mimicking brain tumor or abscess.[25]

The third presentation, subacute encephalopathy, is characterized by diffuse headache and a depressed level of consciousness. This presentation occasionally includes focal deficits or seizures, but intracranial pressure is normal and papilledema is absent. The differential diagnosis includes encephalitis, disseminated intravascular coagulation, and cerebral vasculitis.[25]

The fourth presentation occurs in cavernous sinus thrombosis. In acute cases, a frontal headache is accompanied by chemosis, proptosis, and ophthalmoparesis. Initially unilateral, bilateral ophthalmoparesis may develop.[25]

CVT has a number of unusual presentations, including thunderclap headache. Because CVT can mimic a ruptured intracranial aneurysm (with evidence of SAH), the cerebral venous system should be studied in patients with SAH without arterial causes.[123] Benign thunderclap headache[124] and migraine attacks (with or without aura)[125] can be the presenting symptoms of CVT.[25]

The best current diagnostic tool for CVT is MRI. Only MRI can noninvasively visualize the thrombus itself; the thrombus appears as an increased signal on both TI and T2 images and is usually obvious between day 5 and day 30 after the onset of symptoms.[126–130] MR venography, helical CT venography, or conventional angiography is indicated in the very early (before day 5) or late (after 6 weeks) stages of CVT, as false negative or equivocal MRIs may occur (Figure 13.2).[25]

Before treating CVT, underlying causes such as hypercoagulable states (malignancy, coagulopathy, sepsis, etc.), Behcet's disease, and lupus should be sought. If these are treatable underlying causes, they should be addressed. CVT is treated symptomatically to control seizures and headache and to reduce raised intracranial pressure. Intravenous heparin (dose-adjusted aPTT) is often used, even if a hemorrhagic lesion is present on CT or MRI.[123,131–134]

Headache treatment usually consists of high doses of oral acetaminophen. Aspirin should be avoided because of its interaction with anticoagulants. The prognosis of CVT is unpredictable,[135] with mortality ranging from 33%[121] to 4% (6/160 in Bousser et al's series). There are three main

causes of death: the brain lesion itself (particularly with massive hemorrhagic infarct), intercurrent complications (such as sepsis, uncontrolled seizures, or pulmonary embolism), or the underlying condition (carcinoma, leukemia, septicemia, paroxysmal nocturnal hemoglobinuria, or heart failure).[25]

Spontaneous internal carotid artery dissection

Spontaneous internal carotid artery dissection (ICAD) is an uncommon but not rare cause of headache and acute neurologic deficit in younger patients. Headache, the most common symptom, is usually unilateral and located in the orbital, periorbital, and frontal regions. It is often accompanied by neck pain. The pain is usually moderate to severe and steady or throbbing in nature. Focal cerebral symptoms such as TIA or stroke may precede the headache but frequently follow it by as much as 2 weeks. These symptoms, seen in 60–75% of cases, point to a vascular etiology for the headache. When focal cerebral symptoms are absent, Horner's syndrome, carotid bruit, dysgeusia, and neck pain suggest the diagnosis, which can be confirmed by arteriography, MRI, or carotid ultrasound.[25]

Dissection of the cervical segment of the internal carotid artery is largely a disorder of middle age for a large series. The mean age of onset was 45 years (range 11–74 years); 70% were between the ages of 35 and 50 years.[136]

Spontaneous ICAD usually occurs without risk factors; the role of trivial trauma is uncertain. It has been reported after violent coughing, chiropractic manipulation,[136] noseblowing, sports activities, and even neck-turning.[137] Systemic arteriopathies associated with carotid dissection include cystic medial necrosis, fibromuscular dysplasia, syphilis, and Marfan's and Ehlers–Danlos syndromes. In addition, migraine is a risk factor for dissection. When hemorrhage into the anterior media occurs, subintimal or subadventitial dissection may result. Subintimal dissection causes stenosis and subadventitial dissection produces sac-like outpouchings of adventitia from the vessel wall.[138] The dissection may rupture back through the intima, forming a false lumen. Cerebrovascular symptoms, caused by tight stenosis or, more commonly, by embolization, can lead to stroke or TIA. The pain of ICAD is due to arterial dilation or distention, which stimulates nociceptors in the vessel wall. Electrical stimulation of the carotid bifurcation produces ipsilateral pain in the face and head.[139]

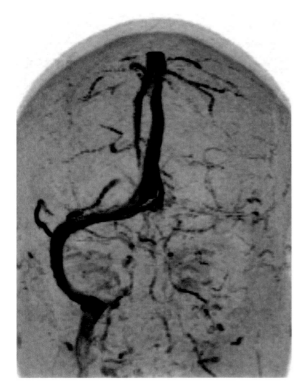

● **Figure 13.2** *Venogram showing lateral sinus thrombosis.*

Clinical features

The IHS has established criteria for the diagnosis of dissection (Table 13.3). The sensitivity and specificity of these criteria has not been established using neuroimaging as the gold standard. Since dissection can occur without Horner's syndrome, arterial bruit, tinnitus, TIA, or stroke, sensitivity is probably low.[106] Pain, the most common symptom of ICAD, usually presents as a unilateral headache that can involve any part of the head, face, or neck. It often has no specific quality and is sudden in onset and variable in severity and location. It can present as carotidynia or as a headache suggestive of SAH with no associated features (Figure 13.3).[106]

Biousse et al[140] studied 67 patients with painful carotid dissection (38 men, 29 women; mean age 63 years). Five

had bilateral extracranial carotid artery dissection. Diagnosis was based on the classical angiographic signs: irregular stenosis, tapered occlusion beginning distal to the cervical bifurcation, and pseudoaneurysm.

Pain was present in 50 patients (75%): headache in 20 patients, neck pain in six patients, facial pain in 11 patients, and a combination of headache and neck pain in 12 patients. In 40 patients (60%), pain was the inaugural symptom of ICAD: headache in 23 patients, facial pain in 10 patients, and neck pain in seven patients; in 10 patients, pain (headache, neck, or facial pain) occurred after another local symptom, such as tinnitus or Horner's syndrome, or after TIA or completed stroke. Headache was unilateral and ipsilateral to the dissection in 20 patients (diffuse in 12 patients, localized in eight patients) and bilateral in 12 patients, two of whom had bilateral extracranial carotid artery dissection. Neck pain and facial pain were always unilateral and ipsilateral to the dissection. Head pain was therefore on the side of the dissection in 38 patients (76%) and bilateral in 12 patients (18%). Pain was considered severe by 35 patients (70%). The pain lasted from 1 hour to 30 days (median 5 days) and usually resolved.[140,141] Cases of persistent pain have been reported,[142] particularly by patients with residual aneurysm.[143]

Migraine was present in 46% of patients with painful ICAD, but in only 18% with nonpainful ICAD. Five patients described the headache of the ICAD as their 'usual migraine'.

In Mokri et al's[144] series of 36 patients with ICAD, 92% initially complained of headache; 85% were unilateral, and the headaches resolved in all but two patients. They were most often periorbital (60%), less often in the ear or mastoid area (39%), frontal area (36%), and temporal area (27%), and least commonly in the face, the occiput, or the angle of the mandible. Headache or neck pain often preceded the onset of cerebral ischemic symptoms by several hours or days. This differs from cases of traumatic carotid dissection, in which focal cerebral ischemic symptoms are the most common.

Retinal or cerebral ischemia is the most common symptom of ICAD. Unilateral head or neck pain in a patient presenting with amaurosis fugax or TIA suggests an ICAD.[24,140,142,143,145–147] Ischemic signs are often delayed and can occur as long as 1 month after the onset of pain.[140] A key element is the presence of ipsilateral local signs associated with the pain in nearly half of patients with ICAD. The most frequent sign is Horner's syndrome, which has long been recognized as suggestive of ICAD.[140,143,145,146,148]

Fisher et al[142] reported on seven patients with persis-

● **Table 13.3** *IHS diagnostic criteria for carotid or vertebral dissection.*

A At least one of the following:
   1 TIA or ischemic stroke in territory of affected artery
   2 Horner's syndrome, arterial bruit, or tinnitus
B Dissection demonstrated by appropriate investigations or surgery
C Headache and cervical pain ipsilateral to arterial dissection

---

THE MOST FREQUENT REGIONS OF HEADACHE AND NECK PAIN ASSOCIATED WITH ICAD

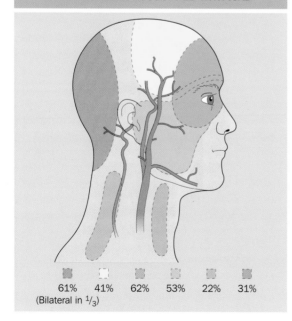

61%　41%　62%　53%　22%　31%
(Bilateral in 1/3)

● **Figure 13.3** *Schematic diagram showing the most frequent regions of headache and neck pain associated with ICAD.*

tent hemiparesis or hemiplegia due to ICAD. All had a TIA or neurologic prodrome of some kind.

Bogousslavsky et al[9] suggested a much greater risk of initial severe infarction resulting from ICAD. Cervical ICAD was found in 2.5% of 1200 consecutive patients seeking treatment for a first stroke, seven of whom died. In this series, carotid dissection did not have its usual benign prognosis, but these patients had associated carotid occlusion and severe ischemic symptoms.

Incomplete Horner's syndrome with ptosis and miosis but not anhidrosis is the third most common sign of ICAD. It occurred in 58% of one series of patients (25)[143] and in 31% of the patients reviewed by Fisher et al.[142] It may persist; in one series it was present in 38% of the patients at late follow-up.[143]

Less common symptoms of ICAD include neck-swelling, tearing, scintillation, syncope, dysgeusia, and ipsilateral tongue paresis from involvement of the hypoglossal nerve and chorda tympani, which course near the internal carotid artery.

ICAD can present with positive visual phenomena that partly resemble migraine visual aura but are associated with features not typical of migraine. In two cases, the visual phenomenon lasted a few days; in a third, it was maximal at onset and did not march.[149]

In Biousse et al's series,[140] associated symptoms included nausea and/or vomiting in 12% of patients, Horner's syndrome in 30%, tinnitus (at times pulsatile) in 16%, TIA in 26%, and completed stroke in 16%. A painful Horner's syndrome was the inaugural symptom of ICAD in 21% of patients.

Radiologic features

The gold standard test for dissection was arteriography. Cervical ICAD typically appears about 2 cm distal to its origin and extends a variable distance, usually terminating at or proximal to the entry of the artery into the petrous bone. Classic positive features on angiography include irregular stenosis ('string sign'), tapered occlusion beginning distal to the cervical bifurcation, and pseudoaneurysm. In a compilation of reports, luminal stenosis was found in 65% of patients, occlusion in 28%, pseudoaneurysm in 26%, luminal irregularity in 13%, distal branch occlusion (emboli) in 13%, intimal flap in 12%, and slow internal carotid artery/middle cerebral artery flow in 11% (Figures 13.4–13.6).[146] High-resolution MRI, especially in the axial planes, can demonstrate the vessel lumina and changes in the arterial wall noninvasively and without contrast (Figure 13.7). This imaging modality is very useful and often alleviates the need for formal angiography. Ultrasound duplex scanning (Table 13.4) is often performed first on an emer-

● Table 13.4 *Duplex sonography: findings suggesting ICAD.[153]*

Indirect findings

No atheromatous plaques visible in carotid bifurcation

Bulb and proximal segment of ICA patent

No flow signal or high-resistance flow pattern (short, only systolic flow peak (stump flow) or bidirectional (reverberating) systolic flow) in proximal ICA

Lack of wall pulsations

Direct signs

Tapering of ICA lumen starting 2 cm distal to bulb

Irregular 'membrane' crossing ICA lumen

Demonstration of true lumen with flow and false (thrombosed) lumen without flow; unlike veins, true and false lumens are noncompressible by probe pressure; flow in false lumen resulting from more distal reentry into true lumen, as frequently found in CCA dissection associated with dissecting aortic aneurysm, is rare

Axial sections show 'membrane' as flap in lumen

Findings at follow-up examinations

Recovery of lumen patency

Flow recovery

Recovery of normal hemodynamics, when combined with TCD

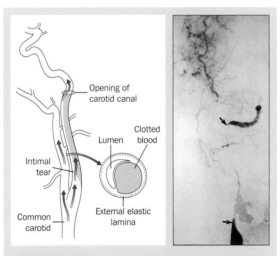

● Figure 13.4 *Carotid angiograph and diagram showing elongated stenosis and abrupt reconstitution of the lumen at the carotid canal.*

gency basis. It can image the arterial lumen as well as the arterial wall and detect intracranial thrombosis. It is noninvasive and can be easily repeated. Early et al[150] reported six patients diagnosed by duplex scanning. Sturzenegger et al[151] found duplex scanning, in combination with transcranial Doppler, to be a useful noninvasive modality for initial

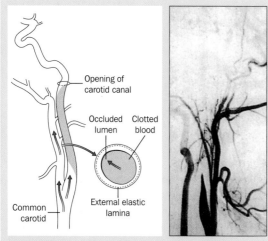

Figure 13.5 *Angiograph and diagram of internal carotid artery dissection in which the intramural hematoma is so enlarged that it has squeezed the true lumen to complete occlusion.*

Figures 13.2–13.5 are reproduced with permission (Rothrock et al[143]).

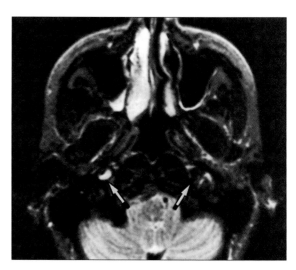

Figure 13.7 *MRI of the head of a patient with unilateral ICAD. The internal carotid artery on the right is normal in size, dark and the region of flow void is round. On the left, the region of flow void is significantly smaller and surrounded by a bright crescent reflecting the intramural hematoma.*

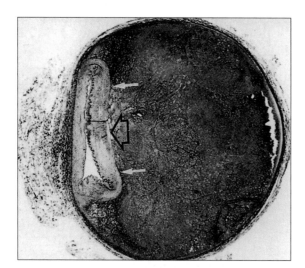

Figure 13.6 *Cross-section of internal carotid artery dissection in which the intramural hematoma is clearly compressed and the true lumen of the vessel has been narrowed.*

diagnosis and an excellent technique for serial follow-up examination. Rothrock et al[152] examined two patients who had ICAD on MRI and carotid duplex examination and found both techniques helpful. Cox et al[153] found MRI useful in two cases of ICAD.

Duplex scanning does have limitations, however (Table 13.5). Since most dissections occur distal to the carotid bifurcation, it is impossible to image a high dissection via duplex scanning. In addition, duplex scanning does not give information about intracerebral dissection or emboli.[150] Additional limitations include its inability to detect aneurysms and to identify the entire length of stenosis. Angiography, MRI, and carotid duplex findings are highly suggestive of, but not specific for, ICAD, unless a double lumen is present. Emboli, temporal arteritis, radiation arteriopathy, and acute atherothrombotic occlusion of the intracranial internal carotid artery can produce a

Table 13.5 *Limitations of duplex sonography.[153]*

Anatomic
Short and/or fat neck, high cervical carotid bifurcation, goitre, calcification of atherosclerotic lesions (sound shadow)
Individual
Restless, agitated patients who continuously swallow air; emphysema; direct examination may be impossible
Methodologic
Occlusion cannot always be demonstrated directly because of its high cervical location
Usually, whole longitudinal extension of wall dissection and especially involvement of intracranial ICA segments (occurring in up to 20%) cannot be detected
Detection of aneurysms is usually not possible
Identification of fibromuscular dysplasia as underlying cause is hardly ever possible

similar angiographic picture, and MRI and carotid duplex may not assist in their differentiation. MRI is pathognomonic if it shows a narrowed lumen with an increase in external diameter and a semilunar-shaped eccentric hypersignal of the vessel wall (mural hematoma).[154] MRA is diagnostic of dissection if it shows sequential narrowing or a lack of arterial signal and an abnormal signal along the length of the dissection site (hematoma) with an increase in the external diameter of the vessel. Combined MRA/MRI has a remarkable diagnostic yield, possibly better than angiography,[155] in extracranial ICAD. For vertebral, basilar artery, or intracranial ICAD, angiography is often required.

Outcome and therapy

Recurrent dissection in a previously dissected and healed vessel is rare. When a patient has had a prior dissection, a new dissection in the uninvolved internal carotid arteries or vertebral arteries is uncommon but not rare. The recurrence rate for second dissections is 2% for the first month and 1% per year for all age groups, more frequent for older patients. Most patients with spontaneous dissections experience excellent clinical and angiographic recovery. A complete or excellent clinical recovery occurs in about 85% of the patients with spontaneous ICAD. Angiographically, stenotic lesions either completely resolve or markedly improve in about 85% of the involved vessels. About 60% of the dissecting aneurysms resolve or diminish in size. Death from massive infarct and edema may occur, but fortunately is quite uncommon (< 5%). Studies that have drawn their cases from acute stroke registries have reported significantly higher death and disability rates. These, however, do not represent the usual disease profile.[156] About 5% of patients with ICAD have severe strokes, and these individuals usually have symptomatic infarction as the initial manifestation. One compilation of 75 cases[149] showed that 75% of patients returned to normal, 16% were left with a minor, nondisabling deficit, and 8% suffered a major deficit or death.

Although the natural history of extracranial spontaneous dissection appears to be relatively benign, a number of medical and surgical therapies have been used to treat these patients. Heparin is the treatment most frequently used. Optimum timing is unclear, but most clinicians delay heparin administration for several days. Worsening ischemic deficit following anticoagulation within several hours of the onset of symptoms has been reported; this may have been related to extension of the medial hemorrhage.[157] Anticoagulants can inhibit thrombosis in an aneurysmal sac. The optimal duration of coagulation has not been established. We often empirically treat with an anticoagulant for 3 months, although data are lacking. Some patients treated with antiplatelet agents, such as aspirin and dipyridamole, have improved, with resolution of the condition and no hemorrhagic complications. For cases refractory to medical therapy, as evidenced by progression or recurrence, acute or delayed surgical intervention may be warranted. Residual dissection, aneurysms, and occlusions appear to be more common with trauma than with spontaneous dissection.[144]

ICAD should be considered when any of the following symptoms are present: painful Horner's syndrome, head pain preceding ischemic symptoms, or unilateral, severe, persistent neck pain of sudden onset with or without headache. Cephalic pain is a frequent symptom of dissection (75%), is often inaugural (60%), and is usually located on the side of the dissection (76%). ICAD can also present with other varieties of head and neck pain, mimicking migraine,[27,62,140,144,148] cluster headache,[140,148] carotidynia,[106] SAH,[106] or Raeder's syndrome.

Carotidynia

'Acute idiopathic carotidynia' is included as a variety of carotid pain and is recognized as a separate entity in the IHS classification with the following four diagnostic criteria:

A	At least one of the following overlying the carotid artery: 1) tenderness, 2) swelling, 3) increased pulsations.
B	Appropriate investigations do not reveal structural abnormality.
C	Pain over the affected side of the neck that may project to the ipsilateral side of the head.
D	A self-limited syndrome of less than 2 weeks' duration.

The term carotidynia was first used by Fay[158] to refer to tenderness of the bifurcation of the carotid artery in some patients with 'atypical facial neuralgia'. Carotidynia now refers to a syndrome characterized by unilateral neck pain and carotid artery tenderness.[159] However, the unilateral neck pain has no specific clinical characteristics or temporal pattern and local tenderness, swelling, and increased pulsations are neither constant nor specific. Carotidynia is not a unique entity but rather a symptom (unilateral neck pain with local tenderness) of many vascular and nonvascular conditions. Recurring attacks of carotidynia with headache that last a few days are probably related to migraine; attacks that last a few minutes suggest chronic paroxysmal hemicrania; and regular daily attacks of 1 or 2 hours' duration suggest cluster headache. Acute self-limited carotidynia may be viral in origin, but carotid dissection must be excluded. Causes of chronic carotidy-nia include carotid artery diseases (occlusion, fibromuscular dysplasia, giant cell arteritis, or carotid endarterectomy), carotid-body tumors, lymphadenitis, pharyngitis, dental infection, local aphthous ulcers, and malignant infiltration.[25,106,159,160]

Angiitis of the central nervous system

Angiitis (vasculitis) is characterized by inflammation of blood vessels. It may be primary or a complication of another disorder, such as infection or carcinoma (secondary angiitis). Angiitis may be restricted to the CNS (isolated angiitis) or part of a systemic illness (systemic angiitis). Headache is a prominent symptom when inflammation affects intracranial blood vessels as in CNS angiitis or extracranial vessels as in temporal arteritis (Table 13.6).

Primary angiitis of the central nervous system

Primary angiitis of the CNS (PACNS; noninfectious granulomatous angiitis, isolated angiitis, primary angiitis, and primary vasculitis of the CNS) is a noninfectious granulomatous angiitis with a predilection for small (200–500 μ) leptomeningeal and intraparenchymal arteries of the CNS with no systemic involvement.[161] It is characterized by fibroid necrosis and infiltration of the vessel walls by lymphocytes, histiocytes, and/or multinucleated giant cells.[162–164] Headache is the most frequent symptom of PACNS, present in 50–67% of reported cases.[25] It is variable in location (but often diffuse), severity (mild to excruciating), and temporal profile (chronic to acute with occasional spontaneous remissions).[165] It can precede other neurologic symptoms by days or weeks, but it never remains isolated.

Headache has very little positive diagnostic value. By contrast, CSF pleocytosis in the absence of headache makes a diagnosis of PACNS less likely. In patients who had a brain biopsy, CSF pleocytosis and headache were the only features that differentiated patients with (36%) and without PACNS: none of the patients who lacked CSF pleocytosis and headache had PACNS; of those who had CSF pleocytosis and/or headache, 49% had PACNS.[166]

A variety of neurologic signs can occur: focal neurologic deficits, cerebellar signs, cranial nerve palsies, generalized or focal seizures, altered cognition, dementia, and disorders of consciousness.[25]

CT and MRI of the brain are usually abnormal in histologically-documented cases, but the findings are non-

Table 13.6 Angiitis of the central nervous system

1. Primary angiitis of the CNS

2. Systemic angiitis with CNS involvement
    - *Large vessel angiitis*
      Giant cell arteritis (temporal arteritis)
      Takayasu's arteritis
    - *Medium vessel angiitis*
      Polyarteritis nodosa
      Kawasaki disease
    - *Small vessel angiitis*
    - With antineutrophil cytoplasmic antibodies
      Wegener's granulomatosis
      Microscopic polyangiitis (microscopic polyarteritis)
      Churg–Strauss syndrome
    - Without antineutrophil cytoplasmic antibodies
      Henoch–Schönlein purpura
      Cryoglobulinemic vasculitis
      Isolated cutaneous leukocytoclastic vasculitis
      Goodpasture's disease

3. Secondary angiitis, due to
    - Infections (viral, bacterial, fungal, rickettsial, mycoplasmal, protozoal)
    - Connective tissue diseases and other systemic diseases (outside angiitis)
    - Drugs and toxics (sympathomimetics, cocaine, radiations)
    - Malignancies

Modified table from Bousser et al[25]

specific: multiple small T2 lesions in both grey and white matter are the most frequent findings, but hemorrhages, mass lesions, leptomeningeal enhancement, or even diffuse, extensive white matter lesions can be seen.[167–174]

CSF is nonspecifically abnormal in 80–90% of histologically-diagnosed cases and in 50–53% of angiographically-diagnosed cases.[165,175,176] The findings usually reflect aseptic meningitis with a modest pleocytosis and elevated protein levels.

The role of angiography is debatable.[165,170,172,177–180] Cases have been diagnosed by angiography alone, but changes attributed to PACNS (alternating areas of stenosis and ectasia in multiple vascular distributions) occur in less than 40–50% of histologically-proven cases,[162,165] and more than half of patients with these classical changes have other conditions, such as distal atheroma or spasm.[162,165]

Histologic confirmation remains the gold standard for the diagnosis of PACNS. Brain biopsy is crucial to rule out other conditions that can mimic PACNS, such as lympho-proliferative diseases, certain infections, and sarcoidosis;[162,164,165] however, its sensitivity is poor since biopsies are negative in as many as 25% of autopsy-documented cases of PACNS.[181] PACNS has a variable prognosis; from death in a few months to slowly progressive with spontaneous remissions. With no treatment, 80% of patients die in the first year and nearly all die in 4 years.[182] There are no controlled trials of PACNS treatment. A small series[169] suggested that aggressive combination of cyclophosphamide (3–5 mg/kg/day) and prednisone (1 mg/kg/day) is beneficial.

Benign angiopathy of the central nervous system

Benign angiopathy of the central nervous system is characterized by the acute onset of headache and other neurologic signs and angiographically by reversible multiple segmental stenosis.[183] When it occurs after delivery it is called postpartum cerebral angiopathy.[25] Headache, a constant feature of this syndrome, is usually severe, diffuse, and pulsatile. It has an acute onset, reaching its maximum in minutes or hours, but it can also be extremely sudden, mimicking SAH or thunderclap headache,[184] or progressive over days or weeks.[185] Headache may be the only symptom of this syndrome, but it is usually associated with nausea and vomiting and frequently with other neurologic signs, such as phonophobia, photophobia, seizures, or focal deficits.

The outcome is generally favorable, with full resolution in 2–16 weeks (usually 4 weeks). CSF is usually normal in contrast to PACNS. Diagnosis is by angiography, which typically shows diffuse, multifocal, segmental narrowings involving large- and medium-sized arteries in the anterior and posterior circulations, with occasional dilated segments (like 'sausage strings') (Figure 13.8).[186] The angiographic pattern of reversible, multifocal, segmental narrowing is thought to be due to a widespread arterial vasoconstriction. It may be due to, or triggered by, many substances or conditions, which often induce acute hypertension. These include pheochromocytoma,[187,188] eclampsia,[189,190] sympathomimetic drugs (amphetamine), ephedrine, phenylpropanolamine,[191] isometheptene, nicotine, ergot alkaloid derivatives, particularly lisuride, and bromocriptine when used to suppress lactation,[192,193] ergonovine, other ergot derivatives,[194] and sumatriptan (in association with cocaine in one case and with dihydroergotamine in another).

There is no accepted treatment: symptomatic treatment includes analgesics and nimodipine, with antiepileptic and antihypertensive drugs added as needed. The role of steroids is uncertain.

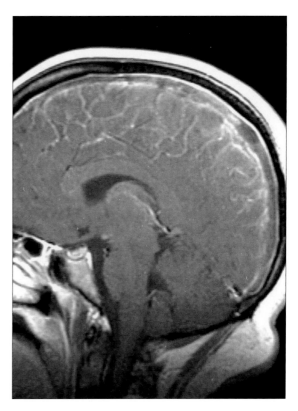

● *Figure 13.8* Superior sagittal sinus thrombosis.

Implications for management, diagnosis, and treatment

The many linkages between headache and stroke have implications for patient management. TIA or stroke can be very similar to migraine aura without headache, creating diagnostic challenges. Episodes of TIA or stroke are often associated with headache; headache may precede or follow the onset of a thromboembolic event.[1] Differentiating TIA or stroke from migraine aura depends on the pattern of symptoms. A history of a slow march of aura symptoms with features that cross vascular territories suggests migraine. The gradual evolution of both positive and negative phenomena (i.e. scintillating scotoma) suggests migraine aura, in contrast to the acute onset of monocular or hemianoptic visual loss seen with stroke. Any patient with migraine and focal neurologic signs or with symptoms that are not consistent with IHS migraine with simple aura requires a neuroimaging study to search for structural disease (i.e. mass lesion, arteriovenous malformation, or stroke).

Epidemiologic studies indicate that migraine is an independent risk factor for stroke (especially in young women). Certainly, migraine patients should be advised not to smoke. Vasoconstrictive medications should be limited or avoided when patients have hemiplegic migraine, basilar migraine, and migraine with prolonged aura. Despite controlled trials that show they are safe and effective, there is some controversy about the use of beta-blockers in migraine with aura. B1-selective blockers, which have no adverse effect on platelet function, can be used in preference to nonselective beta-blockers, which can increase platelet aggregability. We prefer to use calcium-channel blockers, such as verapamil, as preventive treatment for patients with migraine with aura. Divalproex sodium, a Food and Drug Administration-approved migraine medication, is not vasoactive and is an excellent first-choice drug for preventive therapy for migraineurs with aura, especially those for whom vasoactive medications are contraindicated.[195] Topiramate, gabapentin, and lamictal[T] (lamotrigne) are other options.[196]

Possible shared risk factors for migraine and stroke include the APL syndromes, increased platelet aggregability, and mitral valve prolapse. Since these conditions could potentially lead to migrainous infarction, antiplatelet therapy (low-dose aspirin) should be considered if there are no medical contraindications. Aspirin use should also be considered for patients with prolonged or atypical aura. Other cerebrovascular risk factors need to be identified.

● **Table 13.7**   *Risk of stroke.*

General	
Risk of stroke in a female age 20 years	2 per 100 000 women
Risk of stroke on oral contraceptives	3.6 per 100 000 women
Excess stroke risk during pregnancy and 6 weeks' postpartum	8.1 per 100 000 pregnancies
Migraineurs	
Added risk (OR) to a female migraineur under the age of 45 years from:	
Migraine without aura	3
Migraine with aura	6
Oral contraceptives and migraine	13.9
Smoking and migraine	10.2

The use of low-dose estrogen-containing oral contraceptives or hormonal replacement should be avoided if patients are at high risk for stroke, although their use by patients with typical migraine poses only a small absolute risk (Table 13.7). Patients with nonvisual aura symptoms (aphasia, focal sensory motor symptoms, or brainstem symptoms) or prolonged aura require aggressive preventive migraine treatment and an extensive evaluation for coexistent cerebrovascular or other CNS disease. Any change in migraine aura symptoms, especially atypical aura, requires urgent reevaluation, as those symptoms may represent impending stroke rather than migraine.

References

1. Gorelick PB, Hier DB, Caplan LR, Langeberg P. Headache in acute cerebrovascular disease. Neurology 1986; 36: 1445–50.
2. Mitsias P, Ramadan NM. Headache in ischemic cerebrovascular disease. Part II: mechanisms and predictive value. Cephalalgia 1992; 12: 341–4.
3. Mitsias P, Ramadan NM. Headache in ischemic cerebrovascular disease. Part I: clinical features. Cephalalgia 1992; 12: 269–74.
4. Fere C. Contribution à l'étude de la migraine opthalmique. Rev Med (Paris) 1881; 1: 625–47.
5. Caplan LR. Migraine and vertebrobasilar ischemia. Neurology 1991; 41: 55–61.
6. Welch KMA, Levine SR. Migraine-related stroke in the context of the International Headache Society classifications of migraine. Arch Neurol 1990; 47: 458–62.
7. Alvarez J, Matias-Guiu J, Sumalla J. Ischemic stroke in young adults: analysis of etiological subgroups. Acta Neurol Scand 1989; 80: 29–34.
8. Tatemichi TK, Mohr JP. Migraine and stroke. In: Barnett HJM, Mohr JP, Stein BM, Yatsu FM, eds. Stroke: pathophysiology, diagnosis and management. 2nd edn. New York: Churchill-Livingstone, 1992, 761–85.
9. Bogousslavsky J, Despland PA, Regli F. Spontaneous dissection with acute stroke. Arch Neurol 1987; 44: 137–40.
10. Rothrock J, North J, Madden K et al. Migraine and migrainous stroke: risk factors and prognosis. Neurology 1993; 43: 2473–6.
11. Broderick JP, Swanson JW. Migraine-related strokes: clinical profile and prognosis in 20 patients. Arch Neurol 1987; 44: 868–71.
12. Sacquengna T, Andreoli A, Baldrati A et al. Ischemic stroke in young adults: the relevance of migrainous infarction. Cephalalgia 1989; 9: 255–8.
13. Bogousslavsky J, Reglli F, Van Melle G. Migraine stroke. Neurology 1988; 38: 223–7.
14. Collaborative Group for the Study of Stroke in Young Women. Oral contraceptives and stroke in young women. JAMA 1975; 231: 718–22.
15. Henrich JB, Horowitz RI. A controlled study of ischemic stroke risk in migraine patients. J Clin Epidemiol 1989; 42: 773–80.
16. Tzourio C, Iglesias S, Hubert JB et al. Migraine and risk of ischaemic stroke: a case–control study. Br Med J 1993; 307: 289–92.
17. Tzourio C, Iglesias S, Tehindrazanarivelo A et al, for the AICSJ Group. Migraine and ischemic stroke in young women. Stroke 1994; 25: 15.
18. Carolei A, Marini C, DeMatteis G, Italian National Research Council Study Group on Stroke in the Young. History of migraine and risk of cerebral ischaemia in young adults. Lancet 1996; 343: 1503.
19. Baring JE, Herbert P, Romero J et al. Migraine and subsequent risk of stroke in the physicians' health study. Arch

Neurol 1995; 42: 128–34.

20. Tzourio C, Tehindrazanarivelo A, Iglesias S et al. Case–control study of migraine and risk of ischaemic stroke in young women. Br Med J 1995; 310: 830–3.

21. Lidegaard O. Oral contraceptives, pregnancy, and the risk of cerebral thromboembolism: the influence of diabetes, hypertension, migraine, and previous thrombotic disease. Br J Obstet Gynaecol 1995; 102: 153–9.

22. Chang CL, Donaghy M, Poulter N. Migraine and stroke in young women: case–control study. The World Health Organization Collaborative Study of Cardiovascular Disease and Steroid Hormone Contraception. Br Med J 1999; 318: 13–18.

23. Wijman C, Wolf PA, Kase CS et al. Migrainous visual accompaniments are not rare in late life: the Framingham Study. Stroke 1998; 29: 1539–43.

24. Headache Classification Committee of the International Headache Society. Classification and diagnostic criteria for headache disorders, cranial neuralgia, and facial pain. Cephalalgia 1988; 8: 1–96.

25. Bousser MG, Good J, Kittner ST, Silberstein SD. Headache associated with vascular disorders. In: Silberstein SD, Lipton RB, Dalessio DJ, eds. Wolff's Headache and Other Head Pain. 7th edn. New York: Oxford University Press, 2001, 349–92.

26. Bousser MG. Migrainous stroke. Diagnosis and treatment. In: Fieschi C, Fisher M, eds. Prevention of ischemic stroke. London: Martin Dunitz, 1999, 253–64.

27. Bousser MG, Baron JC, Chiras J. Ischemic strokes and migraine. Neuroradiology 1985; 27: 583–7.

28. Fisher CM. An unusual case of migraine accompaniments with permanent sequelae. A case report. Headache 1986; 26: 266–70.

29. Iglesias S, Bousser MG. Migraine et infarctus cerebral. Circ Metab Cerveau 1990; 7: 237–49.

30. Welch KM, Tatemichi TK, Mohr JP. Migraine and stroke. In: Barnett HJ, Mohr JP, Stein BM, Yatsu FM, eds. Stroke, Pathophysiology, Diagnosis, and Management. 3rd edn. Philadelphia: Churchill Livingstone, 1998, 845–67.

31. Welch KMA. Relationships of stroke and migraine. Neurology 1994; 44: 33–6.

32. Varelas PN, Wojman CA, Fayad P. Uncommon migraine subtypes and their relation to stroke. The Neurologist 1999; 5: 135–44.

33. Lauritzen M, Olesen J. Regional cerebral blood flow during migraine attacks by xenon-133 inhalation and emission tomography. Brain 1984; 107: 447–61.

34. Levine SR, Welch KM, Ewing JR, Robertson WM. Asymmetric cerebral blood flow patterns in migraine. Cephalalgia 1987; 7: 245–8.

35. Olesen J. Cerebral and extracranial circulatory disturbances in migraine: pathophysiological implications. Cerebrovasc Brain Metab Rev 1991; 3: 1–28.

36. Joseph R, Welch KMA. Migraine and the platelet. Headache 1987; 27: 375–80.

37. Kalendovsky Z, Austin J, Steele P. Increased platelet aggregability in young patients with stroke. Arch Neurol 1975; 32: 13–20.

38. Kalendovsky Z, Austin JH. 'Complicated migraine'; its association with increased platelet aggregability and abnormal plasma coagulation factors. Headache 1975; 15: 18–35.

39. Ramadan NR, Tietjen GE, Levine SR, Welch KMA. Carotid artery dissection associated with scintillating scotomata. Neurology 1991; 41: 1084–7.

40. Pfaffenrath V, Pöllmann W, Autenreith G, Rosmanith U. Mitral valve prolapse and platelet aggregation in patients with hemiplegic and nonhemiplegic migraine. Acta Neurol Scand 1987; 75: 253–7.

41. Herman P. Migraine and mitral valve prolapse. Arch Neurol 1989; 46: 1165.

42. Brey RL, Hart RG, Sherman DG, Tegeler CH. Antiphospholipid antibodies and cerebral ischemia in young people. Neurology 1990; 40: 1190–6.

43. Tietjen GE, Levine SR, Welch KMA. Migraine and antiphospholipid antibodies. In: Appel SH, ed. Current Neurology. Chicago: Mosley Year Book, 1992, 201–13.

44. Pavlakis SG, Rowland LP, DeVivo DC et al. Mitochondrial myopathies and encephalomyopathies. In: Pavlakis SG, Rowland LP, DeVivo DC, Bonilla F, Divlauro S, eds. Advances in Contemporary Neurology. Philadelphia: FA Davis, 1988, 95–134.

45. Ciafaloni E, Ricci J, Shanske S. MELAS: clinical features, biochemistry, and molecular genetics. Ann Neurol 1992; 31: 391–8.

46. Chabriat H, Vahedi K, Iba-Zizen MT et al. Clinical spectrum of CADASIL: a study of seven families. Lancet 1995; 346: 934–9.

47. Olesen J, Larsen B, Lauritzen M. Focal hyperemia followed by spreading oligemia and impaired activation of RCBF in classic migraine. Ann Neurol 1981; 9: 344–52.

48. Lauritzen M, Olsen TS, Lassen NA, Paulson OB. Changes in regional cerebral blood flow during the course of classic migraine attacks. Ann Neurol 1983; 13: 633–41.

49. Olesen J, Lauritzen M, Tfelt-Hansen PK et al. Spreading cerebral oligemia in classical and normal cerebral blood flow in common migraine. Headache 1982; 22: 242–8.

50. Lauritzen M. Pathophysiology of the migraine aura: the spreading depression theory. Brain 1994; 17: 199–210.

51. Leão AAP. Spreading depression of activity in cerebral cortex. J Neurophysiol 1944; 7: 359–90.

52. Levine SR, Welch KMA, Ewing JR et al. Cerebral blood flow asymmetries in headache-free migraineurs. Stroke 1987; 18: 1164–5.

53. Lagreze HL, Dettmers C, Hartmann A. Abnormalities of interictal cerebral perfusion in classic but not common migraine. Stroke 1988; 19: 1108–11.

54. Launer LJ, Terwindt GM, Nagelkerke NJ, Ferrari MD. Risk factors for stroke in female migraineurs and nonmigraineurs: the GEM study. Neurology 1999; 52: 123.

55. Del Sette M, Angeli S, Leandri M et al. Migraine with aura and right-to-left shunt on transcranial Doppler: a case–control study. Cerebrovasc Dis 1998; 8: 327–30.

56. d'Amico D, Moschiano F, Leone M et al. Genetic abnormalities of the protein C system: shared risk factors in young adults with migraine with aura and with ischemic stroke? Cephalalgia 1998; 18: 618–21.

57. Kontula Y, Ylikorkala A, Miettinen H et al. Arg 506 Factor V mutation (Factor V Leiden) in patients with ischemic cerebrovascular disease and survivors of myocardial infarction. Thromb Hemostas 1995; 73: 558–60.

58. Haan J, Kappelle LJ, deRonde H et al. The Factor V Leiden mutation (R506Q) is not a major risk factor for migrainous cerebral infarction. Cephalalgia 1997; 17: 605–7.

59. Sorani S, Borgna-Pignatti C, Trabetti E et al. Frequency of factor V Leiden in juvenile migraine with aura. Headache 1998; 38: 779–81.

60. Couch JR, Hassanein RS. Platelet aggregability in migraine. Neurology 1977; 27: 843–8.

61. Bousser MG, Baron JC, Mas JL. More on unusual angiographic appearance during an attack of hemiplegic migraine. Headache 1986; 26: 487.

62. Shuaib A. A stroke from other etiologies masquerading as a migraine-stroke. Stroke 1991; 22: 1068–74.

63. d'Anglejan-Chatillon J, Ribeiro V, Mas JL et al. Migraine: a risk factor for dissection of cervical arteries. Headache 1989; 29: 560–1.

64. Moskowitz MA. The neurobiology of vascular head pain. Ann Neurol 1984; 16: 157–68.

65. Schon R, Harrison MJ. Can migraine cause multiple segmental cerebral artery constrictions? J Neurol Neurosurg Psychiatry 1987; 50: 492–4.

66. Laurent B, Michel D, Antoine JC, Montagnon D. Migraine basilaire avec alexie sans agraphie; spasme arteriel a l'arteriographie et effet de la naloxone. Rev Med (Paris) 1984; 40: 663–5.

67. Schroth G, Gerber WD, Langohr HD. Ultrasonic Doppler flow in migraine and cluster headache. Headache 1983; 23: 284–8.

68. Thie A, Spitzer K, Lachenmayer L, Kunze K. Prolonged vasospasm in migraine detected by noninvasive transcranial Doppler ultrasound. Headache 1988; 28: 183–6.

69. Levine SR, Ramadan NM. The relationship of stroke and migraine. In: Adams HP, ed. Handbook of Cerebrovascular Diseases. New York: Marcel Dekker, Inc., 1993, 221–31.

70. Olesen J, Friberg L, Olsen TS et al. Ischemia-induced (symptomatic) migraine attacks may be more frequent than migraine-induced ischemic insults. Brain 1993; 116: 187–202.

71. Welch KMA. Migraine: a behavioral disorder. Arch Neurol 1987; 44: 323–7.

72. Welch KMA, Chabi E, Nell JH et al. Biochemical comparison of migraine and stroke. Headache 1976; 6: 160.

73. Tournier-Lasserve E, Joutel A, Melki J. Cerebral autosomal arteriopathy with subcortical infarcts and leukoencephalopathy maps to chromosomes. Nat Genet 1993; 3: 256–9.

74. Ophoff RA, van Eijk R, Sandkuijl LA et al. Genetic heterogeneity of familial hemiplegic migraine. Genomics 1994; 22: 21–6.

75. Chabriat H, Tournier-Lasserve E, Vahedi K et al. Autosomal dominant migraine with MRI white-matter abnormalities mapping to the CADASIL locus. Neurology 1995; 45: 1086–91.

76. Marchioni E, Galimberti A, Soragna D et al. Familial hemiplegic migraine versus migraine with prolonged aura: an uncertain diagnosis in a family report. Neurology 1995; 45: 33–7.

77. Whitty CW. Familial hemiplegic migraine. J Neurol Neurosurg Psychiatry 1953; 16: 172–7.

78. Harrison MJ. Hemiplegic migraine. J Neurol Neurosurg Psychiatry 1981; 44: 652–3.

79. Baron JC, Serdaru M, Lebrun-Gandrie P et al. Debit sanguine cerebral et consommation d'oxygene locale au cours migraine hemiplegique prolongee. In: Sandoz Editions, ed. Migraine et cephales. Vol. 1. France: Colloque de Marseille, 1983: 33–43.

80. Fitzsimons RB, Wolfenden WH. Migraine coma. Meningitic migraine with cerebral edema associated with a new form of autosomal dominant cerebellar ataxia. Brain 1985; 108: 555–77.

81. Mtinte TF, Miiler-Vahl H. Familial migraine coma: a case study. J Neurol 1990; 237: 59–61.

82. Joutel A, Bausser MG, Biousee V. A gene for familial hemiplegic migraine maps to chromosome 19. Nat Genet 1993; 5: 40–5.

83. Ferro JM, Melo TP, Oliveira V et al. A multivariate study of headache associated with ischemic stroke. Headache 1995; 35: 315–19.

84. Gorelick PB. Ischemic stroke and intracranial hematoma. In: Olesen J, Tfelt-Hansen P, Welch KMA, eds. The Headaches. New York: Raven Press Ltd, 1993.

85. Melo TP, Pinto AN, Ferro JM. Headache in intracerebral hematomas. Neurology 1996; 47: 494–500.

86. Fisher CM, Picard EH, Polak P, Ojemann RG. Acute hypertensive cerebellar hemorrhage: diagnosis and surgical treatment. J Nerve Ment Dis 1965; 140: 38–57.

87. Kase CS, Mohr JP, Caplan LR. Intracerebral hemorrhage. In: Barnett HJ, Mohr JP, Stein BM, Yatsu FM, eds. Stroke: Pathophysiology, Diagnosis, and Management. 3rd edn. New York: Churchill Livingstone, 1998.

88. Ott KH, Kase CS, Ojemann RG, Mohr JP. Cerebellar hemorrhage: diagnosis and treatment. A review of 56 cases. Arch Neurol 1974; 31: 160–7.

89. Silberstein SD. Evaluation and emergency treatment of headache. Headache 1992; 32: 396–407.

90. Leblanc R. The minor leak preceding subarachnoid hemorrhage. J Neurosurg 1987; 66: 35–9.

91. Waga S, Otsubo K, Handa H. Warning signs in intracranial aneurysms. Surg Neurol 1975; 3(1): 15–20.

92. Fontanarosa PB. Recognition of subarachnoid hemorrhage. Ann Emerg Med 1989; 18: 1119–205.

93. Duffy GP. The 'warning leak' in spontaneous subarachnoid hemorrhage. Med J Aust 1983; 1: 514–16.

94. King RB, Saba MI. Forewarnings of major subarachnoid hemorrhage. NY State J Med 1974; 74: 638–9.

95. Bartleson JD, Swanson JW, Whisnant JP. A migrainous syndrome with cerebrospinal fluid pleocytosis. Neurology 1981; 31: 1257–62.

96. Harling DW, Peatfield RC, van Hille PT, Abbott RJ. Thunderclap headache: is it migraine? Cephalalgia 1989; 9: 87–90.

97. Adams HP, Kassell NF, Torner JC, Sahs AL. CT and clinical correlations in recent aneurysmal subarachnoid hemorrhage: a preliminary report of the cooperative aneurysm study. Neurology 1983; 33: 981–8.

98. Silberstein SD, Marcelis J. Headache associated with changes in intracranial pressure. Headache 1992; 32: 84–94.

99. Day JW, Raskin NH. Thunderclap headache: symptom of unruptured cerebral aneurysm. Lancet 1986; 1247–8.

100. Wijdicks EFM, Kerkhoff H, van Gijn H. Long-term follow-up of 71 patients with thunderclap headache mimicking subarachnoid hemorrhage. Lancet 1988; 2: 68–70.

101. Markus HS. A prospective follow up of thunderclap headache mimicking subarachnoid haemorrhage. J Neurol Neurosurg Psychiatry 1992; 54: 1117–18.

102. Hughes RL. Identification and treatment of cerebral aneurysms after sentinel headache. Neurology 1992; 42: 1118–19.

103. Ng PK, Pulst SM. Not so benign 'thunderclap headache'. Neurology 1992; 260: 42.

104. Raps EC, Rogers JD, Galetta SL et al. The clinical spectrum of unruptured intracranial aneurysms. Arch Neurol 1993; 50: 265–8.

105. Leow K, Murie JA. New information on several painful conditions: thunderclap headache mimicking subarachnoid hemorrhage. Neurology Alert 1988; 7: 5–6.

106. Biousse V, Woimant F, Amarenco P et al. Pain as the only manifestation of internal carotid artery dissection. Cephalalgia 1992; 12: 314–17.

107. Tehindrazanarivelo A, Lutz G, Petitjean C, Bousser MG. Headache following carotid endarterectomy: a prospective study. Cephalalgia 1991; 11: 353.

108. Leviton A, Caplan L, Salzmen E. Severe headaches after carotid endarterectomy. Headache 1975; 15: 207–10.

109. Pearce J. Headache after carotid endarterectomy. Br Med J 1976; 2: 85–6.

110. de Marinis M, Zaccaria A, Faraglia V et al. Postendarterectomy headache and the role of the oculosympathetic system. J Neurol Neurosurg Psychiatry 1991; 54: 314–17.

111. Dolan JG, Mushlin AL. Hypertension, vascular headaches, and seizures after carotid endarterectomy. Arch Int Med 1984; 144: 1489–91.

112. Bernstein M, Fleming JF, Deck JH. Cerebral hyperperfusion after carotid endarterectomy: a cause of cerebral hemorrhage. Neurosurg 1984; 15: 50–6.

113. Reigel MM, Hollier LH, Sundt TM et al. Cerebral hyperperfusion syndrome: a cause of neurologic dysfunction after carotid endarterectomy. J Vasc Surg 1987; 5: 628–34.

114. Breen JC, Caplan LR, de Witt LD et al. Brain edema after carotid surgery. Neurology 1996; 46: 175–81.

115. Ille O, Woimant F, Pruna A et al. Hypertensive encephalopathy after bilateral carotid endarterectomy. Stroke 1995; 26: 488–91.

116. Nichols FT, Mawad M, Mohr JP et al. Focal headache during balloon inflation in the internal carotid and middle cerebral arteries. Stroke 1990; 21: 555–9.

117. Martins IP, Baeta E, Paiva T et al. Headaches during intracranial endovascular procedures: a possible model of vascular headache. Headache 1993; 33: 227–33.

118. Marks MP, Marcellus M, Norbash AM et al. Outcome of angioplasty for atherosclerotic intracranial stenosis. Stroke 1999; 30: 1065–9.

119. Ameri A, Bousser MG. Cerebral venous thrombosis. Neurol Clin 1992; 10: 87–111.

120. Bousser MG, Chiras J, Sauron B et al. Cerebral venous thrombosis. A review of 38 cases. Stroke 1985; 16: 199–213.

121. Cantu C, Barinagarrementeria F. Cerebral venous thrombosis associated with pregnancy and puerperium: review of 67 cases. Stroke 1993; 24: 1880–4.

122. Daif A, Awada A, al-Rajeh S et al. Cerebral venous thrombosis in adults. A study of 40 cases from Saudi Arabia. Stroke 1995; 26: 1193–5.

123. Bousser MG, Russell RR. Cerebral venous thrombosis. In: Bousser MG, Russell RR, eds. Major Problems in Neurology. Vol. I. London: Saunders, 1997, 175.

124. de Bruijn SF, Stam J, Kappelle U. Thunderclap headache as first symptom of cerebral venous sinus thrombosis. For the CVST Study Group. Lancet 1996; 348: 1623–5.

125. Newman DS, Levine SR, Curtis VL, Welch KMA. Migraine-like visual phenomena associated with cerebral venous thrombosis. Headache 1989; 29: 82–5.

126. Dormont D, Anxionnat R, Evrard S et al. MRI in cerebral venous thrombosis. J de Neuroradiologie 1994; 21: 81–99.

127. Mattle H, Edelkman RR, Reis MA, Atkinson DJ. Flow quantification in the superior saggittal sinus using magnetic resonance. Neurology 1990; 40: 813–15.

128. Padayachee TS, Bingham JB, Grave MJ et al. Dural sinus thrombosis. Diagnosis and follow-up by magnetic resonance angiography and imaging. Neuroradiol 1991; 33: 165–7.

129. Rippe DJ, Boyko OB, Spritzer CE et al. Demonstration of dural sinus occlusion by the use of MR angiography. Am J Neuroradiol 1990; 11: 199–201.

130. Tsai FY, Wang AM, Matovich VB et al. MR stating of acute dural sinus thrombosis: correlation with venous pressure measurements and implications for treatment and prognosis. Am J Neuroradiol 1995; 16: 1021–9.

131. Einhaupl KM, Villringer A, Meister W et al. Heparin treatment in sinus venous thrombosis. Lancet 1991; 338: 597–600.

132. Villringer A, Mehraein S, Einhdupl KM. Treatment of sinus venous thrombosis beyond the recommendation of anticoagulation. J Neuroradiol 1994; 21: 72–80.

133. Bousser MG. Cerebral venous thrombosis. Nothing, heparin, or local thrombolysis? Stroke 1999; 30: 481–3.

134. de Bruijn SF, Stam J. Randomized, placebo-controlled trial of anticoagulant treatment with low molecular weight heparin for cerebral sinus thrombosis. For the Cerebral Venous Sinus Thrombosis Group. Stroke 1999; 30: 484–8.

135. Barinagarrementeria F, Cantu C, Arredondo H. Aseptic cerebral venous thrombosis: proposed prognostic scale. J Stroke Cerebrovasc Dis 1992; 2: 34–9.

136. Hart RG, Easton JD. Dissections of cervical and cerebral arteries. Neurol Clin 1983; 1: 155–82.

137. Luken MG, Ascherl GF, Correll JW. Spontaneous dissecting aneurysms of the internal carotid arteries. Am J Surg 1971; 122: 549–51.

138. Friedman WA, Day AL, Quisling RG et al. Cervical carotid dissecting aneurysms. Neurosurgery 1980; 7: 207–14.

139. Fay T. Atypical facial neuralgia, a syndrome of vascular pain. Ann Otol Laryngol 1932; 41: 1030–62.

140. Biousse V, d'Angletan JD, Touboul P et al. Headache in 67 patients with extracranial internal carotid artery dissection. Fifth International Headache Congress. Cephalalgia 1991; 11: 349–50.

141. Mas JL, Bousser MG, Hasboun D, Laplane D. Extracranial vertebral artery dissections: a review of 13 cases. Stroke 1987; 18: 1037–47.

142. Fisher CM, Ojemann RG, Robertson GH. Spontaneous dissection of cervicocerebral arteries. J Neurol Sci 1987; 5: 9–19.

143. Mokri B, Sundt TM, Houser OW, Piepgras DG. Spontaneous dissection of the cervical internal carotid artery. Ann Neurol 1986; 19: 126–38.

144. Mokri B, Houser W, Sandok BA, Piepgras DG. Spontaneous dissections of the vertebral arteries. Neurology 1988; 38: 880–5.

145. d'Anglejan Chatillon J, Ribiero V, Mas JL et al. Dissection de l'artère carotide interne extracranienne. Soixante deux observations. Presse Méd 1990; 19: 661–7.

146. Anson J, Crowell RM. Cervicocranial arterial dissection. Neurosurgery 1991; 29: 89–96.

147. Biller J, Hingtgen WL, Adams HP et al. Cervicocephalic arterial dissections. A ten year experience. Arch Neurol 1986; 43: 1234–8.

148. Fisher CM. The headache and pain of spontaneous carotid dissection. Headache 1982; 22: 60–5.

149. Ramadan NM, Tietjen GE, Levine SR, Welch KMA. Scintillating scotomata associated with internal carotid dissection: a report of three cases. Neurology 1991; 41: 1084–7.

150. Early TF, Gregory RT, Wheeler JR et al. Spontaneous carotid dissection: duplex scanning in diagnosis and management. J Vasc Surg 1991; 14: 391–7.

151. Sturzenegger M. Ultrasound findings in spontaneous carotid artery dissection. Arch Neurol 1991; 48: 1057–63.

152. Rothrock JF, Lim V, Press G, Gosink B. Serial magnetic resonance and carotid duplex examinations in the management of carotid dissection. Neurology 1989; 39: 686–92.

153. Cox LK, Bertorini T, Laster RE. Headaches due to spontaneous internal carotid artery dissection: magnetic resonance imaging evaluation and follow up. Headache 1991; 31: 12–16.

154. Ozdoba C, Sturzenegger M, Schroth G. Internal carotid artery dissection: MR imaging features and clinical–radiologic correlation. Radiology 1996; 199: 191–8.

155. Smith HJ, Kerty E, Dahl A. Cervicocranial artery dissection. Detection by Doppler ultrasound and MR angiography. Acta Radiologica 1996; 37: 529.

156. Mokri B. Headache in spontaneous carotid and vertebral artery dissections. In: Goadsby PJ, Silberstein SD, eds. Blue Books of Practical Neurology. Boston: Butterworth-Heinemann, 1997: 327–54.

157. Chapleau CE, Robertson JT. Spontaneous cervical carotid artery

dissection: outpatient treatment with continuous heparin infusion using a totally implantable infusion device. Neurosurgery 1981; 8: 83–7.

158. Fay T. Atypical facial neuralgia. Arch Neurol Psychiatry 1927; 18: 309–15.

159. Biousse V, Bousser MG. The myth of carotidynia. Neurology 1994; 44: 993–5.

160. Vijayan N, Watson C. Raeder's syndrome, pericarotid syndrome and carotidynia. In: Vinken PJ, Bruyn GW, eds. Headache. Vol. 4. Amsterdam: North Holland Publishing Company, 1986, 329–41.

161. Cravioto J, Feigin I. Noninfectious granulomatous angiitis with a predilection for the nervous system. Neurology 1959; 9: 599–609.

162. Chu CT, Gray L, Goldstein LB, Hulette CM. Diagnosis of intracranial vasculitis: a multidisciplinary approach. J Neuropathy Exp Neurol 1998; 57: 30–8.

163. Lie JT. Primary (granulomatous) angiitis of the central nervous system: a clinicopathologic analysis of 15 new cases and a review of the literature. Hum Pathol 1992; 23: 164–71.

164. Parisi JE, Moore PM. The role of biopsy in vasculitis of the central nervous system. Neurology 1994; 14: 341–8.

165. Calabrese LH, Duna GF, Lie JT. Vasculitis in the central nervous system. Arthritis Rheum 1997; 40: 1189–201.

166. Alrawi A, Trobe JD, Blaivas M, Musch D. Brain biopsy in primary angiitis of the central nervous system. Neurology 1999; 53: 858–60.

167. Sudo K, Tashiro K. Idiopathic granulomatous angiitis of the CNS manifesting as white matter disease. Neurology 1998; 51: 1774.

168. Berger JT, Wei T, Wilson D. Idiopathic granulomatous angiitis of the CNS manifesting as white matter disease. Neurology 1998; 51: 1774–5.

169. Cupps TR, Moore PM, Fauci AS. Isolated angiitis of the central nervous system: prospective diagnostic and therapeutic experience. Am J Med 1983; 74: 97–105.

170. Harris KG, Tran DD, Sickels WJ et al. Diagnosing intracranial vasculitis: the roles of MR and angiography. Am J Neuroradiol 1994; 15: 317–30.

171. Stone JH, Pomper MG, Roubenoff R et al. Sensitivities of noninvasive tests for central nervous system vasculitis: a comparison of lumbar puncture, computed tomography, and magnetic resonance imaging. J Rheumatol 1994; 21: 1277–82.

172. Greenan TJ, Grossman RI, Goldberg HI. Cerebral vasculitis: MR imaging and angiographic correlation. Radiology 1992; 182: 65–72.

173. Ehsan T, Hasan S, Powers JM, Heiserman JE. Serial magnetic resonance imaging in isolated angiitis of the central nervous system. Neurology 1995; 45: 1462–5.

174. Finelli PF, Onyiuke HC, Uphoff DF. Idiopathic granulomatous angiitis of the CNS manifesting as diffuse white matter disease. Neurology 1997; 1696–9.

175. Moore PM. Diagnosis and management of isolated angiitis of the central nervous system. Neurology 1989; 39: 167–73.

176. Moore PM. Vasculitis of the central nervous system. Semin Neurol 1994; 14: 313–19.

177. Calabrese LH, Gragg LA, Furlan AJ. Benign angiopathy: a distinct subset of angiographically defined primary angiitis of the central nervous system. J Rheumatol 1993; 20: 2046–50.

178. Koo EH, Massey EW. Granulomatous angiitis of the central nervous system: protean manifestations and response to treatment. J Neurol Neurosurg Psychiatry 1988; 51: 1126–33.

179. Alhalabi M, Moore PM. Serial angiography in isolated angiitis of the central nervous system. Neurology 1994; 44: 1221–6.

180. Vollmer TL, Guarnaccia J, Harrington W et al. Idiopathic granulomatous angiitis of the central nervous system: diagnostic challenges. Arch Neurol 1993; 50: 925–30.

181. Calabrese LH, Furlan AH, Gragg LA, Ropos TH. Primary angiitis of the central nervous system: diagnostic criteria and clinical approach. Cleve J Med 1992; 59: 293–306.

182. Hankey GJ. Necrotizing and granulomatous angiitis of the CNS. In: Ginsberg MD, Bogousslavsky J, eds. Cerebrovascular Disease: Pathophysiology, Diagnosis, and Management. Vol. 2. London: Blackwell Science, 1998: 1647–83.

183. Calabrese LH. Angiographically defined primary angiitis of the CNS: is it really benign? Neurology 1999; 52: 1302.

184. Dodick DW, Brown RD, Britton JW, Huston J. Nonaneurysmal thunderclap headache with diffuse, multifocal, segmental, and reversible vasospasm. Cephalalgia 1999; 19: 118–21.

185. Call GK, Fleming MC, Sealfon S et al. Reversible cerebral segmental vasoconstriction. Stroke 1988; 19: 1159–70.

186. Comabella M, Alvarez-Sabin J, Rovira A, Codina A. Bromocriptine and postpartum cerebral angiopathy. A causal relationship? Neurology 1996; 46: 1754–6.

187. Armstrong FS, Hayes GJ. Segmental cerebral arterial constriction associated with pheochromocytoma. J Neurosurg 1961; 18: 843–6.

188. McColl GJ, Fraser K. Pheochromocytoma and pseudovasculitis. J Rheumatol 1995; 22: 1441–2.

189. Trommer BC, Homer D, Mikhael MA. Cerebral vasospasm and eclampsia. Stroke 1988; 19: 326–9.

190. Will AD, Lewis KL, Hinshaw DB et al. Cerebral vasoconstriction in toxemia. Neurology 1987; 37: 1555–7.

191. LeCoz P, Woimant F, Rougemont D et al. Angiopathies cerebrales benignes et phenylpropanolamine. Rev Neurol 1988; 144: 295–300.

192. Janssens E, Hommel M, Mounier-Vehier F et al. Postpartum cerebral angiopathy possibly due to bromocriptine therapy. Stroke 1985; 26: 128–30.

193. Lucas C, Deplanque D, Salhi A et al. Angiopathie benigne du postpartum: un cas clinicoradiologique associé à la prise de bromocriptine. Rev Med Intern 1996; 17: 839–41.

194. Senter HJ, Lieberman AN, Pinto R. Cerebral manifestations of ergotism, report of a case and review of the literature. Stroke 1976; 7: 88–92.

195. Silberstein SD, Saper J, Mathew N. The safety and efficacy of divalproex sodium in the prophylaxis of migraine headache: a multicentered double-blind, placebo-controlled trial. Headache 1993; 33: 264–265.

196. Hering R, Kuritzky A. Sodium valproate in the prophylactic treatment of migraine: a double-blind study versus placebo. Cephalalgia 1992; 12: 81–4.

chapter 14

Sinus headache and nasal disease

Sinusitis

Sinus infections are much less common today than they were in the preantibiotic era, but they are still frequently overdiagnosed. Acute sinusitis, a relatively uncommon cause of headache in relation to other headache disorders, is due to infection of one or more of the cranial sinuses (Figure 14.1). Acute sinusitis is usually characterized by purulent discharge in the nasal passages and a pain profile determined by the site of infection. Sinusitis is overdiagnosed as a cause of headache because of the belief that pain over the sinuses must be related to the sinuses. In fact, frontal head pain is more often caused by migraine and tension-type headache. It should not follow that if a patient fails to respond to treatment for migraine and tension-type headache one should reconsider the diagnosis of sinus disease. Whether nasal obstruction can lead to chronic headache is very controversial.[1] Paradoxically, sinus disease also tends to be underdiagnosed, as sphenoid sinus infection is frequently missed.[2]

Because sphenoid sinusitis differs from the other forms of sinusitis both in clinical features and treatment, it will be considered separately in this chapter. Although it represents only 3% of sinusitis cases, sphenoid sinusitis is important out of proportion to its prevalence because it is potentially life-threatening.

This chapter discusses the relevant anatomy and pathophysiology of sinusitis, its clinical features, diagnostic testing, and treatment and then describes sphenoidal sinusitis and nasal headache.

Sinusitis, which affects more than 31 million people in the United States, resulted in 16 million physician visits in 1985.[3] By 1994, the National Health Interview Survey estimated that 35 million people were affected.[4] A national health interview survey conducted in the United States between 1990 and 1992 found that chronic sinusitis was the second most frequent disease after orthopedic deformities, with an annual average of 33.1 million cases.[5] The prevalence of acute sinusitis is increasing, according to data from the National Ambulatory Medical Care Survey, from 0.2% of diagnoses at office visits in 1990 to 0.4% of diagnoses at office visits in 1995.[4] About 0.5% of upper respiratory infections in adults are complicated by sinusitis.[6] As many as 38% of patients with symptoms of sinusitis in adult general medicine clinics may have acute bacterial rhinosinusitis. In otolaryngology practices, the prevalence was higher (50–80%). While sinusitis is generally more common in children than adults, frontal and sphenoid sinusitis are rare in children. In the primary care setting, between 6% and 18% of children presenting with upper respiratory infections may have acute bacterial sinusitis.[4] In the preantibiotic era, the sphenoid sinus was involved in as many as 33% of cases of sinusitis. Today its incidence is about 3%.[2]

The maxillary and ethmoid sinuses, both present at birth, are the most common sites of clinical infection in children. The sphenoid sinus develops after the age of 2 years and starts to pneumatize at the age of 8 years. The frontal sinuses develop from the anterior ethmoid sinus at about 6 years of age. The frontal and sphenoid sinuses become clinically important in the teenage years, and they frequently become infected in pansinusitis. Isolated sphenoid sinusitis is rare.[7,8] The clinical diagnosis of sinusitis is usually based on symptoms that suggest maxillary or frontal sinus involvement. Ethmoid sinusitis is frequently a cause of frontal and maxillary sinusitis.[9,10] Obstruction of the osteomeatal complex, the common drainage pathway for the ethmoid, frontal, and maxillary sinuses, is the usual precursor to sinus disease.[11]

Anatomy and physiology

The ethmoid bone, a T-shaped structure that supports the bilateral ethmoid labyrinth, forms the lateral nasal wall. The horizontal limb of the T is formed by the cribriform plate, from which the ethmoid labyrinth is suspended. This is a complex structure with multiple bony septa and the medial projections of the superior and middle turbinates.

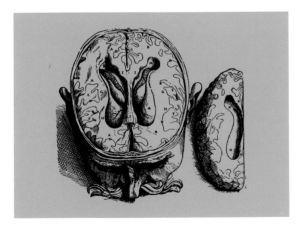

● **Figure 14.1** A view of the Brain from Andreas Vesalins' Fabrica, showing the ventricles.

Lateral to the uncinate process, which is a secondary projection of the ethmoid bone, is the infundibulum, a recess into which the maxillary sinus drains. The infundibulum drains into the hiatus semilunaris, which in turn drains into the middle meatus, which is located between the uncinate process and the middle turbinate. The frontal sinus drains into the frontal recess, which may drain into either the middle meatus or the ethmoidal infundibulum. This region is known as the osteomeatal complex[11] (maxillary sinus ostium, infundibulum, hiatus semilunaris, middle turbinate, ethmoidal bulla, and frontal ostium). The sphenoidal sinus and posterior ethmoidal cells drain into the sphenoethmoidal recess (Figure 14.2).

The primary functions of the nasal passages are to warm, humidify, and filter inspired air. The paranasal sinuses are air-filled cavities that connect with the nasal airway. They are lined with pseudostratified-ciliated epithelial tissue, which is covered by a thin layer of mucus. Large inhaled particulate matter pass over this constantly moving ciliated epithelial layer and are deposited there. The cilia and the mucous layer are in constant motion in a predetermined direction. Mucus and debris are transported towards the ostia by the beating of the cilia and are expelled into the nasal airway.[7,11,12] Any bacterial contamination of the sinuses is effectively cleared by this mechanism. If the sinus ostia are obstructed, mucociliary flow is interrupted. Obstruction causes the oxygen tension within the sinus to decrease and the carbon dioxide tension to increase. This anaerobic, high-carbon-dioxide, stagnant environment can facilitate bacterial growth.[11]

For many years, surgical drainage of the sinuses, avoiding the region of the natural ostia, was the treatment of choice for sinus infections. This procedure alleviated the acute sinus infection but did not prevent reaccumulation of mucus within the sinus. Furthermore, because the normal beat of the cilia transports mucus toward the natural ostium, surgically creating a new ostium at a site distant from the natural ostium fails to direct the flow of mucus to the new opening.[11]

All sinuses normally contain anaerobic bacteria, and more than one-third harbor a mixed environment of anaerobic and aerobic organisms. Ciliary dysfunction and retention of secretions that are commonly the result of ostial obstruction can result in bacterial proliferation and sinus infection. Aerobes that are present in both normal and disease states include the Gram-positive streptococci (alpha, beta, and *Streptococcus pneumoniae*) and *Staphylococcus aureus*, and Gram-negative *Moraxella catarrhalis*, *Haemophilus influenzae*, and *Escherichia coli*. Anaerobic organisms include the Gram-positive peptococci and *Propionibacterium* species. *Bacteroides* and *Fusobacterium* species also play a role in chronic sinusitis.[7,13]

Systemic diseases that predispose to sinusitis include cystic fibrosis, immune deficiency, bronchiectasis, and the immobile cilia syndrome. Local factors include upper respiratory infection (usually viral), allergic rhinitis, overuse of topical decongestants, hypertrophied adenoids, deviated nasal septum, nasal polyps, tumors, and cigarette smoke.[7] The most common predisposing factor is mucosal inflammation from viral upper respiratory infection or allergic rhinitis.[6] The sinuses are involved in nearly 90% of viral upper respiratory infections. In patients with a common cold and no previous history of rhinosinusitis, 87% had maxillary sinus abnormalities, 65% had ethmoid sinus abnormalities, and 30–40% had frontal or sphenoid sinus abnormalities on computed tomography (CT). The abnormalities are most likely due to highly viscid secretions in the sinuses. In 77% of patients, the infundibulum was occluded. In most patients, these abnormalities resolved spontaneously, but some developed secondary bacterial infections.[14] Foreign bodies are a common cause of obstruction in children, and 10% of sinus infections are of dental origin.[6] Loss of immunocompetence due to human immunodeficiency virus (HIV) infection, chemotherapy, posttransplant immunosuppression, insulin-dependent diabetes mellitus, and some connective tissue disorders predispose patients to rhinosinusitis and increases the likelihood of its persistence. Rhinosinusitis is common in the intensive care unit (ICU), since prolonged supine positioning compromises mucociliary clearance and adds to the problems created by mucosal drying from transnasal supplemental oxygenation and sinus ostial obstruction from nasotracheal or nasogastric tubes. Rhinosinusitis occurred in 95.5% of bedridden ICU patients who had a nasogastric or nasotracheal tube in place for at least a

OSTEOMEATAL COMPLEX

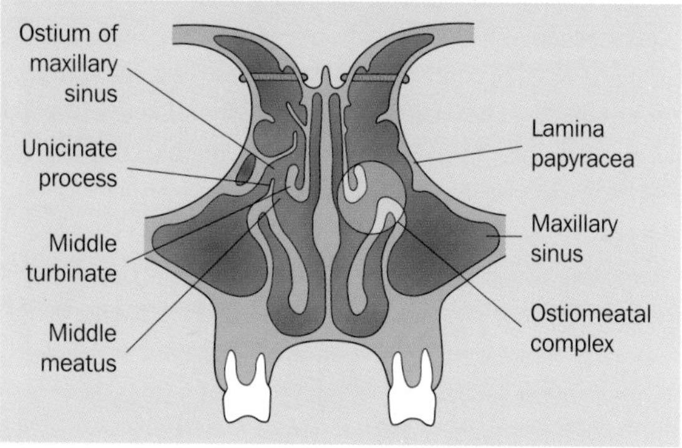

Ostium of maxillary sinus

Unicinate process

Middle turbinate

Middle meatus

Lamina papyracea

Maxillary sinus

Ostiomeatal complex

● **Figure 14.2** *Diagram showing the position of the region known as the osteomeatal complex.*

week.[15] Unobstructed flow through the sinus ostia and its narrow communicating passage within the osteomeatal complex is integral to mucociliary clearance and ventilation. Persistent low-grade inflammation in the ethmoid sinus may cause few localizing symptoms but can predispose to recurrent maxillary and frontal sinus infections.[7,11]

Diagnostic testing

The physical examination may not be helpful, particularly in sphenoid sinusitis. Not all patients are febrile, and sinus tenderness is not always present. Pus is not always seen in sphenoid sinusitis. Kibblewhite et al found purulent exudate in only three of 14 patients.[16] Transillumination of the sinuses has low sensitivity and specificity[17] and routine anterior rhinoscopy performed with a headlight and nasal speculum allows only limited inspection of the anterior nasal cavity.

Standard radiography

Standard X-ray is inadequate for the clinical evaluation of sinusitis because it does not evaluate the anterior ethmoid air cells, the upper two-thirds of the nasal cavity, or the infundibular, middle meatus, or frontal recess air passages.[12]

Neuroimaging

CT is the optimal radiographic study to assess the paranasal sinuses for evidence of disease. The mucosa of the normal, non-infected sinus approximates the bone so closely that it cannot be visualized on CT. Therefore, seeing any soft tissue within a sinus is abnormal.[18] CT may demonstrate mucosal thickening, sclerosis, clouding, or air–fluid levels. Imaging must be performed in the coronal plane to adequately demonstrate the ethmoid complex. It can reveal the extent of mucosal disease in the osteomeatal complex. The test–retest reliability of CT in the assessment of chronic rhinosinusitis was high and stable in a prospective series of patients scheduled for endoscopic sinus surgery.[19] The prevalence of reversible sinus abnormalities on CT in patients with the common cold is high.[14] This suggests that CT may not be specific for bacterial infections.[6] In 100 CT examinations of patients with chronic sinusitis, the middle meatus was involved in 72%. Anterior ethmoid sinus infection was found in every patient who had frontal or maxillary sinusitis. Middle meatal disease was found in the rest of these patients; it extended to, and occluded, the frontal recess in the patients who had frontal sinusitis and extended to, and occluded, the infundibulum in all cases of maxillary mucoperiosteal disease.[3,20]

During the edematous phase of the nasal cycle, normal nasal mucosa on T2-weighted image can resemble pathological change. Despite these problems with specificity, magnetic resonance imaging (MRI) is more sensitive than CT in detecting fungal infection.[12] Maxillary mucosal thickening > 6 mm, complete sinus opacification, and air–fluid levels on neuroimaging correlate to positive sinus cultures.[21] However, 30–40% of the normal population will have mucosal thickening on CT evaluation.[22] The Agency for Healthcare Policy and Research (AHCPR) (1999) meta-analysis of six studies showed that sinus radiography has moderate sensitivity (76%) and specificity (79%) compared with sinus puncture in the diagnosis of acute bacterial rhinosinusitis. CT or MRI is necessary to definitively diagnose sphenoid sinusitis, because plain X-rays are non-diagnostic in about 26% of cases.[23] CT scanning is the gold standard for the diagnosis of sphenoid sinus disease; MRI is an adjunct.

Transillumination, ultrasonography, and anterior rhinoscopy

Transillumination of the sinuses has low sensitivity and specificity.[17] Ultrasonography has lower sensitivity and specificity than sinus X-rays.[17] Routine anterior rhinoscopy performed with a headlight and nasal speculum allows only limited inspection of the anterior nasal cavity.

Diagnostic fiberoptic endoscopy

The flexible fiberoptic rhinoscope allows direct visualization of the nasal passages and sinus drainage areas (osteomeatal complex) and is complementary to CT or MRI. A trained operator can easily perform this procedure, and the patient tolerates it well. Infection is easily diagnosed if purulent material is seen emanating from the sinus drainage region. Mucosal sinus thickening is frequently present in normal, nonsymptomatic patients. In these cases, endoscopy should be positive before a diagnosis of sinusitis can be made.[11,13] Sphenoid sinusitis is an exception to this generalization.

Endoscopy should be considered when a sinus-related problem is suspected in a patient for whom conservative medical treatment fails and whose CT or MRI is inconclusive. Some physicians use endoscopy prior to neuroimaging. Negative neuroimaging and endoscopy usually, but not always, rules out sinus disease.[12]

Castellanos and Axelrod[24] evaluated 246 patients with undiagnosed headache and a negative neurologic evaluation. Ninety-eight had only rhinoscopic evidence of sinusitis, 84 had both rhinoscopic and standard radiographic evidence of sinusitis, and 64 had neither. Patients were treated with antibiotics for 4 weeks, at which time only those patients with rhinoscopic and/or radiologic evidence of sinusitis reported headache improvement. This was an open, uncontrolled study, but repeat rhinoscopic evaluation showed clearing of infection coincident with headache improvement.

Clinical findings

In 1996, the American Academy of Otolaryngology – Head and Neck Surgery standardized the terminology for paranasal infections.[25] The term rhinosinusitis was felt to be more appropriate than sinusitis since rhinitis typically precedes sinusitis, purulent sinusitis without rhinitis is rare, the mucosa of the nose and sinuses are contiguous, and symptoms of nasal obstruction and discharge are prominent in sinusitis.[26] The diagnosis of rhinosinusitis is usually based on symptoms indicating maxillary or frontal sinus involvement. This may occur secondary to, and is frequently a result of, ethmoid disease. Obstruction of the sinus ostia is the usual precursor of sinusitis.[12,20]

Rhinosinusitis is divided into four categories based on the temporal course and the signs and symptoms of the disease (Table 14.1).

Acute rhinosinusitis is sudden in onset, lasts from 1 day to 4 weeks, and there is complete resolution of the symptoms. *Subacute rhinosinusitis* is continuous with acute rhinosinusitis and lasts for 4–12 weeks;[27] recurrent acute rhinosinusitis requires four or more episodes of acute rhinosinusitis, lasting at least 7 days each, in any 1-year period. Chronic rhinosinusitis requires that signs or symptoms persist for 12 weeks or longer and may be punctuated by acute infectious episodes.

● **Table 14.1** *Classification of adult rhinosinusitis*

Classification	Duration	Strong history	Include in differential	Special notes
Acute	≤4 weeks	≥two major factors, one major factor and two minor factors, or nasal purulence on examination	One major factor or ≥two minor factors	Fever or facial pain does not constitute a suggestive history in the absence of other nasal signs or symptoms; consider acute bacterial rhinosinusitis if symptoms worsen after 5 days, persist for >10 days, or are out of proportion to those typically associated with viral infection
Subacute	4–12 weeks	Same as chronic	Same as chronic	Complete resolution after effective medical therapy
Recurrent acute	≥four episodes per year, with each episode lasting ≥7–10 days and no intervening signs and symptoms of chronic rhinosinusitis	Same as acute		
Chronic	≥12 weeks	≥two major factors, one major factor and two minor factors, or nasal purulence on examination	One major factor or ≥two minor factors	Facial pain does not constitute a suggestive history in the absence of other nasal signs or symptoms
Acute exacerbations of chronic	Sudden worsening of chronic rhinosinusitis, with return to baseline after treatment			

Facial tenderness and pain, nasal congestion, and purulent nasal discharge are common manifestations of acute sinus infection. Other 'classic' signs and symptoms include anosmia, pain upon mastication, and halitosis. An upper respiratory infection or a history of such infection may be present.[17] While fever is present in about 50% of adults and 60% of children and headache is common, the symptoms of headache, facial pain, and fever are often of minimal value in the diagnosis of sinusitis. Williams et al[28] looked at the sensitivity and specificity of individual symptoms in making the diagnosis of sinusitis. No single item was both sensitive and specific. Maxillary toothache was highly specific (93%), but only 11% of the patients had this symptom. Logistic regression analysis showed five independent predictions of sinusitis: maxillary toothache (odds ratio (OR) = 2.9), abnormal transillumination (OR = 2.7, sensitivity = 73%, specificity = 54%), poor response to decongestants (OR = 2.4), purulent discharge (OR = 2.9), and colored nasal discharge (OR = 2.2). The data did not support the other textbook findings for sinusitis (an antecedent upper respiratory infection or history of facial pain). 'Headache' had an OR of 1.0, with a 68% sensitivity and 30% specificity. The low specificity is due to lack of descriptive features of the headache. Facial pain and itchy eyes had an OR of 1.0. Fever, sweats, or chills were found in 48%, with an OR of 0.9 (sensitivity 45%, specificity 51%). It has been suggested that highly specific symptoms, such as facial erythema or maxillary toothache, or symptoms that persist for more than 10 days warrant a diagnosis and treatment.[29] The AHCPR evidence report,[4] based on limited evidence, suggested that diagnostic accuracy may be similar to that of sinus radiography when three or four of the following symptoms are present: purulent rhinorrhea with unilateral predominance, local pain with unilateral predominance, bilateral purulent rhinorrhea, and pus in the nasal cavity.

Children with acute and chronic sinusitis almost always present with purulent nasal discharge, which is not characteristic in adults. Fever is infrequent, even with acute sinusitis, and is usually associated with complicated acute sinusitis.[30]

Sinus infection can result in acute suppurative meningitis, subdural or epidural abscess, and brain abscess. In addition, osteomyelitis and subperiosteal abscess can occur. Infection of the ethmoid, and, to a lesser extent, the sphenoid sinuses, is responsible for orbital complications, which include edema, orbital cellulitis, and subperiosteal and orbital abscess.[7] A mucocele is a mucus-containing cyst located in the sinuses. These are most common (and benign) in the maxillary sinus (mucus retention cyst). Those located in the frontal, sphenoid, or ethmoid sinus can enlarge and erode into the surrounding structures. A pyocele is an infected mucocele.[8,31]

Wolff[32] showed that the sinuses themselves are relatively insensitive to pain. The pain associated with sinusitis comes from engorged and inflamed nasal structures: nasofrontal ducts, turbinates, ostia, and superior nasal spaces. Headache associated with paranasal sinus disease usually has a deeper, dull, aching quality combined with a heaviness and fullness. It is seldom associated with nausea and vomiting.

The International Headache Society (IHS) has established criteria for acute sinus headache (Table 14.2).[33] To qualify as acute sinus headache, there must be purulent discharge, abnormal neuroimaging, and simultaneous onset of headache and sinusitis. These criteria may not be valid for sphenoid sinusitis, however, as purulent discharge is often lacking, and headache may precede sinus drainage. Once drainage begins, obstruction is relieved and the headache may begin to abate.

All sinusitis pain is not the same. Maxillary sinusitis pain is most typically located in the cheek, the gums, and the teeth of the upper jaw. Ethmoid sinusitis pain is said to be felt between the eyes. The eyeball may be tender and

---

● **Table 14.2** *IHS criteria for acute sinus headache*

A. Headache location
   1. In acute frontal sinusitis, headache is located directly over the sinus and may radiate to the vertex or behind the eyes;
   2. In acute maxillary sinusitis, headache is located over the antral area and may radiate to the upper teeth or to the forehead;
   3. In acute ethmoiditis, headache is located between and behind the eyes and may radiate to the temporal area;
   4. In acute sphenoiditis, headache is located in the occipital area, the vertex, the frontal region, or behind the eyes.
B. Clinical, laboratory, and/or imaging evidence of an acute sinusitis, e.g. purulent discharge in the nasal passage, either spontaneous or by suction or CT or MRI findings
C. Simultaneous onset of headache and sinusitis
D. Headache disappears after treatment of acute sinusitis

pain may be aggravated by eye movement. Frontal sinusitis pain is felt mainly in the forehead. Sphenoid sinusitis pain is said to be felt in the vertex, but has more general localization. Ethmoid and maxillary sinusitis is usually associated with rhinitis.

Hypertrophic turbinates, atrophic sinus membranes, and nasal passage abnormalities due to septal deflection are other conditions that may cause headache; however, they are not sufficiently validated as a cause of headache. Migraine and tension-type headache are often confused with true sinus headache because of similarity in location. In order to diagnose 'IHS' sinus headache, the above criteria must be strictly fulfilled.

The relationship between headache and subacute and chronic sinus disease is highly controversial. Radiographic evidence of sinus disease is very common and does not establish the headache's etiology.[22] Headache associated with sinus disease is usually continuous, not intermittent. Chronic sinusitis is frequently associated with engorged and swollen nasal mucosa and a purulent or sanguinopurulent nasal discharge. The IHS has not validated chronic sinusitis as a cause of headache or facial pain unless it relapses into an acute stage.[34]

Faleck et al[35] reported that 10% of 150 children and adolescents who presented with chronic, nonprogressive headache, clinically indistinguishable from 'muscle contraction' headache, had radiographic evidence of sinus pathology. None had prominent respiratory symptoms. All improved with treatment directed towards the sinus pathology. Although some had complete sinus opacification, none had endoscopy to show the presence of active disease in the ostia.

Treatment

The following are management goals for the treatment of sinusitis:

- Treat bacterial infection;
- Reduce ostial swelling;
- Drain sinuses;
- Maintain sinus ostia patency.

Uncomplicated sinusitis, other than sphenoid sinusitis, should be treated with a broad spectrum oral antibiotic for 10–14 days. Nasal culture does not correlate to sinus pathogens, thus initial treatment is empiric.[17] Steam and saline prevent crusting of secretions in the nasal cavity and facilitate mucociliary clearance. Locally active vasoconstrictor agents provide symptomatic relief by shrinking inflamed and swollen nasal mucosa. Their use should be limited to 3–4 days to prevent rebound vasodilation. Oral

decongestants should be used if prolonged treatment (> 3 days) is necessary. These agents are α-adrenergic agonists that reduce nasal blood flow without the risk of rebound vasodilation.[17]

Antihistamines are not effective in the management of acute rhinitis. Anti-inflammatory topical corticosteroids may help maintain ostial patency. Treatment failure and recurrent infections are indications for neuroimaging and endoscopy to search for a source of obstruction. Sinus sampling for culture should be considered. Endoscopic nasal surgery may be necessary to reopen and maintain the patency of the sinus ostia and osteomeatal complex.[17]

Complications should be treated with high doses of intravenous antibiotics and surgical drainage, if appropriate, of any enclosed space.

Sphenoid sinusitis

Sphenoid sinusitis, because of its rarity, unique location, and complications, is discussed separately. It is an uncommon infection that accounts for approximately 3% of all cases of acute sinusitis. It is usually accompanied by pansinusitis; it is less common for it to occur alone. In contrast to other paranasal sinus infections, it is frequently misdiagnosed,[23] since the sphenoid sinus is not adequately visualized with routine sinus X-rays and is not accessible to direct clinical examination, even with the flexible endoscope. While sphenoid sinusitis is an uncommon cause of headache, it is potentially associated with significant morbidity and mortality and requires early identification and aggressive management.[2,16,23]

The sphenoid sinus is contained within the body of the sphenoid bone deep in the nasal cavity and is divided in half by the intersphenoid septum. Each sinus communicates with the sphenoethmoidal recess, which is located at the posterior superior aspect of the superior concha. The sphenoidal sinuses are present as minute cavities at birth, and it is not until puberty that their main development occurs.[36]

The roof of the sphenoid sinus is related to the middle cranial fossa and the pituitary gland in the sella turcica; lateral is the cavernous sinus; posterior is the clivus and pons; anterior are the posterior nasal cavity, posterior ethmoid cells, and cribriform plate; and inferior is the nasopharynx. The cavernous sinus (which is lateral to the sphenoid sinus) contains the internal carotid arteries and the IIIrd, IVth, Vth, and VIth cranial nerves. The maxillary division of the Vth nerve may indent the wall of the sphenoid sinus. The sphenoid walls can be extremely thin, and sometimes the sinus cavity is separated from the adjacent structure by just a thin mucosal barrier. Because of the close proximity to the cortical venous system, cranial nerves, and meninges, infection may spread to these structures and present as a central nervous system infection or neurological catastrophe.[2,37]

Symptoms (Table 14.3)

Headache is the most common symptom of acute sphenoid sinusitis: *it is present in all patients who are able to complain about it*. The headache is aggravated by standing, walking, bending, or coughing. It often interferes with sleep and is poorly relieved by opioids. Its location is variable: vertex headache is rare; frontal, occipital, or temporal headache, or a combination of these locations, is most common.

Periorbital pain is common. This is in contrast to the common teaching that retro-orbital or vertex headache is the most common presenting symptom of sphenoid sinusitis.[2,16,23,38–40] Nausea and vomiting frequently occur, but nasal discharge, stuffiness, and postnasal drip are unusual. Fever occurs in over half of patients with acute sphenoid sinusitis.

Diagnosis

The diagnosis of sphenoid sinusitis is frequently delayed. Sphenoid sinusitis should be included in the differential diagnosis of acute or subacute headache. It may be mistaken for frontal or ethmoid sinusitis, aseptic meningitis, brain abscess, or septic thrombophlebitis. It can mimic trigeminal neuralgia, migraine, carotid artery aneurysm, or brain tumor.[2,16,23]

A severe, intractable, new-onset headache that interferes with sleep and is not relieved by simple analgesics should alert one to the diagnosis of sphenoid sinusitis. The headache increases in severity and has no specific location. Pain or paresthesias in the facial distribution of the Vth nerve and photophobia or eye tearing are suggestive of sphenoid sinusitis.[2,16,23,38,39,41]

The physical examination may not be helpful. Not all patients are febrile, sinus tenderness is rarely present, and pus is not always seen, although Lew et al[2] state that a careful examination of the nose and throat often demonstrates pus. Whether this reflects advanced disease or the presence of pansinusitis is uncertain. In a more recent series of 14 patients with acute sphenoid sinusitis, Kibblewhite et al[16] found purulent exudate in only three patients.

Neuroimaging is necessary to definitively diagnose sphenoid sinusitis. All of Kibblewhite's cases were diagnosed by X-ray.[16] Some cases can be diagnosed by plain sinus X-rays, but, because of the superimposition of soft tissues, plain X-rays are nondiagnostic in about 25% of cases.[23] If sphenoid sinusitis is suspected and plain radiographs are nondiagnostic, CT or MRI is indicated (Figure 14.3).

In a high-risk group of 300 patients who were referred with a clinical diagnosis of sinusitis, 68% had abnormal plain radiographs, but none had sphenoid sinus abnormalities, suggesting that the specificity of plain radiographs is very high.[42] The mucosa of the sinus approximates the bone so closely that it cannot be visualized on CT. Therefore, any bulge of soft tissue seen in the sinus is abnormal.[18] Digre et al[43] reviewed 300 CT or MRI radiographic studies. The sphenoid sinus was visualized in all cases. Abnormalities were detected in 7% of routine CT scans, 8% of posterior fossa scans, and 6% of MRI scans. Of the 21 patients with sphenoid abnormalities, 24% in their highly selected sample had important clinical related disease.

● **Table 14.3** *Sphenoid sinusitis*

Symptom	Goldman[21]	Kibblewhite[22]	Lew[2]
Headache or facial pain	12/12	13/14*	30/30**
Pain worse with head movement	12/12	Most	?
Nasal discharge/congestion	6/12	4/14	?
Fever	7/12	8/14	Most
Nausea or vomiting	?	8/14	?
Complications	0/12	8/14	10/14 acute, 3/15 chronic

* Patient comatose; ** 15 acute, 15 chronic

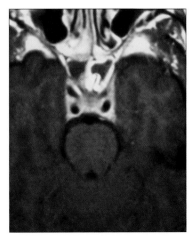

● **Figure 14.3**
MRI or CT neuroimaging can be used to diagnose sphenoid sinusitis.

Complications

Major complications of sphenoid sinusitis include bacterial meningitis,[2] cavernous sinus thrombosis,[2,16,23,37] subdural abscess,[2,16,23] cortical vein thrombosis,[2,16,23] ophthalmoplegia, and pituitary insufficiency.[2,16,23] Sphenoid sinusitis can present as aseptic meningitis owing to the presence of a parameningeal focus.[44] Patients can present with the complications of sphenoid sinusitis, including visual loss mimicking optic neuritis, multiple cranial nerve palsies, or papilloedema. Sudden onset, as a result of cavernous sinus thrombosis, can mimic a subarachnoid hemorrhage.[45]

Øktedalen and Lilleås[46] reported on four patients who were admitted to an infectious disease department with meningitis, sepsis, and orbital cellulitis. Diagnosis was difficult in all cases. All four patients had fever and headache. Three of the four had normal plain sinus radiographs. CT scan diagnosed all cases. Six of Lew et al's[2] 15 acute cases had meningitis, five had cavernous sinus thrombosis, one had cortical vein thrombosis, one had unilateral ophthalmoplegia, and one had orbital cellulitis. Eight of Kibblewhite et al's[16] 14 patients had complications on admission. None of Goldman et al's[23] patients had complications. The difference in the complication rate is a result of selection bias: Goldman et al's[23] patients were retrieved from emergency room records, Lew et al's[2], Øktedalen and Lilleås',[46] and Kibblewhite et al's[16] from inpatient records.

Treatment

Sphenoid sinusitis without complications may be managed with high-dose intravenous antibiotics and topical and systemic decongestants for 10–14 days.[16,23] If the fever (if present) and the headache do not start to improve in 24–48 hours, or if any complications are present or develop, sphenoid sinus drainage is indicated.[23]

Nasal headache

Many rhinologists strongly hold the controversial belief that septal deformation, especially of traumatic origin, may exert pressure on the sensitive structure of the lateral nasal wall, causing referred pain and 'chronic headache'. McAuliffe et al[47] studied the sensitivity of the nasal cavities and paranasal sinuses using touch, pressure, and faradic stimulation. The nasal turbinates and sinus ostia were much more sensitive than the mucosal lining of the septum and the paranasal sinuses. Most of the pain elicited was referred pain. It was of increased intensity, longer duration, and referred to larger areas in subjects who had swelling and engorgement of the nasal turbinates and the sinus ostia.

Schønsted-Madsen et al[1] followed up 444 patients with nasal obstruction, of whom 157 had headache. Treatment consisted of septoplastic surgery, reconstruction of the nasal pyramids, or submucosal conchotomy. The headache was usually localized to the forehead, glabella, or above and around the eyes. Thirty-six patients had constant, 48 daily, 56 weekly, and 17 monthly headache. Fifty-seven patients had mild headache, 66 had moderate headache, and 34 had severe headache. Many of these patients misused analgesics. Eighty per cent of the patients who underwent surgery were relieved of nasal obstruction (the primary reason for surgery), and 60% of the patients who underwent surgery were relieved of chronic headache. If the surgery relieved the nasal obstruction, 80% had headache relief; however, if the surgery failed, only 30% had headache relief.

Clerico[46] reported 10 patients who had intractable migraine, tension-type, or cluster headache without significant nasal or sinus symptoms. Various intranasal and sinus abnormalities, such as anatomic variation or subclinical inflammation, were found on CT or nasal endoscopy. The patients were treated medically and/or surgically, and all improved.[48] Low and Willatt[47] reported 106 patients who had a submucous resection for a deviated nasal septum. Almost half (47.4%) had recurring headaches preoperatively. Postoperatively, 63.6% had complete or partial relief at follow-up for as long as 18 months. While 79.3% of patients had headache relief when evaluated before 1 year, only 46.2% had relief after 1 year.[49]

These studies do not account for the historical relationship between headache onset and the development of nasal obstruction, or for the analgesic or decongestant overuse that may produce daily headache. In addition, any surgical procedure has a powerful placebo effect. The studies do suggest that some patients with nasal obstruction have headache that is relieved by successful medical or surgical treatment. Since migraine prevalence in the population is about 12%, episodic tension-type headache prevalence about 90%, and chronic tension-type headache prevalence about 3%, these data are difficult to interpret. In addition, these studies had no control group and in Clerico's study[46] only responders were reported. In controlled trials of medication, the placebo effect can be quite large.

In a retrospective review of operative notes of 170 patients who underwent functional endoscopic sinus surgery, 50 patients (29%) who had a history of chronic headaches were identified. Thirty-seven met the predetermined inclusion criteria for this study, which were: 1) a history of chronic headaches; 2) rhinologic cause for these headaches suggested by the presence of contact points (documented by nasal endoscopy and/or CT scans); 3) no other origin or cause of headaches after a thorough evaluation; and 4) surgical intervention that included relief of contact points by inferior, middle, and/or superior turbinoplasty. Following surgery, 29 of the 34 patients (85%) in the study group reported a decrease in headache frequency. However, there were many patients who had severe contact points on CT scan and did not complain of headaches. In fact, most patients with headaches and contact points also had concurrent chronic sinusitis, which

served as the primary indication for surgery in this patient population.[50]

Other open studies[51,52] and a review[53] have suggested that headache can be the only clinical presentation of sinus or nasal pathology. These studies do not use IHS criteria for headache or the new diagnostic criteria for sinusitis. With the common involvement of the sinuses on CT with no symptoms of sinusitis it is very difficult to comment favorably on these open trials.

References

1. Schønsted-Madsen U, Stoksted P, Christensen PH, Koch-Henriksen N. Chronic headache related to nasal obstruction. J Laryngol Otol 1986; 100: 165–70.

2. Lew D, Southwick FS, Montgomery WW et al. Sphenoid sinusitis: a review of 30 cases. N Engl J Med 1983; 19: 1149–54.

3. Moss AJ, Parsons VL. Current estimates from the National Health Interview Survey. United States 1985. Vital and Health Statistics 1986; i–iv: 1–182.

4. Agency for Healthcare Policy and Research. Diagnosis and treatment of acute bacterial rhinosinusitis. Summary. 1999;

5. Collins JG. Prevalence of selected chronic conditions: United States, 1990–1992. Vital Health Stat. 1997; 10; 984:1–89.

6. Diaz I, Bamberger DM. Acute sinusitis. Semin Respir Infect 1995; 10: 14–20.

7. Reilly JS. The sinusitis cycle. Otolaryngol Head Neck Surg 1990; 103: 856–62.

8. Kennedy DW. First-line management of sinusitis: a national problem? Overview. Otolaryngol Head Neck Surg 1990; 103: 847–54.

9. Hilding AC. Physiologic basis of nasal operations. Calif Med 1950; 72: 103–7.

10. Messerklinger W. Endoscopy of the nose. Baltimore: Urban and Schwartzenberg, 1978.

11. McCaffrey TV. Functional endoscopic sinus surgery: an overview. Mayo Clin Proc 1993; 68: 675–7.

12. Zinreich SJ. Paranasal sinus imaging. Otolaryngol Head Neck Surg 1990; 103: 863–9.

13. Kennedy DW. Surgical update. Otolaryngol Head Neck Surg 1990; 103: 884–6.

14. Gwaltney JM, Phillips CD, Miller RD et al. Computed tomographic study of the common cold. N Eng J Med 1994; 330: 25–30.

15. Rouby J, Laurent P, Gosnach M et al. Risk factors and clinical relevance of nosocomial maxillary sinusitis in the critically ill. Am J Resp Crit Care Med 1994; 150: 776–83.

16. Kibblewhite DJ, Cleland J, Mintz DR. Acute sphenoid sinusitis: management strategies. J Otolaryngol 1988; 17: 159–63.

17. Stafford CT. The clinician's view of sinusitis. Otolaryngol Head Neck Surg 1990; 103: 870–5.

18. Schatz CJ, Becker TS. Normal CT anatomy of the paranasal sinuses. Radiol Clin North Am 1984; 22: 107–18.

19. Bhattacharyya N. Test–retest reliability of computed tomography in the assessment of chronic rhinosinusitis. Laryngoscope 1999; 109: 1055–8.

20. Zinreich SJ, Kennedy DW, Rosenbaum AE et al. Paranasal sinuses: CT imaging requirements for endoscopic surgery. Radiology 1987; 163: 769–75.

21. Druce HM, Siavin RG. Sinusitis: a critical need for further study. J Allergy Clin Immunol 1991; 88: 675–7.

22. Havas TE, Motbey JA, Gullane PJ. Prevalence of incidental abnormalities on computed tomographic scans of the paranasal sinuses. Arch Otolaryngol 1988; 114: 856–9.

23. Goldman GE, Fontanarosa PB, Anderson JM. Isolated sphenoid sinusitis. Am J Emerg Med 1993; 11: 235–8.

24. Castellanos J, Axelrod D. Flexible fiberoptic rhinoscopy in the diagnosis of sinusitis. J Allergy Clin Immunol 1989; 83: 91–4.

25. Benninger MS, Anon J, Mabry RL. The medical management of rhinosinusitis (review). Report of the Rhinosinusitis Task Force Committee Meeting. Otolaryngol Head Neck Surg 1997; 117: S41–9.

26. Slavin RG. Nasal polyps and sinusitis. JAMA 1997; 278: 1849–54.

27. Lanza DC, Kennedy DW. Adult rhinosinusitis defined. Otolaryngol Head Neck Surg 1997; 117: S1–7.

28. Williams JW, Simel DL, Roberts L, Samsa GP. Clinical evaluation of sinusitis. Ann Intern Med 1992; 117: 705–10.

29. International Rhinosinusitis Advisory Board. Infectious rhinosinusitis in adults: classification, etiology, and management. Ear Nose Throat J 1997; 76: S5–22.

30. Muntz HR, Lusk RP. Signs and symptoms of chronic sinusitis. In: Lusk RP, ed. Pediatric Sinusitis. New York: Raven Press, Ltd, 1992, 1–6.

31. Hilger PA. Diseases of the nose. In: Hilger PA, ed. Boie's Fundamentals of Otolaryngology; a Textbook of Ear, Nose, and Throat Disease. Philadelphia: WB Saunders, 1989, 206–48.

32. Wolff HG. Wolff's headache and other head pain. 1st edn. New York: Oxford University Press, 1948.

33. Headache Classification Committee of the International Headache Society. Classification and diagnostic criteria for headache disorders, cranial neuralgia, and facial pain. Cephalalgia 1988; 8: 1–96.

34. Saunte C, Soyka D. Headache related to ear, nose, and sinus disorders. In: Olesen J, Tfelt-Hansen P, Welch KMA, eds. The Headaches. New York: Raven Press, 1993, 753–7.

35. Faleck H, Rothner AD, Erenberg G, Cruse RP. Headache and subacute sinusitis in children and adolescents. Headache 1988; 28: 96–8.

36. Goss CM. Gray's anatomy of the human body. 27th edn. Philadelphia: Lea & Febiger, 1959.

37. Sofferman RA. Cavernous sinus thrombophlebitis secondary to sphenoid sinusitis. Laryngoscope 1983; 93: 797–800.

38. Deans JAJ, Welch AR. Acute isolated sphenoid sinusitis: a disease with complications. J Laryngol Otol 1991; 105: 1072–4.

39. Nordeman L, Lucid E. Sphenoid sinusitis, a cause of debilitating headache. J Emerg Med 1990; 8: 557–9.

40. Urquhart AC, Fung G, McIntosh WA. Isolated sphenoiditis: a diagnostic problem. J Laryngol Otol 1989; 103: 526–7.

41. Turkewitz D, Keller R. Acute headache in childhood: a case of sphenoid sinusitis.

Pediatr Emerg Care 1987; 3: 155–7.

42. Axelsson A, Jensen A. The roentgenologic demonstration of sinusitis. Am J Roentgenol Rad Ther Neurol Med 1974; 122: 621–7.

43. Digre KB, Maxner CE, Crawford S, Yuh WTC. Significance of CT and MR findings in sphenoid sinus disease. AJNR 1989; 10: 603–6.

44. Brook I, Overturf GD, Steinberg EA, Hawkins DB. Acute sphenoid sinusitis presenting as aseptic meningitis: a pachymeningitis syndrome. Int J Pediatr Otorhinolaryngol 1982; 4: 77–81.

45. Dale BAB, Mackenzie IJ. The complications of sphenoid sinusitis. J Laryngol Otol 1983; 97: 661–70.

46. Øktedalen O, Lilleås F. Septic complications to sphenoidal sinus infection. Scand J Infect Dis 1992; 24: 353–6.

47. McAuliffe GW, Goodell H, Wolff HG. Experimental studies on headache: pain from the nasal and paranasal structures. Res Publ Assoc Res Nerv Ment Dis 1943; 23: 185–206.

48. Clerico DM. Sinus headaches reconsidered: referred cephalgia of rhinologic origin masquerading as refractory primary headaches. Headache 1995; 35: 185–92.

49. Low WK, Willatt DJ. Headaches associated with nasal obstruction due to deviated nasal septum. Headache 1995; 35: 404–6.

50. Parsons DS, Batra PS. Functional endoscopic sinus surgical outcomes for contact point headaches. Laryngoscope 1998; 108: 696–702.

51. Chow JM. Rhinologic headaches. Otolaryngol Head Neck Surg 1994; 111: 211–18.

52. Salman SD, Rebeiz EE. Sinusitis and headache. J Med Libanais 1994; 42: 200–2.

53. Close LG, Aviv J. Headaches and disease of the nose and paranasal sinuses. Sem Neurol 1997; 17: 351–4.

chapter 15

Headache associated with central nervous system infection

Introduction

Headaches are associated with a wide range of infections in both intracranial and extracranial structures. The International Headache Society (IHS) system divides infections into those that are intracranial, those that are extracranial, and those that affect the cranium and associated structures (Table 15.1). This chapter emphasizes selected intracranial and system infections, including meningitis and encephalitis. We discuss issues related to Lyme borreliosis and human immunodeficiency virus (HIV) infection, including the acquired immunodeficiency syndrome (AIDS). These disorders have become increasingly important over the last decade.

Central nervous system (CNS) infections remain a great concern of clinicians worldwide. CNS infections may be announced by headache and headache may remain as a residual problem even after adequate treatment. The importance of CNS infections has recently been increased by AIDS, which may present as, or intercurrently have as a feature, intracranial infections. The IHS defines the clinical problem as headache that occurs at the onset of intracranial infection and disappears after successful treatment of intracranial infection (Table 15.1).[1]

Meningitis

Meningitis refers to an infectious or inflammatory process of the meninges; we will consider infective causes (the inflammatory conditions have been dealt with in a previous

chapter). Meningitis is classified according to the pathogen; it is most commonly viral or bacterial. Other infections are seen mainly in primary or secondary immune deficiency states. Bacterial meningitis was described by Vieusseaux and named 'epidemic cerebrospinal fever' after an outbreak in Switzerland in 1805. 'Aseptic meningitis', a term introduced by Wallgren in 1925, describes a benign and self-limited variant of meningitis that is usually due to a viral infection, with headache a prominent feature of the illness. Quinke, who is responsible for introducing the lumbar puncture in 1881, originally described viral meningitis and encephalitis in 1896.[2] The annual incidence of acute bacterial meningitis in the United States is 5–10 cases per 100 000 population.[3,4] It occurs somewhat more frequently in men than in women.[3–5] Children under the age of 5 years account for most cases, with the highest risk during infancy. Other predisposing factors are sickle cell disease, alcoholism, and AIDS and other immunocompromised states.

Neonatal meningitis is most frequently caused by Group B streptococci, *Listeria*, and *Escherichia coli* and other Gram-negative organisms.[6] In adults, most acute bacterial meningitis is community-acquired.[7] There has been an increase in the incidence of meningococcal infection on college campuses. Until the introduction of *Haemophilus influenza* type B vaccines (Hib) in 1987, *H. influenzae*, *Neisseria meningitides*, and *Streptococcus pneumoniae* were the most common cause of acute bacterial meningitis in adults in the United States, causing approximately 80% of all cases.[4,5] In 1995, the rates of bacterial meningitis (per 100 000) were: *S. pneumoniae* (1.1), *N. meningitides* (0.6), group B streptococcus (0.3), *L. monocytogenes* (0.2), and *H. influenzae* (0.2).[8] At present, the most common causative organisms of community-acquired bacterial meningitis are *S. pneumoniae* and *N. meningitides*. The prevalence of penicillin- and cephalosporin-resistant strains of *S. pneumoniae* has increased. As of 1998, approximately 44% of clinical isolates of *S. pneumoniae* in the United States had intermediate or high levels of resistance to penicillin.[4,9,10] If a cerebrospinal fluid (CSF) leak is present as a result of a skull fracture, pneumococcus is the most common causative organism and skin flora the second most common.[5] *Staphylococcus aureus* and coagulase-negative staphylococci are the predominant meningitis-causing organisms following lumbar puncture for intrathecal

Table 15.1 Classification of headaches associated with infection

7	Headaches associated with non-vascular intracranial disorders
	7.3 Intracranial infections
9	Headaches associated with non-cephalic infections
	9.1 Viral infection
	9.2 Bacterial infection
	9.3 Headache related to other infections
11	Headache or facial pain associated with disorders of the cranium, neck, eyes, ears, nose, sinuses, teeth, mouth or other facial or cranial structures

chemotherapy and invasive neurosurgical procedures, particularly shunting procedures and subcutaneous Ommaya reservoirs.[9] In this era of bioterrorism, it is important to remember that the pulmonary and, less frequently, the cutaneous forms of anthrax can produce fulminant and sometimes hemorrhagic meningitis.

Aseptic meningitis is characterized by headache, low-grade fever, stiff neck, fatigue, and anorexia. The etiologic organisms that may cause this disorder include the enteroviruses (EVs) (echo, coxsackie, polio), arboviruses (herpes simplex virus (HSV) type 2, herpesvirus type 6 (HHV-6)), fungi, Epstein–Barr virus (EBV), varicella-zoster (VZV), *Mycoplasma pneumoniae*, *Borrelia burgdorferi*, and *Treponema pallidum*.[9] Among the viruses, the EVs are the most common causative agents, accounting for 85–95% of all cases.[11,12] HSV type 2 is the most common etiologic agent of Mollaret meningitis (recurrent brief episodes of meningitis alternating with symptom-free intervals).[13]

Clinical features

The clinical features of bacterial and viral meningitis are similar, although bacterial meningitis is generally more clinically fulminant. Headache pathophysiology is described in detail in Chapter 5; however, it is appropriate to comment that the pain is likely to be related to the effects of the agent and, perhaps even more notably, to the host response. Headache is seen in many febrile illnesses, and the headaches of interferons-a,[14] -b,[15] -g,[16] and immunoglobulins[17] suggest that endogenously released substances may play a crucial role in headache generation in CNS infections.

Fever, headache, and stiff neck are the classical triad of meningitis. Nausea, vomiting, photophobia, and lethargy are also common complaints. Lethargy, stupor, or seizure activity is highly suggestive of bacterial meningitis. While the presence of individual symptoms has low sensitivity for the diagnosis of meningitis in adults, the diagnosis is very unlikely in the absence of fever, neck stiffness, and altered mental status. Fever is the most sensitive of the three signs of meningitis, followed by nuchal rigidity and changes in mental status. The absence of these signs (fever, nuchal rigidity, and altered mental status) will help exclude the diagnosis in a low-risk patient.[18] A stiff neck is the pathognomonic sign of meningeal irritation. Nuchal rigidity is present when the neck resists passive flexion. With the patient supine, attempts to passively extend the leg elicit pain when meningeal irritation is present (Kernig's sign). Brudzinski described at least five signs, but his best-known sign is the nape-of-the-neck sign. It is performed with the patient in the supine position and is positive when passive flexion of the neck results in spontaneous flexion of the hips

and knees. Sufferers maintain a flexed posture, with tense neck muscles and head extension.[19] Eye movements are often painful and cranial nerve palsies may be present.[19,20] Reports of seizure activity rates vary significantly, from 5% to 23%,[21-23] 28%[7] to 40%.[9] Seizure activity may occur as part of the initial presentation of bacterial meningitis (76% of patients had seizure within 24 hours in one series),[7] or may occur at any time during the course of the illness.[9] A petechial, purpuric, or erythematous maculopapular rash can occur in meningococcemia, enteroviral meningitis, Rocky Mountain spotted fever, West Nile fever encephalitis, bacterial endocarditis, echovirus type 9 viremia, and pneumococcal or *H. influenzae* meningitis. The most common signs of increased intracranial pressure in bacterial meningitis are an altered level of consciousness and papilledema.

Headache is the most common symptom of bacterial meningitis. It is severe and unremitting, usually generalized (but may be frontally predominant), and may radiate down the neck and back and into the extremities.[24] A thunderclap headache that increases in severity in minutes may be the first symptom of acute bacterial meningitis. Jolt worsening of headache has been reported to have 100% sensitivity for the diagnosis of meningitis in patients with fever and headache. However, in a recent report of 100 cases of acute bacterial meningitis,[7] only 66% of the patients had headache, and headache was less common than fever and nuchal rigidity. Young children usually do not complain of headache.[6,10,19,25] Infants may present with fever and a bulging fontanelle.[6,10,25] The elderly also have fewer headaches than do young adults.[6,20] The signs and symptoms of meningitis may be accompanied by signs involving the original site of infection, such as upper respiratory infection or otitis media.

In *L. monocytogenes* meningitis, clinical presentation with fever is practically the rule and is seen in more than 90% of patients regardless of immune status. Headache is present in three-quarters of patients with CNS disease and obviously is a nonspecific symptom. Meningeal signs are variable, less common, and intensely related to the degree of immunosuppression. Thus, *Listeria* meningitis cannot be excluded on the basis of absence of meningeal signs.[26]

In chronic meningitis, such as tuberculous meningitis, severe headache and fever evolve subacutely and may occur in isolation.[6] Chronic headache that increases in severity over weeks to months, without fever or other neurologic findings, is the most common symptom of cryptococcal meningitis.[27] A picture of chronic infection, in which the patient has a moderate fever, muscle pains, or mild deterioration in cognitive function over time, may be seen. An infection that produces hydrocephalus, such as CNS tuberculosis or a cryptococcal infection may cause progressive ataxia or cognitive decline. More chronic syndromes may be seen with *Brucella* meningitis or Lyme disease. If CNS infection is suspected as the cause of headache, lumbar puncture is often the critical diagnostic test. If acute bacterial meningitis is suspected, rapid initiation of therapy may be life-saving.[1] Lumbar puncture should be performed if bacterial meningitis is suspected and a mass lesion has been ruled out clinically or by neuroimaging. While it is generally the practice to image the brain prior to lumbar puncture to ensure that no mass lesion is present, treatment should not be delayed if acute bacterial meningitis is suspected. Lumbar puncture may be performed without neuroimaging if no contraindications or obstacles are present. Contraindications to lumbar puncture include signs of increased intracranial pressure (papilledema, coma, anisocoria, fixed pupils), focal neurologic signs, suspicion of a CNS mass lesion, a skin infection at the proposed lumbar puncture site, or a coagulopathy that cannot be even temporarily corrected. Obstacles to lumbar puncture include unstable vital signs and the need for ventilatory assistance.

The defining investigation in a suspected case of meningitis is a CSF examination. The CSF opening pressure is usually elevated when meningitis is present. It is essential to obtain an adequate sample. Approximately 6 ml of CSF is sufficient for cell count, glucose and protein concentrations, Gram stain and culture, and latex particle agglutination (LA). The CSF should be sent for Gram stain and culture and examined for glucose (usually < 40 mg/dl or < 50% of the blood glucose), protein (significantly elevated), and cell counts (usually > 1000 cells/mm^3 with polymorphonuclear predominance).[20,28,29] An additional 1 ml of CSF can be sent to the polymerase chain reaction (PCR) laboratory for analysis for viral DNA, as viral encephalitis is the leading disease in the differential diagnosis of bacterial meningitis. As a general rule, Gram stain and culture of CSF obtained 24 hours after the initiation of antimicrobial therapy will be negative if the organism is sensitive to the antibiotic. The CSF should also be sent for specific bacterial antigen and endotoxin assays.[10,28–30] Blood cultures should be drawn, since they are positive in more than 50% of cases of bacterial meningitis.[30,31] The peripheral white blood count (WBC) will probably be elevated, with a predominance of polymorphonuclear cells and immature forms, supporting the diagnosis of a bacterial process. X-rays of the skull and sinuses may reveal a site of infection or portal of entry into the CNS, but they are not routinely used. Likewise, magnetic resonance imaging (MRI) may show meningeal enhancement,[32] but it is seldom necessary in typical cases (Table 15.2).[29]

Due to inadequate sampling, many patients have had multiple lumbar punctures in an attempt to diagnoses meningitis. In addition, antibiotic treatment prior to lumbar puncture can complicate diagnosis. In this setting negative CSF cultures are common; using immunologic testing can facilitate diagnosis. This can be avoided if a microbiological differential diagnosis is carefully formulated, with advice from an infectious disease specialist when chronic meningitis is suspected. Treatment is directed to specific therapy, antibiotic, antiviral or antifungal agents, and supportive measures, such as fluids and antipyretics.

Bacterial meningitis

Bacterial meningitis remains a deadly disease. Rapid assessment is essential and can be life-saving. Bacterial infections present typically with fever, headache, and neck stiffness; the most common causes are listed in Table 15.3. The most common organisms, which cause approximately 80% of all cases of acute bacterial meningitis in adults in the United States, are *H. influenzae*, *N. meningitidis* and *S. pneumoniae*.[4,5] In children, as a result of immunization, meningitis due to *H. influenzae* type B is less common than it used to be. *E. coli* and *Listeria* are together responsible for approximately 10% of bacterial meningitis. Neonatal meningitis is caused by Group B streptococci, *Listeria*, and *E. coli* and other Gram-negative organisms.[4,6,10] If a CSF leak is present secondary to a skull fracture, pneumococcus is the most common causative organism, followed by skin flora.[5] Neurosurgical patients may be affected with a wide variety of organisms, particularly Gram-negative rods.[5,6] Patients who are receiving chemotherapy and are immunosuppressed, those who have lymphoma, leukaemia, and malnutrition, and those with AIDS, may be infected with unusual pathogens. *Mycobacterium tuberculosis* causes both subacute and chronic meningitis, while *Cryptococcus*, *Nocardia*, *Candida*, *Histoplasma*, and coccidiomycosis are common causes of chronic meningitis. Faced with immunocompromised patients, such as those with acquired immunodeficiency from malnutrition, HIV infection, leukaemia, lymphoma, or anticancer treatments, a search for more unusual pathogens is mandatory. Bacterial meningitis may complicate sinusitis, skull fractures, mastoiditis, or local cranial infections, as well as being a manifestation of a primary infection in any site, such as may be seen in osteomyelitis or pneumonia. When a bacterial infection is present, the CNS contains a purulent exudate that is reflected in highly active CSF with neutrophils, protein, and a low glucose compared with a contemporaneous blood glucose level (Table 15.2). The normal WBC count ranges from 0 to 5 mononuclear cells (lymphocytes and monocytes) per mm^3 in uninfected adult CSF.[3] Normal uninfected adult CSF should contain no polymorphonuclear leukocytes;

● Table 15.2 *Differential diagnosis of CSF lymphocytic pleocytosis*

With normal CSF glucose concentration	With decreased CSF glucose concentration
Enteroviruses	Partially treated bacterial meningitis
Mumps virus	*Listeria monocytogenes*
Arthropod-borne viruses	
Herpes simplex virus-1 and –2	*Mycobacterium tuberculosis*
Human immunodeficiency virus	
Influenza virus types A and B	*Cryptococcus neoformans*
Measles, SSPE*	*Coccidioides immitis*
Varicella-zoster virus	*Histoplasma capsulatum*
Cytomegalovirus	*Candida*
	Blastomyces dermatitidis
Treponema pallidum	
Borrelia burgdorferi	Herpes simplex virus-1
Leptospirosis	Mumps virus
	Lymphocytic choriomeningitis virus
Rickettsia rickettsii	
Human monocytic ehrlichiosis	Sarcoidosis
Human granulocytic ehrlichiosis	Leptomeningeal carcinomatosis
Behcet disease	
Migraine	
Vasculitis	
Postinfectious encephalomyelitis	
Nonsteroidal anti-inflammatory agents	
Azathioprine	
Trimethoprim-sulfamethoxazole	
Isoniazid	
Intravenous immune globulin	

*SSPE, subacute sclerosing parencephalitis

however, an occasional polymorphonuclear leukocyte may be seen with a cytocentrifuge. In bacterial meningitis, there are 10–10 000 WBCs/mm^3 in the CSF, with a predominance of polymorphonuclear leukocytes. The LA test has a specificity of 96% for *S. pneumoniae* and 100% for *N. meningitis*. It has a sensitivity of 69–100% for the detection of *S. pneumoniae* and a sensitivity of 33–70% for the detection of bacterial antigens of *N. meningitis* in CSF. The Limulus amebocyte lysate assay is a rapid diagnostic test for

● Table 15.3 *Common causes of acute bacterial infections in the CNS*

Haemophilus influenzae
Neisseria meningitidis
Streptococcus pneumoniae
Streptococcus (group B)
Listeria monocytogenes
Escherichia coli
Staphylococcus (aureus and epidermidis)

the detection of Gram-negative endotoxin in CSF and thus for making a diagnosis of Gram-negative bacterial meningitis. This test is reported to have a sensitivity of 99.5% and a specificity of 86–99.8%.[9]

Three-quarters of patients with *Listeria* meningitis have a CSF pleocytosis (median cell count 585 cells/mm^3 (mean 1 183 cells/mm^3)), with a predominance of neutrophils, frequently mixed with lymphocytes or monocytes. In the remaining cases, lymphocytes or monocytes predominate. Protein elevations in the CSF exceed 199 mg/dl. Glucose levels are in the normal range. CSF cultures are positive in at least 80% of cases of meningitis and meningoencephalitis.[26] Once it is suspected, there should be no delay in treating the infection with antibiotics that would cover the pathogens expected in the community or hospital setting in which the infection was acquired (Tables 15.4 and 15.5).

Nonbacterial infections

Aseptic meningitis is characterized by a severe, rapid-onset headache, fever, malaise, anorexia, phonophobia, photophobia, and nuchal rigidity. There may be altered

● **Table 15.4** *Empiric treatment for meningitis*

Age	Common bacterial pathogens	Empirical antimicrobial therapy*
0–4 weeks	Streptococcus agalactiae, Escherichia coli, Listeria monocytogenes, Kliebsella pneumoniae	Ampicillin plus cefotaxime, or ampicillin plus aminoglycoside
4–12 weeks	S. agalactiae, E. coli, L. monocytogenes, Haemophilus influenzae, S. pneumoniae, Neisseria meninigitides	Ampicillin plus third-generation cephalosporin†
3 months to 18 years	H. influenzae‡, N. meninigitides, S. pneumoniae	Third-generation cephalosporin† ± ampicillin§. or ampicillin plus chloramphenicol
18–50 years	S. pneumoniae, N. meninigitides	Third-generation cephalosporin† ± ampicillin§
>50 years	S. pneumoniae, N. meninigitides, L. monocytogenes, aerobic Gram-negative bacilli	Ampicillin plus third-generation cephalosporin†

*Vancomyclin should be added to empirical regimens when highly penicillin- or cephalosporin-resistant pneumoncoccal meningitis is suspected.

†Cefotaxime or ceftriaxone.

‡Incidence of invasive disease caused by H. influenzae Type B has decreased in countries, such as the United States, in which conjugate vaccines have been introduced.

§Add if meningitis caused by L. monocytogenes is suspected (e.g. in patients with deficiencies in cell-mediated immunity).

● **Table 15.5** *Treatment for common bacterial pathogens*

Micro-organism	Therapy
Haemophilus influenzae Type B	Third-generation cephalosporin*
Neisseria meninigitides	Penicillin G or ampicillin or third-generation cephalosporin*
Streptococcus pneumoniae	Vancomycin plus third-generation cephalosporin*†
Listeria monocytogenes	Ampicillin or penicillin G‡
Streptococcus agalactiae	Ampicillin or penicillin G‡
Escherichia coli	Third-generation cephalosporin*

*Cefotaxime or ceftriaxone.
†Addition of rifampicin may be considered.
‡Addition of aminoglycosdie should be considered.

sensorium, although this rarely progresses to obtundation or coma.[6,33,34] Again, the headache may be less prominent in children. All patients with aseptic meningitis experience a severe, bilateral headache.[35] Generally, although not invariably, non-bacterial intracranial infections follow a more benign clinical course. Many such patients, when first seen with headache, fever, and neck stiffness, are managed with antibiotics, and the diagnosis is questioned when there is no obvious response. The CSF examination, with an excess of lymphocytes, an unremarkable or modestly elevated CSF protein, and a normal ratio of CSF to blood plasma glucose, suggests a non-bacterial infection.

In viral meningitis, the CSF shows a mild pleocytosis (usually < 100 cells/mm³).[6,29,33,34] Early in the course, there may be a predominance of polymorphonuclear cells, but this rapidly shifts to lymphocytic pleocytosis. The CSF pressure and CSF protein are normal or slightly elevated and the glucose is normal or slightly reduced. If the diagnosis is still in doubt, antibiotics should be started and the lumbar puncture repeated after 12 hours to document the shift from polymorphonuclear cells to mononuclear cells. The CSF should be analysed for viral antigens and incubated for viral culture. Acute and convalescent serum viral titers will provide clues to the etiology of the disease. The peripheral WBC may be normal or elevated with a normal differential cell count. In some cases virus can be isolated from other sites, such as the throat and stool.[6] The common viral causes vary between different geographic areas and some common causes are listed in Table 15.6. Aseptic meningitis is usually viral in origin, with the enteroviruses (echo, coxsackie, polio), the mumps virus, and the arboviruses being the most common causative organisms.[3,6,36] Less common viral causes are HIV, lymphocytic choriomeningitis virus, herpes simplex virus type

● **Table 15.6** *Common viral pathogens in meningitis*

Enterovirus	Epstein–Barr virus
Coxsackie A and B	Rubella
Cytomegalovirus	Mumps
Herpes simplex	Adenovirus
Herpes zoster	Human immunodeficiency virus

2, rubella, Epstein-Barr virus, herpes zoster, influenza, parainfluenza, and adenovirus.[6,34,37] The causative virus is isolated in only 11–12% of cases.[3,36]

The PCR is the most promising alternative to viral culture for EV diagnosis. This technique is typically directed at genomic RNA in the highly conserved regions of the 5' non-coding region and designed for reverse transcription combined with PCR (RT-PCR). EV RT-PCR has now been tested in clinical settings by numerous investigators and has been found to be consistently more sensitive than culture and virtually 100% specific; in many laboratories, an accurate diagnosis of EV infection is now available in less than 1 day.[11,38,39] Compared with brain biopsy, the sensitivity of HSV-1 PCR in encephalitis is better than 95% and the specificity approaches 100%.[40] The new technique, microchip electrophoresis of PCR products, reduces analysis time of HSV DNA from 18 hours to less than 110 s per sample, with the same sensitivity and specificity as established methods.[41] If Mollaret meningitis is a consideration, both CSF and serum PCR and HSV antibody should be studied to make a diagnosis of HSV encephalitis.[13]

Other conditions that can resemble aseptic meningitis include fungal meningitis, parameningeal infections, non-infectious conditions (malignant meningitis, sarcoidosis or chemical meningitis from spinal anesthesia, myelography, or intrathecal medications), and bacterial agents that are difficult to culture (such as those causing syphilis (*Treponema palladium*), tuberculosis (*Mycobacterium tuberculosis*), and Lyme disease (*Borrelia burgdorferi*)).[34,37,42] EBV may have a very long chronic course, and it has been suggested that many cases of new daily persistent headache are triggered by an episode of Epstein–Barr infection. An interesting diagnosis of exclusion related to nonbacterial intracranial infections is the clinical syndrome of a migrainous headache, with prolonged aura, neck stiffness, fever, and a lymphocytosis in the CSF.[43] The nature of this syndrome remains to be more clearly elucidated. The subacute aseptic meningitis syndrome may be because of a fungal infection, most frequently *Cryptococcus neoformans*. Fungal meningitis and its possible concomitant brain parenchymal involvement constitute a major diagnostic challenge, since the yield of traditional diagnostic methods, such as culture, may not be positive.

Patients who have cryptococcal meningitis generally have symptoms of headaches and fever, but this is not always the case. Cryptococcal meningitis can present as a subacute dementia. The duration of symptoms, prior to diagnosis, is commonly more than 1–2 weeks, varying from months in nonimmunosuppressed patients to less than a week in severely immunosuppressed patients.[44] Headache and fever are also the most common clinical manifestations in patients who have *Candida* meningitis,[45] the clinical symptoms of which are highly variable and can range from acute to chronic in nature.[46] CNS aspergillosis often presents with the sudden onset of seizure or neurologic deficits.[47]

Noninfectious etiologies of the aseptic meningitis syndrome include sarcoidosis, leptomeningeal carcinomatosis, systemic lupus erythematosus, Wegener's granulomatosis, Behcet's disease, and medications. Aseptic meningitis, characterized by headache, meningismus, and a CSF lymphocytic pleocytosis, may be a recurrent problem in patients who have neurosarcoidosis.[48] Headache is the most frequent complaint in leptomeningeal carcinomatosis and is often associated with nausea, vomiting, and lightheadedness. Neck pain and stiffness are often present, although the meningismus is much less severe than that seen in purulent meningitis patients.[49] The presenting symptoms in Wegener's granulomatosis are typically cough, chest pain, hemoptysis, epistaxis, purulent nasal discharge, and sinus pain.

Most cases of fungal meningitis have a mononuclear pleocytosis in the range of 20–500 cells/mm³. However, in *Aspergillus*, Zygomycetes, *Pseudoallescheria*, or *Blastomyces* fungal meningitis, there is a predominance of polymorphonuclear cells.[44] When eosinophils are detected in the cell count and differential, *Coccidioides immitis* needs to be considered as the cause of the meningitis. CSF protein levels are generally elevated and glucose concentrations are variable but commonly depressed in fungal meningitis. Fungal meningitis is one condition that causes hypoglycorrhachia.[44] Positive cultures are the 'gold standard' for diagnosing fungal meningitis, but they may be negative or slow-growing. To increase the yield of fungal cultures, a large volume of CSF (10–30 ml) is needed. Series of CSF serologic tests for fungal antigens or antibodies should be obtained. CSF lactic acid concentrations are generally elevated during fungal meningitis.[44]

The CSF abnormalities in sarcoidosis are nonspecific and include: 1) lymphocytic pleocytosis; 2) elevated protein concentration; 3) decreased glucose concentration; 4) elevated IgG index and synthesis rate indicative of intrathecal immunoglobulin production; 5) oligoclonal banding; and 6) elevated CSF angiotensin-converting enzyme (ACE).[48] To make a diagnosis of neurosarcoidosis, the following are recommended: 1) chest radiography for bilateral, symmetric hilar and mediastinal lymphadenopathy; 2) serum and CSF ACE; and 3) lymph node, skin, or transbronchial lung biopsy.[9]

A CSF glucose concentration between 45 and 35 mg/dl, in combination with a lymphocytic pleocytosis, an unrelenting headache, stiff neck, fatigue, night sweats, and fever, is highly suspicious for tuberculous meningitis.[50] The CSF glucose concentration rarely falls below 20 mg/dl in cases of tuberculous meningitis.[51] Positive smears for acid-fast bacilli are reported in only 10–40% of cases of tuberculous meningitis in adults. It takes 4–8 weeks to identify the organism with CSF culture, which is positive in approximately 50% of adults.[52] The PCR technique uses the mycobacterial insertion element IS6110 as the DNA marker for *M. tuberculosis* complex organisms. The specificity of the PCR in this setting is reported to be 80–100%, but the sensitivity ranges from 25% to 80%.[51] If *Mycoplasma tuberculosis* is suspected, the initiation of chemotherapy should not await the results of CSF cultures and should not depend on the results of acid-fast bacilli smears. The most common abnormalities on neuroimaging in tuberculous meningitis are meningeal enhancement and hydrocephalus.

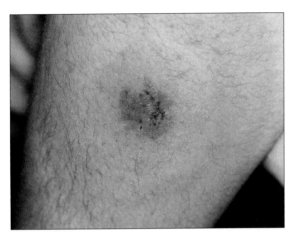

● **Figure 15.1** *Rash of Lyme disease (erythema chronicum migrans).*

Lyme disease

Neuroborreliosis or Lyme disease of the nervous system produces a pleomorphic clinical picture that may include lymphocytic meningitis with or without cranial nerve lesions, encephalomyelitis, encephalopathy, and radiculopathy and neuropathy of either the cranial or peripheral nerves.[53] Lyme borreliosis is a multisystem infection caused by the spirochete *Borrelia burgdorferi*.[54] Early in the illness, patients may have a characteristic cutaneous lesion, erythema migrans (Figure 15.1). Some patients develop disseminated and then chronic infections with prominent neurologic, rheumatologic, and cardiac manifestations. During erythema migrans, headache occurs in 38–54% of patients and presents few diagnostic challenges.[55,56] Headache may also accompany the causally related neurologic syndromes described below. More problematic are the patients who present with headache as an isolated manifestation of Lyme disease.

The American Academy of Neurology (AAN) 'Practice Parameters for the Diagnosis of Patients with Nervous System Lyme Borreliosis (Lyme Disease)' defines four causally related forms of neurologic disease or dysfunction:[57]

- Lymphocytic meningitis with or without cranial neuritis or painful radiculoneuritis or both. This syndrome is common early in the course of Lyme borreliosis. Headache occurs in most patients and is typically bilateral, gradual in onset, and variably associated with migrainous features (throbbing quality, nausea). Meningism is uncommon in patients with Lyme meningitis.[56,58]
- Encephalomyelitis. This monophasic, slowly progressive, unifocal or multifocal inflammatory disease of the CNS occurs in about 0.1% of patients

with Lyme borreliosis.[57] The disorder involves white matter more prominently than grey matter. Headache is common; it is often bilateral, and again variably associated with migrainous features.
- Peripheral neuropathy. The radiculoneuropathy, usually a mononeuropathy multiplex, occurs without meningitis and without evidence of CNS infection. Only a minority of patients complains of headache.[56]
- Encephalopathy. Cognitive complaints and cognitive dysfunction may develop in the absence of evidence of CNS infection. Encephalopathy may be an indirect effect of system infection, mediated by the action of cytokines and neuromodulators on the CNS. Headache may occur in the encephalopathy syndrome.

Occasionally, headache is the most prominent neurologic manifestation of CNS Lyme disease. Halperin et al.[59] reported a woman with chronic headache and a positive CSF Lyme antibody index whose headaches completely resolved after treatment with ceftriaxone. Brinck et al.[60] reported two patients with headaches that resembled chronic tension-type headache. In both cases, the CSF Lyme antibody index was positive and the headaches resolved after intravenous antibiotic therapy. In addition to headaches, the first patient had constant nausea, vomiting, weight loss, and episodes of paresthesias in her fingertips. The second patient had double vision and a progressive paraparesis that evolved over a 2-year period and eventually led to a work-up and diagnosis.

Brinck et al[60] point out that neither of their patients had meningeal signs or fever. Both had headache symptoms that did not fully meet IHS criteria. Both went from having very few headaches to an almost constant headache over several days. They recommend considering a workup for Lyme borreliosis when headaches are atypical, especially if the onset is subacute. Several patients have had positive CSF Lyme antibody indices, which provide strong evidence for CNS infection with *B. burgdorferi*. In these cases, the headaches completely resolved after treatment with ceftriaxone.

Laboratory tests

The appropriate workup for patients with headache and suspected Lyme disease is problematic. Halperin et al[57] recently reviewed the role of laboratory tests for neuroborreliosis. Selected information about selected tests is summarized below.

Serologic testing

Serologic diagnostic tests (enzyme-linked immunosorbent assay (ELISA)) for Lyme and for other infectious agents demonstrate possible exposures to the causative agent, not current active infection.[60] In asymptomatic individuals, serologic tests are positive in 5–10% of the population in endemic areas and in 1% of the population in nonendemic areas.[57,61] Thus, most positive serologic tests in otherwise asymptomatic patients with headache will be false-positives. If serologic testing is performed in individuals with a characteristic Lyme-related illness (a high prior probability of Lyme disease), the positive predictive value goes up.[57]

Western blot

While serologic tests detect antibody, the Western blot test characterizes the specific *B. burgdorferi* antigens. This test serves primarily to confirm a positive ELISA or to identify false-positives.[57] Demonstrating intrathecal antibody production within the CNS relies on the ratio of antibody in CSF to antibody in serum. These procedures have high specificity (95%) and sensitivity (90%), are quite valid, and may even (rarely) be positive despite negative peripheral serologic tests.[62,63]

Culture and polymerase chain reaction

Culture and PCRs are highly specific, but are not always positive.[57,64,65] Serologic tests for Lyme should be used only to support a clinical diagnosis of Lyme disease, not as the basis for making diagnostic or treatment decisions. This test is not useful early in the course of Lyme disease (see below) because of its low early sensitivity. A positive second-step result indicates that there is either serologic evidence of cross-reacting antibodies or past or current infection with *B. burgdorferi*. Centers for Disease Control recommendations call for confirmation of positive or equivocal ELISA results by Western blot.[66] Serologic testing is not needed and not recommended for patients with ery-

thema migrans, due to its low sensitivity. Therefore, serologic testing is unnecessary to support the clinical diagnosis for most patients with Lyme disease who have objective findings.[67] Neither testing nor antibiotic treatment is cost-effective if the pretest probability of Lyme disease is low. Empirical antibiotic therapy is recommended if the pretest probability is high, and two-step testing is recommended if the pretest probability is intermediate.[68] The sensitivity of ELISA kits for serum specimens collected early ranged from 58% to 92%, and late serum specimens all had sensitivities of 77%. Concordance between test kits was very low. Serologic tests do not become positive until weeks after a tick bite.[66] ELISA-based tests that use lysate with the full range of antigens will not distinguish vaccinated from infected individuals when Lyme disease vaccines that use the recombinant *B. burgdorferi* protein are available.[66]

Preliminary recommendations

Routine testing for Lyme disease is not recommended for patients who present with headache. The tests that frequently yield false-positive results would most likely lead to inappropriate evaluation or treatment. If a headache is accompanied by apparent systemic or neurologic manifestations that are suggestive of Lyme disease, we suggest serum antibody testing by ELISA. Evaluation should proceed as recommended in the AAN practice guidelines (as reviewed above).[57] In patients with atypical headaches (e.g. rapid increase to near-daily headache, unusual associated symptoms, or poor response to treatment), serologic testing for Lyme disease should be considered. ELISA should be confirmed by a Western blot for *Borrelia*-specific antigens. Patients who have headache as the sole neurologic manifestation and a positive ELISA and Western blot should be treated with oral doxycycline 100 mg p.o. b.i.d. for 3–4 weeks. If the headache does not remit, lumbar puncture should be considered. In patients with headache and evidence of Lyme-related neurologic disorders/dysfunction (such as encephalopathy, cognitive deficits, and focal deficits), neuroimaging and lumbar puncture for cell count, protein glucose, and Lyme antibody index should be performed. If CNS disease is present, intravenous therapy should be considered, as discussed in the AAN practice guidelines.[57]

Encephalitis

In the United States, the incidence of viral encephalitis is 7.4 per 100 000 per year, with most cases beginning in the summer and early fall.[3,36] The incidence is highest in infancy and gradually drops, to attain a steady rate by the age of 40 years. Males are more often affected than females. HSV is the most commonly recognized cause of acute sporadic encephalitis in the United States and other

● **Table 15.7** *Common causes of encephalitis*

Mumps	Toxoplasmosis
Arbovirus	Epstein–Barr virus
Herpes simplex	Adenovirus
Herpes zoster	

industrialized countries.[68] Japanese encephalitis virus is the most common cause in Asia, with an estimated 50 000 cases and 15 000 deaths annually.[69] Outbreaks of encephalitis include the Nipah virus encephalitis outbreak in Malaysia and Singapore and the West Nile virus encephalitis outbreak in the eastern United States. The outbreak in New York was thought to have infected 8200 people (2.6% of the population); about 1700 had febrile infections, and 59 of these had meningoencephalitis (about 0.7% of all infections).[70]

Encephalitis is an infection involving the brain parenchyma. Encephalitic processes are generally due to viral infections; the common causes are listed in Table 15.7. The causative agent in encephalitis is identified approximately 15% of the time in large population studies.[3,36] In one study of a very select group of patients (summarized by Johnson),[72] the aetiology was determined in two-thirds of the cases. Mumps was isolated 15% of the time, arbovirus 11%, EVs 10%, lymphocytic choriomeningitis virus 9%, and herpes simplex virus 95%. Other causes included EBV, measles, influenza virus, and *Mycoplasma*. The larger studies reported somewhat higher incidences of measles and VZR, especially in children. Measles, mumps, and VZR can cause postinfectious encephalomyelitis as well as infectious encephalitis. HSV encephalitis typically has no identifiable systemic prodrome and may present with behavioral changes or memory disturbance.[34,72] In one series of patients with HSV encephalitis, two-thirds of patients presented with signs of meningeal irritation, almost all with fever, about 90% with focal neurologic deficits, and 61% with seizures. More than one-third of patients were comatose on admission.[73] When there is mass effect, which commonly involves the temporal cortex, a localized headache may be present. Subacute encephalopathy that progresses over several months, with headache, lethargy, and possibly focal neurologic signs, is another presentation of HSV encephalitis.[74] The symptomatology may recur after antiviral therapy, although this is rare and may be due to postinfectious encephalitis.[75]

Encephalitis is characterized by headache, fever, alteration in consciousness, impaired cognition, and sometimes distinct focal neurologic clinical syndromes. Meningeal signs (neck stiffness) may be present; however, headache and impaired consciousness may be the only clinical manifestation. Thunderclap headache alone may be the initial manifestation of encephalitis.[71] The cerebral picture may be predated by a prodrome of feeling generally unwell, with fever, malaise, or myalgia for up to a week prior to the more acute presentation. While some encephalitides are clinically mild, some, such as herpes simplex, can be devastating. Herpes simplex often involves the bilateral temporal cortex and is often accompanied by an abnormal electroencephalogram. Thus, patients with suspected herpes simplex encephalitis require early adequate treatment with antiviral agents. In immunosuppressed patients certain pathogens, such as toxoplasmosis, cryptococcoses, and cytomegalovirus, are more common and must be actively sought.

Encephalitis is associated with almost 100 DNA and RNA viruses (readers are referred to several excellent reviews).[68,76,77] Even with the help of sophisticated molecular techniques, a definitive etiology is identified in only about one-half of cases of infectious encephalitis.[78] In the United States, the most common pathogens are HSV-1, arboviruses, EVs, measles, and mumps. Arbovirus infections occur more frequently in the summer in the northern hemisphere; mumps is more frequent in the winter, and HSV encephalitis occurs all year around.

Diagnosing encephalitis during an epidemic is not difficult; however, a sporadic case may easily be confused with encephalopathy. The presence or absence of fever, headache, and focal neurologic signs help in the diagnosis. Peripheral leukocytosis, CSF pleocytosis, and regional abnormalities on neuroimaging or electroencephalogram favor the diagnosis of encephalitis.[34] The CSF protein may be normal or elevated and the glucose is normal or slightly depressed.[29] The CSF cell count is usually < 200 cells/mm^3, predominantly lymphocytes. In HSV encephalitis, the CSF may be xanthochromic and may contain red blood cells, reflecting the hemorrhagic necrosis taking place in the brain.[29] Antigen may be detected in the CSF.[79] The ability of MRI to detect HSV encephalitis at an earlier stage than CT scanning has made it the imaging procedure of choice;[32,79] however, a brain biopsy may occasionally be needed to establish a definite diagnosis. Virus may be isolated from the brain specimen, but the culture results may not be available for several days. Since aciclovir is effective against only a small number of encephalitides and is not innocuous, the indiscriminate use of this drug must be avoided. If a brain biopsy is going to be performed, the patient can be given aciclovir up to 24 hours before surgery without affecting HSV isolation from the specimen.[34] PCR assays for HSV in the CSF has expedited the diagnosis[80] and may obviate the need for brain biopsy; CSF assays for HSV glycoproteins are also being developed.

Eastern equine encephalitis produces focal radiographic signs on MRI. The characteristic early involvement of the basal ganglia (71%) and thalami (71%) distinguishes it from HSV. The presence of large lesions did not predict a poor outcome.[81]

Human immunodeficiency virus infection and the acquired immunodeficiency syndrome

Of all the conditions that predispose to intracranial infection and thus produce headache, HIV disease is perhaps one of the most challenging. Headache can occur as a primary manifestation of HIV infection in the acute phase of the infection, as part of an HIV meningitis or encephalitis. It may also occur in the setting of AIDS as a manifestation of an opportunistic infection or of CNS lymphoma. CNS toxoplasmosis is the most common nervous system infection in AIDS patients. It usually presents as single or multiple contrast-enhancing parenchymal lesions on CT brain scans. The diagnosis is supported by positive toxoplasmosis titers. The condition generally responds to treatment; biopsy diagnosis is indicated if the brain lesions are atypical, if empirical therapy fails or it there are other atypical features. Meningitis in AIDS can involve all of the common pathogens, but opportunistic infections are frequent. Cryptococcal infection is common and relatively easily diagnosed via CSF examination with India ink stain and cryptococcal antigen testing. Similarly, tuberculous meningitis is often seen in AIDS patients and must be sought diligently with CSF examination using PCR techniques.

Brain abscess

The overall incidence of brain abscess is approximately one per 100 000 population, with peak incidence in childhood and after the age of 60 years.[3] Brain abscesses account for approximately 1 in 10 000 hospital admissions in the United States. Otitis media and mastoiditis have been the most commonly identified underlying conditions in patients in developed countries.[82] In one series, 27% of those affected had multiple abscesses.[83] Brain abscesses are three times more likely to occur in men than women. Risk factors include neurosurgery, penetrating brain trauma, and, particularly in children, otitis media. The risk of brain abscess in cases of otitis media is less than 0.5%.[82]

The signs and symptoms of a brain abscess depend on the location of the abscess and the amount of mass effect it produces. Headache, often hemicranial, is the most common presenting symptom, but an abscess can present with a seizure.[84,85] Focal neurologic signs and altered mental status are common.[83,86] Signs of an antecedent infection, such as otitis media, sinusitis, a dental infection, or endocarditis, may be present. Fever and leukocytosis

are less likely to be present. Nausea and vomiting often begin a week after headache onset.[83] These symptoms may result from increased intracranial pressure, although less than half of patients have papilledema at presentation.[83,87] With a cerebellar abscess, the headache is often suboccipital and there is associated cervical pain and rigidity.[24] In 1893, Sir William Macewen described the successful treatment of brain abscess by surgical drainage. The development of antibiotics, advances in neurosurgical techniques, and the use of CT scanning and MRI have all contributed to the significant reduction in mortality that has occurred.[83,89]

Brain abscesses may be caused by aerobic or anaerobic bacteria and often contain multiple organisms that come from the source of the infection.[83,86,88] Those arising from otitis media, mastoiditis, or sinusitis contain aerobic or anaerobic streptococci, S. aureus, and Bacteroides. Those arising from open head trauma or neurosurgery are associated with streptococci, staphylococci, or Gram-negative rods. Bacterial endocarditis yields abscesses with S. aureus or Streptococcus viridans. Pulmonary infections are associated with staphylococci, streptococci, Actinomyces, Gram-negative rods, or Fusobacterium, and, less commonly, Nocardia (especially in an immunocompromised host).[83,86] Abscess formed by Candida, Aspergillus, or Toxoplasma may also be found in an immunocompromised host. Overall, there is a high incidence of S. milleri isolated from brain abscesses of all causes.[83,87]

Neuroimaging is the diagnostic procedure of choice for brain abscesses. The CT scan shows a central area of decreased attenuation surrounded by a ring of intense contrast enhancement, which may then be surrounded by edema.[32,83,86,88] The presence of gas within the lesion supports the diagnosis. Prior to capsule formation, a low-density region, reflecting early cerebritis, may be seen. MRI may be superior to CT scanning in its ability to detect early cerebritis, edema, minor hemorrhage, and disruption of the blood–brain barrier,[32,84] but this imaging procedure is not always readily available. Since a brain tumor, a cerebral infarct, and radiation necrosis may appear identical to an abscess on CT scan, diagnostic (and therapeutic) neurosurgical intervention is often necessary,[86,88] although with the growing availability of MRI, diagnostic intervention is seldom necessary. The abscess should be incised and its contents drained and sent for bacterial culture and biopsy. Routine blood tests are rarely helpful in the diagnosis of a brain abscess; the peripheral WBC is usually normal or only slightly elevated. Blood cultures should be performed if endocarditis is suspected.

A brain abscess must be differentiated from a brain tumor. Their appearance on CT may help differentiate them, although both may 'ring-enhance'. A brain abscess with early cerebritis may produce fever, headache, and meningeal signs that mimic meningitis. A subdural hematoma or empyema can mimic a brain abscess. A history of closed head trauma and the appearance of the lesion on imaging studies will help distinguish between these entities. When there is no history of fever or prior infection, a brain abscess may be confused with a cerebral infarction or a subdural hematoma; imaging studies will differentiate between them.

Headache treatment

The headache associated with intracranial infections should resolve with treatment of the underlying condition. Until the infection has cleared, the headache can be treated with nonopioid analgesics or, if it is severe, with opioids, bearing in mind that the use of narcotics may obscure certain aspects of the neurologic examination (e.g. level of consciousness, pupillary size). If the headache persists long after the infection and its complications have resolved, the patient may require evaluation and treatment of a chronic type of headache. The evaluation includes neuroimaging to rule out the sequelae of intracranial infections, such as obstructive or communicating hydrocephalus, residual cerebral edema, or mass effect. Once these entities have been excluded, a lumbar puncture may be necessary to rule out increased intracranial pressure, even in the absence of papilledema. Treatment of the residual headache is described in Chapter 8.

References

1. Headache Classification Committee of the International Headache Society. Classification and diagnostic criteria for headache disorders, cranial neuralgia, and facial pain. Cephalalgia 1988;8:1–96.
2. Silberstein SD. Headache associated with meningitis, encephalitis, and brain abscess. La Jolla: Arbor, 1997.
3. Nicolosi A, Hauser WA, Beghi E, Kurland LT. Epidemiology of central nervous system infections in Olmsted County, Minnesota. J Infect Dis 1986;154:399–408.
4. Schlech WF. The epidemiology of bacterial meningitis. Antibiot Chemother 1992;45:5–17.
5. Schlech WF, Ward JI, Band JD et al. Bacterial meningitis in the United States, 1978 through 1981. JAMA 1985;253:1749–54.
6. Franke E. The many causes of meningitis. Postgrad Med J 1987;82:175–88.
7. Hussein SH, Shafran SD. Acute bacterial meningitis in adults: a 12-year review. Medicine (Baltimore) 2000;79:360–8.
8. Schuchat A, Robinson K, Wenger JD et al. Bacterial meningitis in the United States in 1995 (for the Active Surveillance Team). N Eng J Med 1997;337:970–6.
9. Roos KL. Acute bacterial meningitis. Sem Neurol 2000;20:293–306.
10. Lipton JD, Schafermeyer RW. Evolving concepts in pediatric bacterial meningitis – Part I: Pathophysiology and diagnosis. Ann Emerg Med 1993;22:1602–15.
11. Rotbart HA. Diagnosis of enteroviral meningitis with the polymerase chain reaction. J Ped 1990;117:85–9.
12. Sawyer MH, Holland D, Aintablian N et al. Diagnosis of enteroviral central nervous system infection by polymerase chain reaction during a large community outbreak. Pediatr Infect Dis J 1994;3:177–82.
13. Roos KL. Pearls and pitfalls in the diagnosis and management of central nervous system infectious diseases. Sem Neurol 1998;18:185–96.
14. Schiller JH, Hank J, Storer B. A direct comparison of immunologic and clinical effects of interleukin 2 with and without-alpha in humans. Cancer Res 1993;53:1286–92.
15. Yung WK, Castellanos AM, VanTassel P et al. A pilot study of recombinant interferon beta (IFN-beta ser) in patients with recurrent glioma. J Neuro Oncol 1990;9:29–34.
16. Gluszko P, Undas A, Amenta S et al. Administration of gamma interferon in human subjects decreases plasminogen activation and fibrinolysis without influence in C1 inhibitor. J Lab Clin Med 1994;123:232–40.
17. Watson JD, Gibson J, Joshua DE, Kronenberg H. Aseptic meningitis associated with high dose intravenous immunoglobulin therapy. J Neurol Neurosurg Psychiatry 1991;54:275–6.
18. Attia J, Hatala R, Cook DJ, Wong JG. Does this adult patient have acute meningitis? JAMA 1999;282:175–81.
19. Isenberg H. Bacterial meningitis: signs and symptoms. Antibiot Chemother 1992;45:79–95.
20. Carpenter RR, Petersdorf RG. The clinical spectrum of bacterial meningitis. Am J Med 1962;33:262–75.
21. Durand ML, Calderwood SB, Weber DJ et al. Acute bacterial meningitis in adults. N Eng J Med 1993;328:21–8.
22. Sigurdardottir B, Bjornsson OM, Jensdottir KE et al. Acute bacterial meningitis in adults. A 20-year overview. Arch Intern Med 1997;157:425–30.
23. Pfister HW, Feiden W, Einhaupl KM. Spectrum of complications during bacterial meningitis in adults: results of a clinical study. Arch Neurol 1993;50:578–81.
24. De Marinis M, Kurdi AA, Welch KMA. Headache associated with intracranial infection. In: Olesen J, Tfelt-Hansen P, Welch KMA, eds. The Headaches. New York: Raven Press, 1993, 697–704.
25. Lipton JD, Schafermeyer RW. Evolving concepts in pediatric bacterial meningitis – Part II. Current management and therapeutic research. Ann Emer Med 1993;22:1619–29.
26. Bartt R. Listeria and atypical presentations of Listeria in the central nervous system. Sem Neurol 2000;20:361–73.
27. Tjia TL, Yeow YK, Tan CB. Cryptococcal meningitis. J Neurol Neurosurg Psychiatry 1985;48:853–8.
28. Benson CA, Harris AA, Levin S. Acute bacterial meningitis: general aspects. In: Vinken PJ, Bruyn GW, Klawans HL, Harris AA, eds. Handbook of Clinical Neurology: Microbial Disease. Amsterdam: Elsevier Science Publishers, 1988, 1–19.
29. Fishman RA. Cerebrospinal fluid in diseases of the nervous system. 2nd edn. Philadelphia: WB Saunders Company, 1992.
30. Oliver LG, Harwood-Nuss AL. Bacterial meningitis in infants and children: a review. J Emerg Med 1993;11:555–64.
31. Pohl CA. Practical approach to bacterial meningitis in childhood. Am Fam Physicians 1993;47:1595–603.
32. Smith RR. Neuroradiology of intracranial infection. Pediatr Neurosurg 1992;18:92–104.
33. Lepow ML, Coyne N, Thompson LB et al. The clinical, epidemiologic and laboratory investigation of aseptic meningitis during the four-year period, 1955–1958. N Eng J Med 1962;266:1188–93.
34. Davis LE. Acute viral meningitis and encephalitis. In: Kennedy PGE, Johnston RT, eds. Infections of the Nervous System. London: Butterworths, 1987, 155–76.
35. Lamonte M, Silberstein SD, Marcelis JF. Headache associated with aseptic meningitis. Headache 1995;35:520–6.

36. Beghi E, Nicolosi A, Kurland LT et al. Encephalitis and aseptic meningitis, Olmsted County Minnesota. 1950–1981. I. Epidemiology. Ann Neurol 1984;16: 283–94.

37. Connolly KJ, Hammer SM. The acute aseptic meningitis syndrome. Infect Dis Clin North Am 1990;4:599–622.

38. Byington CL, Taggart EW, Carroll KC, Hillyard DR. A polymerase chain reaction-based epidemiologic investigation of the incidence of nonpolio enteroviral infections in febrile and afebrile infants 90 days and younger. Pediatrics 1999;103:E27.

39. Hamilton MS, Lackson MA, Abel D. Clinical utility of polymerase chain reaction testing for enteroviral meningitis. Pediatr Infect Dis J 1999;18:533–8.

40. Zunt JR, Marra CM. Cerebrospinal fluid testing for the diagnosis of central nervous system infection. Neurol Clin 1999;17: 675–89.

41. Hofgartner WT, Huhmer AF, Landers JP, Kant JA. Rapid diagnosis of herpes simplex encephalitis using microchip electrophoresis of PCR products. Clin Chem 1999;45:2120–8.

42. Bharucha NE, Bhaba SK, Bharucha EP. Infections of the nervous system. B. Viral infections. In: Bradley WG, Daroff RB, Fenichel GM, Marsden CD, eds. Neurology in Clinical Practice. Stoneham: Butterworth-Heinnman, 1991, 1085–97.

43. Pachner AR, Steere AC. The triad of neurological manifestation of Lyme disease: meningitis, cranial neuritis, and radiculoneuritis. Neurology 1985;35: 47–53.

44. Gottfredsson M, Perfect J. Fungal meningitis. Sem Neurol 2000;20: 307–22.

45. Casado JL, Quereda C, Oliva J et al. Candida meningitis in HIV-infected patients: analysis of 14 cases. Clin Infect Dis 1997;25:673–6.

46. Voice RA, Bradley SF, Sangeorzan JA, Kauffman CA. Chronic candidal meningitis: an uncommon manifestation of candidiasis. Clin Infect Dis 1994;19:60–6.

47. Beal MF, O'Carroll CP, Kleinman GM, Grossman RI. Aspergillosis of the nervous system. Neurology 1982;32:473–9.

48. Stern BJ, Krumholz A, Johns C. Sarcoidosis and its neurological manifestations. Arch Neurol 1985; 42:909–17.

49. Wasserstrom WR, Glass JP, Posner JB. Diagnosis and treatment of leptomeningeal metastases from solid tumors: experience with 90 patients. Cancer 1982;49:759–72.

50. Roos KL. Mycobacterium tuberculosis meningitis and other etiologies of the aseptic meningitis syndrome. Sem Neurol 2000;20:329–35.

51. Starke JR. Tuberculosis of the central nervous system in children. Sem Ped Neurol 1999;6:318–31.

52. Garcia-Monco JC. Central nervous system tuberculosis. Neurol Clin 1999;17:737–59.

53. Schraeder PL, Burns RA. Hemiplegic migraine associated with an aseptic meningeal reaction. Arch Neurol 1980; 37:377–9.

54. Steere AC. Lyme disease. N Engl J Med 1989;321:586–96.

55. Berger BW. Cutaneous manifestations of Lyme borreliosis. Rheum Dis Clin North Am 1989;15:635–47.

56. Scelsa SN, Lipton RB, Sander H, Herskoviz S. Headache characteristics in hospitalized patients with Lyme disease. Headache 1995;35:125–30.

57. Halperin JJ, Logigian EL, Finel MF, Pearl RA. Practice parameters for the diagnosis of patients with nervous system Lyme borreliosis (Lyme disease). Neurology 1996;46:619–27.

58. Hansen K, Lebech A. The clinical and epidemiological profile of Lyme neuroborreliosis in Denmark 1985–1990. Brain 1992;115:399–423.

59. Halperin JJ, Luft BJ, Anand AK. Lyme neuroborreliosis central nervous system manifestations. Neurology 1989;39: 753–9.

60. Brinck T, Hansen K, Olesen J. Headache resembling tension-type headache as the single manifestation of Lyme neuroborreliosis. Cephalalgia 1993;13: 207–9.

61. Luger SW. Serologic tests for Lyme disease. Arch Intern Med 1990;150:761–8.

62. Steere AC, Taylor E, Wilson ML et al. Longitudinal assessment of the clinical and epidemiologic features of Lyme disease. J Infect Dis 1986;154:295–300.

63. Steere AC, Berardi VP, Weeks KB et al. Evaluation of the intrathecal antibody response to *Borrelia burgdorferi* as a diagnostic test for Lyme neuroborreliosis. J Infect Dis 1990;161:1203–9.

64. Hansen K, Lebech AM. Lyme neuroborreliosis: a new sensitive diagnostic assay for intrathecal synthesis of *Borrelia burgdorferi* – specific immunoglobulin G, A and M. Ann Neurol 1991;30:197–205.

65. Karlsson M, Hovind HK, Svenungsson B, Stiernstedt G. Cultivation and characterization of spirochetes from cerebrospinal fluid of patients with Lyme borreliosis. J Clin Microbiol 1990;28: 473–9.

66. Brown SL. Role of serology in the diagnosis of Lyme disease. JAMA 1999; 282:62–6.

67. Wormser GP. Lyme disease serology problems and opportunities. JAMA 1999; 282:79–80.

68. Nichol G, Dennis DT, Steere AC et al. Test treatment strategies for patients suspected of having Lyme disease: a cost-effectiveness analysis. Ann Int Med 1998;128:37–48.

69. Roos KL. Encephalitis. Neurol Clin 1999;17:813–33.

70. Solomon T, Cardosa MJ. Emerging arboviral encephalitis. Newsworthy in the West but much more common in the East. Br Med J 2000;321:1484–5.

71. Mostashari F, Bunning ML, Kitsutani PT et al. Epidemic West Nile encephalitis, New York, 1999: results of a household-based seroepidemiological survey. Lancet 2001;358:261–4.

72. Johnson RT. Viral infections of the nervous system. New York: Raven Press, 1982.

73. Silberstein SD. Evaluation and emergency treatment of headache. Headache 1992;32:396–407.

74. Young CA, Humphrey DM, Ghadiali EJ et al. Short-term memory impairment as a presentation of herpes simplex. encephalitis. Neurology 1992;42:260–1.

75. Kennedy PGE. A retrospective analysis of forty-six cases of herpes simplex encephalitis seen in Glasgow between 1962 and 1965. Q J Med 1988;68: 533–40.

76. Johnson RT. Acute encephalitis. Clin Inf Dis 1996;23:219–44.

77. Whitley RJ, Kimberlin DW. Viral encephalitis. Ped Rev 1999;20:192–8.

78. Studahl M, Bergstrom T, Hagberg L. Acute viral encephalitis in adults – a prospective study. Scand J Infect Dis 1998;30: 215–20.

79. Sage JL, Weinstein MP, Miller DC. Chronic encephalitis possibly due to herpes simplex virus: two cases. Neurology 1985;35:1470–2.

80. Lakeman FD, Koga J, Whitley RJ. Detection of antigen to herpes simplex virus in cerebrospinal fluid from patients with herpes simplex encephalitis. J Infect Dis 1987;155:1172–8.

81. Deresiewicz RI, Thaler SJ, Hsu L, Zamani AA. Clinical and neuroradiographic manifestations of eastern equine encephalitis. N Engl J Med 1997; 336:1867–74.

82. Townsend GC, Scheld WM. Infections of the central nervous system. In: Townsend GC, Scheld WM, eds. Advances in Internal Medicine. St Louis: Mosby Yearbook, 1998, 403–47.

83. Chun CH, Johnson JD, Hofstetter M, Raff MJ. Brain abscess. A study of 45 consecutive cases. Medicine (Baltimore) 1986;65:415–31.

84. Takahashi M. Infections of the central nervous system. Curr Opin Neurol Neurosurg 1992;5:849–53.

85. Rowley AH, Whitley RJ, Lakeman FD, Wolinsky SM. Rapid detection of herpes-simplex-virus DNA in cerebrospinal fluid patients with herpes simplex encephalitis. Lancet 1990;335:440–1.

86. Kaplan K. Brain abscess. Med Clin N Amer 1985;69:345–60.

87. Movali A, Dinubile MJ. Brain abscess. In: Vinken PJ, Bruyn GW, Klawans HL, Harris AA, eds. Handbook of Clinical Neurology: Microbial Disease. Amsterdam: Elsevier Science Publishers, 1988:143–66.

88. Nicolosi A, Hauser WA, Musicco, Kurland LT. Incidence and prognosis of brain abscess in a defined population: Olmsted County, Minnesota. Neuroepidemiology 1991;10:122–31.

chapter 16

Pregnancy, breast-feeding and headache

Pregnancy

Headaches continue to occur when a woman becomes pregnant, but a different emphasis is necessary. Migraine, tension-type headache, and other primary headaches occur during pregnancy, as do the conditions that mimic them: vasculitis, brain tumor, and occipital arteriovenous malformations (AVM).[1] Other headache disorders that occur during pregnancy include sinusitis, meningitis, idiopathic intracranial hypertension, and subarachnoid hemorrhage (SAH), and these require neuroimaging or lumbar puncture to diagnose (Table 16.1).[2–5]

Diagnostic testing serves to exclude organic causes of headache, to confirm the diagnosis, and to establish a baseline before treatment. If neurodiagnostic testing is indicated, the study that will provide the most information with the least fetal risk is the study of choice.

Most drugs are not clearly teratogenic, but our knowledge about the effects they have on the growing fetus is still insufficient. While medication use should be limited during pregnancy, it is not absolutely contraindicated. The risk of status migrainosus, for example, to both the fetus and the mother may be greater than the potential risk of the medication. Nonpharmacological treatment would be the ideal solution, but this approach often is less effective than the pharmacological approach. However, analgesics such as acetaminophen (paracetamol) and narcotics can be used on a limited basis. Because of the potential risk to the fetus, preventive pharmacological therapy is a last resort.

Neurodiagnostic testing: radiology

The effect of radiation on the developing conceptus is a major concern during pregnancy. At the time of implantation, the most common radiation effect is death of the conceptus, with a threshold of $\geqslant 5$ rad. Radiation exposure during embryogenesis and organogenesis may result in developmental anomalies or growth retardation, with threshold doses of $\geqslant 5$ rad. A radiation dose of > 15 rad may result in severe deformities. The dose to the uterus from a skull or cervical spine film is < 1 mrad, $\leqslant 1000$ mrad from a thoracic spine series, and 1500 mrad from a lumbar spine series.[6] A standard head or cervical spine computed tomography (CT) exposes the uterus to < 1 mrad, and thoracic CT exposure is about 20 mrad. However, the dose from a lumbar spine CT is approximately 700 mrad.[6]

The radiation dose for a typical cervical or intracranial angiogram is < 1 mrad. Fluoroscopy delivers 1 rad per minute to the skin.[6] Unless an aneurysm, an AVM, or vasculitis is suspected, there is little reason to perform angiography when a patient has a normal neurologic examination, a normal CT or magnetic resonance imaging (MRI), and a history consistent with a benign primary headache disorder, particularly if she is pregnant.

The potential risk of MRI in pregnancy is still controversial. Magnetic resonance magnets induce an electric field and raise the core temperature by $< 1\,°C$. While high body temperature may increase the incidence of neural tube defects, the effects of MRI are unknown. Gadolinium, a contrast agent used with MRI, crosses the placental barrier and is excreted through the fetal kidneys. Although no illeffects have been demonstrated, gadolinium injection should be avoided, as should CT contrast.[6]

Head CT is relatively safe during pregnancy and is the study of choice for head trauma and possible nontraumatic subarachnoid, subdural, or intraparenchymal hemorrhage. For all other nontraumatic or non hemorrhagic craniospinal pathology, MRI is preferred. One should use MRA first to evaluate any suspected vascular pathology, but when necessary, angiography is reasonably safe for the pregnant patient (Table 16.2). Potential indications for CT or MRI in headache investigation during pregnancy include the first headache of the patient's life; an abrupt onset (thunderclap) headache; a change in the frequency, severity, or clinical features of the headache attack; an abnormal neurologic examination; a progressive or new daily persistent headache; neurologic symptoms that do

● **Table 16.1** *Headache disorders and pregnancy*

Less common	As common	More common
Migraine	Idiopathic intracranial hypertension	Stroke
	Tension-type headache	Cerebral venous thrombosis
	Sinusitis	Eclampsia
	Meningitis	Subarachnoid haemorrhage
	Vasculitis	Pituitary tumour
	Brain tumour	Choriocarcinoma

● **Table 16.2** Guidelines for neuroimaging the patient who is or may be pregnant*

- Determine the necessity and the potential risks of the procedure
- If possible, perform the examination during the first 10 days postmenses, or if the patient is pregnant, delay the examination until the third trimester or preferably postpartum
- Pick the procedure with the highest accuracy balanced by the lowest radiation
- Use MRI if possible
- Avoid direct exposure to the abdomen and pelvis
- Avoid contrast agents
- Do not avoid radiologic testing purely for the sake of the pregnancy
- If significant exposure is incurred by a pregnant patient, consult a radiation biologist
- Consent forms are neither required nor recommended

*Adapted from R.B. Schwartz's Neurodiagnostic Imaging of the Pregnant Patient that appeared in 'Neurologic complications of pregnancy'.[6]

not meet the criteria of migraine with typical aura; persistent neurologic defects; definite EEG evidence of a focal cerebral lesion; an orbital or skull bruit suggestive of AVM; and new comorbid partial (focal) seizures.[3] In each case a judgment must be made about the risk of not diagnosing the condition compared with the minor risk of radiation.

Mechanisms

Rising or sustained high estrogen levels have been proposed as the mechanism of the migraine relief that often occurs during pregnancy; this mechanism, however, cannot explain the worsening or new appearance of

migraine that sometimes occurs.[7] The rapid fall of estrogen levels may be responsible for menstrual and postpartum migraine. Women with a prior history of migraine are more likely to have migraine in the postpartum period.[8] Migraine relief during pregnancy is not dependent on adequate 'protective' levels of progesterone.

Course of migraine during pregnancy

Approximately 60–70% of migraineurs will improve during pregnancy, while some women without prior migraine will experience their first migraine headache (Table 16.3). A smaller group of migraineurs finds that their headaches either worsen, particularly in the first trimester, or remain unchanged. The true incidence of migraine in pregnancy is unknown. Most reported cases have been migraine with aura or prolonged aura. Case reports[7,9] of migraine that occur for the first time during pregnancy emphasize the presence of focal neurologic symptoms (migraine with aura), probably because patients with these dramatic presentations are more likely to be referred to a neurologist (Table 16.3).

In Lance and Anthony's study, migraine improved in 58% of pregnant women, while 42% worsened or had no change.[10] Sixty-four percent of women with menstrual migraine had relief during pregnancy, compared with 48% relief in those without menstrual migraine (Table 16.4).

In Bousser et al's series of 131 pregnancies, preexisting migraine improved or disappeared in 77.9% of patients, worsened in 7.6%, was unchanged in 8.4%, and was variable in 6.1%.[11] Migraine appeared for the first time in 16 women. Disappearance or improvement did not differ significantly in migraine with or without aura, but

● **Table 16.3** Migraine and pregnancy

Parameter	Lance (1966)	Callaghan (1968)	Somerville (1970)	Bousser (1990)	Granella et al. (1993)	Rasmussen (1993)	Chen and Leviton (1994)	Maggioni et al. (1995)
Women studied		200	200	703	1300	975	55,000	428
History of migraine and pregnancies	120	41	38	116	943	80	484	80
Number of pregnancies	252	200	200	147	943		484	?
New migraine during pregnancy	0	33/41 (80%)	7/38 (18%)	16/147 (11%)	12 (1.3%)	?	0	1/428
New migraine postpartum				?	42 (4.5%)	?	0	?
Prior migraine	252	8	31	131	571	80	484	91
Prior migraine improved	145/252 (58%)	4 (50%)	24/31 (77%)	102/131 (78%)	384/571 (67.3%)	48%	382/484 (79%)	80%
Prior migraine unchanged or worsened	107/252 (42%)	3 (38%)	7/31 (23%)	29/131 (22%)	187/571 (32.7%)	52%	102/484 (21%)	20%
Type series	R, H	R, H	R, H	R, O	R, H	R, POP	P, O	R, H

H = headache or neurologic; P = prospective; R = retrospective; POP = population base

Table 16.4 *Menstrual migraine and migraine improvement with pregnancy*

Menstrual/non-menstrual	Lance (1966)	Bousser (1990)
Menstrual		
Disappeared or improved	64%	86%
Worsened	36%	7%
Non-menstrual		
Disappeared or improved	48%	60%
Worsened	52%	15%

worsening was much more common in migraine with aura. Women with menstrual migraine showed the most improvement (Table 16.4). Granella et al found significant improvement in 17.4% of patients and worsening in 3.5%.[12] Women whose migraine began at menarche had a higher remission rate (36.4% vs. 13.9%) than women whose headaches began at other times. Migraine began during pregnancy in 1.3% of patients and postpartum in 4.5%.

Rasmussen found 49% of pregnant women had significant improvement or disappearance of their headache, and only 4% worsened.[13] Chen and Leviton found that 17% had a complete remission, and another 62% showed some improvement with pregnancy.[14] Maggioni et al found one new case of migraine without aura that began during pregnancy.[15] Of the migraineurs, 80% had at least a 50% decrease in attack frequency, usually after the first trimester.

Outcome of pregnancy in migraineurs

Miscarriage, toxemia, congenital anomalies, and stillbirth are not increased in migraineurs when compared with national averages or controls.[16] However, in Chancellor and Wroe's small series,[7] four of nine patients developed complications, including two who developed preeclampsia. Olesen et al have recently reported that, in Denmark, women with migraine are more likely to have low birth weight children than women without migraine (odds ratio (OR) 3.0).[17]

Postpartum migraine

Postpartum headache (PPH) occurs in about 39% of women and is most frequent on days 3–6 postpartum.[8] PPH is commonly associated with a personal or family history of migraine (58% of migraineurs developed PPH). PPH, while less severe than patients' typical migraine, was bifrontal, prolonged, and associated with photophobia, nausea, and anorexia. Newly occurring frequent headache occurred in 3.6% of women and migraine in 1.4% of 11 701 women by 3 months' postpartum.[18] Two of Wright

and Patel's cases of focal neurologic signs associated with migraine presented postpartum.[9] Both patients had a history of migraine with aura. Migraine frequently restarts in the postpartum period and can begin de novo.

Another cause of headache in the postpartum period is postdural puncture headache owing to a spinal anesthetic or an accidental dural puncture.[19] After spinal anesthesia, nonpostdural puncture headaches occur in 5–16% of patients. Headache also occurs in 25% of parturients who have no neuroaxial anesthetic intervention. Maternal cortical vein thrombosis, an unusual complication of pregnancy, occurs between the first and third weeks' postpartum.[20] Subdural hematoma is a rare complication of a spinal anesthetic or accidental dural puncture complicating an epidural anesthetic.[21–25] Spontaneous subarachnoid hemorrhage owing to aneurysms and AVMs occurs with an incidence of 1–5 per 10 000 pregnancies, which is higher than the incidence for the general population. A postpartum headache may be the harbinger of a serious medical event. Misdiagnosing a postdural puncture headache and placing an epidural blood patch can cloud and confuse further neurologic workups.[21,26]

Treatment
Risk of drug treatment (Table 16.5)
The recognition of the teratogenicity of aminopterin and thalidomide and the rubella epidemic of 1963–1964 resulted in extremely conservative drug use during

Table 16.5 *Definitions and drug effects*

Spontaneous abortion:	Death of the conceptus. Most due to chromosomal abnormality.
Embryotoxicity:	The ability of drugs to kill the developing embryo.
Congenital anomalies:	Deviation from normal morphology or function.
Teratogenicity:	The ability of an exogenous agent to produce a permanent abnormality of structure or function in an organism exposed during embryogenesis or fetal life.
Fetal effects:	Growth retardation, abnormal histogenesis (also congenital abnormalities and fetal death). The main outcome of fetal drug toxicity during the second and third trimesters of pregnancy.
Perinatal effects:	Effects on uterine contraction, neonatal withdrawal, or haemostasis.
Postnatal effects:	Drugs may have delayed long-term effects: delayed oncogenesis, and functional and behavioural abnormalities.

pregnancy. In 1977, the Food and Drug Administration (FDA) developed a policy against phase I and early phase II testing in pregnant women or in women of child-bearing potential, and many practitioners now avoid drug treatment in pregnancy even when it is indicated. The FDA has tested over 3000 drugs and only 20 are known human teratogens. Knowledge about the birth defect risks from drug exposure is insufficient despite the fact that 67% of women take drugs during pregnancy and 50% take them during the first trimester.[27]

Most drugs cross the placenta and have the potential to adversely affect the fetus. Although studies have not absolutely established the safety of any medication during pregnancy, some are believed to be relatively safe (Tables 16.8–16.17).[28–31]

In 1966, the FDA replaced the Multigeneration Continuous Feeding Reproductive Study with a three-segment design, identified as Segment I (Fertility and General Reproductive Performance), Segment II (Teratology), and Segment III (Perinatal and Postnatal Evaluations), for testing drugs. These studies were designed to detect agents that specifically interrupt reproduction. More than 3300 chemicals have been tested; of these, 37% are teratogenic. These studies frequently used very high doses of drugs, which then produced maternal toxicity, not fetal teratogenicity. Currently 19 drugs, or drug groups, and two chemicals have been established as human teratogens. Negative results in other species cannot predict a lack of teratogenicity in humans, and drugs that are teratogenic at high doses in these species may not be teratogenic in humans at lower doses.[32] Thalidomide, which has no teratogenic effect in mice and rats, has profound teratogenic effects in humans.[28,33]

A negative pregnancy test is often a condition of enrollment in a study, while post-enrollment pregnancy can lead to termination of participation. This poses a problem for pregnant women who are sick and in need of treatment. If a drug has not been tested in pregnant women during the research phase, information is lacking about the safety and efficacy of the drug for the women as well as the fetus.[34] The Institute of Medicine Committee on Research in Women made the controversial recommendation to consider pregnant and lactating women eligible for enrollment in clinical studies on a routine basis.[34] This report reversed the existing exclusion of pregnant women and the severely restricted enrollment of women of 'child-bearing potential' from most clinical studies. With regard to enrollment, the Committee recommended that women who are or may become pregnant in the course of a study should be viewed as any other potential research subject.

If women of childbearing age participate in clinical

trials, more information will be gained about the risks of birth defects, but uncertainty will still persist. If a drug is associated with a very high level of birth defects (e.g. thalidomide), very few exposures need to be followed to detect this risk; if a drug is associated with a slight increase in birth defects, approximately 300 exposed pregnancies need to be followed to detect a doubling of risk; and if a drug is associated with an increase of a rare specific defect (e.g. 1/1000), approximately 10 000 exposed pregnancies need to be followed to detect a doubling of risk.[27]

The World Health Organization surveyed drug utilization during pregnancy. Eighty-six percent of 14 778 pregnant women took medication, each receiving an average of 2.9 prescriptions. Over-the-counter drugs were not considered. Of a total of 37 309 prescriptions, 73% were given by obstetricians, 12% by general practitioners, and 5% by midwives. In another study, 40% of pregnant women at Parkland Memorial Hospital in Dallas took some type of medication other than iron or vitamin supplements, and as many as 20% used an illicit drug or alcohol.[35] Discharges of drug-using parturient women increased by 576% and discharges of drug-affected newborns in the United States between 1979 and 1990 increased by 456%. While no medication is absolutely safe, some are believed to be relatively safe.[27]

Adverse drug effects depend on the dose and route of administration, concomitant exposures, and the timing of the exposure relative to the period of development (Table 16.6), which consist of the preimplantation period, embryogenesis, and fetal development. The preimplantation period lasts from conception to 1 week postconception, during which time the conceptus is relatively protected from drugs.[35] Embryogenesis is the time of organogenesis, which occurs from the time of implantation to 60 days' postconception.[35] Most congenital malformations arise during this time. Placental transport is not well established until the fifth week after conception. This protects the embryo from maternal drugs. The final phase, fetal development, follows embryogenesis. As the fetus

● **Table 16.6** *Periods of development*

Preimplantation period
Conception to one week postconception
Conceptus is relatively protected from drugs
Embryogenesis
Time of organogenesis
From implantation to 60 days postconception
Fetal development
Follows embryogenesis

grows in size, structural changes, such as neuronal arrangement, also occur. Malformations can develop at this time in normally formed organs due to their necrosis and reabsorption.[35]

Death to the conceptus, teratogenicity, fetal growth abnormalities, perinatal effects, postnatal developmental abnormalities, delayed oncogenesis, and functional and behavioral changes can result from drugs or other agents (Table 16.5). According to the Perinatal Collaborative Project, which is a prospective and concurrent epidemiological study of more than 50 000 pregnancies, many drugs have little or no human teratogenic risk.[36]

Spontaneous abortion

Nearly half of early pregnancies spontaneously abort, most because of chromosomal abnormalities. Prior to the time of organogenesis, exposure to a potential teratogen or toxic drug has an all-or-none effect. An exposure around the time of conception or implantation may kill the conceptus, but if the pregnancy continues, congenital anomalies do not increase.

Developmental defects

Developmental defects may result from genetic or environmental causes or from interactions between them. Teratogenic drug effects are generally visible anatomic malformations but are defined as the production of a permanent alteration of structure or function in an organ due to intrauterine exposure (Figure 16.1). These effects are dose-

and time-related, with the fetus at greatest risk during the first trimester of pregnancy. Drug exposure accounts for only 2–3% of birth defects; approximately 25% are genetic, and the causes of the remainder are unknown. The incidence of major malformations either incompatible with survival (e.g. anencephaly) or requiring major surgery (e.g. cleft palate or congenital heart disease) is approximately 2–3% in the general population. If all minor malformations are included (ear tags or extra digits), the rate may be as high as 7–10%. The risk of malformation after drug exposure must be evaluated against this background rate. The classic teratogenic period in the human is a critical 6 weeks, lasting from approximately 31 days to 10 weeks from the last menstrual period. A teratogenic effect is dependent on the timing of the exposure as well as the nature of the teratogen. Early exposure, when the heart and central nervous system are forming, may result in an anomaly, such as congenital heart disease or neural tube defect, while later exposure may result in malformation of the palate or ear. Once the teratogenic period has passed, the major risk of congenital anomaly is gone, but other abnormalities can occur. These include fetal effects, neonatal effects, and postnatal effects.

Fetal effects

Fetal effects include damage to normally formed organs, damage to systems undergoing histogenesis, growth retardation, or fetal death. Of these, growth retardation is the most common fetal effect.

Neonatal and postnatal effects

Adverse drug effects include withdrawal, neonatal hypoglycemia, and disorders of uterine contracture and hemostasis. Chronic exposure to psychoactive medications, such as alcohol, during the second and third trimester may cause mental retardation, which may not be recognized until later in life.

Delayed oncogenesis

Exposure to diethylstilboestrol as late as 20 weeks' gestation may cause reproductive organ anomalies that are not recognized until after puberty.

Maternal physiology (Table 16.7)[37]

Profound structural and physiological changes occur during pregnancy. The uterus rapidly increases in size, transforming from an almost-solid structure weighing 70 g into a relatively thin-walled, muscular organ large enough to accommodate the fetus, placenta, and amniotic fluid.[38] Uterine growth depends on estrogen and, to a lesser extent, progesterone, during the first few months of pregnancy. After 12 weeks, growth results from the pressure

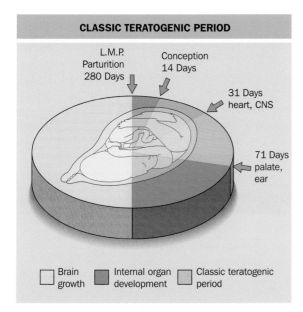

CLASSIC TERATOGENIC PERIOD

L.M.P. Parturition 280 Days

Conception 14 Days

31 Days heart, CNS

71 Days palate, ear

☐ Brain growth ■ Internal organ development ☐ Classic teratogenic period

● *Figure 16.1* *The fetus is at greatest risk from tetatogenic drug effects during the first trimester of pregnancy.*

● Table 16.7 *Physiological changes during pregnancy*

Parameter	Change	Potential implications for toxicology
Extracellular volume	↑4–6 litres	Dilution of substances in circulation
Plasma volume	↑by 40%	Same
Plasma renin/ aldosterone	↑↑	Renal retention/ excretion
Renal blood flow	↑ 30–50%	Same
Glomerular filtration rate	↑30–50%	Same
Sodium and calcium retention	↑↑	Retention of other divalent cations
Cardiac output	↑by 40%	Increased sensitivity to cardiotoxins (?)
Increased blood flow to skin	↑	↑Dermal uptake
Food intake	↑70 kcal/day (average)	Increased dose
Energy demand*	↑~300 kcal/day	Increased dose and metabolic shift
Lipid stores*	↑~3–4 kg over pregnancy	Same
Oxygen consumption*	↑51 ml O2/min	Metabolic shift (?)
Basal metabolic rate	↑13%	Metabolic shifts
Hepatic triglyceride synthesis	↑	Redistribution

*Dependent on nutrition, activity levels, and gestational state.
Table adapted from Metcalfe et al.[37]

exerted by the expanding products of conception. Cell and tissue growth are dependent on increased synthesis of polyamines (including spermine and spermidine and their immediate precursor, putrescine).[38]

Metabolic changes occur in response to the rapidly-growing fetus and placenta. Weight gain, due to increased blood volume and extravascular extracellular fluid and increased size of the uterus and its contents and the breasts, averages about 11 kg, with about 1 kg occurring during the first trimester.[38] Water retention (about 6.5 litres by term) is a normal occurrence, mediated, in part, by a fall in plasma osmolality of 10 mOsm/kg, due to a resetting of the osmoreceptor. The fetus, placenta, and amniotic fluid contain about 3.5 litres of water. Another 3.0 litres of water results from increased maternal blood volume and the increase in uterine and breast size. Near term, blood volume is about 45% above baseline. Weight loss during the first 10 days postpartum averages about 2 kg.[38]

While pregnancy is potentially diabetogenic, a healthy pregnant woman's fasting plasma glucose concentration may fall due to increased plasma insulin levels. Progesterone, when administered to a non-pregnant adult in an amount similar to that produced during pregnancy, results in an increased basal insulin concentration and a response to an oral glucose challenge similar to that of a normal pregnant woman. Additionally, estradiol induces hyperinsulinism in both control and ovariectomized rats.[38]

Lipid, lipoprotein, and apolipoprotein plasma concentrations increase during pregnancy. There is a positive correlation between lipid concentrations and levels of estradiol, progesterone, and human placental lactogen.

The kidneys barely increase in size during pregnancy.[39] Early in pregnancy, at the beginning of the second trimester, the glomerular filtration rate and renal plasma flow increase by about 50%.[40,41] The elevated glomerular filtration rate persists to term, whereas the renal plasma flow decreases during late pregnancy.[41] The human liver does not increase in size during pregnancy, and we are not certain whether or not hepatic blood flow increases.

These profound physiological changes that occur during pregnancy can alter drug pharmacokinetics: plasma volume increases by half, cardiac output increases by 30–50%, and renal plasma flow and glomerular filtration rate increase by 40–50%. Serum albumin decreases by 20–30%, resulting in decreased drug binding and increased drug clearance. Increased extracellular fluid and adipose tissue increases the volume of drug distribution. Drug metabolism may also be increased, modulated, in part, by the high concentration of sex hormones.[42]

● Table 16.8 *FDA risk categories*

Category A:	Controlled human studies show no risk
Category B:	No evidence of risk in humans, but there are no controlled human studies
Category C:	Risk to humans has not been ruled out
Category D:	Positive evidence of risk to humans from human and/or animal studies
Category X:	Contraindicated in pregnancy.

● Table 16.9 *TERIS risk rating*

- Undetermined (C)
- None (A)
- None–minimal (A)
- Minimal (B)
- Minimal–small (D)
- High (X)

Equivalent FDA ratings in parentheses.

Drug risk categories

The FDA lists five categories of labelling for drug use in pregnancy (Table 16.8).[43] These categories provide therapeutic guidance, weighing the risks as well as the benefits of the drug. An alternate rating system is TERIS, an automated teratogen information resource wherein ratings for each drug or agent are based on a consensus of expert opinion and the literature (Table 16.9).[44] TERIS was designed to assess the teratogenic risk to the fetus from a drug exposure. A recent study found that the FDA categories have little, if any, correlation to the TERIS teratogenic risk. This discrepancy results in part from the fact that the FDA categories were designed to provide therapeutic guidance. The TERIS ratings are useful for estimating the teratogenic risks of a drug that a women is exposed to but were not designed to provide therapeutic guidance.[45]

A woman's risk of having a child with a neural tube defect is associated with early pregnancy red cell folate levels in a continuous dose–response relationship.[46] Low serum and red blood cell folate levels are associated with spontaneous abortion and fetal malformations in animals and in humans.[47–50] Treatment with some drugs, including phenytoin, carbamazepine, and barbiturates, can impair folate absorption. Valproic acid does not produce folate deficiency, but it may interfere with folinic acid production by inhibiting glutamate formyl transferase.[51] In a small study, women with epilepsy who were taking phenytoin needed 1 mg of folate supplementation a day to maintain a normal serum level.[52] The current guidelines suggest increasing folic acid intake by 4 mg, which would result in a 48% reduction in neural tube defects.[47] Supplementing this by fortifying food with folate would benefit all women.

Headache treatment

The major concerns in managing the pregnant patient are the effects of both medication and migraine on the fetus. Because of the possible risk of injury to the fetus, medication use should be limited; however, it is not contraindicated during pregnancy.[27] Because migraine usually improves after the first trimester, many women can manage their headaches with this reassurance and non-pharmacological treatments (rest, ice packs, massage, and, at times, biofeedback).[27] Some women, however, will continue to have severe, intractable headaches, sometimes associated with nausea, vomiting, and possible dehydration. Not only are these conditions disruptive to the patient, they may pose a risk to the fetus that is greater than the potential risk of the medications used to treat the pregnant patient.[27]

● **Table 16.10** *Some therapeutic medications*

Drug class		Fetal risk	
		FDA	**TERIS**
Simple analgesics	Aspirin	C (D)	None–minimal
	Acetaminophen	B	None
	Caffeine	B	None–minimal
NSAIDs	Ibuprofen	B (D)	None–minimal
	Indomethacin	B (D)	None
	Naproxen	B (D)	Undetermined
Opoids	Butorphanol	C (D)	None–minimal
	Codeine	C (D)	None–minimal
	Meperidine	B (D)	None–minimal
	Methadone	B (D)	None–minimal
	Morphine	B (D)	None–minimal
	Propoxyphene	C (D)	None–minimal
Ergots	Ergotamine	X	Minimal
	Dihydroergotamine	X	Undetermined
Cortico-steroids	Dexamethasone	C	None–minimal
	Prednisone	B	None–minimal
Barbiturates	Butalbital	C (D)	None–minimal
	Phenobarbital	D	None–minimal
Benzo-diazepam	Chlordiazepoxide	D	None–minimal
	Clonazepam	D	Uncertain
	Diazepam	D	None–minimal
Triptans	Almotriptan	C	Undetermined
	Eletriptan	C	Undetermined
	Frovatriptan	C	Undetermined
	Naratriptan	C	Undetermined
	Rizatriptan	C	Undetermined
	Sumatriptan	C	Undetermined
	Zolmitriptan	C	Undetermined

* Risk factor if used at end of third trimester given in parentheses.

● **Table 16.11** *Neuroleptics/antiemetics*

Drug class		Fetal risk	
		FDA	**TERIS**
Antihi-stamines	Cyclizine (Marezine)	B	Undetermined
	Cyproheptadine	B	Undetermined
	Dimenhydrinate (Dramamine)	B	None–minimal
	Meclizine (Antivert)	B	None–minimal
Neuroleptics	Phenothiazines		
	Chlorpromazine (Thorazine)	C	None–minimal
	Prochlorperazine (Compazine)	C	None
	Butyrophenones Haloperidol	C	None–minimal
	Metoclopramide (Reglan)	B	None–minimal
Other	Emetrol	B	Unknown
	Doxylamine succinate	–	None
	Vitamin B$_6$ (pyridoxine)	B	None
	Ondansetron	B	Unknown
	Granisetron	B	Unknown

Symptomatic treatment, designed to reduce the severity and duration of symptoms, is used to treat an acute headache attack (Tables 16.10, 16.11). For headaches that do not respond to nonpharmacological treatment, symptomatic drugs are indicated. The nonsteroidal anti-inflammatory drugs (NSAIDs), acetaminophen (paracetamol) (alone or with codeine), codeine alone, or other opioids can be used during pregnancy. Aspirin in low, intermittent doses is not a significant teratogenic risk, although large doses, especially if given near term, may be associated with maternal and fetal bleeding. Barbiturate and benzodiazepine use should be limited. Ergotamine, dihydroergotamine, and all triptans should be avoided.

Symptoms associated with migraine, such as nausea and vomiting, can be as disabling as the headache pain itself. In addition, some medications that are used to treat migraine can produce nausea. Metoclopramide, which decreases the gastric atony seen with migraine and enhances the absorption of co-administered medications, is extremely useful in migraine treatment. Mild nausea can be treated with phosphorylated carbohydrate solution (Emetrol) or doxylamine succinate and vitamin B6 (pyridoxine). More severe nausea may require the use of injections or suppositories. Trimethobenzamide, chlorpromazine, prochlorperazine, and promethazine are available orally, parenterally, and by suppository and can all be used safely. We frequently use promethazine and prochlorperazine suppositories. Corticosteroids can occasionally be utilized. Some use prednisone in preference to dexamethasone (which crosses the placenta more readily).

Severe acute attacks of migraine should be treated aggressively.[27] We start intravenous fluids for hydration and then use prochlorperazine 10 mg intravenously to control both nausea and head pain. This can be supplemented by intravenous opioids or intravenous corticosteroids. This is an extremely effective way of handling status migrainosus during pregnancy.

The GlaxoSmithKline pregnancy registries[53] (observational, case-registration, and follow-up studies) were designed to detect evidence of teratogenicity associated with specific medications. After prenatal exposure to the registry medication, pregnancies are registered prospectively, through voluntary reports by healthcare providers. The published risk of birth defects in the general population range is 3–5%, and the risk in women with epilepsy is 6–9%. The proportions of outcomes with birth defects (after first trimester exposure) in the sumatriptan Pregnancy Registry (1996–October 1998) are 3.8% (7/183), (95% confidence interval (CI), 1.7–8.0%). The naratriptan registry has insufficient data for analysis. No excess risk and no pattern of defects has been observed. A small excess risk still cannot be ruled out.

Some 2.5% of fertile Danish women use sumatriptan and continue to use it during pregnancy. Olesen et al[17] analysed data from the Pharmacoepidemiological Prescription Database of North Jutland county from 1991 to 1996. Women exposed to sumatriptan during pregnancy were identified (n = 34), and, using logistic regression models, their pregnancy outcome was compared with two groups of pregnant women: (1) healthy women (n = 15 955) and (2) migraine controls (n = 89), defined as migraine patients who did not redeem prescriptions for migraine treatment during pregnancy. The risk of preterm delivery was elevated among women exposed to sumatriptan compared with migraine controls (OR 6.3, 95% CI 1.2–32.0) and healthy women (OR 3.3, 95% CI 1.3–8.5). The odds ratio for having a newborn with a low birth weight was increased (OR 3.0, 95% CI 1.3 to 7.0) for all migraine patients who delivered at term (n = 115) compared with the outcome of healthy pregnancies.

Preventive treatment

Increased frequency and severity of migraine associated with nausea and vomiting may justify the use of preventive medication. This treatment option should be used with the consent of the patient and her partner after the risks have been explained. Preventive therapy is designed to reduce the frequency and severity of headache attacks. Consider preventive medications when patients experience at least three or four prolonged, severe attacks a month that are particularly incapacitating or unresponsive to symptomatic therapy and may result in dehydration and fetal distress. Beta-adrenergic blockers, such as propranolol, have been used under these circumstances, although adverse effects on the fetus, including intrauterine growth retardation, have been reported. If the migraine is so severe that drug treatment is essential, the patient should be told of the risks posed by all the drugs that are used (Table 16.12). If the patient has a coexistent illness that requires treatment, one drug that will treat both disorders should be used. For example, propranolol can be used to treat hypertension and migraine, and fluoxetine can be used to treat comorbid depression.

Drug exposure

If a woman inadvertently takes a drug while she is pregnant or becomes pregnant while on medication, it is important to determine the dose, timing, and duration of the exposure(s). One must ascertain the patient's past and present state of health and the presence of mental retardation or chromosomal abnormalities in the family and, using a reliable source of information (such as TERIS), determine if the drug is a known teratogen (although for many drugs this is not possible).[33,35,44,54]

● **Table 16.12** *Guidelines for prophylactic treatment*

Drug class	Dose	Fetal risk	
		FDA	**TERIS**
β-blockers			
Atenolol	50–120 mg/day	C	Undetermined
Metoprolol	50–100 mg/day	B	Undetermined
Nadolol	40–240 mg/day	C	Undetermined
Propranolol	40–320 mg/day	C	Undetermined
Timolol	10–30 mg/day	C	Undetermined
Antidepressants			
Tricyclics			
Amitriptyline	10–250 mg/day	D	None–minimal
Doxepin	10–150 mg/day	C	Undetermined
Nortriptyline HCl	10–100 mg/day	D	Undetermined
Protriptyline	10–40 mg/day	C	Undetermined
SSRIs			
Fluoxetine	10–80 mg/day	B	None
Paroxetine	10–50 mg/day	C	Undetermined
Sertraline	50–200 mg/day	B	Unknown
Citalopram	20–60 mg/day	C	Undetermined
Calcium-channel blockers			
Verapamil	240–720 mg/day	C	Undetermined
Nifedipine	30–180 mg/day	C	Undetermined
Diltiazem	120–360 mg/day	C	Undetermined
Flunarizine	5–10 mg/day		
Serotonin agonists			
Methysergide	2–8 mg/day in divided doses up to 14 mg/day	D	Undetermined
Methylergonovine maleate (Methergine)	0.2–0.4 mg q.i.d.	C	Undetermined
Pizotifen	1–6 mg/day		
Anticonvulsants			
Divalproex sodium	500–3000 mg/day	D	Small–moderate
Topiramate	50–300 mg/day	C	Uncertain
Gabapentin	600–2400 mg/day	C	Uncertain

If the drug is teratogenic or the risk is unknown, have the obstetrician confirm the gestational age by ultrasound. If the exposure occurred during embryogenesis, high-resolution ultrasound can be performed to determine whether damage to specific organ systems or structures has occurred. If the high-resolution ultrasound is normal, it is reasonable to reassure the patient that the gross fetal structure is normal (within the 90% sensitivity of the study).[35] However, fetal ultrasound cannot exclude minor anomalies or guarantee the birth of a normal child. Delay in achieving developmental milestones, including cognitive development, is a potential risk, especially for children born to epileptics, that cannot be predicted or diagnosed prenatally. The obstetrician should discuss the results of these studies with the mother and her partner; formal prenatal counselling may be helpful in uncertain cases.[35]

Breast-feeding

Milk is a suspension of fat and protein in a carbohydrate-mineral solution. A nursing mother secretes 600 ml milk/day that contains sufficient protein, fat, and carbohydrate to meet the nutritional demands of the growing and developing infant.[29] The transport of a drug into milk depends on its lipid solubility, molecular weight, degree of ionization, protein binding, and the presence or absence of active secretion. Species differences in the composition of milk can result in differences in drug transfer. Since human milk has a much higher pH (pH usually > 7.0) than cows' milk (pH usually < 6.8), bovine drug transfer data may not be accurate in humans.

Many drugs can be detected in breast milk at levels that are not of clinical significance to the infant. The concentration of drug in breast milk is a variable fraction of the maternal blood level. The infant dose is usually 1–2% of the maternal dose, which is usually trivial. Any exposure to a toxic drug or potential allergen may be inappropriate. Drug concentration in breast milk depends on the drug characteristics (pKa, lipid solubility, molecular weight, protein binding) and the breast milk characteristics (composition and volume). Breast milk derives its unique physicochemical properties from the active transport of electrolytes and the formation and excretion of lactose and proteins by glandular epithelial cells in the breast with passive diffusion of water. The volume produced depends on nutritional factors, the amount of milk removed by the suckling infant, and the increase in mammary blood flow that occurs with breast-feeding. Volume production slowly increases from an average of 600 ml/day to 800 ml/day by the time the infant is 6 months old, and undergoes a diurnal variation, with the greatest quantity occurring in the morning. For the first 10 days of production, milk composition is characterized by a gradual increase in fat and lactose from a milk that is higher in protein content (colostrum).

Since most drugs are either weak acids or bases, the transfer across a biological membrane will be greatly influenced by the ionization characteristics (pKa) and pH differences across the membrane. Because the pH of breast milk (7.0) is slightly lower than that of plasma (7.4), there is a tendency towards ion-trapping of basic compounds.

Classification of drugs used during lactation

The American Academy of Pediatrics Committee on Drugs has reviewed drugs in lactation and categorized the drugs as shown in Table 16.13.[55] When prescribing drugs to lactating women, the guidelines in Table 16.14 should be followed.[55]

Table 16.13 Drug categories and breastfeeding[55]

- Contraindicated
- Require temporary cessation of breast feeding
- Effects unknown but may be of concern
- Use with caution
- Usually compatible

Table 16.14 Prescribing guidelines and breastfeeding[55]

- Is the drug necessary?
- Use the safest drug (e.g. acetaminophen (paracetamol) instead of aspirin).
- If there is a possibility that a drug may present a risk to the infant (e.g. phenytoin, phenobarbital), consider measuring the blood level in the nursing infant.
- Drug exposure to the nursing infant may by minimized by having the mother take the medication just after completing a breast feeding.

Table 16.15 Drugs and breast feeding[55]

Drug class		Breast feeding
Simple analgesics	Aspirin	Caution*
	Acetaminophen	Compatible
	Caffeine	Compatible
	NSAID	Compatible
Opioids		Compatible
Barbiturates		Caution**
Benzodiazepam		Concern***
Antihistamines	Cyproheptadine	Contraindicated
Neuroleptics	Phenothiazines	
	Chlorpromazine	Concern
	Prochlorperazine	Compatible
	Metoclopramide	Concern

* Metabolic acidosis, platelet function abnormality;
** Sedation;
*** Effects unknown but of concern.

Table 16.16 Drugs and breast feeding[55]

Ergot/triptans	Breast feeding
Ergotamine	Contraindicated
Dihydroergotamine	Contraindicated
Methylergonovine maleate	Caution
Methysergide	Caution
Triptans	Caution

Table 16.17 Drugs and breast feeding[55]

Drug class		Breast feeding
Antihypertensives	Beta-blockers	Compatible
	Adrenergic blockers	Compatible
	Calcium-channel blockers	Compatible
Antidepressants	Tricyclic antidepressants	Concern
	Selective serotonin reuptake inhibitors	Caution
Other drugs	Carbamazepine	Compatible
	Valproic acid	Compatible
	Corticosteroids	Compatible
	Bromocriptine	Contraindicated

The migraineur who is breast-feeding should avoid bromocriptine, ergotamine, and lithium, and use triptans, benzodiazepines, antidepressants, and neuroleptics cautiously. Acetaminophen (paracetamol) is compatible with breast-feeding and is preferred to aspirin (Tables 16.15–16.17). Moderate caffeine use is compatible with breast-feeding. However, accumulation may occur in infants whose mothers use excessive amounts. Opioid use is compatible with breast-feeding. Phenobarbital has caused sedation in some nursing infants, and it should be given to nursing mothers with caution.

References

1. Silberstein SD. Migraine and pregnancy. Neurol Clin 1997; 15: 209–31.
2. Silberstein SD, Saper JR, Freitag F. Migraine: diagnosis and treatment. In: Silberstein SD, Lipton RB, Dalessio DJ, eds. Wolff's Headache and Other Head Pain. 7th edn. New York: Oxford University Press, 2001: 121–237.
3. Silberstein SD. Evaluation and emergency treatment of headache. Headache 1992; 32: 396–407.
4. Fox MV, Harms RW, Davis DH. Selected neurologic complications of pregnancy. Mayo Clin Proc 1990; 65: 1595–618.
5. Hainline B. Headache. Headache 1994; 12: 443–60.
6. Schwartz RB. Neurodiagnostic imaging of the pregnant patient. In: Devinsky O, Feldmann E, Hainline B, eds. Neurologic Complications of Pregnancy. New York: Raven Press, 1994: 243–8.
7. Chancellor MD, Wroe SJ. Migraine occurring for the first time in pregnancy. Headache 1990; 30: 224–7.
8. Stein GS. Headaches in the first postpartum week and their relationship to migraine. Headache 1981; 21: 201–5.
9. Wright GD, Patel MK. Focal migraine and pregnancy. Br Med J 1986; 293: 1557–8.
10. Lance JW, Anthony M. Some clinical aspects of migraine. Arch Neurol 1966; 15: 356–61.
11. Bousser MG, Ratinahirana H, Darbois X. Migraine and pregnancy: a prospective study in 703 women after delivery. Neurology 1990; 40: 437 (Abstract).
12. Granella F, Sances G, Zanferrari C et al. Migraine without aura and reproductive life events: a clinical epidemiologic study in 1300 women. Headache 1993; 33: 385–9.
13. Rasmussen BK. Migraine and tension-type headache in a general population: precipitating factors, female hormones, sleep pattern, and relation to lifestyle. Pain 1993; 53: 65–72.
14. Chen TC, Leviton A. Headache recurrence in pregnant women with migraine.

Headache 1994; 34: 107–10.

15. Maggioni F, Alessi C, Maggino T et al. Primary headaches and pregnancy. Cephalalgia 1995; 15: 54 (Abstract).

16. Wainscott G, Volans GN. The outcome of pregnancy in women suffering from migraine. Postgrad Med J 1978; 54: 98-102.

17. Olesen C, Steffensen FH, Sorensen HT et al. Pregnancy outcome following prescription for sumatriptan. Headache 1999; 40: 20–4.

18. MacArthur C, Lewis M, Knox EG. Health after childbirth. Brit J Obstet Gyn 1991; 98: 1193–204.

19. Ponder TM. Differential diagnosis of postdural puncture headache in the parturient. Clin Forum Nurse Anesthetists 1999; 10: 145–54.

20. Ravindran RS, Zandstra GC, Viegas OJ. Postpartum headache following regional analgesia: a symptom of cerebral venous thrombosis. Can J Anesth 1989; 36: 705–7.

21. Cohen JE, Godes J, Morales B. Postpartum bilateral subdural hematomas following spinal anesthesia: a case report. Surg Neurol 1997; 47: 6–8.

22. Eerola M, Kaukinen L, Kaukinen S. Fatal brain lesion following spinal anesthesia. Acta Anesthesiol Scand 1981; 25: 115–16.

23. Jonsson LO, Einarsson P, Olsson GL. Subdural hematoma and spinal anesthesia. Anesthesia 1983; 38: 144–64.

24. Pavlin DJ, McDonald JS, Child B et al. Acute subdural hematoma: an unusual sequela to lumbar puncture. Anesthesiology 1979; 51: 338–40.

25. Edelman JD, Wingard DW. Subdural hematomas after lumbar dural puncture. Anesthesiol 1980; 52: 166–7.

26. Bader AM. Neurologic and neuromuscular disease. In: Chestnut DH, ed. Obstetric anesthesia, principles and practice. St. Louis: Mosby Year Book, 1994: 920–41.

27. Pitkin RM. Drug treatment of the pregnant woman: the state of the art. Proceedings from the Food and Drug Administration Conference on Regulated Products and Pregnant Women. Virginia, November, 1995.

28. Blake DA, Niebyl JR. Requirements and limitations in reproductive and teratogenic risk assessment. In: Niebyl JR, ed. Drug Use in Pregnancy. 2nd edn. Philadelphia: Lea & Febiger, 1988: 1–9.

29. Briggs GG, Freeman RK, Yaffe SJ. Drugs in Pregnancy and Lactation. 5th edn. Baltimore: Williams & Wilkins, 1994.

30. Niebyl JR. Teratology and drugs in pregnancy and lactation. In: Winters R, ed. Danforth's Obstetrics and Gynecology. 6th edn. New York: Lippincott, 1990.

31. Rayburn WF, Lavin JP. Drug prescribing for chronic medical disorders during pregnancy: an overview. Am J Obstet Gynecol 1986; 155: 565–9.

32. Cavagnaro JA. Traditional reproductive toxicology studies and their predictive value. Food and Drug Administration Conference on regulated products and pregnant women. November 7–8, 1994.

33. Silberstein SD. Headaches, pregnancy and lactation. In: Yankowitz J, Niebyl JR, eds. Drug therapy in pregnancy. 3rd edn. Philadelphia: Lippincott Williams and Wilkins, 2001: 231–46.

34. Macklin R. Ethical conflicts and practical realities. Proceedings from the Food and Drug Administration Conference on regulated products and pregnant women. November 7–8, 1994.

35. Gilstrap LC III, Little BB, eds. Drugs and Pregnancy. New York: Elsevier, 1992: 23–9.

36. Heinonen OP, Sloan S, Shapiro S. Birth defects and drugs in pregnancy. Littleton: Publishing Sciences Group, 1977.

37. Metcalfe J, Stock MK, Barron DH. Maternal physiology during gestation. In: Knobel E, Neill J, eds. The Physiology of Reproduction. New York: Raven Press, 1988: 2145–74.

38. Cunningham FG, MacDonald PC, Leveno KJ et al. Maternal adaptations to pregnancy. In: Cunningham FG, MacDonald PC, Leveno KJ, Gant NF, Gilstrap LC, eds. Williams Obstetrics. 19th edn. Connecticut: Appleton and Lange, 1993: 209–46.

39. Bailey RR, Rolleston GL. Kidney length and ureteric dilatation in the puerperium. Br J Obstet Gynecol 1971; 78: 55–61.

40. Chesley LC. Renal function during pregnancy. In: Carey HM, ed. Modern trends in human reproductive physiology. London: Butterworth, 1963.

41. Dunlop W. Serial changes in renal haemodynamics during normal human pregnancy. Br J Obstet Gynecol 1981;
88: 1–9.

42. Chaudhuri G. Pharmacokinetics in pregnancy. Proceedings of the Food and Drug Administration Conference on regulated products and pregnant woman. November 7–8, 1994.

43. Medical Economics Company. Physicians' Desk Reference. 55th edn. 2001.

44. Friedman JM, Polifka JE. Teratogenic effects of drugs: a resource for clinicians (TERIS). Baltimore: Johns Hopkins University Press, 1994.

45. Friedman JM, Little BB, Brent RL et al. Potential human teratogenicity of frequently prescribed drugs. Obstet Gynecol 1990; 75: 594–9.

46. Daly LE, Kirke PN, Molloy A et al. Folate levels and neural tube defects: implications for prevention. JAMA 1995; 274: 1698–702.

47. Ogawa Y, Kaneko S, Otani K, Fukushima Y. Serum folic acid levels in epileptic mothers and their relationship to congenital malformations. Epilepsy Res 1991; 8: 75–8.

48. Jordan RL, Wilson JG, Shumacher HJ. Embryotoxicity of the folate antagonist methotrexate in rats and rabbits. Teratology 1977; 15: 73–80.

49. Dansky LV, Andermann E, Rosenblatt D et al. Anticonvulsants, folate levels, and pregnancy outcome: a prospective study. Ann Neurol 1987; 21: 176–82.

50. Reynolds EH. Anticonvulsants, folic acid and epilepsy. Lancet 1973; 1: 1376–8.

51. Wegner C, Nau H. Alteration of embryonic folate metabolism by valproic acid during organogenesis: implications for mechanism of teratogenesis. Neurology 1992; 42: 17–24.

52. Berg MG, Stumbo PJ, Chenard CA et al. Folic acid improves phenytoin pharmacokinetics. J Am Diet Assoc 1995; 95: 352–6.

53. Reiff-Eldridge R, Heffner CR, Ephross SA et al. Monitoring pregnancy outcomes after prenatal drug exposure through prospective pregnancy registries: a pharmaceutical company commitment. Am J Obstet Gynecol 2000; 182: 159–63.

54. Shepard TH. Catalog of teratogenic agents. 8th edn. Baltimore: Johns Hopkins University Press, 1973.

55. American Academy of Pediatrics Committee on Drugs. The transfer of drugs and other chemicals into human milk. Pediatrics 1994; 93: 137–50.

chapter 17

Geriatric headache

Introduction

Age is an important factor in the diagnosis and treatment of headache disorders. Headache prevalence varies with age.[1] Although less common in the elderly, headache is still a significant problem, with 10% of women and 5% of men reporting severe headaches at the age of 70 years.[2,3] Etiology also varies with age. The incidence of primary headache disorders declines dramatically while the incidence of secondary headache disorders (such as mass lesions and temporal arteritis) increases with advancing age. Some secondary headache disorders, such as giant cell arteritis (GCA; temporal arteritis), occur almost exclusively in the elderly (Table 17.1).[4] At least one primary headache disorder, the hypnic headache syndrome, is much more common in the elderly. Older patients are also more likely to have comorbid medical illness.[5]

Frequent headache was found in 11% of elderly women and 5% of elderly men who participated in a health screening program.[6,7] These patients commonly had other medical disorders.[8] Table 17.2 summarizes the major causes of headaches that begin late in life, divided into secondary and primary headache disorders. Headaches that begin after the age of 65 years are more likely to be due to serious conditions.[1,7] Systemic illnesses or medications that produce headache become increasingly common with advancing age. Mass lesions and GCA have potentially devastating, but often avoidable, consequences. For these reasons, more testing is indicated when older patients present with headache, particularly if the headaches are atypical, of recent onset, or associated with neurologic findings. A full evaluation is indicated to identify or exclude secondary headaches.[9]

The initial evaluation of an elderly patient with a new-onset headache should be directed toward identifying or excluding secondary headaches. A new-onset headache or the onset of a new type of headache in a patient who is over 50 years of age requires neuroimaging (computed tomography (CT) or magnetic resonance imaging (MRI)) and an erythrocyte sedimentation rate (ESR) as part of the initial work-up to identify or rule out structural lesions and GCA. A careful review of systemic illness and medications that may cause headache and additional work-up may be necessary to identify potential causes of secondary headache. After secondary causes of headache have been excluded, the primary headache disorder should be identified and treated. Although the common primary headache disorders (migraine, cluster headache, and tension-type headache (TTH)) usually begin earlier in life, their prevalence in the elderly is significant and they may have unusual presentations. For example, migraine aura without headache is common (it is called late-life migraine accompaniments).

In this chapter, we will discuss the major secondary headache disorders as they present in later life. The discussion of primary headache disorders will emphasize the diagnostic and treatment dilemmas encountered in elderly patients.

● **Table 17.1** Headache prevalence as a function of age

Decrease in prevalence	Equally common	Increase in prevalence	Typically only in the elderly
Migraine	?Cluster headache	Intracranial lesions	Giant cell arteritis
Tension-type headache		Medication-induced (except rebound)	Hypnic headache
		'Metabolic headache' anemia hypoxia hypercalcemia hyponatremia chronic renal failure	Headache of Parkinson's disease
		Cerebrovascular disease	

Modified from ref. 7.

● **Table 17.2** Common causes of headache beginning in late life

Secondary headache disorders	Primary headache disorders
Mass lesions	Migraine
Giant cell arteritis	Tension-type headache
Medication-related headaches	Cluster headache
Trigeminal neuralgia	Hypnic headache
Postherpetic neuralgia	
Systemic disease	
Disease of the cranium, neck, eyes, ears and nose	
Cerebrovascular disease	
Parkinson's disease	

Secondary headache disorders in the elderly

Mass lesions

Brain tumors (primary and metastatic) and subdural hematomas (SDH) occur with increased frequency in the elderly.[10,11] In the International Headache Society (IHS) criteria, mass lesions are included in the category called 'headache associated with nonvascular intracranial disorders'. The most frequent primary brain tumors are gliomas, meningiomas (especially common in elderly women) (Figure 17.1), and pituitary adenomas.[10,11] The most frequent metastatic tumors are lung and breast cancer, followed by malignant melanomas and carcinomas of the kidney and gastrointestinal tracts.[10]

Pain patterns resulting from primary and metastatic tumors vary because pain is generated by diverse mechanisms and depends upon the tumor location and the pattern of radiation. The headache profile most often resembles that of TTH; the 'brain tumor triad' of severe pain, early morning awakening, and nausea occurs in only 17% of all patients with brain tumors.[12] Headaches can antedate the development of focal neurologic features; thus, early detection requires neuroimaging procedures in elderly patients with new-onset headaches.

Chronic SDHs, grouped by the IHS with 'headaches associated with vascular disorders',[9] often act as mass lesions and may present with headache symptoms similar

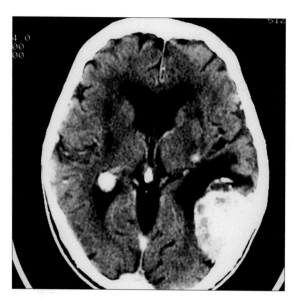

● *Figure 17.1* *CT of the brain illustrates meningioma arising in the left parietal region of an elderly woman. Because meningiomas arise from the dura mater, the tumors typically have a dural base as illustrated here.*

to those of brain tumors. The elderly are at greater risk for SDHs, owing, in part, to brain atrophy; this decreases the support of bridging veins, increasing the risk for venous tears with minor head injury. Because SDHs are extra-axial (outside the brain parenchyma), they are less likely to produce early neurologic deficits. Even large lesions may produce headache with no focal neurologic dysfunction. Some patients present with headache and confusion or a fluctuating level of consciousness. SDH may present long after trauma. Unfortunately, the history of an antecedent head injury is often absent, sometimes because the patient has forgotten the incident.

Giant cell arteritis

GCA is a systemic vasculitis that primarily affects medium-sized arteries. Signs and symptoms include headache, visual loss, fatigue, and myalgias. Rare before the age of 50 years, the incidence of GCA increases dramatically after the age of 50 years, occurring in 10 per 100 000 population per year, with women affected three times more often than men.[4,13,14] Salvarani et al[15] estimated the age-adjusted incidence for individuals aged 50 years or older to be 24.2 per 100 000 women and 8.2 per 100 000 men. In another report, incidence estimates increased by age and were 200 per 100 000 individuals aged 50 years and older, and 1100 per 100 000 individuals aged 85 years and older.[16] In a Swedish population study, the average annual incidence of GCA among individuals older than 50 years was 22.2 per 100 000 and the incidence increased with age.[17] In fact, the higher prevalence of GCA (1.5%) in one large autopsy series suggests that the disorder may be either unrecognized or clinically occult in many cases.[18]

GCA should be considered in any elderly patient who has new-onset headaches or a substantial change in headache pattern. Headache, the most frequent symptom, is prominent in 70–90% of patients, and is the initial symptom in a third.[19] The pain can be intermittent or constant; it is characteristically throbbing, continuous, and located over the temples or (less commonly) the occipital area. Often there is associated scalp tenderness, especially over inflamed arteries. As a consequence, local pressure, such as wearing a hat or resting the head on a pillow, may exacerbate the pain (Table 17.3).[20,21]

GCA produces a broad range of signs and symptoms. Polymyalgia rheumatica, whose symptoms include muscle pain and joint stiffness, occurs in 50% of patients with GCA.[19,20] Other common symptoms include fever, weight loss, night sweats, jaw (masseter) claudication (principally with chewing), amaurosis fugax (which may be bilateral in half of patients), permanent blindness (often without

Table 17.3 *Symptoms and signs in giant cell arteritis*

Headache

Fatigue

Myalgia

Arthralgia

Depressed mood

Jaw claudication

Features of the temporal artery
- tenderness
- induration
- diminished or absent pulse

warning) or partial visual loss (often due to anterior ischemic optic atrophy).[22] GCA should be included in the differential diagnosis of amaurosis fugax.[23] Dysphoric mood, anorexia, and weight loss are common in GCA and may lead to the primary diagnosis of depression. Patients or physicians may mistakenly relate the onset of symptoms to a coincidental painful life event.

Visual loss is the most feared complication of GCA, occurring in 7–60% of untreated patients, with a pooled incidence of 36% in 819 cases.[24] Visual loss is usually sudden and irreversible; however, gradual visual loss and recovery of vision with treatment have been reported.[25–29] Visual loss is usually due to ischemic optic neuropathy secondary to arteritis of the short posterior ciliary arteries (the blood vessels that supply the anterior optic nerve).[21,25,26,30,31] Visual loss may also occur secondary to posterior ischemic optic neuropathy, central retinal artery occlusion or bilateral occipital lobe infarction.[21,24,27,30,31] In untreated cases, monocular visual loss may be followed by loss of vision in the other eye.[10,25]

Other ischemic symptoms can occur. Jaw (or masseter) claudication is characterized by the gradual onset of pain resulting from chewing for several minutes.[24] This gradual onset contrasts with the rapid onset of lancinating pain with chewing that characterizes trigeminal neuralgia. Temporomandibular joint dysfunction is typified by the rapid onset of a dull ache. Ischemia of the extraocular muscles and/or the oculomotor nerves may produce diplopia owing to ocular motor paresis. Coronary, mesenteric, hepatic, and renal artery ischemia have also been reported. Aortic arch syndrome may occur with rupture.[32]

Stroke and transient ischemic attack (TIA) can occur in GCA. Stroke is usually associated with extracranial thrombus formation at sites of inflammation in the internal carotid or vertebral arteries, leading to distal embolization or propagation of extracranial clot. Intracranial vasculitis is

rare, perhaps because cerebral arteries lose their internal elastic lamina (which is the site of pathology) after they pass through the dura mater.[33]

The history and physical examination may support the diagnosis of GCA. The relationship between specific clinical features and the likelihood of a positive biopsy has been extensively studied. One way of expressing the likelihood of GCA is a statistic termed the likelihood ratio (LR). For example, jaw claudication is associated with a LR of 4.2 for a positive biopsy. This means that patients with jaw claudication are 4.2 times more likely to have a positive biopsy than those who do not have jaw claudication. Diplopia substantially increases the probability of positive biopsy results (LR = 3.4). No single sign or symptom is absolutely required for the diagnosis of GCA. As a consequence, clinical suspicion should be driven more by the features that are present than by the features that are absent.[34] Induration and tenderness of the temporal or occipital scalp arteries are the most common signs of GCA (Figure 17.2). The visual fields and visual acuity should be carefully assessed. In patients without visual loss, the funduscopic examination is often normal. In acute anterior ischemic optic neuropathy, optic disc edema and visual loss may occur.[24,30] Altitudinal defects and central scotomas breaking into the periphery are frequent. In posterior ischemic optic neuropathy, the normal initial funduscopic examination is replaced over weeks by optic disc pallor.[31] Diplopia is rare, and, when present, is usually due to ischemia of the extraocular muscle, the cranial nerves, or both. True cranial nerve palsy is rare. Arterial bruits or diminished pulses are present in one-third of patients. Synovitis makes the diagnosis less likely, while

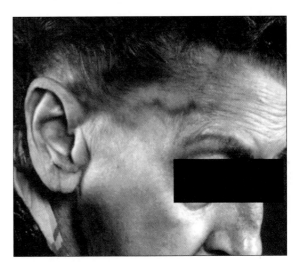

Figure 17.2 *Prominent temporal artery in a patient with giant cell arteritis. (Reproduced from ref. 90, with permission.)*

beaded, prominent, enlarged, and tender temporal arteries each increase the likelihood of positive biopsy results. Beaded, prominent, or enlarged arteries confer the highest positive LRs of any clinical or laboratory feature and substantially increase the probability that a patient with suspected GCA will have positive biopsy results. These findings increase the chance of having GCA, but vary in sensitivity, from 16% (beaded temporal artery) to 65% (any temporal artery abnormality).[34]

The most consistent laboratory abnormality is an elevation of the Westergren ESR. In one series, 41% of patients had a value > 100 mm/h and 89% had a value > 50 mm/h. Elevated C-reactive protein, mild liver function abnormalities, and mild anemia are also common. GCA occasionally is diagnosed despite a normal ESR. In some cases, a normal ESR at presentation is followed by an elevated ESR as the disease progresses.[25,28,35] The ESR may be reduced in patients who are taking aspirin, nonsteroidal anti-inflammatory drugs (NSAIDs), or systemic steroids, leading to a false-negative test. ESR test results alter the likelihood of positive biopsy results. A normal ESR (LR = 0.2) or an ESR of less than 50 mm/h (LR = 0.35) make positive biopsy results unlikely, but setting the ESR threshold at 100 mm/h is less efficient, as patients with an ESR less than 100 mm/h have an LR (0.8) that only slightly lowers the likelihood of disease. Among patients who are clinically suspected of disease, those with an ESR greater than 100 mm/h have an increased likelihood of biopsy-proven GCA (LR = 1.9).[34]

Temporal artery biopsy is the diagnostic gold standard and should be performed within 48 hours of initiating steroid treatment, if possible. Diagnostic yield on biopsy can be optimized by selecting a clinically symptomatic arterial segment based on tenderness, induration, or a diminished pulse. If the biopsy appears negative (and this can occur, because the disease can be patchy), multiple sections should be examined to improve yield. GCA is characterized pathologically by skip lesions; affected and unaffected segments may be adjacent. If the biopsy is negative and the index of suspicion remains high, a second contralateral temporal artery biopsy is sometimes diagnostic.[32]

In patients who have the characteristic GCA profile and an elevated ESR, treatment should be initiated promptly while awaiting the results of the temporal artery biopsy (Figure 17.3). A short course of steroids prior to biopsy should not produce false-negative results. The major goal of treatment is to prevent sudden, irreversible visual loss. Initial doses of prednisone range from 60 to 80 mg daily, and some experts give intravenous corticosteroids as the first dose. If a patient presents with an acute neurologic

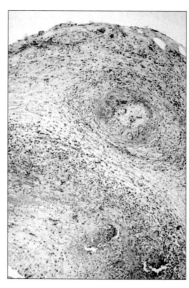

● *Figure 17.3*
Micrograph of a temporal artery biopsy in a patient with giant cell arteritis. (Reproduced from ref. 116, with permission.)

syndrome or a rapidly worsening neurologic status, whether it be visual loss, mononeuritis multiplex, or acute encephalopathy, treatment may begin empirically with an intravenous pulse over several days (1000 mg methylprednisolone per day), or with a very high oral dose of steroids (up to 120 mg prednisone).[19] The headache and systemic symptoms typically remit shortly after treatment is started. After several weeks of therapy, the prednisone dose can be gradually reduced. The patient should take a maintenance dose that controls symptoms for 6 months to 1 year. Steroids commonly produce minor side-effects and may produce major side-effects. Steroid therapy is often complicated by gastrointestinal side-effects, osteoporosis, steroid myopathy, and weight gain, among other ill-effects.

Trials of other immunosuppressant drugs, including azathioprine,[36] methotrexate,[37] cyclophosphamide,[38] and dapsone,[39] have been attempted for their steroid-sparing effects. Limited experience suggests that cyclophosphamide may be the most consistently effective immunosuppressant other than corticosteroids,[38–40] and may permit more rapid steroid tapering when instituted following a relapse.

Medication and headache

Medications are an important cause of headache in the elderly (Table 17.4). Drugs may initiate a new type of headache or exacerbate a preexisting headache disorder.[41] Because a drug is associated with a headache does not prove that it has a causal role for a particular patient, nor does it preclude the need to evaluate other causes. The IHS groups medication-overuse headaches under the rubric 'headaches associated with substances or their withdrawal'.[9] Drugs may initiate a new type of headache or exacerbate a preexisting headache disorder.[41] In addition, medication withdrawal headaches may occur. Preexisting headaches triggered by medication are properly classified as primary, not secondary, headache disorders.[9]

When medications trigger a preexisting headache disorder, the headaches that are provoked are usually similar to the preexisting headaches. Perhaps the most important pharmacologic triggers of headaches are alcohol and nitrate compounds, but antihypertensives are also common culprits in this age group. Nitroglycerin can induce both migraine and cluster attacks. Hormonal replacement therapy and food additives, such as monosodium glutamate, aspartate, caffeine, and tyramine, may all increase headache frequency.[42–46]

Medication overuse headaches (rebound headaches), which are very common in headache subspecialty practices, are still common in the elderly.[47,48] The typical patient with chronic (transformed) migraine associated with medication overuse has a prior history of episodic migraine. Over the years, medication use and headache frequency increase, while the severity of the pain and associated features (e.g. nausea or photophobia) decrease. Finally, nearly continuous headaches, which may be without prominent migrainous features, and superimposed interval headaches with typical migrainous features may occur. Medication that was initially administered as a headache treatment may become a cause of headache. The drugs that cause rebound include opioids, analgesics, caffeine, barbiturate-containing products, ergotamine, and triptans (Table 17.4).

Trigeminal neuralgia

Trigeminal neuralgia is the most common neuralgic syndrome in the elderly, with a peak incidence of 155 cases per million and a female : male ratio of 3 : 2 (Table 17.5).[49] Trigeminal neuralgia is typically unilateral, but it can be bilateral in 4% of patients.[50] It is characterized by brief paroxysms of unilateral pain, similar to a spasm or an electric shock, in the distribution of one or more divisions of the trigeminal nerve. The mandibular or maxillary branches of the nerve are most frequently involved. The pain may be provoked by stimulation of specific parts of the face or by stimuli, such as washing, shaving, talking, or brushing the teeth. The pain may precipitate facial muscle spasms, which resulted in the condition's earlier name, tic douloureux. Between paroxysms, a sustained, deep, dull ache may be present.[51]

Pretrigeminal neuralgia, is a dull, continuous, aching-type pain in the jaw. It may be provoked by pressure about the face or mouth and may evolve into true trigeminal neuralgia. These nonspecific clinical features may lead to dental evaluation and procedures. Hence, dental procedures may be a response to pretrigeminal neuralgia rather than a cause of trigeminal neuralgia.[52]

The etiology of trigeminal neuralgia varies with age (Table 17.6). When trigeminal neuralgia begins in the twenties and thirties, causes include demyelinating disease (multiple sclerosis), compression of the trigeminal nerve root at its exit foramen (e.g. myeloma or metastatic carcinoma of the sphenoid bone), and other mass lesions, such as meningiomas, acoustic neuromas, trigeminal neuromas, cholesteatomas, chordomas, aneurysms (especially of the basilar artery), and other vascular abnormalities.

In the elderly, trigeminal neuralgia most often results

● **Table 17.4** Selected medications reported to cause headaches

Amantadine	Monoamine oxidase inhibitors
Calcium-channel blockers	Nonsteroidal antiinflammatory agents
Caffeine	
Cimetidine	Nitrates
Corticosteroids	Nicotinic acid
Cyclophosphamide	Phenothiazines
Dipyridamole	Ranitidine
Estrogens	Sympathomimetic agents
Ethanol	Tamoxifen
Hydralazine	Theophyllines (thioxanthines)
Indomethacin (Indometacin)	Tetracyclines
L-Dopa	Trimethoprim

● **Table 17.5** Idiopathic trigeminal neuralgia[9]

Diagnostic criteria
A Paroxysmal attacks of facial or frontal pain which last a few seconds to less than 2 minutes.
B Pain has at least 4 of the following characteristics:
1 Distribution along one or more divisions of the trigeminal nerve.
2 Sudden, intense, sharp, superficial, stabbing, or burning in quality.
3 Pain intensity severe.
4 Precipitation from trigger areas, or by certain daily activities such as eating, talking, washing the face or cleaning the teeth.
5 Between paroxysms the patient is entirely asymptomatic.
C No neurologic deficit.
D Attacks are stereotyped in the individual patient.
E Exclusion of other causes of facial pain by history, physical examination, and special investigations.

Table 17.6 *Causes of trigeminal neuralgia*

A Decreased facial sensation
- Intracranial aneurysms
- Giant cell arteritis
- Intracranial tumors
- Dental mandibular malignancy
- Cranial malignancy

B Normal facial sensation
- Idiopathic trigeminal neuralgia (due to vascular compression)
- Multiple sclerosis
- Dental pathology
- Dental procedures

from neurovascular compression of the trigeminal nerve owing to abnormal arterial loops near the trigeminal nerve root entry zone. Vascular compression leads to demyelination and aberrant neuronal activity, which may produce sensitization in the trigeminal nucleus caudalis.[53] Other causes of trigeminal neuralgia in the elderly are the same as in young adults, as outlined above.

The diagnosis of trigeminal neuralgia is established by its typical clinical features. The physical examination is normal except for positive trigger points. Diagnostic studies are generally normal. Impaired sensation in the distribution of the Vth nerve suggests a structural, demyelinating, or compressive trigeminal nerve lesion (Table 17.6). The initial evaluation should include MRI, with special attention to the region of the cerebellopontine angle and the exit foramen of the trigeminal nerve. Majoie et al[54] assessed the diagnostic yield of MRI in patients who had symptoms

and signs related to the trigeminal nerve. A normal examination and trigeminal neuralgia symptoms alone were highly correlated with a negative MRI study. Impaired sensation, subjective feelings of facial numbness, other positive neurologic signs and symptoms, progression of symptoms and signs, and symptoms that had been present for less than 1 year correlated with an abnormal MRI. Trigeminal evoked potentials may also be a valuable diagnostic aid in the search for underlying compressive lesions of the trigeminal nerve. Sundaram et al[55] demonstrated abnormal trigeminal evoked potentials in all patients with trigeminal neuralgia resulting from known intracranial mass lesions, suggesting that trigeminal evoked potentials should be considered in the normal work-up of patients who have trigeminal neuralgia and negative MR imaging. If the evoked potential responses are abnormal, then nerve compression is still the most likely cause of the patient's trigeminal neuralgia symptoms.

Medical therapy is initiated in the absence of structural disease (Table 17.7). Carbamazepine is one of the best drugs for the tic of trigeminal neuralgia and is the first-line agent used by most physicians. To avoid neurotoxicity, carbamazepine should be started at a low dose (100 mg one to two times a day). The dose can be increased by 100–200 mg every 3 days until pain relief is achieved. The usual maintenance dose is between 400 and 800 mg a day; most patients remain on less than 1200 mg a day, although some need a dose of 1500 mg a day or more. Carbamazepine is highly effective. It delivers pain relief in up to 80% of individuals, both initially and short-term. Over time, however, fewer responders continue to have sustained relief. Phenytoin was the first effective drug for trigeminal neuralgia but is now a second- or third-line agent. The starting dose of phenytoin is 200 mg a day. The

Table 17.7 *Drug treatment of trigeminal neuralgia*

Drug	Bioavailability (%)	Time to maximum concentration (h)	Half-life (h)	Time to steady-state concentration (days)*	Therapeutic 'target' range (mmol/l)
Baclofen	–	3–8	3–4	1	–
Carbamazepine	>70	2–8	11–27	5	24–43
Clonazepam	100	1–2	24–48	12	30–270
Lamotrigine	100	2–3	18–30	8	4–16
Oxcarbazepine	100	1–2	14–26	7	5–110
Phenytoin	98	4–8	15–20	14	20–80
Valproic acid	99	1–4	6–17	5	200–700

Note: modified from Ref. 61.

usual target dose is between 300 and 500 mg a day given in three divided doses. Phenytoin, in its parenteral form, can be utilized as acute therapy for trigeminal neuralgia in the Emergency Department. Baclofen is a GABA analog that can be used alone or in combination with phenytoin or carbamazepine. As monotherapy, baclofen is started at 5–10 mg three times a day. The dose can be increased by 5–10 mg every other day until pain is relieved. The normal maintenance dose is between 50 and 60 mg a day in four to six divided doses. When baclofen is combined with other medication, the dosage of each drug needed for pain relief is often lower than what was needed as monotherapy.

Clonazepam was found to be effective in 65% of individuals with trigeminal neuralgia.[56] Clonazepam should be started at an initial dose of 0.5 mg three times a day and increased by 0.5 mg every 3–5 days until pain relief is obtained. The normal therapeutic dosing range is between 1.5 and 8 mg a day.

Valproic acid was studied by Peiris et al[57] in an open label study using 600–1200 mg a day. Thirteen of 20 patients had a good response. Four responders required combination therapy to achieve pain relief. The initial dose of valproic acid is 250–500 mg a day, increasing by 125–250 mg a week, up to 1500 mg a day, or higher if tolerated.

Lamotrigine, a sodium channel modulator, is a new oral agent for trigeminal neuralgia. Lamotrigine should be started at 25 mg a day and the dose increased by 25 mg every third day, up to 400 mg a day. Individuals respond between 150–400 mg a day.

Gabapentin is anecdotally effective for trigeminal neuralgia.[58] Gabapentin is started at 300 mg a day and increased by 300 mg every other day until pain relief is achieved. Most limit the dose to 4000 to 5000 mg a day.

Oxcarbazepine, a keto derivative of carbamazepine, has obtained US Food and Drug Administration (FDA) approval for the treatment of epilepsy. It is probably equal or superior to carbamazepine in the treatment of trigeminal neuralgia. Oxcarbazepine should be started at a dose of 150–300 mg and increased every third day in 150–300 mg increments until there is pain relief (the total dose needed is usually less than 1200 mg a day). Oxcarbazepine's adverse event profile is better than carbamazepine's.

Topiramate, a novel antiepileptic, was shown to be successful in treating refractory trigeminal neuralgia in multiple sclerosis patients. In an open-label, consecutive case series, five patients became completely pain-free on topiramate. Four patients had pain relief with 200 mg, while a single patient needed 300 mg.[59]

Rules for Medical Therapy in Trigeminal Neuralgia (adapted from Rozen et al[60])

1. Do not overtreat.
2. Chronic anticonvulsant therapy can cause cognitive impairment.
3. Many trigeminal neuralgia patients become less responsive to medication with time.
4. Minimize medication side-effects by carefully titrating doses throughout the day.
5. Monotherapy is preferable, but polypharmacy is acceptable.
6. Oxcarbazepine, lamotrigine, and gabapentin may be more effective and better tolerated than carbamazepine and phenytoin.

If medication fails to control symptoms adequately, ablative procedures should be considered. Alcohol or glycerol injections may be used, with more proximal injections producing better long-term results. Gasserian ganglion injections have a 5-year recurrence rate of 41–86%. Retrogasserian glycerol injections can produce mild facial numbness, but painful dysesthesia (impairment of any sense, especially touch) is rare and anesthesia dolorosa (pain in an area or region that is anesthetized) is absent. Mean recurrence time varies from 6 to 47 months. Radiofrequency and percutaneous bulbar gangliolysis provides relief in 82–100% of patients, with a recurrence rate of 9–28%. Major complications are rare: loss of corneal reflex occurs in 70% of patients; masseteric weakness occurs in approximately half of patients, but this improves over a 3–6-month period.[61] Minor paresthesias (abnormal sensation, i.e. burning, prickling) occur in about 10% of patients, but anesthesia dolorosa is rare.

The Janetta procedure (microvascular decompression), performed via an occipital craniotomy, removes any aberrant blood vessels from the trigeminal nerve root. Long-term benefit is reported in over 80% of patients, with recurrence rates of 1–6%. Surgical mortality is 1% and serious morbidity 7%. Gamma knife radiosurgery, a form of stereotactic radiosurgery, is one of the newest therapeutic techniques for trigeminal neuralgia. The normal radiation dose received is 70–80 Gy. Young et al[62] examined 51 patients after gamma knife radiosurgery; 74.5% were completely pain-free after the procedure. A 50–90% decrease in facial pain was seen in another 13.7% of patients, while in 11.1% the procedure failed. A disadvantage of gamma knife radiosurgery is that onset to pain relief may be slow. There is also no long-term follow-up of gamma knife radiosurgery in trigeminal neuralgia. Gamma knife surgery may have a higher complication rate than has been appreciated previously owing to delayed onset and underreporting.[63] We start with less invasive procedures, such as percutaneous glycerol injection and radiofrequency rhizotomy, and reserve microvascular decompression for refractory patients.[61]

Glossopharyngeal neuralgia

Glossopharyngeal neuralgia (Table 17.8) is much less common than trigeminal neuralgia. Glossopharyngeal neuralgia and trigeminal neuralgia occur in combined form in 10% of patients. Unilateral pain occurs in the distribution of the glossopharyngeal and vagus nerves in and around the ear, jaw, throat, tongue, or larynx. Radiation from the oropharynx to the ear is common. Paroxysms of jabbing or electric pain last for about 1 minute and may be accompanied by deep, continuous pain between paroxysms. Patients may have as many as 30–40 attacks a day and may be awakened from sleep by the attacks.[64]

Chewing, talking, yawning, coughing, or swallowing cold liquids may trigger paroxysms of pain. Stimulation of the external auditory canal and postauricular area may also provoke pain. In approximately 2% of cases, syncope (secondary to bradycardia or asystole) and seizures (from cerebral ischemia) have occurred. Atropine prevents syncope, suggesting a vagal afferent mechanism.[65]

The diagnosis of glossopharyngeal neuralgia is based on history. The neurologic examination is usually normal. Other disorders are ruled out by history, physical examination, and diagnostic testing. The assumed cause of glossopharyngeal neuralgia is nerve compression from aberrant blood vessels. Symptomatic causes of a glossopharyngeal neuralgia-like syndrome include cerebellopontine angle tumor, nasopharyngeal carcinoma, carotid aneurysm, peritonsillar abscess, and compression from an osteophytic stylohyoid ligament lateral to the glossopharyngeal nerve.[66]

The best diagnostic test is anesthetization of the tonsil and pharynx, which can temporarily terminate a painful paroxysm and confirm the diagnosis. Pharmacotherapy is identical to the approach outlined for trigeminal neuralgia (Table 17.7). Surgical treatment involves intracranial sectioning of the glossopharyngeal nerve and the upper rootlets of the vagus nerve at the jugular foramen.[66]

Postherpetic neuralgia (Table 17.9)

Postherpetic neuralgia, a significant cause of head pain in the elderly, is defined by the presence of pain after the eruption of herpes zoster.[67] Acute herpes zoster often begins with paresthesias and pain in the affected region, followed 4 or 5 days later by a vesicular eruption. Most patients have a deep aching or burning pain, paresthesias, and dysesthesia. Some patients also report electric shock-like pains. Typical involvement in the head occurs unilaterally in the distribution of the ophthalmic or maxillary divisions of the trigeminal nerve, or at the occipitocervical junction.[67] Ophthalmic herpes may be associated with diplopia due to involvement of cranial nerves III, IV, and VI. Geniculate herpes is associated with facial palsy (cranial nerve VII). Vesicles are often seen in the external auditory canal.

Many people have persistent pain after the eruption clears. Opinions vary on how long the pain must persist before the term 'postherpetic neuralgia' is applied. Most authors favor intervals varying from 1 to 6 months. Age is a risk factor for postherpetic neuralgia; it occurs in 5% of patients with acute zoster under the age of 40 years, 50% of those in their sixties, and 75% of those in their seventies. Postherpetic neuralgia may be more common when the acute attack of zoster is intense. Other risk factors include diabetes mellitus, an ophthalmic location for the eruption, and immunological compromise.[67]

The pain of postherpetic neuralgia has three components:

- constant, deep burning and pain;
- repetitive stabs and needle-pricking sensations; and
- superficial, sharp or radiating pain or itching provoked by light touch.

● Table 17.8 *Idiopathic glossopharyngeal neuralgia*

Diagnostic criteria

A Paroxysmal attacks of facial pain which last a few seconds to less than two minutes.

B Pain has at least 4 of the following characteristics:

  1 Unilateral location

  2 Distribution within the posterior part of the tongue, tonsillar fossa, pharynx, or beneath the angle of the lower jaw, or in the ear

  3 Sudden, sharp, stabbing, or burning in quality

  4 Pain intensity severe

  5 Precipitation from trigger areas or by swallowing, chewing, talking, coughing, or yawning

C No neurologic deficit.

D Attacks are stereotyped in the individual patient.

E Other cause of pain ruled out by history, physical and special investigations.

● Table 17.9 *Chronic postherpetic neuralgia*

Diagnostic criteria

A Pain is restricted to the distribution of the affected cranial nerves or divisions thereof.

B Pain persists more than 6 months after the onset of herpetic eruption.

The prominence of each of these components varies among individuals. Sleep is often interrupted. Postherpetic neuralgia is a deafferentation pain syndrome sometimes accompanied by increased sympathetic activity. The pain typically remits, and after 3 years, 56% of patients are free of troublesome pain.[68]

Topical therapies, such as compresses of Burrow's solution, colloidal oatmeal, or calamine lotion are used to treat acute zoster. Oral glucocorticoids may speed the resolution of acute zoster pain,[69] but it is not clear if they prevent postherpetic neuralgia.[67] Antiviral agents may attenuate acute herpes zoster in immunocompromised patients. A 21-day course of acyclovir (aciclovir) may ameliorate pain in the acute phase, but it has not been proven to reduce the risk of postherpetic neuralgia.[67] Famcyclovir (famciclovir), an antiviral drug, may shorten the duration of postherpetic neuralgia. The most effective treatment of the pain of acute herpes zoster is neuroblockade, but it is uncertain if this will reduce postherpetic neuralgia.[67]

Postherpetic neuralgia should be treated as soon as the diagnosis is made. Amitriptyline is commonly used, but nortriptyline or desipramine may be preferable, since they have fewer anticholinergic side-effects. Capsaicin, a topical agent that depletes substance P, is helpful, but the burning pain that sometimes accompanies its application may limit its usefulness. Topical NSAIDs may be useful. Local anesthetic preparations have been used with some success. Peripheral and central surgical techniques are of little, if any, value.

Headaches associated with systemic disease

Headache can be a symptom of a systemic disease, some of which are more common in the elderly. The IHS groups these disorders as 'headaches associated with noncephalic infections' and 'headaches associated with metabolic diseases'.[9] Infections are the most common systemic cause of headaches. Systemic viral and bacterial infections may produce headaches that are not necessarily age-related. Lyme disease and other spirochetes can produce chronic headache, usually with associated abnormalities on neurologic examination.[70] Headache may be associated with both acute Epstein–Barr virus infection and chronic fatigue syndrome.

Other systemic diseases that can cause headaches include acute, but not chronic, hypertension, hypercalcemia, severe anemia, and both renal disease and its treatment (dialysis). Hypoxia or hypercarbia are more common in the elderly and may produce headache regardless of cause, such as obstructive sleep apnea (e.g. primary pulmonary disorders, sleep apnea or high alti-

tude). Involvement of the mediastinum during the course of pacemaker insertion or by tumor may produce pain referred to the head through the autonomic nervous system.[71,72] Angina may present with exertional headache without thoracic pain, an entity called cardiac cephalgia.[73]

Headache associated with disorders of the cranium, neck, eyes, ears, and nose

Primary disorders of the cranial bones are rare. Abnormalities of the cervical spine have been reported to produce anterior or posterior head pain, perhaps by direct involvement of the cervical nerve roots or indirect involvement of the descending tract of the trigeminal nerve. The existence of cervicogenic headache as a distinct neurologic disorder is controversial. The IHS recognizes a narrowly defined disorder termed 'headache associated with disorder of the cervical spine'.[9]

Typical clinical features of headache of cervical origin include:

- occipital or suboccipital pain, sometimes reproduced or augmented by suboccipital pressure;
- neck tenderness and muscle spasms that may produce limitation of movement, unusual postures, or pain with neck movement; and
- sensory abnormalities in the distribution of the upper cervical roots.

These headaches are usually unilateral.[9,74] On imaging, cervical spine abnormalities are similar to those found in age-matched control subjects without pain complaints. Upper cervical spine radiographic abnormalities are common in the elderly, thus, the positive predictive value of any given abnormality is low.[74] Many patients diagnosed with what has been called cervicogenic headache meet criteria for migraine or TTH. It seems clear that, in addition to the many other trigger factors for migraine, cervical spine disease may be a particularly problematic one in the elderly.

Primary open-angle glaucoma, which is the most common cause of glaucoma, is rarely painful. Miotic eye-drops, such as pilocarpine, used in its treatment may produce brow ache. Acute angle closure glaucoma is less common; acute attacks produce intense eye pain that radiates widely; it is often associated with a red eye, corneal cloudiness, and nausea. Laser iridotomy is curative. Secondary angle closure glaucoma resulting from diabetes or carotid insufficiency may produce a deep, boring, unrelenting pain associated with a red eye and poor vision.[75] Intermittent angle closure glaucoma consists of multiple, self-aborting episodes of angle closure with resultant intermittent eye pain. The typical signs and symptoms of angle closure glaucoma are often absent between episodes, making the diagnosis difficult. In chronic angle closure glaucoma, the intraocular pressure does not change rapidly, and is therefore an unlikely cause of eye and head pain on the basis of intraocular pressure alone.

Inflammation or infection can produce headache. Middle or external ear infection can usually be diagnosed on routine examination.[76] Acute sinusitis produces headache, usually associated with sinus tenderness, purulent nasal discharge, and, perhaps, fever.[77] The pattern of pain referral varies with the infected sinus. Nasopharyngeal malignancies may cause the sensation of nasal congestion and pain behind the nose. If this condition is suspected, an otolaryngologic examination is warranted.

Infection of the teeth or the mucous membranes of the mouth may cause pain in the adjacent areas of the mouth or face and can also produce pain beyond the site of disease, evoking head and facial pain.

Headaches associated with other neurologic disorders

Several other neurologic disorders, including cerebrovascular disease, postherpetic neuralgia and Parkinson's disease, may produce headache in the elderly. Cerebrovascular disease may give rise to headaches before, during, or after the onset of stroke or TIA.[9] The headaches may occur with large vessel thrombotic stroke (20–40%), embolic stroke (20–40%), lacunar infarction (18%), subarachnoid hemorrhage (> 95%), or intracerebral hemorrhage (80%). Headaches associated with stroke have been described in a series of studies.[78–80] Headache may also occur following carotid endarterectomy.[81,82]

Parkinson's disease

The association between Parkinson's disease[83] and headache is controversial. In one series, headache occurred in 41% of Parkinson's disease patients and 13% of controls. Another controlled series found no difference in headache prevalence.[84] Possible headache mechanisms include comorbid depression and muscle rigidity. In one study of early morning occipital headache in patients with Parkinson's disease, the headache failed to improve with treatment directed at muscle spasm, but it did improve with levodopa.[85] These headaches may also respond to amitriptyline.[86]

Primary headache disorders in the elderly

Migraine headache

Migraine prevalence peaks in mid-adult life, near the age of 40 years, but migraine continues to occur even in elderly patients. Migraine prevalence is 5% in women and 2% in men over the age of 70 years. However, in a recently published Italian community survey, the prevalence of migraine was 13.8% in women and 7.4% in men 65 years of age or older.[87] Migraine incidence also declines: only 2% of all migraine cases begin after the age of 65 years.[88] Thus, caution is advised when making the diagnosis of new-onset migraine in the elderly.

In one study, only one of 193 patients with headache beginning after age 65 years had migraine.[4] Cull,[89] however, collected ten patients with migraine onset after the age of 60 years, two of whom had strokes on CT. The ratio of migraine with aura to migraine without aura was reversed (86%:14%) among new-onset migraine patients over the age of 40 years. Whether this is because of referral patterns or biological factors is uncertain.

Anecdotal information and clinic-based reports suggest that headache characteristics may change with advancing age. Several patterns have been described. Migraine attacks may remit or evolve into chronic migraine, with or without medication overuse.[47,90] Migraine with aura may transform into a periodic neurologic deficit, with little or no headache pain.[91,92] This phenomenon of 'aura without headache' has been termed late-life migraine accompaniments.[91,92]

Features of late-life migraine accompaniments are listed in Table 17.10. The features most consistent with migrainous accompaniments are: scintillations or other visual displays; a slow evolution of the neurologic deficit,

---

● **Table 17.10** *Migraine accompaniments*

- Gradual appearance of focal neurologic symptoms — spread or intensification over a period of minutes.
- Positive visual symptoms characteristic of 'classic' migraine, specifically fortification spectra (scintillating scotoma), flashing lights, dazzles.
- Previous similar symptoms associated with a more severe headache.
- Serial progression from one accompaniment to another.
- The occurrence of two or more identical spells.
- A duration of 15 to 25 minutes.
- Occurrence of a 'flurry' of accompaniments.
- A generally benign course without permanent sequelae.

typically over a period of minutes; and the serial progression from one symptom to another.[91,92] Fisher stressed that it is best to regard the diagnosis as one of exclusion. The neurologic examination and neuroimaging studies are normal. Alternative diagnoses include cerebral thrombosis, embolism, TIA, carotid or vertebral dissection, subclavian steal syndrome, epilepsy, thrombocythemia, polycythemia, hyperviscosity syndrome, and lupus. Patients with late-life migraine accompaniments have normal angiograms and rarely develop permanent neurologic deficits.

Medications that older patients commonly take can exacerbate preexisting migraine or precipitate new migraine-like headaches. Common offenders include nitroglycerin compounds and estrogen replacement therapy.[93] Reducing the dose of the offending agent may ameliorate the headaches.

Acute migraine treatments that should be prescribed with caution to elderly patients include:

- Ergot alkaloids and the triptans (sumatriptan, rizatriptan, naratriptan, zolmitriptan, frovatriptan, and almotriptan), which may exacerbate preexisting hypertension, coronary artery disease, peripheral vascular disease, or cerebrovascular disease, and in some instances provoke ischemic complications, including angina, myocardial infarction, or claudication.[94–96]
- NSAIDs, which may cause more peptic ulcer disease in elderly patients than in younger ones and can potentially interact with anticoagulants, hypoglycemics, digoxin, antihypertensive agents, and diuretics.[97,98] They may cause cognitive side-effects and are associated with an increased risk of gastrointestinal bleeding.
Antiemetic agents, such as metoclopramide (metochlopramide) and chlorpromazine, which can cause extrapyramidal syndromes.[24]
- Benzodiazepines and barbiturates, which may cause excessive sedation; the long-acting benzodiazepines, in particular, may cause excessive side-effects due to slowed metabolic clearance.

Preventive treatments cause more side-effects in the elderly than in younger patients.[1,5,98,99] The distribution and excretion of many medications are altered in elderly patients, generally resulting in higher blood levels for a given dose of drug.[97,100] Elderly patients are also more sensitive to anticholinergic, orthostatic, sedative, and cardiac side-effects. For these reasons, medication should be started at a lower dose and increased slowly in the elderly.

- Tertiary amine tricyclic antidepressants (amitriptyline and doxepin), which are potent anticholinergic agents, may exacerbate glaucoma, produce visual blurring, and cause cognitive problems. Use instead agents with minimal anticholinergic and sedative side-effects, such as nortriptyline, which is a secondary amine.
- Selective serotonin reuptake inhibitors, although not as effective for migraine prophylaxis, are well tolerated by the elderly.
- Methysergide and methylergonovine may cause cardiac ischemia because they are vasoconstrictors, so they are relatively contraindicated.[98]
- Divalproex sodium, topiramate, and gabapentin have a particularly good benefit-to-side-effect profile.
- The use of unconventional therapies such as riboflavin and botulinum A toxin may be considered.

The principles of migraine treatment outlined in Chapter 6 apply to the elderly.

Nonpharmacologic treatment in the elderly, as in all patients, is attractive because it avoids medications that may present risks or cause excessive side-effects. Eliminating triggers, avoiding excess caffeine, and maintaining a proper diet and regular sleep pattern are strategies that are useful in all patients. The most important nonpharmacologic approach involves identifying and treating comorbid medical and psychiatric conditions. The use of botulinum A toxin should be considered for patients in this age group.

Tension-type headache

Tension-type headache (TTH) can begin at any age, but its onset is most common prior to the fourth decade. Headache prevalence declines with increasing age; headache severity decreases in the women who continue to report headaches, but does not change in men.[7,101] In approximately 10% of patients, TTH begins after the age of 50 years. One community-based study reported a 27% prevalence rate in subjects over the age of 65 years.[6] Medical disorders that are common in the elderly may be mistaken for TTH, inflating prevalence estimates and leading to misdiagnosis in individual cases. The differential diagnosis includes mass lesions, GCA, visual acuity problems, and chronic migraine.[5,102]

Treatment of TTH should be modified in elderly patients. Combination analgesics contain sedatives or caffeine and their use should be limited, as overuse may cause dependence and more side-effects. Preventive therapy should be administered when a patient has frequent headaches that produce disability or may lead to acute medication overuse. Antidepressants, the medication of choice, should be started at a very low dose and increased slowly every 3–7 days.[98] Selective serotonin reuptake inhibitors may be preferable to tricyclics.

Cluster headache

Cluster headache typically begins between the ages of 20 and 50 years, although onset in the eighth decade has been reported.[88] Both the episodic and chronic varieties of cluster may occur for the first time in the elderly. Cluster attacks may recur after many years of remission, or persist into senescence. Long-duration disease helps account for the continued presence of cluster headache in the elderly, despite its low incidence at advanced age. Of the many medications utilized in this age group, sublingual or transdermal nitroglycerin are potent precipitators of cluster attacks.[88]

Pharmacological treatment of cluster headache in the elderly[103–106] is influenced by the presence of coexistent medical conditions and their treatments. In the absence of chronic obstructive pulmonary disease, oxygen inhalation may be the safest and most effective method of aborting attacks. The other mainstays of abortive treatment, sumatriptan, dihydroergotamine, or ergotamine compounds, must be used very cautiously,[94–96] even in the absence of peripheral vascular disease, coronary heart disease, or hypertension.

We do not recommend methysergide for elderly patients. Verapamil, lithium, and prednisone should be used with caution. Divalproex sodium is well tolerated.

Hypnic headaches

The hypnic headache syndrome is a rare primary headache disorder of the elderly.[107–109] The initial description of the syndrome was a bilateral, throbbing headache without associated autonomic features that lasted from 15 to 60 minutes and recurred once to three times nightly, often during rapid eye movement (REM) sleep. At the time of this writing, a total of 37 patients with the disorder have been described. The disorder has a female predominance (26 females, 11 males), with a sex ratio of 2.36 : 1. Although most patients are elderly, the age of onset ranges from 40 to 82 years (mean 66 years; median 66 years). Headaches occur at a consistent time each night, usually between 1:00 and 3:00 AM, and may on rare instances occur during a daytime nap.[110] The headaches begin abruptly, are diffuse and throbbing, and spontaneously resolve in 15–180 minutes. In 10 patients (27%), the headache was hemicranial.[110–113] No associated autonomic symptoms accompany the pain, but nausea, photophobia, and phonophobia may rarely be present. The

● **Table 17.11** *Suggested IHS diagnostic criteria for hypnic headache*[9]

4.7 Hypnic headache
A Headaches occur at least 15 times per month for at least one month.
B Headaches awaken patient from sleep.
C Attack duration of 5–60 minutes.
D Pain is generalized or bilateral.
E Pain not associated with autonomic features.
F At least one of the following: • There is no suggestion of one of the disorders listed in groups 5–11. • Such a disorder is suggested but excluded by appropriate investigations. • Such a disorder is present, but the first headache attacks do not occur in close temporal relation to the disorder.

Modified from Goadsby and Lipton (Brain 1997; 120: 193–209).

headaches may be associated with REM sleep (Table 17.11).[107]

Hypnic headache must be differentiated from a mass lesion, which may also present with nocturnal pain, and from GCA. Cluster headaches also present with nocturnal attacks, but can be differentiated from hypnic headaches by their unilaterality, their periorbital and temporal location, and their prominent autonomic features.

After excluding organic disease with an imaging procedure and an ESR, treatment with lithium carbonate at a dose of 300 mg at bedtime usually produces a prompt remission. If headaches recur, higher doses of lithium may be required. Lithium should be used with caution in the elderly, especially in the presence of renal disease, dehydration, or diuretic therapy. Alternative treatments, such as bedtime doses of caffeine, flunarizine, indomethacin (indometacin), atenolol, and a combination of ergotamine tartrate, belladonna, and caffeine, have been reported to treat this syndrome.[110,112,113]

The exploding head syndrome

The exploding head syndrome is not associated with pain but can be confused with hypnic headache.[114,115] Patients, more often women, typically complain of either a 'loud bang' or an 'explosion,' which invariably occurs at night and typically in the twilight stage as the patient is falling asleep. Age of onset is variable, but no decade is spared, with most patients reporting their first attack after the age of 50 years.[115] There is no treatment except reassurance that it is a benign syndrome.

Conclusions

The approach to the elderly patient with a new-onset headache begins with a systematic search for an underlying cause. If one is identified, treatment should address both the underlying cause and the specific pain syndrome. If secondary headaches are excluded, a specific primary headache disorder should be diagnosed. Treatment goals include pain prevention, pain relief, and optimal functioning and quality of life.

References

1. Young WB, Silberstein SD. Headache in the elderly. In: Pathy MS, ed. Principles and Practice of Geriatric Medicine. 3rd edn. England: John Wiley & Sons Ltd, 1998, 733–46.
2. Stewart WF, Lipton RB, Celentano DD, Reed ML. Prevalence of migraine in the United States. Relation to age, income, race, and other sociodemographic factors. JAMA 1992; 267: 64–9.
3. Lipton RB, Stewart WF, Diamond S et al. Prevalence and burden of migraine in the United States: data from the American Migraine Study II. Headache 2001; 41: 646–57.
4. Hauser KA, Ferguson RH, Holley KE. Temporal arteritis in Rochester, Minnesota. Mayo Clin Proc 1971; 46: 597–602.
5. Baumel B, Eisner LS. Diagnosis and treatment of headache in the elderly. Med Clin N Amer 1991; 75: 661–75.
6. Solomon G, Kunkel RS, Frame J. Demographics of headache in elderly patients. Headache 1990; 30: 273–6.
7. Edmeads J. Headache in the elderly. In: Olesen J, Tfelt-Hansen P, Welch KMA, eds. The Headaches. 2nd edn. Philadelphia: Lippincott Williams & Wilkins, 2000, 947–52.
8. Cook NR, Evans DA, Funkenstein H et al. Correlates of headache in a population-based cohort of elderly. Arch Neurol 1989; 46: 1338–44.
9. Headache Classification Committee of the International Headache Society. Classification and diagnostic criteria for headache disorders, cranial neuralgia, and facial pain. Cephalalgia 1988; 8: 1–96.
10. Salcman M, Kaplan R. Intracranial tumors in adults. In: Moossa A, Robson M, Schimpff S, eds. Comprehensive Textbook of Oncology. Baltimore: Williams and Wilkins, 1986, 617–29.
11. Schoenberg B. Nervous System. In: Schotterfeld D, Joseph F, eds. Cancer Epidemiology and Prevention. Philadelphia: WB Saunders, 1982, 968–83.
12. Forsyth PA, Posner JB. Headaches in patients with brain tumors. A study of 111 patients. Neurology 1993; 43: 1678–83.

13. Bengtsson BA, Malmvall BE. Giant cell arteritis. Acta Med Scand 1982; Suppl 658: 1–102.
14. Machado EB, Michet CJ, Ballard DJ et al. Trends in incidence and clinical presentation of temporal arteritis in Olmsted County, Minnesota, 1958–1985. Arthritis Rheum 1988; 31: 745–9.
15. Salvarani C, Gabriel SE, O'Fallon WM, Hunder GG. The incidence of giant cell arteritis in Olmsted County, Minnesota: apparent fluctuations in a cyclic pattern. Ann Int Med 1995; 123: 192–4.
16. Lawrence RC, Helmick CG, Arnett FC, et al. Estimates of the prevalence of arthritis and selected musculoskeletal disorders in the United States. Arthritis Rheum 1998; 41: 778–99.
17. Petursdottir V, Johansson H, Nordborg E, Nordborg C. The epidemiology of biopsy-positive giant cell arteritis: special reference to cyclic fluctuations. Rheumatology 1999; 38: 1208–12.
18. Ostberg G. Temporal arteritis in a large necropsy series. Ann Rheum Dis 1971; 30: 224–35.
19. Caselli RJ, Hunder GG. Giant cell arteritis and polymyalgia rheumatica. In: Silberstein SD, Lipton RB, Dalessio DJ, eds. Wolff's Headache and Other Head Pain. 7th edn. New York: Oxford University Press, 2001, 525–38.
20. Solomon S, Cappa KG. The headache of temporal arteritis. Am Geriatr Soc 1987; 35: 163–5.
21. Chisolm H. Cortical blindness in cranial arteritis. Br J Ophthalmol 1975; 59: 332–3.
22. Caselli RJ, Hunder GG, Whisnant JP. Neurologic disease in biopsy-proven giant cell (temporal) arteritis. Neurology 1988; 38: 352–9.
23. Keltner JL. Giant-cell arteritis: signs and symptoms. Ophthalmology 1982; 89: 1101–10.
24. Goodman BW. Temporal arteritis. Am J Med 1979; 67: 839–52.
25. Graham E. Survival in temporal arteritis. Trans Ophthalmol Soc UK 1980; 100: 108–10.
26. Boghen DR, Glaser JS. Ischemic optic neuropathy: the clinical profile and natural history. Brain 1975; 92: 689–708.

27. Lipton RB, Solomon S, Wertenbaker C. Gradual loss and recovery of vision in temporal arteritis. Arch Intern Med 1985; 145: 2252–3.
28. Schneier HA, Weber AA, Ballen PH. The visual prognosis in temporal arteritis. Ann Ophthalmol 1971; 3: 1215–30.
29. McLeod D, Oji EO, Kohner EM. Fundus signs in temporal arteritis. Br J Ophthalmol 1978; 62: 591–4.
30. Wagner KP, Hollenhorst RW. The ocular lesions of temporal arteritis. Surv Ophthalmol 1976; 20: 247–60.
31. Hayreh SS. Posterior ischemic optic neuropathy. Ophthalmologica 1981; 182: 29–41.
32. Wall M, Corbett JJ. Arteritis. In: Olesen J, Tfelt-Hansen P, Welch KM, eds. The Headaches. 2nd edn. Philadelphia: Lippincott Williams & Wilkins, 2000, 797–806.
33. Goodwin J. Temporal arteritis. In: Vinken PJ, Bruyn GW, eds. Handbook of Clinical Neurology. Amsterdam: North Holland, 1980, 313–47.
34. Smetana GW, Shmerling RH. Does this patient have temporal arteritis? J Am Med Assoc 2002; 287: 92–101.
35. Wong RL, Korn JH. Temporal arteritis without an elevated erythrocyte sedimentation rate: case report and review of the literature. Am J Med 1986; 80: 959–64.
36. de Silva M, Hazleman BL. Azathioprine in giant cell arteritis/polymyalgia rheumatica: a double-blind study. Ann Rheum Dis 1986; 45: 136–8.
37. Krall PL, Mazenec DJ, Wilke WS. Methotrexate for corticosteroid-resistant polymyalgia rheumatica and giant cell arteritis. Cleve Clin Med J 1989; 56: 253–7.
38. de Vita S, Tavoni A, Jeracitano G et al. Treatment of giant cell arteritis with cyclophosphamide pulses. J Int Med 1992; 232: 373–5.
39. Demaziere A. Dapsone in the long-term treatment of temporal arteritis. Am J Med 1989; 87: 3.
40. Caselli RJ, Hunder GG. Giant cell (temporal) arteritis and cerebral vasculitis. In: Johnson RT, Griffin JW, eds. Current Therapy in Neurologic Disease. 4th edn. St. Louis: BC Decker, 1993, 196–201.

41. Mathew NT, Reuveni U, Perez F. Transformed or evolutive migraine. Headache 1987; 27: 102–6.

42. Lipton RB, Reuveni U, Cohen JS, Solomon S. Aspartamine as a trigger of migraine. Headache 1989; 29: 90–3.

43. Peatfield RC, Glover V, Littlewood JT et al. The prevalence of diet-induced migraine. Cephalalgia 1984; 4: 179–83.

44. Dalton K. Food intake prior to a migraine attack: study of 2313 spontaneous attacks. Headache 1975; 15: 188–93.

45. Selby G, Lance JW. Observation on 500 cases of migraine and allied vascular headaches. J Neurol Neurosurg Psychiatry 1960; 23: 23–32.

46. Bergh VV, Anery WK. Trigger factors in migraine: a study conducted by the Belgian migraine society. Headache 1987; 27: 191–6.

47. Silberstein SD, Lipton RB. Chronic daily headache including transformed migraine, chronic tension-type headache, and medication overuse. In: Silberstein SD, Lipton RB, Dalessio DJ, eds. Wolff's Headache and Other Head Pain. 7th edn. New York: Oxford University Press, 2001, 247–82.

48. Wang SJ, Fuh JL, Lu SR et al. Chronic daily headache in Chinese elderly: prevalence, risk factors and biannual follow-up. Neurology 2000; 54: 314–19.

49. Penman J. Trigeminal neuralgia. In: Vinken PJ, Bruyn GW, eds. Handbook of Clinical Neurology. Amsterdam: North Holland, 1968, 296–322.

50. White JC, Sweet WH. Pain and the neurosurgeon: a 40-year experience. Springfield, IL: Charles C Thomas, 1969.

51. Dalessio DJ. Diagnosis and treatment of cranial neuralgias. Med Clin N Amer 1991; 75: 605–15.

52. Fromm GH, Graff-Radford SB, Terrence CF, Sweet WH. Pretrigeminal neuralgia. Neurology 1990; 40: 1493–5.

53. Terrence CF, Jensen TS. Trigeminal neuralgia and other facial neuralgias. In: Olesen J, Tfelt-Hansen P, Welch KM, eds. The headaches. 2nd edn. Philadelphia: Lippincott Williams & Wilkins, 2000, 929–38.

54. Majoie CB, Hulsmans FJ, Castelijns JA et al. Symptoms and signs related to the trigeminal nerve: diagnostic yield of MR imaging. Radiology 2000; 209: 557–62.

55. Sundaram PK, Hegde AS, Chandramouli BA, Das BS. Trigeminal evoked potentials in patients with symptomatic trigeminal neuralgia due to intracranial mass lesions. Neurology 1999; 47: 94–7.

56. Court JE, Kase CS. Treatment of tic douloureaux with a new anticonvulsant (clonazepam). J Neurol Neurosurg Psychiatr 1976; 39: 297–9.

57. Peiris JB, Perera GL, Devendra SV, Lionel ND. Sodium valproate in trigeminal neuralgia. Med J Aust 1980; 2: 278.

58. Sist T, Filadora V, Miner M, Lema M. Gabapentin for idiopathic trigeminal neuralgia: report of two cases. Neurology 1997; 48: 1467.

59. Din MU, Zvartan-Hind M, Gilari A et al. Topiramate relieved refractory trigeminal neuralgia in multiple sclerosis patients (abstract). Neurology 2000; 54: A60.

60. Rozen TD, Capobianco DJ, Dalessio DJ. Cranial neuralgias and atypical facial pain. In: Silberstein SD, Lipton RB, Dalessio DJ, eds. Wolff's Headache and Other Head Pain. 7th edn. New York: Oxford University Press, 2001; 509–24.

61. Zakrzewska JM. Trigeminal neuralgia. In: Zakrzewska JM, ed. Major Problems in Neurology. London: WB Saunders Company, Inc., 1995, 108–70.

62. Young RF, Vermeulen SS, Grimm P et al. Gamma knife radiosurgery for treatment of trigeminal neuralgia: idiopathic and tumor related. Neurology 1997; 48: 608–14.

63. Okun MS, Stover NP, Subramanian T et al. Complications of gamma knife surgery for Parkinson disease. Arch Neurol 2002; 58: 1995–2002.

64. Silberstein SD, Lipton RB, Dalessio DJ. Overview, diagnosis, and classification of headache. In: Silberstein SD, Lipton RB, Dalessio DJ, eds. Wolff's Headache and Other Head Pain. 7th edn. New York: Oxford University Press, 2001, 6–26.

65. Rushton JG, Stevens JC, Miller RH. Glossopharyngeal (vagoglossopharyngeal) neuralgia. Arch Neurol 1981; 38: 201–5.

66. Bruyn GW. Glossopharyngeal neuralgia. In: Vinken PJ, Bruyn GW, Klawans HL, eds. Handbook of Clinical Neurology. Amsterdam: Elsevier, 1985, 459–73.

67. Kost RG, Straus SE. Postherpetic neuralgia pathogenesis, treatment, and prevention. N Eng J Med 1996; 335: 32–42.

68. De Moragas JM, Kierland RR. The outcome of patients with herpes zoster. Arch Dermatol 1957; 75: 193–6.

69. Whitley RJ, Weiss H, Gnann J. The efficacy of steroid and acyclovir therapy of herpes zoster in the elderly (abstract). J Invest Med 1995; 45: 252A.

70. Scelsa SN, Lipton RB, Sander H, Herskoviz S. Headache characteristics in hospitalized patients with Lyme disease. Headache 1995; 35: 125–30.

71. Das G. Pacemaker headaches. Pace 1984; 7: 802–7.

72. Moran JF. Headache following pacemaker implantation. JAMA 1985; 254: 1511–12.

73. Lipton RB, Lowenkopf T, Bajwa ZH et al. Cardiac cephalalgia: a malignant form of exertional headache. Neurology 1997; 49: 813–16.

74. Edmeads JG. Disorders of the neck: cervicogenic headache. In: Silberstein SD, Lipton RB, Dalessio DJ, eds. Wolff's Headache and Other Head Pain. 7th edn. New York: Oxford University Press, 2001, 447–58.

75. Gobel H, Martin TJ. Ocular disorders. In: Olesen J, Tfelt-Hansen P, Welch KM, eds. The headaches. 2nd edn. Philadelphia: Lippincott Williams & Wilkins, 2000, 899–904.

76. Birt D. Headache and head pains associated with diseases of the ear, nose and throat. Med Clin N Amer 1978; 62: 523–31.

77. Joseph DJ, Renner G. Head pain from diseases of the ear, nose and throat. Neurol Clin 1983; 1: 399–414.

78. Edmeads J. The headaches of ischemic cerebrovascular disease. Headache 1979; 19: 345–9.

79. Portenoy RK, Abissi CJ, Lipton RB et al. Headache in cerebrovascular disease. Stroke 1984; 25: 1009–12.

80. Fisher CM. Headache in cerebrovascular disease. In: Vinken PJ, Bruyn GW, eds. Handbook of Clinical Neurology. New York: Elsevier, 1968, 124–58.

81. Leviton A, Caplan L, Salzmen E. Severe headaches after carotid endarterectomy. Headache 1975; 15: 207–10.

82. Leviton A. Post carotid-endarterectomy 'hemicrania'. Headache 1985; 15: 13–17.

83. Nishikawa S, Harada H, Takahashi K, Shimomura T. Clinical study on headache in patients with Parkinson's disease. Clin Neurol Neurosurg 1982; 22: 403–8.

84. Lorentz IT. A survey of headache in Parkinson's disease. Cephalalgia 1989; 9: 86.

85. Indo T, Takahashi A. Early morning headache of Parkinson's disease: a hitherto unrecognized symptom? Headache 1987; 27: 151–4.

86. Indaco A, Carrieri PB. Amitriptyline in the treatment of headache in patients with Parkinson's disease: a double-blind placebo controlled study. Neurology 1988; 38: 1720–2.

87. Prencipe M, Casini AR, Ferretti C et al. Prevalence of headache in an elderly population: attack frequency, disability, and use of medication. J Neurol Neurosurg Psychiatry 2001; 70: 377–81.

88. Raskin NH. Headache. 2nd edn. New York: Churchill-Livingstone, 1988.

89. Cull RE. Investigation of late-onset migraine. Scott Med J 1995; 40: 50–2.

90. Saper J. Daily chronic headache. Neurol Clin 1990; 8: 891–901.

91. Fisher CM. Late life migraine accompaniments as a cause of unexplained transient ischemic attacks. Can J Neurol Sci 1980; 7: 9–17.

92. Fisher CM. Late-life migraine accompaniments–further experience. Stroke 1986; 17: 1033–42.

93. Silberstein SD, Merriam GR. Sex hormones and headache. In: Goadsby PJ, Silberstein SD, eds. Headache. Newton: Butterworth-Heinemann, 1997, 143–73.

94. Sanders-Bush E, Mayer SE. 5-Hydroxytryptamine (serotonin): receptor agonists and antagonists. In: Hardman JG, Limbird LE, Goodman-Gilman A, eds. Goodman and Gilman's The Pharmacological Basis of Therapeutics. 10th ed. New York: McGraw-Hill, 2001, 269–90.

95. Medical Economics Company. Physicians' Desk Reference. 55th edn. 2001.

96. Galer B, Lipton R, Solomon S. Myocardial ischemia related to ergot alkaloids: a case report and literature review. Headache 1991; 31: 446–50.

97. Schrier RW. Geriatric medicine. Philadelphia: WB Saunders, 1990, 91–103.

98. Silberstein SD, Saper JR, Freitag F. Migraine: Diagnosis and treatment. In: Silberstein SD, Lipton RB, Dalessio DJ, eds. Wolff's Headache and Other Head Pain. 7th edn. New York: Oxford University Press, 2001, 121–237.

99. Edmeads J, Takahashi A. Headaches in the elderly. In: Olesen J, Tfelt-Hansen P, Welch KMA, eds. The Headaches. New York: Raven Press, Ltd., 1993, 809–13.

100. Cassel C, Riesenberg D, Sorenson L, Walth J. Geriatric Medicine. New York: Springer-Verlag, 1990.

101. Alders EEA, Hentzen A, Tan CT. A community-based prevalence study on headache in Malaysia. Headache 1996; 36: 379–84.

102. Tomsak R. Ophthalmologic aspects of headache. Med Clin N Amer 1991; 75: 693–706.

103. Mokri B, Sundt T, Houser W. Spontaneous internal carotid dissection, hemicrania, and Horner's syndrome. Arch Neurol 1979; 36: 677–80.

104. Kudrow L. Diagnosis and treatment of cluster headaches. Med Clin N Amer 1991; 75: 579–94.

105. Dodick DW, Campbell JK. Cluster headache: diagnosis, management, and treatment. In: Silberstein SD, Lipton RB, Dalessio D, eds. Wolff's Headache and Other Head Pain. 7th edn. New York: Oxford University Press, 2001, 283–309.

106. Dodick DW, Rozen TD, Goadsby PJ, Silberstein SD. Cluster headache. Cephalalgia 2000; 20: 787–803.

107. Raskin NH. The hypnic headache syndrome. Headache 1988; 28: 534–6.

108. Newman LC, Lipton RB, Solomon S. The hypnic headache syndrome. In: Rose FC, ed. New advances in headache research. 2nd edn. London: Smith-Gordon, 1991, 31–4.

109. Newman LC, Lipton RB, Solomon S. The hypnic headache syndrome. Neurology 1990; 40: 1904–5.

110. Dodick DW, Mosek AC, Campbell JK. The hypnic ('alarm clock') headache syndrome. Cephalalgia 1998; 18: 152–65.

111. Gould JD, Silberstein SD. Unilateral hypnic headache: a case study. Neurology 1997; 49: 1749–51.

112. Ivanez V, Soler R, Barreiro P. Hypnic headache syndrome: a case with good response to indomethacin. Cephalalgia 1998; 18: 225–6.

113. Morales-Asin F, Mauri JA, Iniquez C et al. The hypnic headache syndrome: report of three new cases. Cephalalgia 1998; 18: 157–8.

114. Pearce JM. Exploding head syndrome. Lancet 1988; 2: 270–1.

115. Pearce JM. Clinical features of the exploding head syndrome. J Neurol Neurosurg Psychiatry 1989; 52: 907–10.

116. Goadsby PJ, Silberstein SD (eds). Headache. Newton: Butterworth-Heinemann, 1997.

Index